Roberto Kaitsas, Maria Giacinta Paolone

Orthodontics and Periodontology

Combined treatments and clinical synergies

edra

Original title

R. Kaitsas, M.G. Paolone Ortodonzia e Parodontologia. Trattamenti combinati e sinergie cliniche

ISBN: 978-88-214-5366-3

Book Publishing Manager: Costanza Smeraldi
Paper, Printing and Binding Manage: Paolo Ficicchia
Cover: Roberta Venturieri
Translation: Roberto Kaitsas, Maria Giacinta Paolone
Copyediting: ALTER EDOM s.r.l., Noventa Padovana (PD), Italy

ISBN: 978-88-214-5532-2
eISBN: 978-88-214-5533-9

Edra S.p.A.
Via G. Spadolini 7, 20141 Milano
Tel. 02 881841
www.edizioniedra.it

Printed by "Printer Trento" S.r.l., Trento (Italy), September 2021

(*) Edra S.p.A. a LSWR GROUP company.

Authors

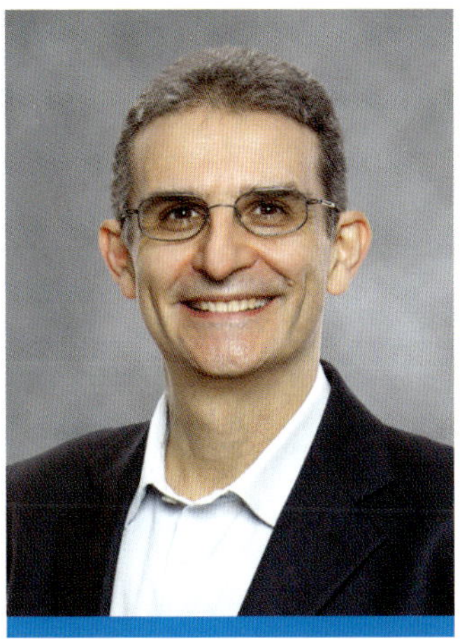

Roberto Kaitsas

Private Practice in Rome (Italy)
Graduate in Dentistry, Catholic University of the Sacred Heart, Rome (Italy)
Postgraduate in Oral Surgery, University of Rome "La Sapienza"
Specialization Course in Endodontics, University of Rome "La Sapienza"
Co-author of *Manual of Oral Surgery*, 2011, Edra SpA
Author of the paragraph on periodontal-restorative relationships in *Restauri Diretti nei Settori Posteriori* , by S. Scolavino and G. Paolone
Italian Academy of Osseointegration (formerly Italian Society of Oral Surgery and Implantology), Active Member
Italian Society of Endodontics (Società Italiana di Endodonzia), Active Member
European Society of Endodontology, Certified Member
European Board of Oral Surgery Societies, Certified
He is Tutor for the Education Group for the IAO (Italian Academy of Osseointegration)

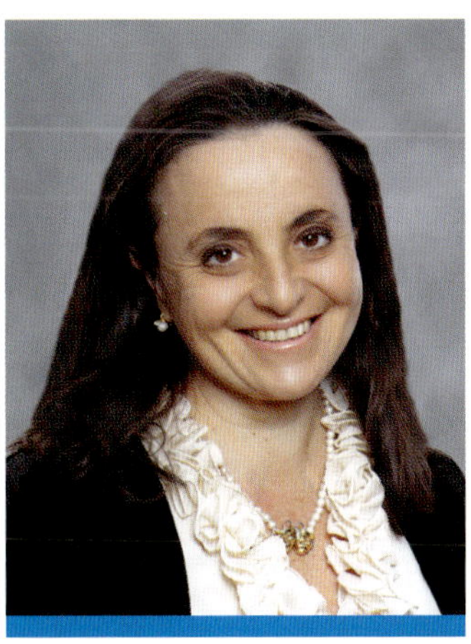

Maria Giacinta Paolone

Private Practice in Rome (Italy)
Graduate in Dentistry, Catholic University of the Sacred Heart, Rome (Italy)
Postgraduate in Orthodontics, Catholic University of the Sacred Heart, Rome (Italy)
European Board of Orthodontics, Certified
Italian Board of Orthodontics, Certified
Angle Society of Europe, Active Member
Tweed Foundation for Orthodontic Research, Regular Member
World Society of Lingual Orthodontics, Active Member
Italian Society of Orthodontics (Società Italiana di Ortodonzia), Active Member
Italian Academy of Orthodontics, Effective Member
College Europeen d'Orthodontie, Membre Titulaire
European Society of Lingual Orthodontics, Active Member
American Association Orthodontists, International Member
World Federation of Orthodontists, Member
Adjunct Professor, Catholic University of the Sacred Heart, Rome (Italy), Postgraduate School in Orthodontics, 2019-2021

Forewords

Dentistry, interdisciplinarity, synergies.

These are the three words from which this text originates, around which it develops and which lead to clinical success.

Dentistry is a specialty that has some peculiarities and, among others, interdisciplinarity is the one that distinguishes it better. Success in dentistry can be achieved only through the synergistic interaction between different disciplines and with a global vision of the patient, taking into account their needs and medical clinical picture.

This book is an example of how orthodontic clinics can merge with periodontal clinics and oral surgery clinics to achieve the best possible treatment for each individual patient.

I have known Roberto Kaitsas for many years, first as an Active Member of the Italian Society of Oral Surgery and then as a Fellow of the European Board of Oral Surgery Societies, and I am aware that he has put all his energy into completing this text, which will be for many clinicians a knowledge base and guidance in the complicated world of the clinic.

I wish the Authors a brilliant editorial success.

Antonio Barone
Lecturer and Head of Implantology and Oral Surgery
Dpt. of Surgical Pathology, Medical, Molecular, and Critical Area
Director of the Master in Oral Implantology, University Hospital, University of Pisa (Italy)
Adjunct Professor, Dpt. Oral and Maxillofacial Surgery, SUNY, Buffalo, USA
Past President of the Italian Society of Oral Surgery and Implantology
Past President European Federation Oral Surgery Societies
Past President International Bone, Biomaterials and Beyond Academy

The interdisciplinary treatments in orthodontics are an area of interest and depth that have been growing for several decades. The key for success is undoubtedly tied to the professional ability based on deep knowledge and expertise of the principles of the various disciplines, but excellence is achieved with the ability to apply this knowledge and skills in perfect harmony between the different professionals. For this reason I can think of no better than the great family team consisting of Maria Giacinta Paolone and Roberto Kaitsas, who can lead us by the hand to deal with the diagnosis and treatment of cases that require both an orthodontic and periodontal approach.

Giovanni Biondi
Former Member of the Board of Directors,
Tweed International Foundation
for Orthodontic Research and Education, Tucson, AZ, USA

Who is Maria Giacinta? A former student who become a friend. How to define her: serious, applied, determined. In her book, all clinical requirements have one answer: "put the cases on the table". I am proud of you and thank you for all your help.

Joseph Felix Giordanetto
French Board (BFO) certified
Past President of the European College of Orthodontics (CEO)
Tweed International Foundation Instructor
for Orthodontic Research and Education, Tucson, AZ, USA

The perio-ortho relationships have always been a fascinating chapter in the vast world of interdisciplinary dentistry.

Writing the presentation of a book on this subject would already be rewarding for anyone but, in this case, it is more than that because the Authors are talented colleagues, who are not only a professional couple but also in their lives. A couple who has been able to cultivate their passions and grow their professionalism in perfect harmony, combining skills and knowledge in a wise way.

With this volume, the result of years of a careful and disciplined profession, Roberto and Maria Giacinta lead us into perio-ortho relationships overcoming the field of simple definitions and of the enounced principles and entering what is the clinical world, made of complex cases, treated and followed in perfect synthesis between scientific evidence and clinical experience.

The text deals with rigor and with an extensive and accurate clinical documentation one of the most fascinating and rich clinical and biological potential issues.

The book comes out in a period in which the new classification of periodontitis has clearly and unequivocally defined the importance of the interdisciplinarity in the treatment of patients with stage IV disease, with particular regard to the effects of occlusal trauma.

The integration of orthodontic treatment becomes not more and not only a niche treatment, but the response needed to correct the effects of periodontitis. A therapy that, to be successful, requires the perfect integration between periodontist and orthodontist.

I am sure that this book, rich in documentation and in excellent clinical cases, not only will be a valid study of the concepts that govern the perio-ortho relationships, but it will also be able to give the reader practical information and clinical tips of great clinical utility, because they are based on the experience gained in the field, an element that makes this text indispensable for those who want to deal with the interdisciplinary treatment of complex cases.

To the Authors go not only the compliments, but also the thanks for sharing their daily clinical practice with the dental community in such a generous way.

Thank you.

Luca Landi
Graduate in Dentistry, Catholic University of the Sacred Heart, Rome (Italy)
Post-graduate in Periodontology (CAGS),
Boston University Goldman School of Dental Medicine
Certified from the American Board of Periodontology and Implantology
Active Member of the American Academy of Periodontology (AAP)
and of the Academy of Osseointegration (AO)
Active Member of the Italian Society of Periodontology and Implantology (SIdP),
of which he is President in the 2020-2021 biennal period

La gestion des traitements orthodontiques de l'adulte necessite le plus souvent une prise en charge pluridisciplinaire (parodontologie, chirurgie orale, chirurgie implantaire, prothese) qui augmente la complexite de ces traitements et oblige a un travail d'equipe gere par l'orthodontiste.

L'ouvrage du Dr Paolone explique de maniere claire, detaillee et precise comment integrer dans nos plans de traitement orthodontique ces differentes disciplines pluridisciplinaires.

Le Dr Paolone illustre son propos d'exemples de cas difficiles traits en orthodontie linguale par ses mains expertes.

Pour l'orthodontiste, ce livre vient enrichir nos champs de competence et apporte une immense et precieuse contribution scientifique et clinique qui justifie a elle seule l'acquisition de ce livre.

J'admire la competence scientifique du Dr Paolone et son talent d'orthodontiste.

Je souhaite a ce livre d'etre diffuse et apprecie comme il le merite.

Patricia Obach Dejean
French Board (BFO) and European Board (EBO) certified
Past President of the European College of Orthodontics (CEO)
Past President of the French Federation of Orthodontics (FFO)
Past Director of the European Board examiners
Past Chairman of the Scientific Committee
of the Angle society of Europe (ASE) and Active Member
Visiting Professor Postgraduate in Orthodontics
at Toulouse University (2011-2015)

The clinical orthodontist must understand and respect the physiological environment of the dentition – the alveolar housing and the surrounding tissues, i.e. the periodontium. The fundamental concept of dimensions of the dentition must be understood by all orthodontists. The teeth must not be moved out of the periodontal structures – bone and soft tissues – that support them. This book acknowledges and addresses these fundamental truths of both specialties.

James L. Vaden
Professor and Chairman of the Department of Orthodontics,
University of Tennessee, 1999-2010
Adjunct clinical professor at the University of Michigan
in Ann Arbor, 1991-2000
Past President and Director American Board of Orthodontics
Co-Director of the Tweed Study Course in Tucson, AZ, USA

Preface

The idea for this book was born from a desire to share twenty-years of teamwork and to communicate how this interaction can guide us towards a new diagnostic and therapeutic approach in the execution of combined treatments. Together we learned to observe the patient not only from an orthodontic or periodontal perspective but also on a surgical-periodontal-orthodontic point of view that is always integrating and evolving. The diagnosis and subsequent orthodontic treatment plan requires a daily periodontal integration both in adults and in the growing age, such as the periodontal diagnosis and treatment plan must be integrated with an orthodontic vision.

This book includes a collection of clinical cases, ideas, biomechanical applications, surgical techniques, periodontal strategies, treatment plans observed under an integrated view and developed under the study of literature, our constant guide and to which all our treatment plans refer. We consider it important to describe the one that can be considered our workflow which is not mono-specialist, but trying to pay attention on how the relationship between the two disciplines is biunivocal. The patient's risk assessment in already ortho-perio overt patients and the early detection, even in the adolescent patient, often whose only dental reference is the orthodontist, allows the interception of future risk factors of periodontal disease and mucogingival problems. Synergy between the two specialties means dealing with ortho-perio timing to standardize a protocol work and interrelation among the different disciplines with a mutual and daily updating and strengthening among clinicians, so that tradition marries with new technologies.

Roberto Kaitsas and Maria Giacinta Paolone

Acknowledgments

To Paola Sammaritano, Elena Mezzetti, Costanza Smeraldi and all the Edra staff for the support, guidance, professionalism, advices and patience that have accompanied us on this journey.

To Massimo Gagliani for his precious suggestions.

To Gaetano Paolone for living with us in a single group, in the clinic and in the family.

To Vassilios Kaitsas who raised us professionally as children and for his continuous support.

To our assistants, to always be with us in the daily life of clinical passion.

To Stefano Corso, our precious photographer, for making us "beautiful" and "iconographic".

To our patients and their smiles.

Gaetano Paolone
Contribution to Chapter 10
Private Practice in Rome (Italy)
Italian Academy of Restorative Dentistry (Accademia Italiana di Conservativa), Active Member
Italian Academy of Esthetic Dentistry, Active Member
American Academy Restorative Dentistry (AARD), Associate Member
AIC Secretary 2018-2019, member of the AIC 2020-2022 Scientific Commetee
Author and co-author of scientific publications in national and international journals
Adjunct Professor Restorative Dentistry, Università Vita-Salute San Raffaele, Milan, since 2014
Lecturer at the Master in Esthetics and Restorative Dentistry, University of Bologna
Visiting Professor, University of Montpellier, France

Table of contents

To Francesco and Raffaella, so that they always look for the light of freedom, dream and knowledge

To my parents

To my brother

To my husband Roberto and his smile

Maria Giacinta

To Raffaella and Francesco, that their thirst for knowledge never stops and always continues to grow as the universe

To my parents

To my sister

To my wife Maria Giacinta and her patience

Roberto

"Perio-Guided" orthodontic treatment plan

Introduction

Orthodontics is a periodontal therapy because it works on the dentoalveolar complex because of the existence of the periodontal ligament and has this peculiarity in common with periodontology. The orthodontic treatment plan in a periodontal patient must therefore be periodontally guided. This is true for every patient. It is important to carry out a diagnostic and therapeutic revolution in every orthodontic treatment plan, not only in patients that are typically affected by the periodontal disease, but also in the apparently healthy patient. Clinicians need a daily protocol to detect and identify the existence of a latent pathology and risk factors in more susceptible patients, adults and children, who might develop periodontal disease in the future[1].

The concept of gingival unit and periodontal attachment must be part of the daily orthodontic treatment plan[2], in each phase of the therapy, re-evaluation and follow-up. Orthodontics and Periodontology must integrate and share their protocols to customize a treatment based on an individual periodontal risk assessment and management[3] and allow the interdisciplinary team to have a targeted treatment plan.

Literature states that orthodontic treatment, if carried out under strict plaque control with healthy periodontal tissues, does not lead to a worsening of the periodontal disease[4-12], even in the presence of a reduced periodontal support[13,14] and aggressive periodontitis[15]. It is therefore possible to orthodontically move teeth with reduced but healthy periodontal tissue, without destructive effects on the periodontal attachment level[16]. Histological findings that orthodontic forces do not *per se* convert gingivitis into periodontal destruction[17] confirm clinical findings that there is no contraindication to orthodontic treatment for periodontally compromised patients[8].

Perio-patients with Stage III or IV[18,19] periodontitis are now treated by a team involving an orthodontist and periodontist to improve the chances of saving and restoring a deteriorated dentition since orthodontics is not a contraindication in the presence of reduced periodontal support[20,21], confirming that orthodontics becomes a periodontal therapy itself.

Orthodontic diagnosis integrated by periodontal data

Periodontal health must be analysed by the interdisciplinary team at the very beginning of the therapy and re-evaluated during orthodontic treatment in order to influence the treatment plan, timing, sequence, duration and type of forces to be used in orthodontic mechanics[7,22]. The periodontally-guided orthodontic approach is easy to understand when the patient is affected by a periodontal pathology, and is referred to the orthodontist by periodontists or prosthodontists. However, not every orthodontic patient is always a pure ortho-patient, and, on the other hand, not every periodontal patient can be an orthodontic one.

A patient's request for orthodontics is often an opportunity to discover periodontal defects that can reveal a different therapeutic approach and other treatment priorities beyond the simple required alignment. This diagnosis must be realized early in everyday treatments and must be part of daily screening even in interdisciplinary non-electively orthodontic treatments. A simple diastema (📷 1.1) can hide a much more complex reality that can be intercepted by periodontal probing and the patient shifts from orthodontic to periodontal relevance (📷 1.2 and 1.3). Similarly, the request for an orthodontic correction by a patient for a single tooth (📷 1.4 and 1.5) could, once evaluated from the periodontal point of view, require treatments that are not primarily orthodontic (📷 1.6-1.9). This can happen only if the periodontal probe is used routinely during the first orthodontic appointment. The Orthodontist must reappropriate the use of the periodontal probing and consider the probe an essential daily ally in the initial screening and then refer the patient to the periodontist for the definitive periodontal evaluation.

The orthodontist is used to define a treatment goal and to afford a malocclusion with references that are defined by the commissions of the Boards and National and International Societies, such as marginal, crestal, pits alignment, dental and skeletal class relationships[23]. It is essential to integrate this data into a periodontal perspective. In 1997 Mathews and Kokich pointed out the concept that the orthodontist should incorporate a periodontal screening recording (PSR) in the first appointment[24-26] and that if there were no coincidence between the levelling of dental marginal ridges and bone levels, the real guide to bracket positioning should not be the marginal ridge but the level of the bone defect[23]. Compared to conventional orthodontic education, the real limit of the dentition must be brought back to a periodontal level not only in adults but also in growing patients. If incisal edges and marginal ridges are not physiological guides for the positioning of adjacent teeth than the reference becomes the bone level. Therefore, once the bone has been levelled, the Orthodontist can contribute to the right position of the dental relationships, dental classes, morphology of the coronal vertical and crown-root relationships opening the way to restorative dentistry for the correction of residual morphological deficiencies[23].

It is important not to undertake a treatment until after having obtained the periodontal probing, evaluation and diagnosis from the periodontist[27] and not to be afraid to include vertical bitewings, apart from the Panoramic Rx, in the first appointment if interproximal bone defects are detected in order to integrate the data obtained with palpation, periodontal probing and occlusal observation[23,24]. The conventional treatment plan and its development, therefore, must be carried out not only on classical criteria and data, but integrated with periodontal records and the diagnosis and responsibility in patient management must be shared[27].

For orthodontists, at first, it might not seem easy to give up the ideal goals of occlusal and skeletal treatment and overturn the logic of the therapeutic plan and consequent goals. Nevertheless, it may not be spontaneous for the periodontal-restorative team to visualize a final result modified by a possible orthodontic contribution in severely compromised teeth. This collaboration is only achievable through dialogue, symbiosis and ongoing re-evaluation among specialists about the limits, sequences, treatment goals and therapeutic approaches and tools. The visualization of the aforementioned objectives and therapeutic sequences, which Kokich anticipated with the concept of "Create the Vision"[28] and "the art of seeing" proposed by Zachrisson[29] where "you can only correct what you see", reaffirms the importance of how the dialogue and the visualization of the objectives in a group by conventional or virtual set-

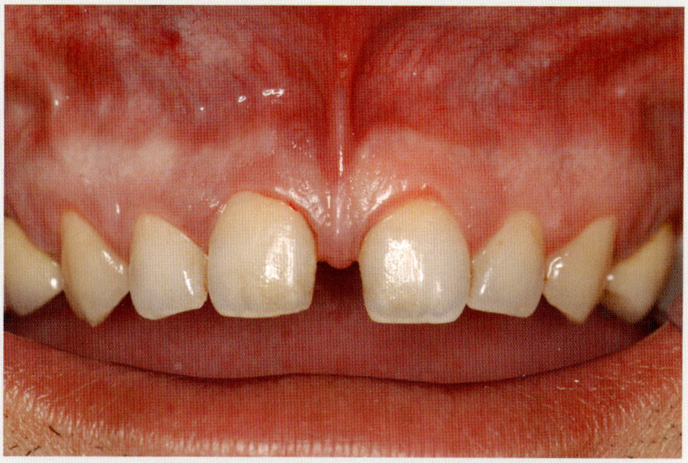

1.1 Diastema. Patient's request: orthodontic closure of the diastema.

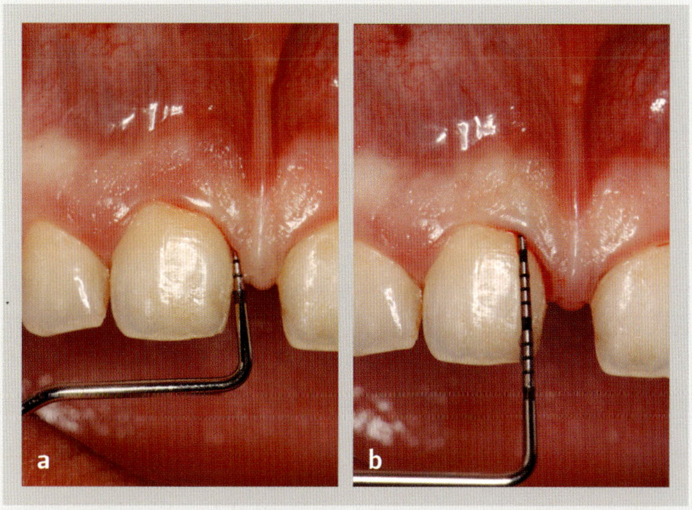

1.2 Periodontal probing of the papilla.

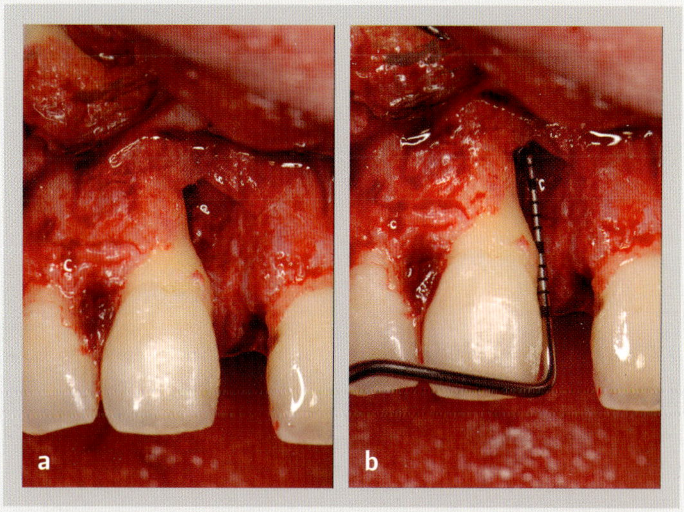

1.3 Surgical view of the intraosseous bone defect associated with the diastema.

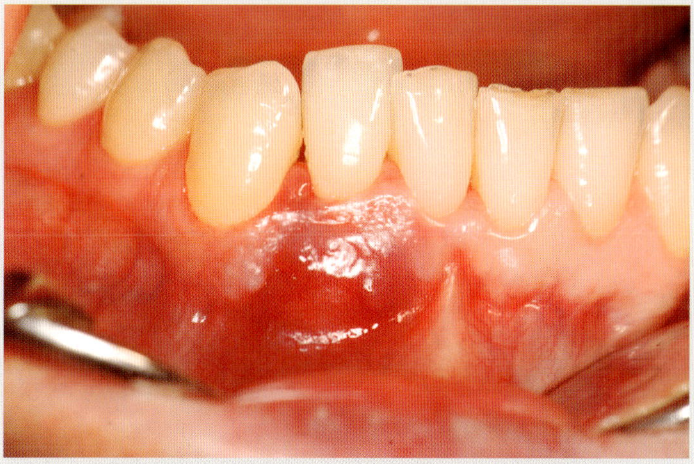

1.4 Lower incisor crowding. Patient's request: orthodontic correction of the dental extrusion and crowding.

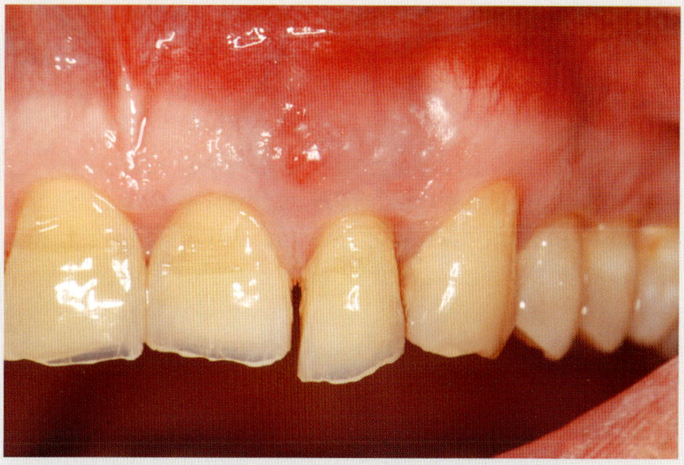

1.5 Upper lateral incisor extrusion. Patient's request: extrusion correction.

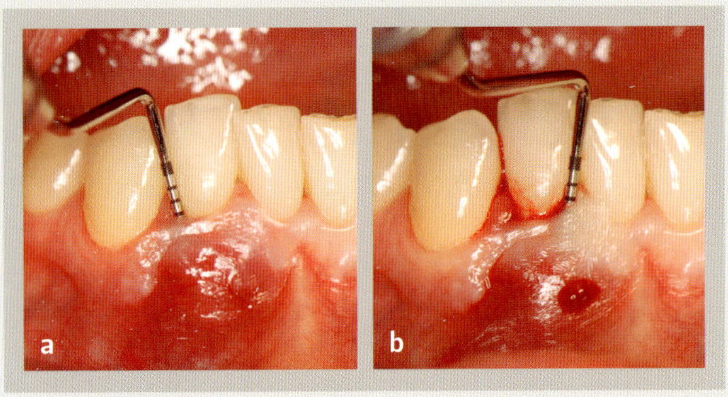

1.6 Periodontal probing on the distal and mesial aspect of the tooth.

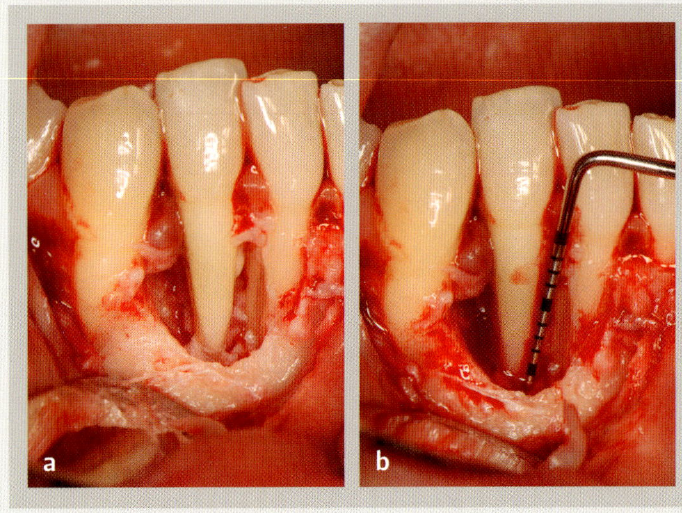

1.7 Surgical view of the huge bone defect associated with the crowding.

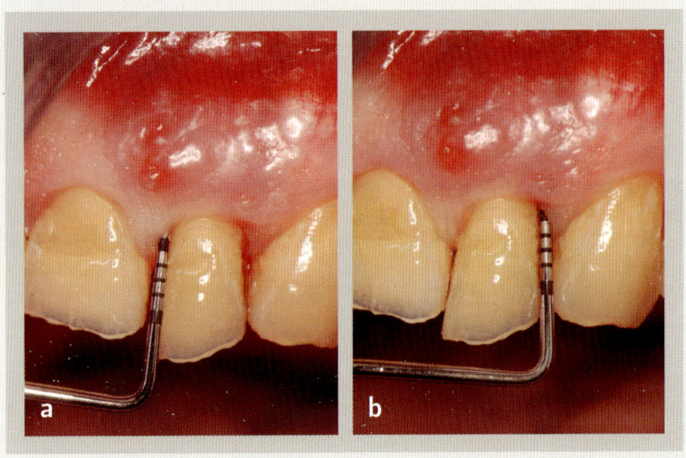

1.8 Periodontal probing on the mesio - and disto - vestibular aspect of the tooth.

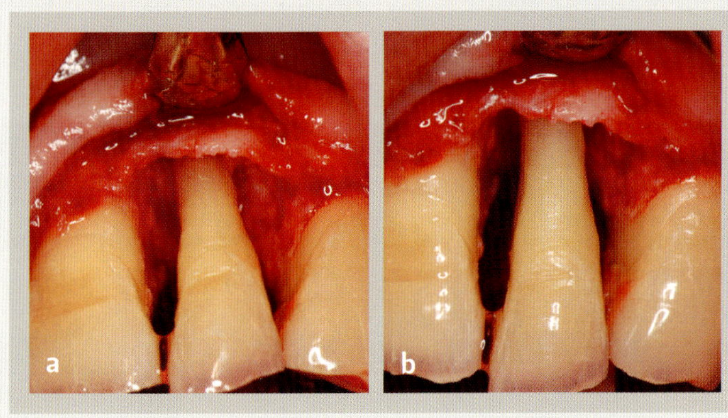

1.9 Surgical view of the funnel-shaped bone defect around the tooth.

up must be common (e.g. model cast or virtual set-up, cephalometric tracing, periodontal probing)[28]. It is important to shift adult and perio patients from an idealistic objective treatment plan typical of growing patients to biological, economic, occlusal and restorative ones[28,30,31]. In ortho-perio patients, even limited tooth movement can help to prevent or intercept disease progression and be part of periodontal therapy[32]. These patients very often present very complex oral rehabilitation problems that require not only practical but also comfortable and esthetically acceptable solutions[33].

Recognizing and identifying patients with periodontal disease in orthodontic routine remains a key to successful treatment, stability and long-term maintenance of the teeth; in the same way it is essential that the periodontist considers the hypothesis of orthodontic treatment as an integral part of the periodontal therapeutic plan, as we can see in Chapter 3. The combined therapeutic strategy, hygiene compliance, type of mechanics, severity of the malocclusion and duration of treatment must be evaluated by both specialists[34].

All patients who require an oral rehabilitation must be informed that in a rehabilitative solution, implants included, an orthodontic contribution can offer alternatives, a different predictability, a different surgical approach. In the same way every orthodontic patient has the right to have a periodontal diagnosis at any age the treatment is performed, to assess the individual risk factor and the therapeutic follow-up[2].

Orthodontics can be a component of the treatment whose aim is remodeling and reconstructing the alveolar process either combined with other dental specializations or alone, with a role on trophism, on the morphology of the alveolar bone and on the positioning of the teeth in the alveolar process[35,36].

The awareness and knowledge of the objectives and results to be achieved and what are the biological costs of the treatment in interdisciplinary patients must be clear from the very beginning[37]. Sometimes, due to periodontal, skeletal and bone boundaries and due to the need to limit the time of the treatment, the type and the direction of forces in a reduced periodontium, the objectives to reduce bone defects, to increase the dental longevity, to facilitate oral hygiene and to improve the esthetic and psychological well-being of the patient, impose a compromise in obtaining class I ideals to which orthodontists have been trained, while the objective of obtaining a stable occlusion remains undiscussed[37]. Orthodontic dental movement is a reconstruction process of the occlusion with the morphological remodeling of the bone. The team's approach is essential in organizing a treatment plan that allows the orthodontist to favourably change the morphology of a defect because the shape of the defect is a critical factor in the predictability of regenerative processes[38].

The orthodontic treatment, being itself capable of modifying the bone morphology, often reaching a minor surgical reduction, can restore a topography of the alveolar ridge, improve the periodontal architecture, distribute along the major axis of the teeth occlusal forces, contribute to the position in the natural alveolar housing[2], correct crowding[39] and contact point distortion which during dental eruption could have reduced the archwire length and enhanced the formation of pockets bringing the plaque into subgingival position[40] and resolve secondary malocclusions due to spontaneous dental migration because of loss of bone support in periodontal disease[41,42]. Orthodontics can provide reconstructive and rehabilitative dentistry with the correct intra- and inter-arch dimensions for each individual patient[28] and, through the three-dimensional bone level guide, carry out the positioning of the brackets and participate to the planning of future reconstructive and occlusal detailing[24]. Therefore, positioning and root parallelism on an alveolar or skeletal basis should not be read on a typical orthodontical point of view, but should be integrated with the patient's periodontal-restorative situation[23].

For all these reasons orthodontic treatment can and must be guided by a periodontal vision and diagnosis.

REFERENCES

1. Ong MM, Wang HL. Periodontic and orthodontic treatment in adults. *Am J Orthod Dentofacial Orthop.* 2002;122(4):420-428.
2. Palomo L, Paolomo JM, Bissada NF. Salient periodontal issues for the modern biologic Orthodontist. *Semin Orthod.* 2008;14(4):229-245.
3. Palomo L. Treatment in the age of periodontal risk management. *Semin Orthod.* **2019;25(2):109.**
4. Zoizner R, Arbel Y, Yavnai N et al. Effect of orthodontic treatment and comorbidity risk factors on interdental alveolar crest level: A radiographic evaluation. *Am J Orthod Dentofacial Orthop.* 2018;154(3):375-381.
5. Papageorgiou SN, Papadelli AA, Eliades T. Effect of orthodontic treatment on periodontal clinical attachment: a systematic review and meta-analysis. *Eur J Orthod.* 2018;40(2):176-194.
6. Cardaropoli D, Gaveglio L, Abou-Arraj RV. Orthodontic movement and periodontal bone defects: Rationale, timing, and clinical implications. *Semin Orthod.* 2014;20(3):177-187.
7. Feng X, Oba T, Oba Y, Moriyama K. An interdisciplinary approach for improved functional and esthetic results in a periodontally compromised adult patient. *Angle Orthod.* 2005;75(6):1061-1070.
8. Re S, Corrente G, Abundo R, Cardaropoli D. Orthodontic treatment in periodontally compromised patients: 12-year report. *Int J Periodontics Restorative Dent.* 2000;20(1):31-39.
9. Nelson PA, Artun J. Alveolar bone loss of maxillary anterior teeth in adult orthodontic patients. *Am J Orthod Dentofacial Orthop.* 1997;111(3):328-334.
10. Boyd RL, Leggott PJ, Quinn RS et al. Periodontal implications of orthodontic treatment in adults with reduced or normal periodontal tissues versus those of adolescents. *Am J Orthod Dentofacial Orthop.* 1989;96(3):191-198.

11. **Artun J, Urbye KS.** The effect of orthodontic treatment on periodontal bone support in patients with advanced loss of marginal periodontium. *Am J Orthod Dentofacial Orthop.* 1988;93(2):143-148.

12. **Ericsson I, Thilander B, Lindhe J, Okamoto H.** The effect of orthodontic tilting movements on the periodontal tissues of infected and non-infected dentitions in dogs. *J Clin Periodontol.* 1977;4(4):278-293.

13. **Nakamura Y, Gomi K, Oikawa T et al.** Reconstruction of a collapsed dental arch in a patient with severe periodontitis. *Am J Orthod Dentofacial Orthop.* 2013;143(5):704-712.

14. **Gkantidis N, Christou P, Topouzelis N.** The orthodontic-periodontic interrelationship in integrated treatment challenges: a systematic review. *J Oral Rehabil.* 2010;37(5):377-390.

15. **Zafiropoulos GG, di Prisco MO, Deli G et al.** Maintenance after a complex orthoperio treatment in a case of generalized aggressive periodontitis: 7-year result. *J Int Acad Periodontol.* 2010;12(4):112-122.

16. **Polson A, Caton J, Polson AP et al.** Periodontal response after tooth movement into intrabony defects. *J Periodontol.* 1984;55(4):197-202.

17. **Eliasson LA, Hugoson A, Kurol J, Siwe H.** The effects of orthodontic treatment on periodontal tissues in patients with reduced periodontal support. *Eur J Orthod.* 1982;4(1):1-9.

18. **Tonetti MS, Greenwell H, Kornman KS.** Staging and grading of periodontitis: framework and proposal of a new classification and case definition [published correction appears in *J Clin Periodontol.* 2019 Jul;46(7):787]. *J Clin Periodontol.* 2018;45 (Suppl 20):S149-S161.

19. **Tonetti MS, Greenwell H, Kornman KS.** Staging and grading of periodontitis: framework and proposal of a new classification and case definition [published correction appears in *J Periodontol.* 2018 Dec;89(12):1475]. *J Periodontol.* 2018;89(Suppl 1):S159-S172.

20. **Cardaropoli D, Gaveglio L.** The influence of orthodontic movement on periodontal tissues level. *Semin Orthod.* 2007;13(4):234-245.

21. **Cardaropoli D, Re S, Manuzzi W et al.** Bio-Oss collagen and orthodontic movement for the treatment of infrabony defects in the esthetic zone. *Int J Periodontics Restorative Dent.* 2006;26(6):553-559.

22. **Hazan-Molina H, Levin L, Einy S, Aizenbud D.** Aggressive periodontitis diagnosed during or before orthodontic treatment. *Acta Odontol Scand.* 2013;71(5):1023-1031.

23. **Kokich VG.** Excellence in finishing: modifications for the perio-restorative patient. *Semin Orthod.* **2003;9(3):184-203.**

24. **Mathews DP, Kokich VG.** Managing treatment for the orthodontic patient with periodontal problems. *Semin Orthod.* 1997;3(1):21-38.

25. **Lindhe J, Nyman S.** Long-term maintenance of patients treated for advanced periodontal disease. *J Clin Periodontol.* 1984;11(8):504-514.

26. **Lindhe J, Svanberg G.** Influence of trauma from occlusion on progression of experimental periodontitis in the beagle dog. *J Clin Periodontol.* 1974;1(1):3-14.

27. **Kokich VG.** Don't start without the charting. *Am J Orthod Dentofacial Orthop.* **2011;139(Suppl 4):S14.**

28. **Kokich VG.** Esthetics: the orthodontic-periodontic restorative connection. *Semin Orthod.* **1996;2(1):21-30.**

29. **Zachrisson BU, Amat P.** La recherche de l'excellence en orthodontie de l'adulte: entretien avec Bjørn U. Zachrisson [The search for excellence in adult orthodontics; an interview with Bjørn U. Zachrisson]. *Orthod Fr.* 2014;85(4):301-26.

30. **Kokich VG, Spear MF.** Guidelines for managing the orthodontic-restorative patient. *Semin Orthod.* 1997;3(1):3-20.

31. **Reichert C, Hagner M, Jepsen S, Jäger A.** Interfaces between orthodontic and periodontal treatment: their current status. *J Orofac Orthop.* 2011;72(3):165-186.

32. **Vanarsdall RL.** Orthodontics and periodontal therapy. *Periodontol 2000.* **1995;9(1):132-149.**

33. **Machuca G, Martínez F, Machuca C, Bullón P.** A combination of orthodontic, periodontal, and prosthodontic treatment in a case of advanced malocclusion. *Int J Periodontics Restorative Dent.* 2003;23(5):499-505.

34. **Geisinger ML, Abou-Arraj RV, Souccar NM et al.** Decision making in the treatment of patients with malocclusion and chronic periodontitis: scientific evidence and clinical experience. *Semin Orthod.* 2014;20(3):170-176.

35. **Fontenelle A.** Concetti parodontali dello spostamento dentale guidato. *S.I.D.O. Syllabus.* **1992;2.**

36. **Melsen B, Agerbaek N.** Orthodontics as an adjunct to rehabilitation. *Periodontol 2000.* 1994;4(1):148-159.

37. **Janson M, Janson G, Murillo-Goizueta OE.** A modified orthodontic protocol for advanced periodontal disease in Class II division 1 malocclusion. *Am J Orthod Dentofacial Orthop.* 2011;139(Suppl 4):S133-S144.

38. **Cao T, Xu L, Shi J, Zhou Y.** Combined orthodontic-periodontal treatment in periodontal patients with anteriorly displaced incisors. *Am J Orthod Dentofacial Orthop.* 2015;148(5):805-813.

39. **Mihram WL, Murphy NC.** The orthodontist's role in 21st century periodontic-prosthodontic therapy. *Semin Orthod.* 2008;14(4):272-289.

40. **Waerhaug J.** Eruption of teeth into crowded position, loss of attachment, and downgrowth of subgingival plaque. *Am J Orthod.* 1980;78(4):453-459.

41. **Williams S, Melsen B, Agerbaek N, Asboe V.** The orthodontic treatment of malocclusion in patients with previous periodontal disease. *Br J Orthod.* 1982;9(4):178-184.

42. **Thilander B.** Indications for orthodontic treatment in adults. *Eur J Orthod.* **1979;1(4):227-241.**

"Ortho-Guided" periodontal treatment plan. Ortho-Perio Risk Assessment (OPRA)

Introduction

The periodontal treatment plan main aim is the elimination of bacterial infection and prevention of the recurrence of periodontal disease. These can be obtained by the creation of an environment that can be cleaned in an accurate way in order to host as few pathogens as possible. The therapy is individualised because it depends on the type, severity and the morphology of the defect which remains after initial periodontal therapy[1,2]. On the other hand, keeping the periodontal tissues out of inflammation is a challenge for most patients of any age.

"Every orthodontic intervention has a periodontal dimension"[3]. This statement enhances how much periodontal environment has an influence on orthodontic treatment because orthodontics depends on root length and shape (2.1), alveolar bone width and height (2.2) and gingival phenotype (2.3). As a matter of fact, orthodontic movements are related to the interaction of teeth with their periodontal support tissues[4].

Periodontal patients show various orthodontic problems that require treatment[5]. In order to have the best results from both the specialties we must start with the identification of periodontal problems that eventually can become more complex during orthodontic treatment and the detection of problems that can have benefit from orthodontic therapy[6]. Specific periodontal evidences (bone topography, atrophic edentulous ridges, sinus morphology, frenulum attachment, PPD [Periodontal Probing Depth], CAL [Clinical Attachment Loss]), make it necessary to modify the orthodontic treatment in these patients taking into account various aspects: the simplification of oral hygiene, the modification of biomechanics, the absence of growth in adult patients and the difference in anchorage for the reduction of periodontal bone support[7]; in these patients there is a risk for future periodontal problems and breakdown that can cause tooth loss, often associated with complex malocclusions[8].

Orthodontics is a tool capable of repositioning the tooth with its whole periodontal tissue in the desired position within the limits of the anatomical and phenotypic potential. Under this approach a new kind of periodontal treatment can be developed and the orthodontist can and "must" participate to this therapy. Periodontal tissues can be moulded at their leisure and must not be considered by orthodontists a limitation that distracts

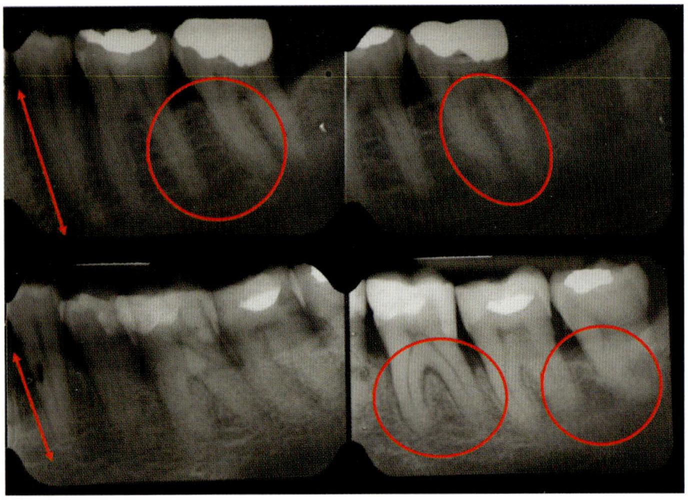

2.1 Difference between root shape and length.

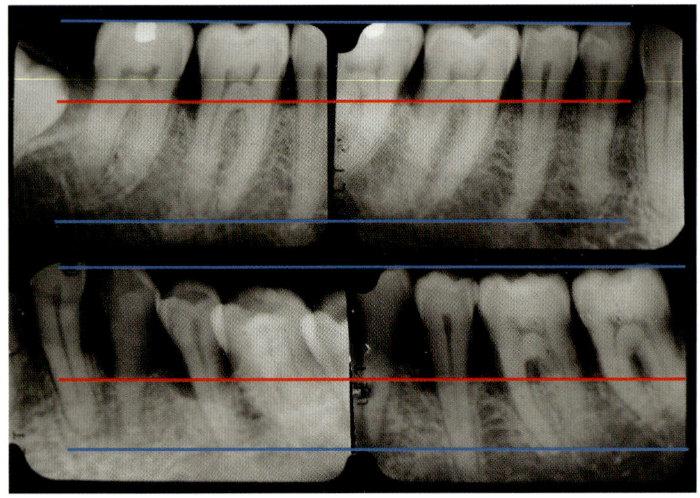

2.2 Difference between bone width and height.

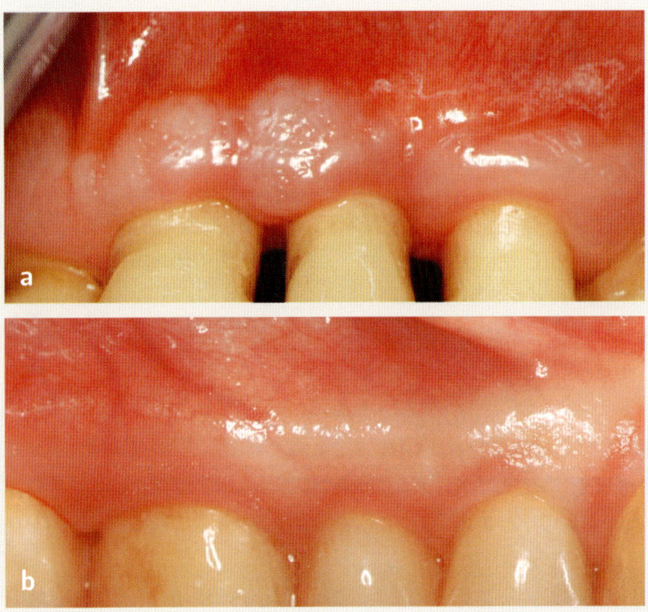

2.3 Difference between thick and thin phenotype.

from the mechanics passion, but great opportunity. "Alveolar-topography engineering" has to be considered as parodontology with an orthodontic component[9]. The possibility of saving and rehabilitating compromised teeth depends not only on the number of teeth that remain in the arch and their periodontal status and degree of destruction, but also from the morphology of the aveolar process and the position of the teeth in this. Orthodontic forces induce a remodeling of the periodontal tissue during tooth movement[8]. From this point of view orthodontics can be seen as an alternative or as a component of treatment, which may be seriously compromised without orthodontics itself[10].

Orthodontics, according to the periodontal vision, must have as guideline the tissues on which periodontology works. The first ones are hard tissues, an important element of tooth stability that in resective surgery procedures are remodelled for the treatment of the periodontal disease sequelae. The second ones are soft tissues where mucogengival surgery has a plastic tissutal action, which is very important for esthetics. Hard and soft tissues will guide orthodontics to model the environment around the teeth in order to modify and relocate tissues where treatment plan needs. Controlled tooth movement seems to have a positive, but extremely variable effect, on support tissue. The correction of different orthodontic problems such as tipped molars, traumatic deepbite, PTM (Pathological Tooth Migration) and diastema can be beneficial to perio-patients reaching a periodontal stability and can enhance the choice for orthodontics[11]. The objective of the ortho-perio treatment must be evaluated under different factors: esthetics, function, risks correlated to orthodontic movement, biomechanical considerations and periodontal prognosis[3].

The functional levelling of the teeth, apart from solving esthetic problems, can direct occlusal forces along the tooth axis in order to improve the periodontal architecture and to position teeth in relation to the tooth housing. Modification of the housing of the teeth in the alveolar bone can improve the width and the height of the keratinized tissue and an axial charge on teeth can enhance cortical bone[6]. Orthodontic treatment does not have a worsening effect on the periodontal status even in patients with a severe or aggressive periodontitis without tissue inflammation[12]. In a recent study on the efficacy of the combined ortodontic-periodontal treatment some Authors[13] state that, after the combined treatment, all the periodontal indexes (PPD, PI [Plaque Index], CAL, BOP [Bleeding On Probing]) improve considerably without significant differences compared to healthy patients showing a quicker recovery in comparison to the conventional periodontal treatment.

Ortho-perio cooperation is not limited to a reciprocal scientific exchange of knowledge but reinforces the patient's motivation and the long-term stability in clinical results. Patient's compliance, motivation and oral hygiene care are universally recognised as important factors in evaluating what kind of impact orthodontic movement can have on periodontal status. Regular monitoring of adults with a predisposition to periodontal breakdown during tooth movement is mandatory. The importance of maintaining periodontal health must be clear from the very beginning of the periodontal therapy and during the whole orthodontic treatment and must continue during all the patient's "dental" life[14]. This strategy must be used as a preventive routine during orthodontic fixed mechanics[6]. Very often going back to periodontal health allows the patient to recover and improve motivation and compliance to oral hygiene that had been lost for a compromised esthetics and gingival situation[15].

Microbiology and orthodontics

The main reason for plaque accumulation in orthodontic patients is the presence on the teeth of retentive surfaces such as fixed appliances[8,16,17], even if the use of orthodontic appliances is not correlated to the worsening of periodontal conditions[18]. A bad oral hygiene increases the plaque formation that brings to the modification of the oral environment concerning the quantity, the flow and the composition of saliva including its buffer capacity, pH, and this can produce gingival hyperplasia and bleeding on probing[19]. We will analyze now in which way the different orthodontic appliances can modify the microbial plaque in terms of quality and quantity.

Orthodontic appliances

The application of an orthodontic appliance can indirectly contribute to the exacerbation of tissue inflammation, because it appears to be a complication in the execution of normal hygiene procedures, increasing bacterial aggregation. On the other hand, the real problem is not the bacterial aggregation *per se*, but the possibility of the transition of the subgingival plaque in a more periodontopathogenic bacterial flora which may encourage the conversion from gingivitis to parodontitis[5]. The bacterial adhesion, colonisation and growth on different surfaces depend on various factors which are related to the properties of the materials, their surface morphology, their shape and positioning. They are also linked to the patient's characteristics, with a particular reference to their oral hygiene[20] and their compliance to the orthodontic appliance[14]. This leads to plaque accumulation[14,21,22] and its maturation[23], which increases during the first 6 months of treatment[24]. Microbiological indexes tend to normalize 6 months after the fixed appliance removal[25]. Various studies have tried to quantify the plaque accumulation with different appliances (self-legating brackets, metallic ligatures, elastomeric ligatures) to understand if there are any differences between the different devices.

Despite inconclusive results, bonding instead of banding molars seems to be the safest solution[5,8], notwithstanding the fact that the composite residues increase plaque retention[12] and that the bonding material can have an impact on adhesion and maturation of the bacterial biofilm because of the characteristics of the material such as the surface rugosity, the tooth-material interface, factors which protect the biofilm from the mechanical removal[26]. This leads, in 2-3 weeks, to the presence of a mature plaque on the excesses of composite and along the composite/tooth surface gap where bacteria accumulate[27]. This requires the complete and preventive accurate removal of the composite excesses around the brackets. In fact, the meticulous plaque control and the continuous and repeated motivation to professional and domestic oral hygiene procedures and to the biofilm control in periodontal therapy since the very first steps of the orthodontic treatment, increase periodontal results reducing negative consequences being essential factors for success in ortho-perio treatments[14,28].

Fixed appliances increase the quantity of acidogenic biofilm increasing the risk of gingivitis[29-31]. The accumulation of plaque can create the conditions for a transition from a subgengival plaque to a more periodontopathogenic one[32,33] with an increase in anaerobic gram-negative[34]. This does not happen before one week, because the composition and the width of the emerging biofilm do not provide the necessary condition of anaerobiosis at this depth. Later there are significant modifications in the composition of the biofilm. This increased adhesion of the bacteria is due to: 1) wider metallic surfaces with greater niches where the biofilm adheres in an easier way; 2) increase in performing a good oral hygiene level; 3) bacteria species which adhere to other bacterial colonies creating special populations that are structured in communities of biofilm; 4) biofilm of mixed bacterial communities which are thicker and more stable than monospecies biofilm[19].

Microbiological studies on the composition of subgingival plaque in patients with brackets show significant modifications[35-37], with an increase after the application of the brackets in the experimental group compared to the controls concerning periodontopathogenic bacteria such as *Porphyromonas gingivalis*, *Prevotella intermedia/Prevotella nigrescens*, *Tannerella forsythia* and *Fusobacterium*; also superinfections can be found from *Enterobacter cloacae*, *Klebsiella oxytoca*, *Klebsiella pneumonia* and *Serratia marcescens*[38]. It is particularly interesting to underline that during the initial phase the anaerobic condition of the emerging biofilm analysed at the fixed appliance and not in the periodontal pockets could be sufficient to promote the growth of anaerobic bacteria that can cause periodontitis: *Tannerella forsythia*, *Treponema denticola* and *Porphyromonas gingivalis*[19]. These species, together with *Prevotella nigrescens*, are more present in orthodontic patients than in patients that did not have orthodontic treatments, even if they did not show a serious periodontal disease[39].

Several Authors[40-43] state that orthodontic appliances, in the long-term, can contribute to a (unfortunate but predictable) qualitative alteration in bacterial subgingival biofilm, which progressively becomes more perio-pathogenic showing an increase in the presence of *Actinobacillus actinomycetemcomitans* (today called *Aggregatibacter actinomycetemcomitans*), which however does not seem to be a serious risk factor for the deterioration of the periodontal conditions during the 3 years of observation[44]. Research with DNA probes have revealed that periodontopathogenic bacteria (*Actinobacillus actinomycetemcomitans*, *Porphyromonas gingivalis*, *Prevotella intermedia*, *Tannerella forsythia*, *Eikenella corrodens*, *Fusobacterium nucleatum*, *Treponema denticola* and *Campylobacter rectus*) increase 6 months after orthodontic treatment but return to the same level after 12 months of therapy[24,33], and remain stable at the 2-year follow-up, when all the values normalize[32]. According to different Authors, an important care would consist of the most accurate reduction of the wire loops and elastomeric ligatures and in the immediate removal of the excess of the bonding, giving preference to the self-ligating brackets[45] or to metal ligatures more than elastomeric ones, which seem to favour a greater plaque retention and a greater gingival bleeding[46-48]; there are not real differences in PI, GI (Gingival Index), PPD, BOP and in the presence of *S. mutans* between self-ligating and conventional brackets[45,49-53]. Van Gastel et al.[54] have shown that the bracket design has a significant impact on bacterial load and on periodontal parameters, but 1 year later the microbiological and periodontal situation does not show a statistically significant difference[55].

Bands

The use of the bands causes plaque retention and bacterial colonization[56-59]. Although bands and cement can cause tissue inflammation, it is an inadequate oral hygiene care that contributes to the development of gingival inflammation[57]. At a microbiological level, bands bring an increase in the percentage of spirochaetes, movable rods, filaments and fusiforms[60], lattobacilli, anaerobics and *Prevotella intermedia*, and a decrease in facultative anaerobes [61].

Aligners

Regarding the composition and the microbial diversity of the plaque, aligners do not show different effects from fixed appliances. For this reason, the simplification of the procedures of oral hygiene, rather than changes in the microbiota, can be the reason for the easy maintenance of oral health in patients wearing aliners[62]. In fact it is reported that in these patients the microbial structure, including *Firmicutes*, *Bacteroides*, *Fusobacteria* and *Actinobacteria*, does not change significantly before and 6 months after the use of aligners. The improvement seems to happen thanks to the enhancement of the awareness and motivation to oral hygiene[63], which is a key factor in every orthodontic treatment.

Lingual appliances

Lingual orthodontic appliances (brackets included) show an higher plaque retention compared to the vestibular ones[64], with a consequent hard control of oral hygiene[65]; however, different studies do not agree and do not refer differences between lingual and vestibular brackets[34,58,60] and show that a significant impact does not exist on periodontal indexes (PPD and BOP) and on the microbiological count of streptococci, anaerobic and bacterial colonies[66]. After the completion of orthodontic therapy, the greatest part of the inflammatory conditions results are reversible[23] without permanent disruptive effects on deep periodontal tissues[17,40,44,45,67] even if the microbial colonization remains high with respect to controls[24].

Conclusions

All these microbial changes that happen in orthodontic patients remind the orthodontist to pay particular attention to bonding and banding and to avoid sub- or peri-gingival positioning of brackets and bands[8]. It can be concluded that orthodontic fixed appliances are not a risk factor for the induction of the disease, but can, however, facilitate a temporary condition of plaque build-up and gengivitis[45,68].

Clinical effects of orthodontics on tissues

Fixed appliances have a major impact on periodontal conditions, which can vary in relation to the specific patient, site and appliance characteristics. Changes that may occur are[25,31,54]:

1. *Increase in PPD and BOP.* Patients treated orthodontically show an average increase in PPD of 0.35 mm (0.03-0.72 mm), a value with minimal clinical importance, compared to untreated patients[49,69]. This value tends to normalize 3 months after the removal of the fixed appliance[25]. According to Bollen et al.[70] orthodontic patients show a 0.13 mm loss of alveolar bone and a 0.23 mm of PPD; according to Nelson and Artun[71] only 2.5% of all the patients showed a bone loss greater than 2 mm, confirming that orthodontic treatment is not contraindicated in the periodontal patient, that it does not cause irreversible destruction of the periodontal tissue and that it does not increase the incidence of periodontal diseases. Sadowsky and BeGole[72] demonstrated that pocket depth is not significantly different between orthodontically and non-orthodontically treated groups. The same situation happens for the average loss of periodontal attachment and for gingival recessions[36]. An increase in PPD could be due to moderate gingival hyperplasia without significant attachment loss[5]. Papageorgiou et al.[73], in a recent meta-analysis, found that orthodontic treatment is associated with an average clinical attachment loss of 0.11 mm, which is neither statistically nor clinically significant, demonstrating that a similar amount of clinical attachment loss, with the same statistical and clinical significance, occurred in the control patients group. The authors, by meta-regression tool, indicated that clinical attachment loss is inversely related to the mean age of the patients and that older patients showed less attachment loss; this has been attributed to the fact that adolescents have a worse plaque control during treatment, resulting in increased PPD and gingival inflammation[73].
2. *Increased volume of crevicular fluid.*
3. *Change from aerobic to anaerobic microbial species* as described above.
4. *Increase in GI and GBI (Gingival Bleeding Index)*, which tend to decrease within the first 3-6 months with the establishment of good oral hygiene. In a recent systematic review the authors[23], together with Reichardt et al.[19], confirmed that the use of orthodontic appliances, in particular fixed ones, can promote the increase of inflammation in periodontal tissues, increasing the periodontal parameters (BOP, PI, GI) probably as a consequence of the effect of the plaque retention by the brackets, an event that complicates the maintenance of a standard oral hygiene[52].

Clinical parameters[17] (PI, GI, GBI, PPD) gradually increase from week 4 to a maximum peak at 3 months[67] after the placement of the fixed orthodontic appliance, decreasing then up to 6 months and stabilizing together with gingival inflammation during the whole duration of the treatment[74]. This is due to the fact that, after a rapid initial qualitative and quantitative change in the microbial composition at the beginning of the therapy, a new equilibrium is formed which remains stable for the entire duration of the application of the orthodontic appliance[19]. In conclusion, orthodontic treatment is characterized by minimal and temporary clinical and microbiological changes (increased plaque accumulation, difficulty in maintaining oral hygiene) which do not lead to modifications in the patient's periodontal status[75]. Since a small number of patients may present a significant risk of irreversible periodontal destruction, special attention should be paid to initial periodontal therapy and accurate monitoring should be realized during treatment[49].

Long-term ortho-perio treatment

We have seen how orthodontic treatment can assist periodontal therapy. But, in the long-term, how does this association behave? Can orthodontic treatment promote long-term periodontal health for these patients? Can patients who have undergone orthodontic treatment have overall a better oral health during their lifetime? If the patient undergoing orthodontic treatment has less periodontal inflammation over time, is orthodontic treatment justified to achieve long-term oral health stability[76]?

Even in the presence of aggressive forms, orthodontic-periodontal treatment does not lead to a worsening of the periodontal disease if it is kept under strict periodontal control.

Several authors evaluated the long-term stability of ortho-perio treatment with the analyses of case reports. Feu et al.[77] confirmed the stability at a radiographic level with negative BOP, showing furthermore a modification of the infraosseous defect dimensions and the realization of a more maintainable modified architecture and more favorable periodontal bone levels around the periodontal affected teeth. Zafiropoulos et al.[78] and Derton et al.[79], 7 years after orthodontic-periodontal treatment, confirmed these considerations radiologically with periodontal probing. Boyer et al.[80] showed that long-term periodontal orthodontic treatment, at an average time of 16 years, enhances stable bone gain improving results over time; periodontal health can be preserved with strict oral hygiene, dental alignment, arch harmonization and correction of tooth migration, confirming that combined orthodontic treatment enhances the benefits of periodontal treatment alone. Roccuzzo et al.[81] observed at a 10-year follow-up in 36 regenerated and orthodontically moved sites with carefully controlled infection, that orthodontic treatment did not reduce the long-term benefits of regenerative periodontal treatment even when the disease had caused a huge tissue destruction. Aimetti et al.[82], in a retrospective study with patients with stage IV periodontitis in supportive periodontal therapy for 11.6 ± 1.6 years after the end of periodontal therapy, who underwent orthodontic treatment for 4 to 36 months, stated that the orthodontic movement did not have important effects on reduced but healthy periodontium in patients enrolled in a rigorous periodontal maintenance program who completed active therapy with a proper plaque and inflammation control (FMPS [Full- Mouth Plaque Score] - FMBS [Full- Mouth Bleeding Score] <20%) and without residual pockets (PPD ≤4 mm). This allowed not to have a loss of the level of clinical attachment due to a recurrence of periodontitis.

Two important conclusions can be drawn from the literature data: periodontal treatment, before any orthodontic treatment, must achieve complete stability and periodontal health conditions must be maintained in the long-term with an adequate supportive therapy program. Orthodontic-periodontal treatment has an immediate and long-lasting clinical effect and allows patients to have stable esthetics and function restored (📷 2.4-2.6; see Chapter 4, *Clinical case 1)*.

Risk assessment of the ortho-perio patient

As happens in the routine approach for the periodontal patient, a focused risk assessment of disease progression must also be performed for the ortho-perio patient[83], analyzing the conditions that could worsen

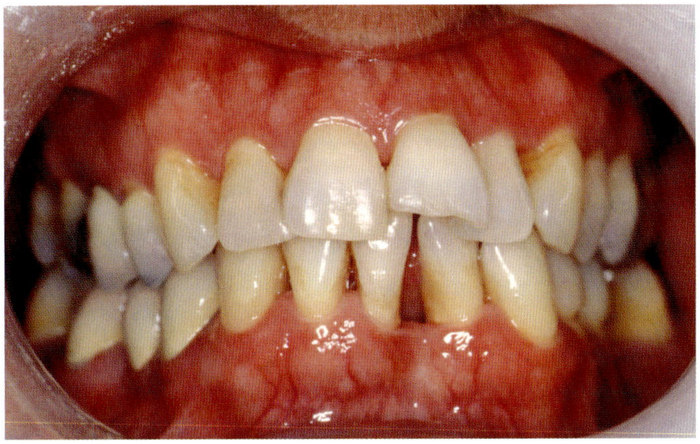

2.4 Ortho-perio patient: initial recordings. Start of treatment.

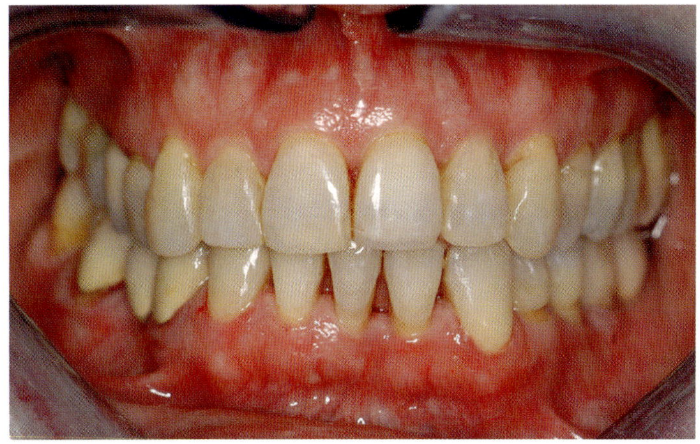

2.5 Long-term Ortho-perio treatment stability. 3 year follow-up.

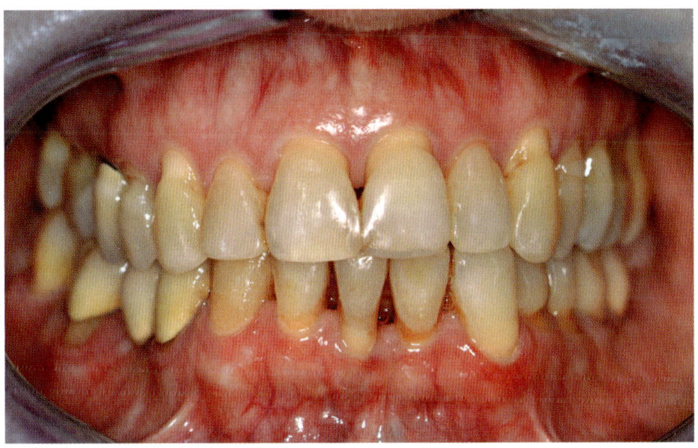

2.6 Long-term Ortho-perio treatment stability. 10 year follow-up.

during combined treatment and considering the factors that could cause orthodontic and periodontal problems during and after interdisciplinary treatment. The clinician must identify susceptible patients and implement strategies to prevent attachment loss and gingival recessions[2].

A thorough periodontal risk assessment should be performed to intercept and to try to prevent and avoid undesirable consequences during and after orthodontic treatment[14]. The activity and prognosis of periodontal disease for each individual patient require careful individual risk assessment and it influences the indications and outcomes of orthodontic treatment[3]. There is a small portion of high-risk patients who are more likely to develop adverse effects for what concerns attachment loss, so it is important to carry out meticulous monitoring and a careful risk assessment before and during treatment to early identify and reduce these risks[49].

This protocol must be carried out not only in orthodontic-periodontal adult patients: the young age of patients, in fact, must not deceive and induce the orthodontist to treat adolescent patients while considering them free from risk of periodontal disease. In fact, patients aged from 13 to 18 years old may host infection and show a periodontal attachment loss which is normally not found at their age[6]. Cappelli et al.[84] determined that the 25.7% of students in a study of Hispanic patients, showed early-onset periodontitis (EOP), where 1.7% were diagnosed as localized juvenile periodontitis (A/N - The definition reported in the article does not follow the current classification). These data must alert the orthodontist, because the adolescent population could present periodontal problems which do not manifest[6].

The clinical importance of a risk assessment profile determines the need for its "inclusion" in the treatment plan. This means that the treatment must be planned and carried out in relation to specific factors and the therapeutic plan must be modulated to try to prevent complications. The risk assessment must be reassessed over time and the patient placed in a long-term supportive therapy program that is scheduled and modified in relation to this new risk profile.

Before assessing the combined orthodontic- periodontal risk it is mandatory to perform the periodontal risk assessment.

Tab. 2.1 Table with summary of mean evaluation models of Periodontal Risk Assessment

Assessment model	Risk factors
Continuous Multilevel Risk Assessment (Lang and Tonetti[85])	3 levels factors : PATIENT (diabetes, stress, compliance, smoking history, bone loss/age, FMBS - FMPS, PPD ≥ 5 mm); TOOTH (tooth malposition, mouth breathing, tooth malformation, furcation lesions, iatrogenic factors, residual periodontal support, mobility); SITE (BOP, PPD, probing technique - dimension and placement of probe, crudeness of the measurement scale, probing force, gingival tissue condition, suppuration)
PRC (Page et al.[86,97])	11 factors (age, smoking history, diabetes, previous periodontal surgery, BOP, furcation involvement, subgingival restorations, vertical intrabony defects, root calculus, PPD, radiographic bone loss)
PRA (Lang and Tonetti[88])	6 factors (% BOP, PPD ≥5mm, number loss teeth, % bone loss/age, systemic and/or genetic conditions, environmental factors like smoking habits)
Modified PRA (Chandra[90])	8 factors (% BOP, PPD ≥5mm, CAL/age, smoking habits, diabetes, dental status-systemic factors interplay, psychosocial factors)
3-level Method Assessment Approach (Rotundo and Pini Prato[97])	PATIENT (FMBS - FMPS, PPD ≥ 5 mm, mm radiographic bone loss, N. lost teeth, N. of systemic diseases with immune response deficiencies, N. cigarettes/day, age, microbial pattern); TOOTH (mobility, crown/root ratio, furcation lesion, aberrant fillings/margin crowns, tooth malposition: mesial tipping, rotation, inclination); SITE (recession, PPD, degree of inflammation: BOP and suppuration)
PRAS (Leininger et al.[91])	6 factors (BOP, PPD ≥5mm, radiographic bone loss/age, systemic condition, smoking habits)
PerioRisk (Trombelli et al.[94-96])	5 factors (BOP, PPD ≥5mm, radiographic bone loss/age, smoking habits, diabetes)
DentoRisk (Lindskog et al.[92,93])	20 factors (systemic predictors/local predictors)

Perio Risk Assessment and periodontal risk factors. When evaluating the prognostic factor of a periodontal patient, several factors are taken into consideration. Various Authors have tried to develop models or methods for assessing such factors that can modify prognosis, continuously monitoring the patient's condition and drawing up individual risk models for each patient, such as Lang's and Tonetti's Continuous Multilevel Risk Assessment[85], the Page's PRC (Periodontal Risk Calculator)[86,87], the Lang's and Tonetti's PRA (Periodontal Risk Assessment)[88] aimed at patients included in a support therapy program, the Renvert's PPRD (Periodont Pentagon Risk Diagram)[89], the Chandra's modified PRA[90], the Leininger's PRAS (Periodontal Risk Assessment Diagram Surface)[91], the Lindskog's DentoRisk[92.93], the Farina and Trombelli's simplified PerioRisk[94-96], which we use in clinical cases of this text, and the Rotundo and Pini Prato's stratified three-level method[97]. The factors that are taken into account by these models are listed in 2.1.

Ortho-Perio Risk Assessment (OPRA)

We will now analyze the additional factors for compiling the Ortho-Perio Risk Assessment (OPRA).

Pre-existing factors

1. *Periodontal risk assessment*: it is assessed with the methods used in periodontology already described above (see 2.1).
2. *Family history*: a positive family history of previous periodontal disease should be noted also in adolescents and children.
3. *Dental factors*: apical root resorption[98], previous decays and carioreceptivity, timing and causes of dental loss, aptitude of the child and his family to maintain oral hygiene and/or positive dental history from neglected hygiene.
4. *Gingival phenotype*: the various gingival phenotypes respond differently to treatment. Thin phe-

notypes show a reduced resistance to mechanical stress and inflammation and may be related to the development of recessions[14].

5. *Number of recessions present*[99,100].
6. *Presence of crowding*: crowding complicates hygiene procedures and facilitates the conversion of the present plaque into a periopathogenic one.

Orthodontic considerations

1. *Morphology of the future contact point and interproximal bone septum*: prediction of a suitable bone septum and a broad and stable interdental contact[101,102].
2. *Estimated time of orthodontic therapy*: indicative estimated treatment time.
3. *Tooth movement*: tooth movement cannot be performed without limits. Some factors influence the extension of orthodontic movement, such as alveolar bone anatomy, skeletal pattern, pressure by the soft tissues, level of the periodontal attachment, neuromuscolar forces and teeth/lips relationship. Normally it is thought that the limits in orthodontic movement are defined by strict physiologic and anatomic limits that, if violated, can produce alteration of the periodontal tissue and of the alveolar bone support[103,104]. As a result, great dental movements exceeding the "envelope of discrepancy" can be integrated with orthognatic surgery or corticotomy and/or the Periodontally Accelerated Osteogenic Orthodontics (PAOO)[105-108]. It is not clear, however, how much these boundaries can be exceeded before tissue injures passing from a healthy state to a condition of disease[11]. Wennström et al.[109] stated that as long as the tooth moves within the "envelope" of the alveolar process (genetically and/or functionally predetermined[5]), the risk of dangerous side effects on the marginal tissue is minimal[14]. It is recommended to keep the teeth as much as possible within the dentoalveolar process especially in patients who perform aggressive brushing[11]. The movement of the tooth outside the alveolar bone can lead to dehiscence and fenestration, with consequent gingival recessions[7]. The *envelope of discrepancy* of Proffit[103] (2.7), an observation also present in the concept of the limit of the dentition of Tweed[104], indicates that there are some millimetric limits to the dental movement, distinguishing: the only dental movement whose limit is orthodontic and periodontal (inner circle, pink), the possible actions by orthopedic and orthodontic treatments in growing patients (middle circle, light blue) and the limits of actions with combined orthodontic-surgical treatment in the three planes of space (outer circle, orange). The envelopes for the transverse dimension in the upper and lower premolar areas are smaller than the ones for the incisors in the antero-posterior plane of space[2]. In Chapter 7 we will see in detail what it is reported by the literature.
   - *Anterior/variation in incisor inclination*: in Chapter 7 we will see how an orthodontic increase in the lower incisor inclination on mandibular plane up to 8,9° does not show a correlation with an increase in the risk of recession development[110] and a proclination >10° shows an association with the onset of recessions[111] up to 25%[112].
   - *Lateral/torque variation:* transversal correction can be obtained in greater safety conditions with a torque movement, respecting the physiological thickness of the tissues[113,114], avoiding expansions[2].
   - *Risk of the apex contact with the cortical bone plates:* movement of the apex of the mandibular incisor towards the cortical bone plates increases the risk of vertical bone loss[115].
   - *Direction of movement towards/outside the alveolar housing*: the movement towards the alveolar housing protects periodontal tissues[116].

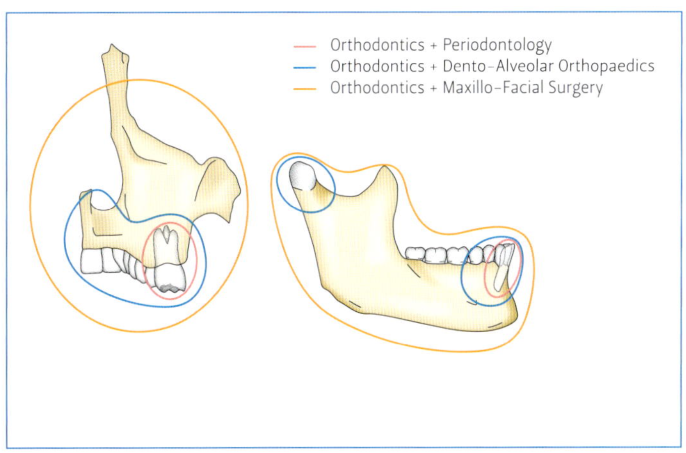

2.7 Anatomic boundaries and therapeutic tasks.

Tab. 2.2 Ortho-Perio Risk Assessment (OPRA)

Pre-existing factors			
	Low	**Medium**	**High**
Periodontal risk assessment	0	2	3
	Absent	**Present**	
Family history	0	1	
History and dental factors			
· Cause of tooth loss			
	Absent	**Present**	
– Decay	0	1	
– Periodontal disease	0	3	
· Abscess of deciduous teeth – neglected hygiene	0	1	
· Apical root resorption	0	2	
	Thick	**Thin**	
Gingival phenotype	0	2	
	n <2	**2< n <5**	**n >5**
Number of recessions	1	2	3
	n <5 mm	**5< n <7 mm**	**n >7 mm**
Dental crowding	1	2	3
Orthodontic considerations			
	<6 months	**6< months <12**	**>12 months**
Length of orthodontic treatment	1	2	3
	Reachable	**Unreachable**	
Future contact point morphology	0	2	
Proper interproximal bone septum	0	2	
Dental movement	**n <5°**	**5°< n <8,9°**	**n >10°**
· Anterior: variation of the incisor inclination	1	2	3
	Absent	**Present**	
· Lateral: torque variation	0	1	
· Lateral: expansion variation	0	3	
· Apical contact risk on the cortical bone plates	0	3	
	Towards	**Outside**	
· Direction of the movement towards/outside the alveolar "housing"	0	3	
TOTAL			

We propose our risk assessment called OPRA (Ortho-Perio Risk Assessment) (■ 2.2) which is a daily screening support for the orthodontist, in cooperation with the periodontist[117] in the early detection and identification of patients at risk, as a diagnostic, prognostic and therapeutic reference and help in combined treatments, in pure orthodontic treatments, in adults and growing patient orthodontic therapies.

An OPRA with a value ranging from 0 to 10 indicates a low risk factor, a value between 11 to 25 indicates a medium risk, while a value between 26 and 40 shows a high risk.

REFERENCES

1. Zasciurinskiene E, Lindsten R, Slotte C, Bjerklin K. Orthodontic treatment in periodontitis-susceptible subjects: a systematic literature review. *Clin Exp Dent Res.* 2016;2(2):162-173.
2. Vanarsdall RL. Orthodontics and periodontal therapy. *Periodontol 2000.* 1995;9(1):132-149.
3. Diedrich P, Fritz U, Kizinger G. Interrelationship between periodontics and adult orthodontics. *Perio.* 2004;1(3):143-149.
4. Harshita N, Kamath DG, Kadakampally D. Perio-Ortho Interactions. A review. *J Pharm Sci & Res.* 2018; 10(5):1053-1056.
5. Gkantidis N, Christou P, Topouzelis N. The orthodontic-periodontic interrelationship in integrated treatment challenges: a systematic review. *J Oral Rehabil.* 2010;37(5):377-390.
6. Palomo L, Palomo JM, Bissada NF. Salient periodontal issues for the modern biologic Orthodontist. *Semin Orthod.* 2008;14(4):229-245.
7. Johal A, Ide M. Orthodontics in the adult patient, with special reference to the periodontally compromised patient. *Dent Update.* 1999;26(3):101-108.
8. Reichert C, Hagner M, Jepsen S, Jäger A. Interfaces between orthodontic and periodontal treatment: their current status. *J Orofac Orthop.* 2011;72(3):165-186.
9. Mihram WL, Murphy NC. The orthodontist's role in 21st century periodontic-prosthodontic therapy. *Semin Orthod.* 2008;14(4):272-289.
10. Melsen B, Agerbaek N. Orthodontics as an adjunct to rehabilitation. *Periodontol 2000.* 1994;4(1):148-159.
11. Antoun JS, Mei L, Gibbs K, Farella M. Effect of orthodontic treatment on the periodontal tissues. *Periodontol 2000.* 2017;74(1):140-157.
12. Czochrowska EM, Rosa M. The orthodontic/periodontal interface. *Semin Orthod.* 2015;21(1):3-14.
13. Zhang J, Zhang AM, Zhang ZM et al. Efficacy of combined orthodontic-periodontic treatment for patients with periodontitis and its effect on inflammatory cytokines: A comparative study. *Am J Orthod Dentofacial Orthop.* 2017;152(4):494-500.
14. Gorbunkova A, Pagni G, Brizhak A et al. Impact of orthodontic treatment on periodontal tissues: a narrative review of multidisciplinary literature. *Int J Dent.* 2016;2016:4723589.
15. Nakamura Y, Gomi K, Oikawa T et al. Reconstruction of a collapsed dental arch in a patient with severe periodontitis. *Am J Orthod Dentofacial Orthop.* 2013;143(5):704-712.
16. Ousehal L, Lazrak L, Es-Said R et al. Evaluation of dental plaque control in patients wearing fixed orthodontic appliances: a clinical study. *Int Orthod.* 2011;9(1):140-155.
17. Ristic M, Vlahovic Svabic M, Sasic M, Zelic O. Clinical and microbiological effects of fixed orthodontic appliances on periodontal tissues in adolescents. *Orthod Craniofac Res.* 2007;10(4):187-195.
18. Gomes SC, Varela CC, da Veiga SL et al. Periodontal conditions in subjects following orthodontic therapy. A preliminary study. *Eur J Orthod.* 2007;29(5):477-481.
19. Reichardt E, Geraci J, Sachse S et al. Qualitative and quantitative changes in the oral bacterial flora occur shortly after implementation of fixed orthodontic appliances. *Am J Orthod Dentofacial Orthop.* 2019;156(6):735-744.
20. Papaioannou W, Makou M. Changes in the oral microbiota during orthodontic treatment. In: Eliades T, Katsaros C. *The ortho-perio patient: clinical evidence & therapeutic guidelines.* Batavia, IL. Quintessence Publishing Co; 2019:33-42.
21. Glans R, Larsson E, Øgaard B. Longitudinal changes in gingival condition in crowded and noncrowded dentitions subjected to fixed orthodontic treatment. *Am J Orthod Dentofacial Orthop.* 2003;124(6):679-682.
22. Alexander SA. Effects of orthodontic attachments on the gingival health of permanent second molars. *Am J Orthod Dentofacial Orthop.* 1991;100(4):337-340.
23. Verrusio C, Iorio-Siciliano V, Blasi A et al. The effect of orthodontic treatment on periodontal tissue inflammation: A systematic review. *Quintessence Int.* 2018;49(1):69-77.
24. Papageorgiou SN, Xavier GM, Cobourne MT, Eliades T. Effect of orthodontic treatment on the subgingival microbiota: A systematic review and meta-analysis. *Orthod Craniofac Res.* 2018;21(4):175-185.
25. van Gastel J, Quirynen M, Teughels W et al. Longitudinal changes in microbiology and clinical periodontal parameters after removal of fixed orthodontic appliances. *Eur J Orthod.* 2011;33(1):15-21.
26. Quirynen M, Bollen CM. The influence of surface roughness and surface-free energy on supra- and subgingival plaque formation in man. A review of the literature. *J Clin Periodontol.* 1995;22(1):1-14.
27. Sukontapatipark W, el-Agroudi MA, Selliseth NJ et al. Bacterial colonization associated with fixed orthodontic appliances. A scanning electron microscopy study. *Eur J Orthod.* 2001;23(5):475-484.
28. Han JY. A comparative study of combined periodontal and orthodontic treatment with fixed appliances and clear aligners in patients with periodontitis. *J Periodontal Implant Sci.* 2015;45(6):193-204.
29. Topaloglu-Ak A, Ertugrul F, Eden E et al. Effect of orthodontic appliances on oral microbiota - 6 month follow-up. *J Clin Pediatr Dent.* 2011;35(4):433-436.
30. Kim K, Heimisdottir K, Gebauer U, Persson GR. Clinical and microbiological findings at sites treated with orthodontic fixed appliances in adolescents. *Am J Orthod Dentofacial Orthop.* 2010;137(2):223-228.
31. van Gastel J, Quirynen M, Teughels W et al. Longitudinal changes in microbiology and clinical periodontal variables after placement of fixed orthodontic appliances. *J Periodontol.* 2008;79(11):2078-2086.
32. Ghijselings E, Coucke W, Verdonck A et al. Long-term changes in microbiology and clinical periodontal variables after completion of fixed orthodontic appliances. *Orthod Craniofac Res.* 2014;17(1):49-59.
33. Thornberg MJ, Riolo CS, Bayirli B et al. Periodontal pathogen levels in adolescents before, during, and after fixed orthodontic appliance therapy. *Am J Orthod Dentofacial Orthop.* 2009;135(1):95-98.
34. Atack NE, Sandy JR, Addy M. Periodontal and microbiological chang-

es associated with the placement of orthodontic appliances. A review. *J Periodontol.* 1996;67(2):78-85.

35. **Yáñez-Vico RM, Iglesias-Linares A, Ballesta-Mudarra S et al.** Short-term effect of removal of fixed orthodontic appliances on gingival health and subgingival microbiota: a prospective cohort study. *Acta Odontol Scand.* 2015;73(7):496-502.

36. **Thomson WM.** Orthodontic treatment outcomes in the long term: findings from a longitudinal study of New Zealanders. *Angle Orthod.* 2002;72(5):449-455.

37. **Petti S, Barbato E, Simonetti D'Arca A.** Effect of orthodontic therapy with fixed and removable appliances on oral microbiota: a six-month longitudinal study. *New Microbiol.* 1997;20(1):55-62.

38. **Naranjo AA, Triviño ML, Jaramillo A et al.** Changes in the subgingival microbiota and periodontal parameters before and 3 months after bracket placement. *Am J Orthod Dentofacial Orthop.* 2006;130(3):275.e17-22.

39. **Lee SM, Yoo SY, Kim HS et al.** Prevalence of putative periodontopathogens in subgingival dental plaques from gingivitis lesions in Korean orthodontic patients. *J Microbiol.* 2005;43(3):260-265.

40. **Sallum EJ, Nouer DF, Klein MI et al.** Clinical and microbiologic changes after removal of orthodontic appliances. *Am J Orthod Dentofacial Orthop.* 2004;126(3):363-366.

41. **Perinetti G, Paolantonio M, Serra E et al.** Longitudinal monitoring of subgingival colonization by Actinobacillus actinomycetemcomitans, and crevicular alkaline phosphatase and aspartate aminotransferase activities around orthodontically treated teeth. *J Clin Periodontol.* 2004;31(1):60-67.

42. **Paolantonio M, Festa F, di Placido G et al.** Site-specific subgingival colonization by Actinobacillus actinomycetemcomitans in orthodontic patients. *Am J Orthod Dentofacial Orthop.* 1999;115(4):423-428.

43. **Mattingly JA, Sauer GJ, Yancey JM, Arnold RR.** Enhancement of Streptococcus mutans colonization by direct bonded orthodontic appliances. *J Dent Res.* 1983;62(12):1209-1211.

44. **Paolantonio M, Pedrazzoli V, di Murro C et al.** Clinical significance of Actinobacillus actinomycetemcomitans in young individuals during orthodontic treatment. A 3-year longitudinal study. *J Clin Periodontol.* 1997;24(9 Pt 1):610-617.

45. **Elkordy SA, Palomo L, Palomo JM, Mostafa YA.** Do fixed orthodontic appliances adversly affect the periodontium? A systematic review of systematic reviews. *Semin Orthod.* 2019;25(2):130-157.

46. **Alves de Souza R, Borges de Araújo Magnani MB, Nouer DF et al.** Periodontal and microbiologic evaluation of 2 methods of archwire ligation: ligature wires and elastomeric rings. *Am J Orthod Dentofacial Orthop.* 2008;134(4):506-512.

47. **Türkkahraman H, Sayin MO, Bozkurt FY et al.** Archwire ligation techniques, microbial colonization, and periodontal status in orthodontically treated patients. *Angle Orthod.* 2005;75(2):231-236.

48. **Forsberg CM, Brattström V, Malmberg E, Nord CE.** Ligature wires and elastomeric rings: two methods of ligation, and their association with microbial colonization of Streptococcus mutans and lactobacilli. *Eur J Orthod.* 1991;13(5):416-420.

49. **Papageorgiou SN, Eliades T.** Clinical evidence on the effect of orthodontic treatment on the periodontal tissues. In: Eliades T, Katsaros C. *The ortho-perio patient: clinical evidence & therapeutic guidelines.* Batavia, IL. Quintessence Publishing Co; 2019:161-173.

50. **Yan X, Wang T, Su H.** Effects of a self-ligating appliance for orthodontic treatment of severe adult periodontitis. *J Oral Sci.* 2019;61(2):200-205.

51. **Arnold S, Koletsi D, Patcas R, Eliades T.** The effect of bracket ligation on the periodontal status of adolescents undergoing orthodontic treatment. systematic review and meta-analysis. *J Dent.* 2016;54(1):13-24.

52. **Nalçaci R, Özat Y, Çokakoğlu S et al.** Effect of bracket type on halitosis, periodontal status, and microbial colonization. *Angle Orthod.* 2014;84(3):479-485.

53. **Pandis N, Papaioannou W, Kontou E et al.** Salivary Streptococcus mutans levels in patients with conventional and self-ligating brackets. *Eur J Orthod.* 2010;32(1):94-99.

54. **van Gastel J, Quirynen M, Teughels W et al.** Influence of bracket design on microbial and periodontal parameters in vivo. *J Clin Periodontol.* 2007;34(5):423-431.

55. **van Gastel J, Teughels W, Quirynen M et al.** Longitudinal changes in gingival crevicular fluid after placement of fixed orthodontic appliances. *Am J Orthod Dentofacial Orthop.* 2011;139(6):735-744.

56. **Diedrich P, Rudzki-Janson I, Wehrbein H, Fritz U.** Effects of orthodontic bands on marginal periodontal tissues. A histologic study on two human specimens. *J Orofac Orthop.* 2001;62(2):146-156.

57. **Boyd RL, Baumrind S.** Periodontal considerations in the use of bonds or bands on molars in adolescents and adults. *Angle Orthod.* 1992;62(2):117-126.

58. **Diamanti-Kipioti A, Gusberti FA, Lang NP.** Clinical and microbiological effects of fixed orthodontic appliances. *J Clin Periodontol.* 1987;14(6):326-333.

59. **Hamp SE, Lundström F, Nyman S.** Periodontal conditions in adolescents subjected to multiband orthodontic treatment with controlled oral hygiene. *Eur J Orthod.* 1982;4(2):77-86.

60. **Huser MC, Baehni PC, Lang R.** Effects of orthodontic bands on microbiologic and clinical parameters. *Am J Orthod Dentofacial Orthop.* 1990;97(3):213-218.

61. **Ong MA, Wang HL, Smith FN.** Interrelationship between periodontics and adult orthodontics. *J Clin Periodontol.* 1998;25(4):271-277.

62. **Wang Q, Ma JB, Wang B et al.** Alterations of the oral microbiome in patients treated with the Invisalign system or with fixed appliances [published correction appears in *Am J Orthod Dentofacial Orthop.* 2020 Jan;157(1):4]. *Am J Orthod Dentofacial Orthop.* 2019;156(5):633-640.

63. **Zhao R, Huang R, Long H et al.** The dynamics of the oral microbiome and oral health among patients receiving clear aligner orthodontic treatment. *Oral Dis.* 2020;26(2):473-483.

64. **Lombardo L, Ortan YÖ, Gorgun Ö et al.** Changes in the oral environ-

ment after placement of lingual and labial orthodontic appliances. *Prog Orthod.* 2013;14:28.

65. Rummel V, Wiechmann D, Sachdeva RC. Precision finishing in lingual orthodontics. *J Clin Orthod.* 1999;33(2):101-113.

66. Sfondrini MF, Debiaggi M, Zara F et al. Influence of lingual bracket position on microbial and periodontal parameters in vivo. *J Appl Oral Sci.* 2012;20(3):357-361.

67. Liu H, Sun J, Dong Y, et al. Periodontal health and relative quantity of subgingival Porphyromonas gingivalis during orthodontic treatment. *Angle Orthod.* 2011;81(4):609-615.

68. Cerroni S, Pasquantonio G, Condò R, Cerroni L. Orthodontic fixed appliance and periodontal status: an updated systematic review. *Open Dent J.* 2018;12(1):614-622.

69. Boyd RL, Leggott PJ, Quinn RS, Eakle WS, Chambers D. Periodontal implications of orthodontic treatment in adults with reduced or normal periodontal tissues versus those of adolescents. *Am J Orthod Dentofacial Orthop.* 1989;96(3):191-198.

70. Bollen AM, Cunha-Cruz J, Bakko DW et al. The effects of orthodontic therapy on periodontal health: a systematic review of controlled evidence. *J Am Dent Assoc.* 2008;139(4):413-422.

71. Nelson PA, Artun J. Alveolar bone loss of maxillary anterior teeth in adult orthodontic patients. *Am J Orthod Dentofacial Orthop.* 1997;111(3):328-334.

72. Sadowsky C, BeGole EA. Long-term effects of orthodontic treatment on periodontal health. *Am J Orthod.* 1981;80(2):156-172.

73. Papageorgiou SN, Papadelli AA, Eliades T. Effect of orthodontic treatment on periodontal clinical attachment: a systematic review and meta-analysis. *Eur J Orthod.* 2018;40(2):176-194.

74. Lu H, Tang H, Zhou T, Kang N. Assessment of the periodontal health status in patients undergoing orthodontic treatment with fixed appliances and Invisalign system: A meta-analysis. *Medicine (Baltimore).* 2018;97(13):e0248.

75. Lemos MM, Cattaneo PM, Melsen B et al. Impact of treatment with full-fixed orthodontic appliances on the periodontium and the composition of the subgingival microbiota. *J Int Acad Periodontol.* 2020;22(3):174-181.

76. Consolaro A. In adults: 47.2% have periodontitis! How about in orthodontic patients? *Dental Press J Orthod.* 2013;18(1):3-5.

77. Feu D, Menezes FC, Augusto Mendes Miguel J, Cardoso Abdo Quintão C. Orthodontic treatment in the severely compromised periodontal patient. *J Orthod.* 2012;39(4):303-313.

78. Zafiropoulos GG, di Prisco MO, Deli G et al. Maintenance after a complex orthoperio treatment in a case of generalized aggressive periodontitis: 7-year result. *J Int Acad Periodontol.* 2010;12(4):112-122.

79. Derton N, Derton R, Perini A et al. Orthodontic treatment in periodontal patients: a case report with 7 years follow-up. *Int Orthod.* 2011;9(1):92-109.

80. Boyer S, Fontanel F, Danan M et al. Severe periodontitis and orthodontics: evaluation of long-term results. *Int Orthod.* 2011;9(3):259 273.

81. Roccuzzo M, Marchese S, Dalmasso P, Roccuzzo A. Periodontal regeneration and orthodontic treatment of severely periodontally compromised teeth: 10-year results of a prospective study. *Int J Periodontics Restorative Dent.* 2018;38(6):801-809.

82. Aimetti M, Garbo D, Ercoli E et al. Long-term prognosis of severely compromised teeth following combined periodontal and orthodontic treatment: a retrospective study. *Int J Periodontics Restorative Dent.* 2020;40(1):95-102.

83. Palomo L. Orthodontic treatment in the age of periodontal risk management. *Semin Orthod.* 2019;25(2):109.

84. Cappelli DP, Ebersole JL, Kornman KS. Early-onset periodontitis in Hispanic-American adolescents associated with A. actinomycetemcomitans. *Community Dent Oral Epidemiol.* 1994;22(2):116-121.

85. Lang NP, Tonetti MS. Periodontal diagnosis in treated periodontitis. Why, when and how to use clinical parameters. *J Clin Periodontol.* 1996;23(3):240-250.

86. Page RC, Krall EA, Martin J et al. Validity and accuracy of a risk calculator in predicting periodontal disease. *J Am Dent Assoc.* 2002;133(5):569-576.

87. Page RC, Martin J, Krall EA et al. Longitudinal validation of a risk calculator for periodontal disease. *J Clin Periodontol.* 2003;30(9):819-827.

88. Lang NP, Tonetti MS. Periodontal risk assessment (PRA) for patients in supportive periodontal therapy (SPT). *Oral Health Prev Dent.* 2003;1(1):7-16.

89. Renvert S, Ohlsson O, Persson S et al. Analysis of periodontal risk profiles in adults with or without a history of myocardial infarction. *J Clin Periodontol.* 2004;31(1):19-24.

90. Chandra RV. Evaluation of a novel periodontal risk assessment model in patients presenting for dental care. *Oral Health Prev Dent.* 2007;5(1):39-48.

91. Leininger M, Tenenbaum H, Davideau JL. Modified periodontal risk assessment score: long-term predictive value of treatment outcomes. A retrospective study. *J Clin Periodontol.* 2010;37(5):427-435.

92. Lindskog S, Blomlöf J, Persson I et al. Validation of an algorithm for chronic periodontitis risk assessment and prognostication: analysis of an inflammatory reactivity test and selected risk predictors. *J Periodontol.* 2010;81(6):837-847.

93. Lindskog S, Blomlöf J, Persson I et al. Validation of an algorithm for chronic periodontitis risk assessment and prognostication: risk predictors, explanatory values, measures of quality, and clinical use. *J Periodontol.* 2010;81(4):584-593.

94. Trombelli L, Minenna L, Toselli L et al. Prognostic value of a simplified method for periodontal risk assessment during supportive periodontal therapy. *J Clin Periodontol.* 2017;44(1):51-57.

95. Trombelli L, Farina R, Ferrari S et al. Comparison between two meth-

ods for periodontal risk assessment. *Minerva Stomatol.* 2009;58(6):277-287.

96. **Farina R, Ferrari S, Pasetti P et al.** Comparison between two methods for periodontal risk assessment. Abstracts of the 6th International Congress of the European Federation of Periodontology (Europerio 6), Stockholm June 4-6 2009. *J. Clin Periodontol.* 2009;36(S9):82(abstr. #157).
97. **Rotundo R, Pini Prato GP.** A new computerised method for evaluating risk profiles of periodontal patients. *Perio.* 2007;4(2):139-149.
98. **Al-Qawasmi RA, Hartsfield JK Jr, Everett ET et al.** Genetic predisposition to external apical root resorption. *Am J Orthod Dentofacial Orthop.* 2003 Mar;123(3):242-52.
99. **Serino G, Wennström JL, Lindhe J, Eneroth L.** The prevalence and distribution of gingival recession in subjects with a high standard of oral hygiene. *J Clin Periodontol.* 1994;21(1):57-63.
100. **Löe H, Anerud A, Boysen H.** The natural history of periodontal disease in man: prevalence, severity, and extent of gingival recession. *J Periodontol.* 1992;63(6):489-495.
101. **Kim T, Miyamoto T, Nunn ME et al.** Root proximity as a risk factor for progression of alveolar bone loss: the Veterans Affairs Dental Longitudinal Study. *J Periodontol.* 2008;79(4):654-659.
102. **Waerhaug J.** Eruption of teeth into crowded position, loss of attachment, and downgrowth of subgingival plaque. *Am J Orthod.* 1980;78(4):453-459.
103. **Proffit WR, Fields HW, Larson B, Sarver DM.** *Contemporary orthodontics.* 6th Ed. St. Louis, Missouri, Elsevier; 2018.
104. **Tweed CH.** The diagnostic facial triangle in the control of treatment objectives. *Am J Orthod.* 1969;55(6):651-657.
105. **Mandelaris GA, Richman C, Kao RT.** Surgical considerations and decision making in surgically facilitated orthodontic treatment/periodontally accelerated osteogenic orthodontics. *Clin Adv Periodontics.* 2020;10(4):213-223.
106. **Watahiki J, Ono R, Maeda M et al.** Optimized Periodontal Regeneration for Orthodontics (O-PRO): a case series. *Int J Periodontics Restorative Dent.* 2020;40(6):835-842.
107. **Singh S, Jayan B.** Comparative evaluation of Periodontally Accelerated Osteogenic Orthodontics (PAOO) versus conventional orthodontic tooth movement in adult patients with bimaxillary dentoalveolar protrusion. *Int J Periodontics Restorative Dent.* 2019;39(4):571-577.
108. **Kamal AT, Malik DES, Fida M, Sukhia RH.** Does periodontally accelerated osteogenic orthodontics improve orthodontic treatment outcome? A systematic review and meta-analysis. *Int Orthod.* 2019;17(2):193-201.
109. **Wennström JL, Lindhe J, Sinclair F, Thilander B.** Some periodontal tissue reactions to orthodontic tooth movement in monkeys. *J Clin Periodontol.* 1987;14(3):121-129.
110. **Ruf S, Hansen K, Pancherz H.** Does orthodontic proclination of lower incisors in children and adolescents cause gingival recession?. *Am J Orthod Dentofacial Orthop.* 1998;114(1):100-106.
111. **Antonarakis GS, Joss CU, Triaca A et al.** Gingival recessions of lower incisors after proclination by orthodontics alone or in combination with anterior mandibular alveolar process distraction osteogenesis. *Clin Oral Investig.* 2017;21(8):2569-2579.
112. **Pernet F, Vento C, Pandis N, Kiliaridis S.** Long-term evaluation of lower incisors gingival recessions after orthodontic treatment. *Eur J Orthod.* 2019;41(6):559-564.
113. **Zachrisson BU, Amat P.** La recherche de l'excellence en orthodontie de l'adulte: entretien avec Bjørn U. Zachrisson [The search for excellence in adult orthodontics; an interview with Bjørn U. Zachrisson]. *Orthod Fr.* 2014;85(4):301-326.
114. **Engelking G, Zachrisson BU.** Effects of incisor repositioning on monkey periodontium after expansion through the cortical plate. *Am J Orthod.* 1982;82(1):23-32.
115. **Garlock DT, Buschang PH, Araujo EA et al.** Evaluation of marginal alveolar bone in the anterior mandible with pretreatment and posttreatment computed tomography in nonextraction patients. *Am J Orthod Dentofacial Orthop.* 2016;149(2):192-201.
116. **Wennström JL.** Mucogingival considerations in orthodontic treatment. *Semin Orthod.* 1996;2(1):46-54.
117. **Kye W, Davidson R, Martin J, Engebretson S.** Current status of periodontal risk assessment. *J Evid Based Dent Pract.* 2012;12(3 Suppl):2-11.

The role of orthodontics in the periodontal treatment plan

Introduction

Orthodontics, taking an active part in periodontal treatment in the interdisciplinary patient[1], plays a synergic and adjuvant role in every periodontal problem. Although orthodontics is not one of the conventional periodontal actions to control inflammation and outcomes of periodontal disease in a conventional periodontal treatment plan, one of the most sensible means of optimizing local environmental factors is orthodontic movement. Orthodontics can be used to modify the site-specificity of the disease, correcting local etiological factors such as misplaced teeth that predispose to plaque accumulation and bone defects in order to improve long-term maintenance[2].

Using the same pattern proposed in literature for the periodontal risk assessment (patient/tooth/site) we can define at which level orthodontics can be applied to modify the prognosis, reduce the risk and facilitate the therapy, reiterating that the main contraindication to combined treatment is the lack of inflammation control before and/or during orthodontic movement[2].

"Patient" level

At the "Patient" level (Tab. 3.1) orthodontics can modify the anatomy of the dental position of the entire archwire.

Tab. 3.1 "Patient" level

Alignment and better access to oral hygiene (Fig. 3.1)
Correction of the levels of the gingival margins (Fig. 3.2)
Optimization of adjacent tooth position prior to implant placement (Fig. 3.3-3.5)
Optimization of the position of the dental abutments and parallelism before prosthetic rehabilitation (Fig. 3.6 and 3.7)

Alignment and better access to oral hygiene

The most immediate corrective action realized by orthodontics is dental alignment to eliminate crowding and misplaced teeth that can make oral hygiene procedures harder, with the creation of morphologically homogeneous dental arches. The optimization of interdental spaces makes it possible to have areas that would otherwise be unreachable[2] for home and professional oral hygiene care[3-6]. This allows a more stable and less subject to plaque accommodation morphology of the interproximal contact point. At the periodontal level, in fact, a worsening of prognosis is reported in patients with misplaced teeth[7]. This data is confirmed by the fact that the reduced prevalence of periodontitis in patients orthodontically treated can be associated with dental alignment[3]. Enhancing hard and soft tissue morphology (an advantage that is also

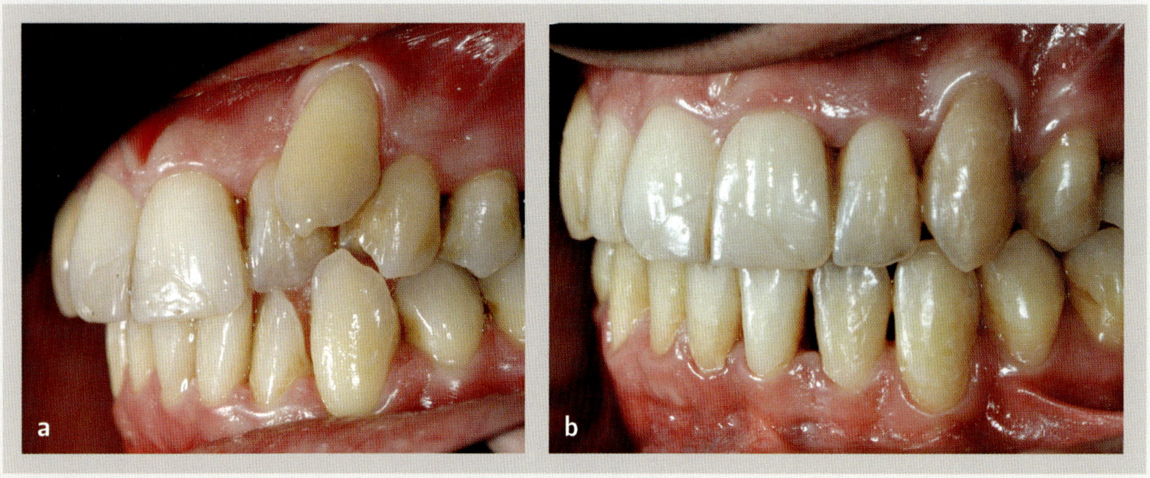

3.1 Dental crowding solution with consequent simplification oral hygiene management.

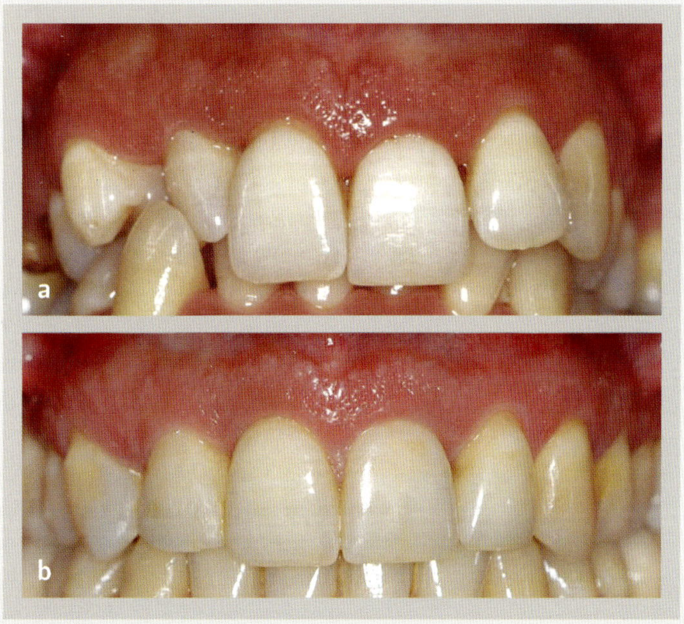

3.2 Correction of the gingival margins on natural teeth.

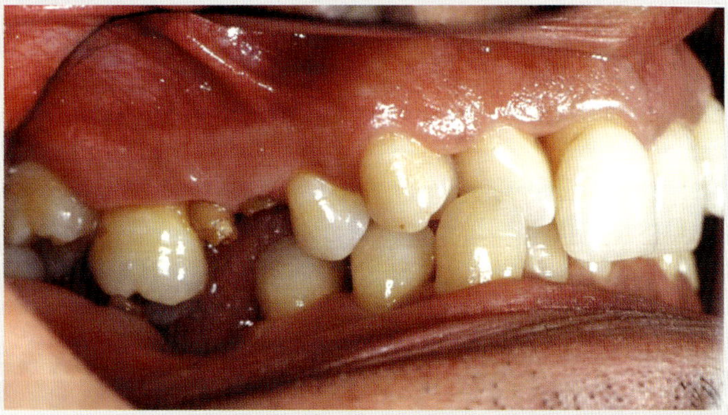

3.3 Patient with multiple edentulous sites. Request for an implant-prosthetic rehabilitation. Start of treatment.

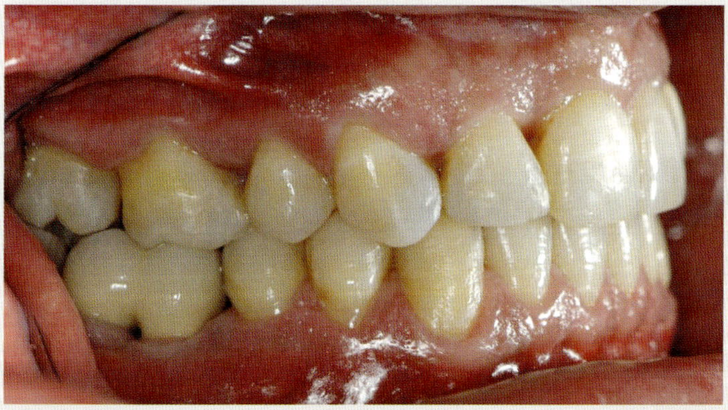

3.4 Patient after optimization of the dental position. End of treatment.

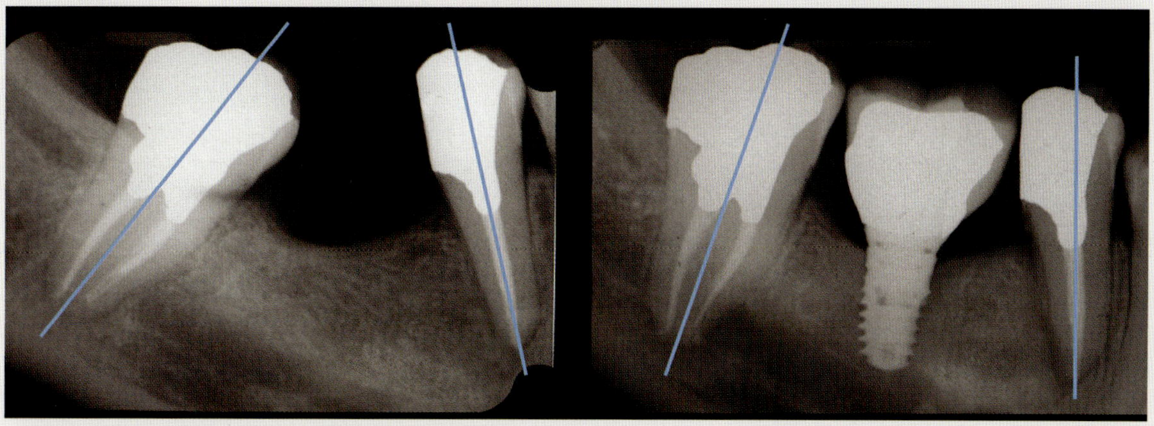

3.5 Molar uprighting movement for space recovery and better implant placement.

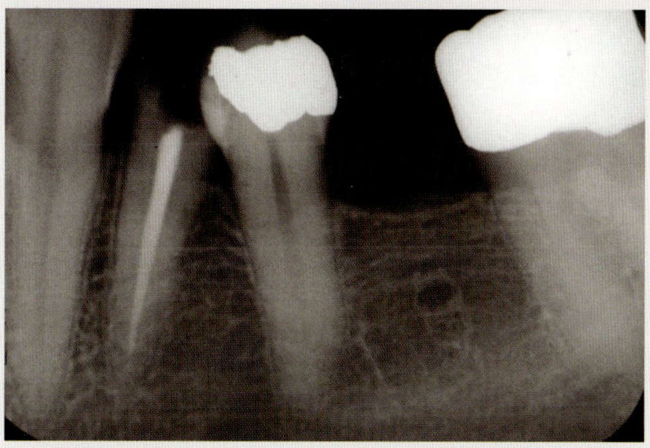

3.6 Non-parallel dental abutment pre-rehabilitation.

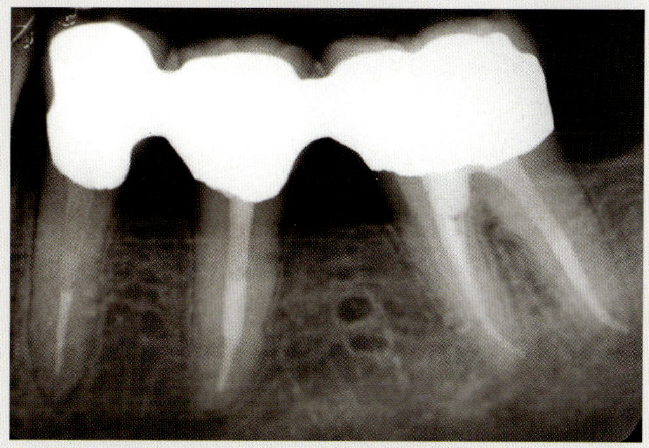

3.7 X-ray follow-up after Fixed Partial Denture application of the case showed in 3.6 after the orthodontic parallelization of the abutments and root movement in the edentulous ridge.

found at the "Site" level) improves the patient's periodontal status[4] and reduces the operative morbidity of the eventual subsequent mechanical and surgical therapy[8]. Furthermore, the improvement of esthetics increases self-esteem and self-awareness, thus promoting all procedures for maintaining oral health.

Correction of the levels of the gingival margins

Orthodontic correction of the gingival margins is important for the esthetic result of the natural teeth and restorative dentistry[9]. Orthodontic treatment can improve this esthetic relationship between the levels of the gingival margins to avoid gingival recontouring, which may require bone removal with subsequent root exposure, and less conservative prosthetic treatments on the teeth.

Optimization of the adjacent teeth position before implant placement

In a prosthetic rehabilitation, teeth can be moved and redistributed to allow better implant positioning, and insert fewer implants or no implants at all (see 3.3-3.5) In this way orthodontists can manage the space closure with the natural dentition reducing an eventual risk of any future peri-implantitis, taking into account that this risk is increased in patients with a history of periodontal disease[10,11]. The orthodontic treatment, therefore, allows to maintain the integrity of the dental arch using the same teeth[12].

Optimization of the position of dental abutments and parallelism before prosthetic rehabilitation

When a conventional prosthetic rehabilitation needs to be carried out where natural teeth must be used as prosthetic abutments, teeth can be orthodontically positioned to increase the parallelism between the abutments in all the three planes of the space, improving the prosthetic restoration[8] (see 3.6 and 3.7), reducing root canal therapy and bone surgery, creating physiological spaces for pontics, improving crown/root ratio, correcting soft and hard tissue morphology and creating correct embrasures with a more favourable distribution of the teeth[2].

"Tooth" level

At the "Tooth" level (3.2) orthodontics can modify the relationships between the dental elements in order to improve their position and their relationship with the tissues.

Tab. 3.2 "Tooth" level

Correction of Pathologic Tooth Migration (PTM) (3.8 and 3.9)
Closing of diastema (3.10)
Better adaptation of the soft tissues to the gingival margins and in the embrasure spaces (3.11 and 3.12)
Dental extrusion and intrusion (3.13)
Alignment of the interdental bone level (3.14)

Correction of Pathologic Tooth Migration (PTM)

Correction of PTM is described in Chapter 4.

Closure of the diastema and better adaptation of the soft tissues to the gingival margins and in the embrasures

The orthodontic closure of the diastemas can contribute to the repositioning of the contact point in relation to the bone ridge[13,14] for a possible filling of the interdental papilla. This movement facilitates the modification of the size of the clinical dental crowns, increases the emergence profile and allows a better adaptation of the soft tissues to the gingival marginal levels and embrasures, improving esthetics (see Chapter 10, *Clinical case 1*).

Dental extrusion and intrusion

The extrusive movement, as described in Chapter 8, during combined orthodontic-periodontal therapies can enhance the results of periodontal treatment, reducing, eliminating or modifying the nature of the defect resulting from periodontal disease[15]. The extrusion reduces the probing depth, changes the periodontal structure and allows occlusal movements of the periodontal tissue, increasing in this way the height of the bone tissue. Orthodontic extrusion, combined with other surgical procedures, provides easier and more predictable results[16] and creates better periodontal conditions due to physiological and microbiological changes in the dental microenvironment. The more everted sulcus and the plaque which becomes supragingival being no more subgingival, reduce the pathogenicity and the negative efects on the gingival tissues[17]. These positive effects are antagonistic to the negative ones of an intrusive movement without plaque control; in this kind of movement the supragingival plaque becomes subgingival, with the possibility of creating or amplifying intraosseous defects and a loss of periodontal attachment[18]. In periodontal patients, intrabony defects can be treated by an extrusive movement, with an improvement of the vertical component and a reduction of probing depth, keeping inflammation under strict control before and during the whole movement[19]. A proximal intraosseous defect in the presence of elongated, tipped and migrated single-rooted teeth can be solved by the orthodontic movement[20]. Before carrying out any intrusion, however, it is important to evaluate the anatomy of the periodontal support of the elements to be intruded and of the adjacent teeth, and their relationship with the cemento-enamel junction, in order not to deepen any present intrabony defects and not to worsen the bone morphology (see 3.13 and 5.7).

Alignment of the interdental bone level

Some cases of altered bone morphology are corrected by means of periodontal surgery. Orthodontics can provide a different bone alignment approach. The tooth movement allows, with selective movements of ex-

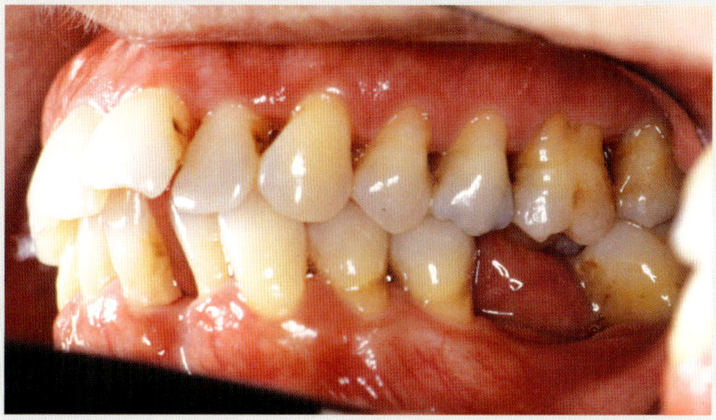

3.8 Correction of the PTM (Pathologic Tooth Migration). Start of treatment.

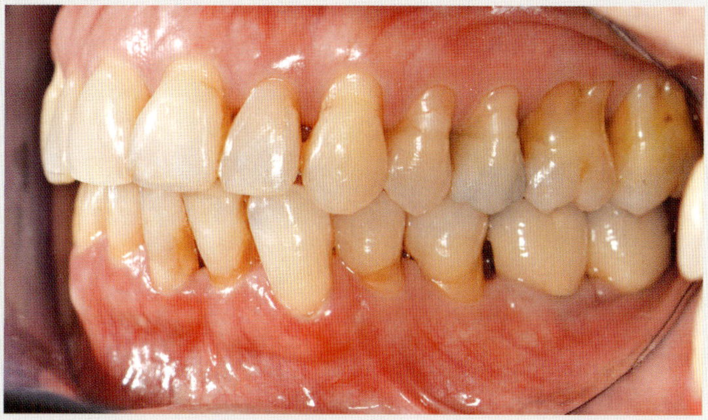

3.9 Correction of the PTM (Pathologic Tooth Migration). End of treatment.

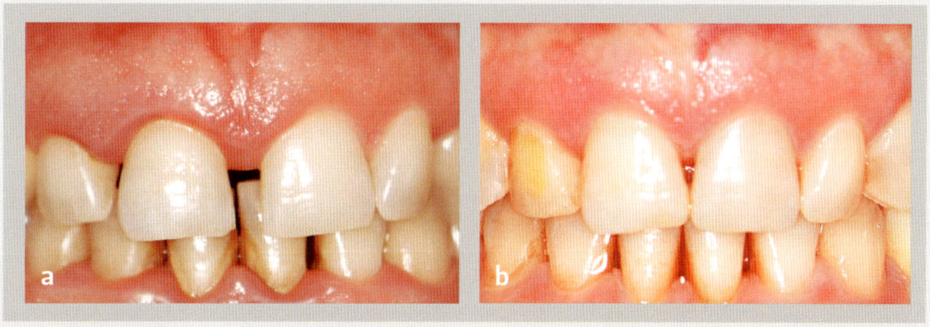

3.10 Diastema closure.

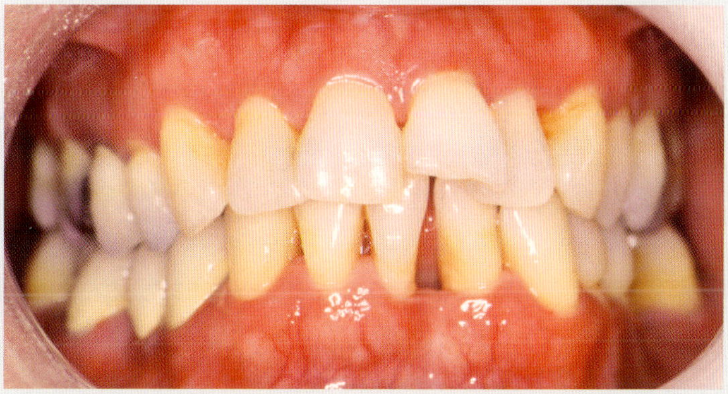

3.11 Better adaptation of the soft tissues to gingival margins and embrasure spaces. Start of treatment.

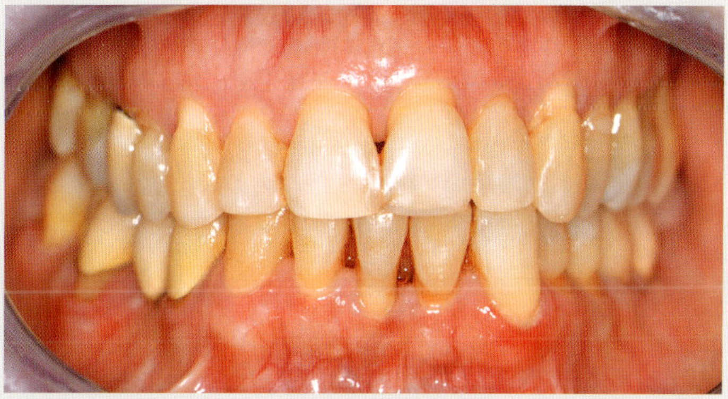

3.12 Better adaptation of the soft tissues to gingival margins and embrasure spaces. End of treatment.

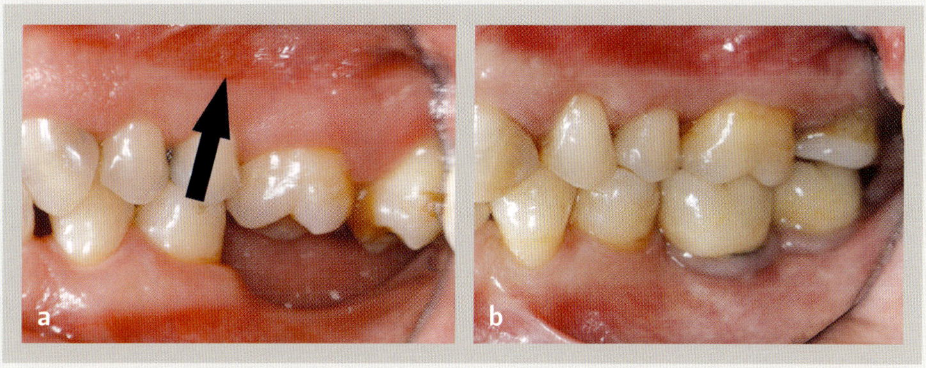

3.13 Intrusion movement of the upper molars for recovering the lower restorative-prosthetic space.

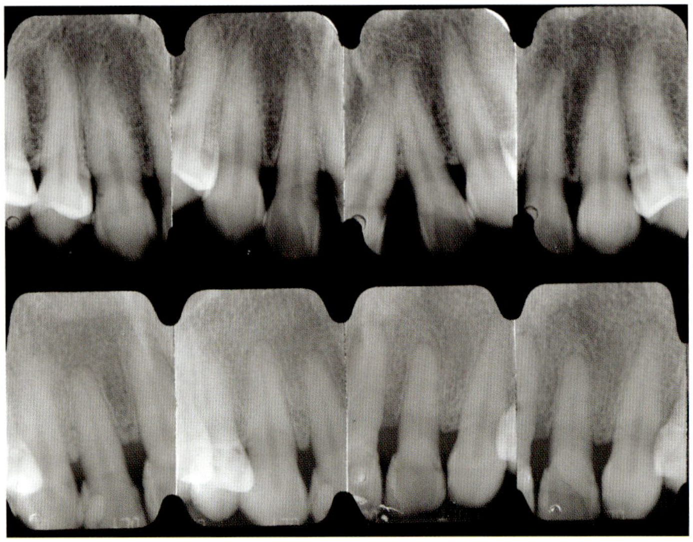

3.14 Bone levelling. X-ray pre- and post-treatment.

trusion, intrusion, tipping and torque, a regularization of the bone level using the bone level itself and not the dental position as a guide, as described in Chapter 6.

"Site" level

At the "Site" level (3.3) orthodontics can modify the local site-specificity of the periodontal problem to improve prognosis, reduce or enhance the predictability of corrective (regenerative or resective) periodontal surgical techniques and implant procedures.

Improvement of crestal, interdental and interradicular bone structures

Interradicular bone structures benefit from orthodontic treatment[8], both at the coronal and at the root level, correcting crowding and uprighting molars. At the coronal level, orthodontics realigns the non-physiological gingival morphology where there is a modified microbial plaque with an increase in periodontal pathogenic species such as spirochetes, mobile rods, *Fusobacterium* and *Capnocytophaga, Campylobacter rectus* and *Peptostreptococcus micros*[21], with improvement of the bacterial flora as it can be found in the uprighting of the mesially tipped molar[2], where bacteria such as *Bacteroides forsythus, Porphyromonas gingivalis, Prevotella intermedia and Actinobacillus actinomycetemcomitans* decrease significantly. The same results were found in another study on *Bacteroides* using DNA probes at the same sites[2]. Furthermore,

Tab. 3.3 "Site" level

Improvement of crestal, interdental and interradicular bone structures (tipped teeth and root proximity). Uprighting - crowding (see 3.5, 3.14 and 3.15)
Elimination of furcation defects by moving the separated roots (3.16)
Development of the implant site (3.17) and recovery of the pre-restorative tooth structure (3.18)

in crowding, since the gingival margins show a non-physiological contour with consequent reduced interproximal areas, the structure of the interproximal gingiva is altered, causing compression and deformation of the papilla with a reduction of the connective stroma. The orthodontic movement modifies these spaces in these altered areas, returning the tissue size to a more physiological shape.

At the root level, tooth movement leads to an increase in the distance in thin alveolar septa. In some conditions, in fact, these septa can present a reduction of the cancellous bone and of the vascularization up to the total absence of bone tissue; therefore, only connective tissue remains between the roots, with the fusion of the periodontal ligaments of the adjacent teeth. These topographical conditions become an area of high risk of crestal bone loss since even a simple uncontrolled inflammation leads to a loss of periodontal attachment[8], because an adequate space between the teeth is necessary for the maintenance of gingival health[22]. Root proximity, in fact, is an important local risk factor for the loss of alveolar bone and for the breakdown of periodontal health where there is a very thin interproximal septum. In the presence of an interradicular distance of adjacent teeth of less than 0.8 mm, the clinician should expect an increased risk of alveolar bone loss[23]. In the anterior teeth, the marginal periodontal breakdown is less directly correlated to the thickness of the interradicular bone[22,24]; the greatest risk of interproximal septal bone loss occurs in the posterior region at the molar level[22,24], where this risk is probably greater for the same amount of root proximity. The presence of narrow interproximal spaces due to the short arch length or the small size of the teeth can become a problem for both the periodontist and the prosthodontist. The apical shifting of the dentogingival complex due to this proximity leads to the formation of niches that are favourable to the proliferation of the biofilm out of the reach of home and professional oral care. This compromises the resistance of the interproximal bone, reducing its vascularity. The laminae durae proximity of two elements reduces the cancellous bone and vascular support. If the patient is susceptible to periodontal disease, this thin bone is easier to be lost. The enlargement of the interproximal bone, the prerogative of orthodontic mechanics, and the restoration of the contact points lead to great local benefits in terms of resistance to the disease. The treatment of interproximal tissue constrictions and modifications of the contact points/embrasures is a correct periodontal motivation for orthodontic treatment and the elimination of crowding. For the periodontally-oriented orthodontist it is the periodontal motivation that drives them to perform targeted and minimal orthodontical treatment, and this opportunity becomes even more important for patients even when a complete treatment is not justified[1].

Elimination of furcation defects by moving the separated roots

The treatment of the furcation defects remains one of the most complex clinical problems in periodontology, in terms of cost/benefit ratio, and for what concerns the interaction with the orthodontic movement, where positive effects are obtained through combined treatments[20]. Orthodontics improves the prognosis of procedures of root separation by moving the root abutments to the most appropriate positions and, even in regenerative surgery, allows orthodontic movement without affecting the neoformation of tissue[25,26]. The main consideration, therefore, is not so much the fact that orthodontics can treat furcation defects, but the consideration that the orthodontic movement does not worsen the results of a possible regenerative treat-

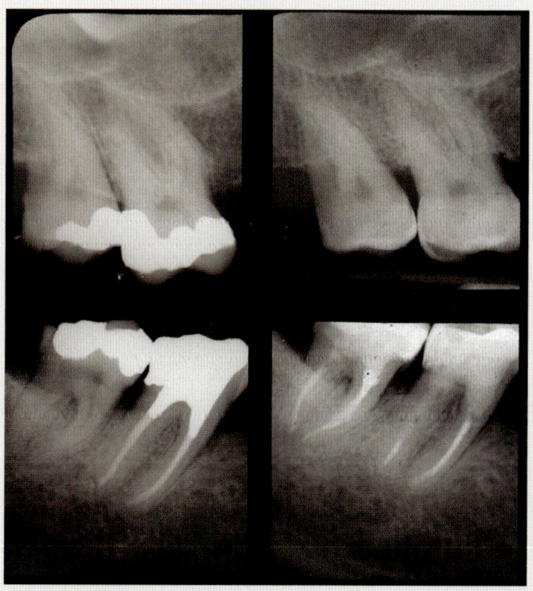

3.15 Improvement of interdental crestal bone structures with the increase of interradicular septa between 1.6-1.7 and 4.7-4.8.

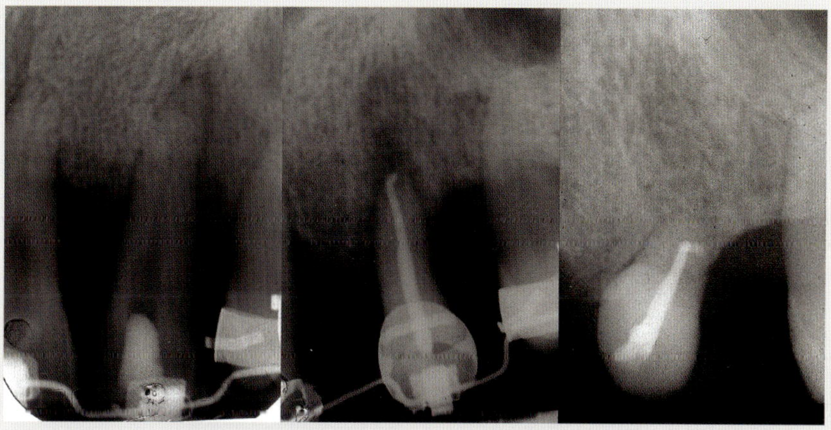

3.17 Implant site development to regenerate bone tissue.

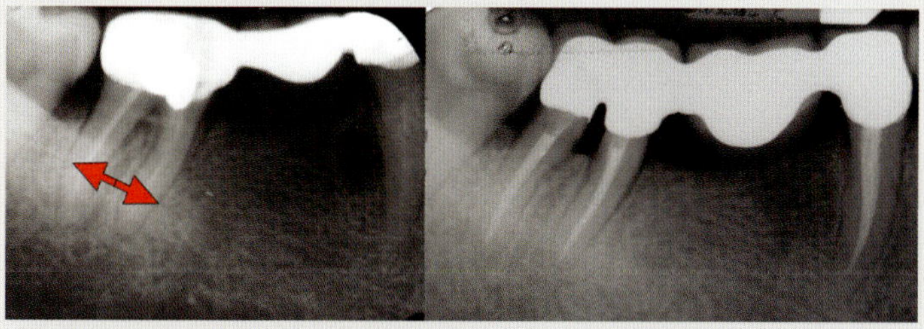

3.16 Orthodontic movement of the separated roots to solve the furcation involvement.

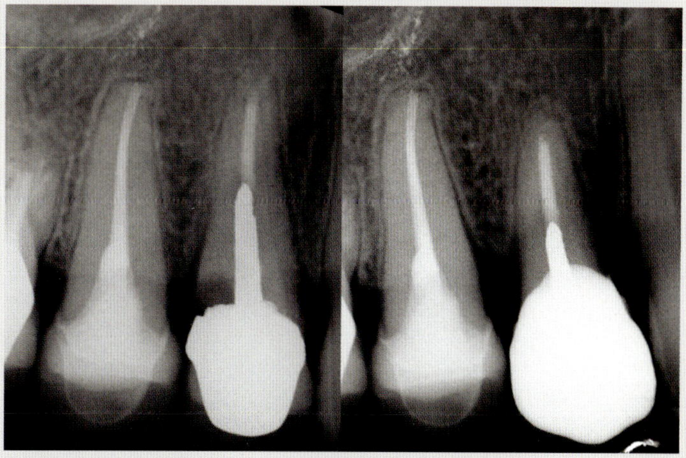

3.18 "Dental" orthodontic extrusion to recover healthy tooth prerestorative structure.

ment in a furcation; for this reason, teeth can be moved without compromising predictability. It must always be kept in mind that with orthodontic movement there can be a worsening of furcation problems if the movement is performed in the presence of inflammation without having carried out a complete periodontal treatment before orthodontic therapy[27].

Implant site development and pre-restorative dental structure recovery

Implant site development and pre-restorative dental structure recovery of the compromised tooth are discussed in Chapter 8.

REFERENCES

1. Mihram WL, Murphy NC. The orthodontist's role in 21st century periodontic-prosthodontic therapy. *Semin Orthod.* 2008;14(4):272-289.
2. Vanarsdall RL. Orthodontics and periodontal therapy. *Periodontol 2000.* 1995;9(1):132-149.
3. Sim HY, Kim HS, Jung DU et al. Association between orthodontic treatment and periodontal diseases: Results from a national survey. *Angle Orthod.* 2017;87(5):651-657.
4. Zhang J, Zhang AM, Zhang ZM et al. Efficacy of combined orthodontic-periodontic treatment for patients with periodontitis and its effect on inflammatory cytokines: a comparative study. *Am J Orthod Dentofacial Orthop.* 2017;152(4):494-500.
5. Nakamura Y, Gomi K, Oikawa T et al. Reconstruction of a collapsed dental arch in a patient with severe periodontitis. *Am J Orthod Dentofacial Orthop.* 2013;143(5):704-712.
6. Melsen B, Agerbaek N, Markenstam G. Intrusion of incisors in adult patients with marginal bone loss. *Am J Orthod Dentofacial Orthop.* 1989;96(3):232-241.
7. McGuire MK, Nunn ME. Prognosis versus actual outcome. II. The effectiveness of clinical parameters in developing an accurate prognosis. *J Periodontol.* 1996;67(7):658-665.
8. Diedrich P, Fritz U, Kizinger G. Interrelationship between periodontics and adult orthodontics. *Perio.* 2004;1(3):143-149.
9. Gkantidis N, Christou P, Topouzelis N. The orthodontic-periodontic interrelationship in integrated treatment challenges: a systematic review. *J Oral Rehabil.* 2010;37(5):377-390.
10. Dreyer H, Grischke J, Tiede C et al. Epidemiology and risk factors of peri-implantitis: A systematic review. *J Periodontal Res.* 2018;53(5):657-681.
11. Papapanou PN, Sanz M, Buduneli N et al. Periodontitis: Consensus report of workgroup 2 of the 2017 World Workshop on the Classification of Periodontal and Peri-Implant Diseases and Conditions. *J Periodontol.* 2018;89(Suppl 1):S173-S182.
12. Agrawal N, Kallury A, Khurana R et al. Interdisciplinary management of aggressive periodontitis. *J Clin Orthod.* 2015;49(9):597-605.
13. Cardaropoli D, Gaveglio L, Abou-Arraj RV. Orthodontic movement and periodontal bone defects: Rationale, timing, and clinical implications. *Semin Orthod* 2014;20(3):177-187.
14. Tarnow DP, Magner AW, Fletcher P. The effect of the distance from the contact point to the crest of bone on the presence or absence of the interproximal dental papilla. *J Periodontol.* 1992;63(12):995-996.
15. Alsahhaf A, Att W. Orthodontic extrusion for pre-implant site enhancement: principles and clinical guidelines. *J Prosthodont Res.* 2016;60(3):145-155.
16. de Barros LA, de Almeida Cardoso M, de Avila ED et al. Six-year follow-up of maxillary anterior rehabilitation with forced orthodontic extrusion: achieving esthetic excellence with a multidisciplinary approach. *Am J Orthod Dentofacial Orthop.* 2013;144(4):607-615.
17. van Venrooy JR, Yukna RA. Orthodontic extrusion of single-rooted teeth affected with advanced periodontal disease. *Am J Orthod.* 1985;87(1):67-74.
18. Ericsson I, Thilander B, Lindhe J, Okamoto H. The effect of orthodontic tilting movements on the periodontal tissues of infected and non-infected dentitions in dogs. *J Clin Periodontol.* 1977;4(4):278-293.
19. Iino S, Taira K, Machigashira M, Miyawaki S. Isolated vertical infrabony defects treated by orthodontic tooth extrusion. *Angle Orthod.* 2008;78(4):728-736.
20. Rotundo R, Bassarelli T, Pace E et al. Orthodontic treatment of periodontal defects. Part II: a systematic review on human and animal studies. *Prog Orthod.* 2011;12(1):45-52.
21. Chung CH, Vanarsdall RL, Cavalcanti EA et al. Comparison of microbial composition in the subgingival plaque of adult crowded versus non-crowded dental regions. *Int J Adult Orthodon Orthognath Surg.* 2000;15(4):321-330.
22. Artun J, Osterberg SK, Kokich VG. Long-term effect of thin interdental alveolar bone on periodontal health after orthodontic treatment. *J Periodontol.* 1986;57(6):341-346.
23. Kim T, Miyamoto T, Nunn ME et al. Root proximity as a risk factor for progression of alveolar bone loss: the Veterans Affairs Dental Longitudinal Study. *J Periodontol.* 2008;79(4):654-659.
24. Artun J, Kokich VG, Osterberg SK. Long-term effect of root proximity on periodontal health after orthodontic treatment. *Am J Orthod Dentofacial Orthop.* 1987;91(2):125-130.
25. da Silva VC, Cirelli CC, Ribeiro FS et al. Intrusion of teeth with class III furcation: a clinical, histologic and histometric study in dogs. *J Clin Periodontol.* 2008;35(9):807-816.
26. da Silva VC, Cirelli CC, Ribeiro FS et al. Orthodontic movement after periodontal regeneration of class II furcation: a pilot study in dogs. *J Clin Periodontol.* 2006;33(6):440-448.
27. Burch JG, Bagci B, Sabulski D, Landrum C. Periodontal changes in furcations resulting from orthodontic uprighting of mandibular molars. *Quintessence Int.* 1992;23(7):509-513.

Ortho-periodontal diagnostics

Introduction

The request for orthodontic treatment in adults is increasing. Consequently, the interrelationships with other disciplines, first of all periodontology, allow to involve orthodontics in the periodontal treatment plan and periodontal contribution in the orthodontic treatment plan[1,2]. The increase in the number of adult patients, where the prevalence of periodontal disease increases with age[3], requires an awareness and a diagnostic protocol that must be shared between professionals. The orthodontist, therefore, takes an active part in the diagnosis by evaluating the periodontal conditions and sharing them at the diagnostic level with the periodontist[1].

It is important to immediately detect cases of periodontal disease where periodontal tissues might appear relatively normal at early stages and a simple clinical inspection does not always reveal the severity and the extent of the disease[4]. Even in growing and adolescent patients that start orthodontic treatment, it is important to make an early diagnosis of any periodontal pathology before starting tooth movements. Very often it is the orthodontist who is the first practitioner to visit these patients at a clinical and radiographic level and who makes an early diagnosis[5]. In an orthodontic-periodontal treatment, any periodontal pathology which is not detected early can lead to an exacerbation of a latent periodontal disease and can limit, to the point of completely failing, the goal of the combined treatment. Paradoxically, treating adult patients could be less risky than treating patients in growing age, because in adults the disease is more evident and manifest, where both the clinician and the patient are aware of any systemic problems, such as smoking, diabetes, connective and endocrine disorders[3].

Notes on the new classification

In 2017, the EFP/AAP Workshop met in Chicago to write the new classification of periodontal disease. The importance of this new classification, as far as periodontitis is concerned, introduces the assessment of the *staging* and the *grading* of the periodontal disease. In 4.1 and 4.2 there is a summary of the main characteristics of periodontitis and in 4.1-4.3 an example of this classification is shown. For further information, please refer to the publications with the classification and subsequent updates[6-8].

Tab. 4.1 Staging of periodontitis according to the new AAP (American Academy of Periodontology) – EFP (European Federation of Periodontology) classification[7,8]

<table>
<tr><th rowspan="2"></th><th colspan="3">Severity</th><th rowspan="2">Complexity (local)</th><th rowspan="2">Extent and distribution</th></tr>
<tr><th>Interdental clinical attachment loss (CAL) at site of greatest loss</th><th>Radiographic bone loss</th><th>Teeth loss due to periodontitis</th></tr>
<tr><td>STAGE I</td><td>1–2 mm</td><td>Third coronal (<15%)</td><td rowspan="2">No tooth loss due to periodontitis</td><td>Max PD ≤4 mm
Mostly horizontal bone loss</td><td rowspan="4">Describe for each stage the extension as localized (<30% teeth involved), generalized or molar/incisor pattern</td></tr>
<tr><td>STAGE II</td><td>3–4 mm</td><td>Third coronal (15–33%)</td><td>Max PD ≤5 mm
Mostly horizontal bone loss</td></tr>
<tr><td>STAGE III</td><td>≥5 mm</td><td rowspan="2">Extending to mid-third of root and beyond</td><td>Tooth loss due to periodontitis ≤4</td><td>In addition to Stage II complexity:
• PD ≥6 mm
• vertical bone loss ≥3 mm
• furcation involvement Class II or III
• moderate ridge defect</td></tr>
<tr><td>STAGE IV</td><td>≥5 mm</td><td>Tooth loss due to periodontitis ≥5</td><td>In addition to Stage III complexity:
Need for complex rehabilitation due:
• masticatory dysfunction
• secondary occlusal trauma (mobility ≥2)
• severe ridge defect
• bite collapse, drifting, flaring
• less than 20 remaining teeth (10 opposing pairs)</td></tr>
</table>

Tab. 4.2 Grading of periodontitis according to the new AAP (American Academy of Periodontology) – EFP (European Federation of Periodontology) classification[7,8]

<table>
<tr><th rowspan="2"></th><th colspan="3">Primary criteria</th><th colspan="2">Grade modifiers</th></tr>
<tr><th colspan="2">Direct evidence of progression</th><th>Indirect evidence of progression</th><th colspan="2">Risk factors</th></tr>
<tr><td></td><td>Longitudinal data (radiographic bone loss or clinical attachment loss, CAL)</td><td>% BL/Age</td><td>Clinical Case Phenotype</td><td>Smoking</td><td>Diabetes</td></tr>
<tr><td>Grade A: slow rate</td><td>Evidence of no bone loss over 5 years</td><td><0.25</td><td>Great biofilm deposits with low destruction</td><td>Non-smoker</td><td>Normoglycemic/No diagnosis of diabetes</td></tr>
<tr><td>Grade B: moderate rate</td><td>Evidence of bone loss <2mm over 5 years</td><td>0.25–1</td><td>Destruction related to biofilm deposits</td><td><10 cig./day</td><td>HbA1c <7% with diabetes</td></tr>
<tr><td>Grade C: rapid rate</td><td>Evidence of bone loss >2mm over 5 years</td><td>>1</td><td>Destruction in excess not related to biofilm deposits</td><td>≥10 cig./day</td><td>HbA1c ≥7% with diabetes</td></tr>
</table>

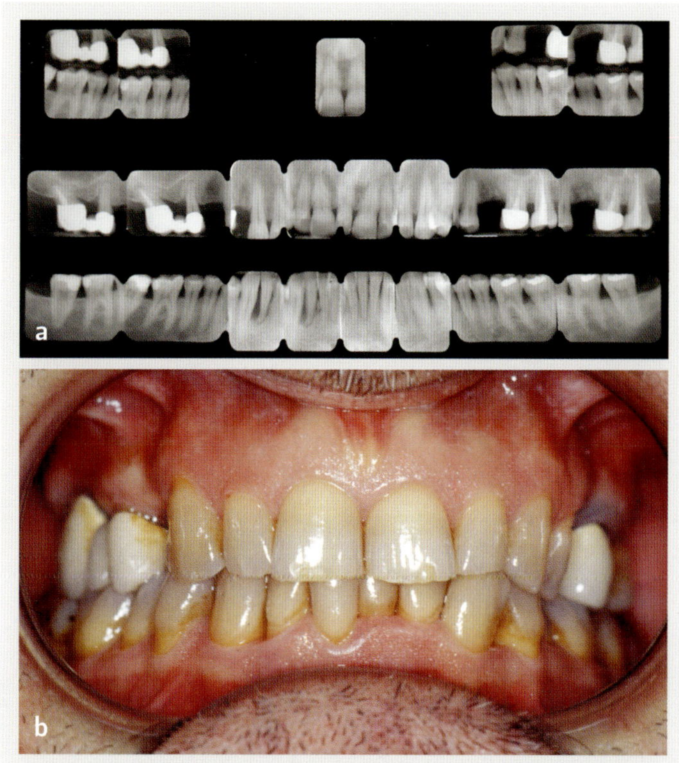

4.1 Clinical and radiographic exam of a case of periodontitis Stage II.

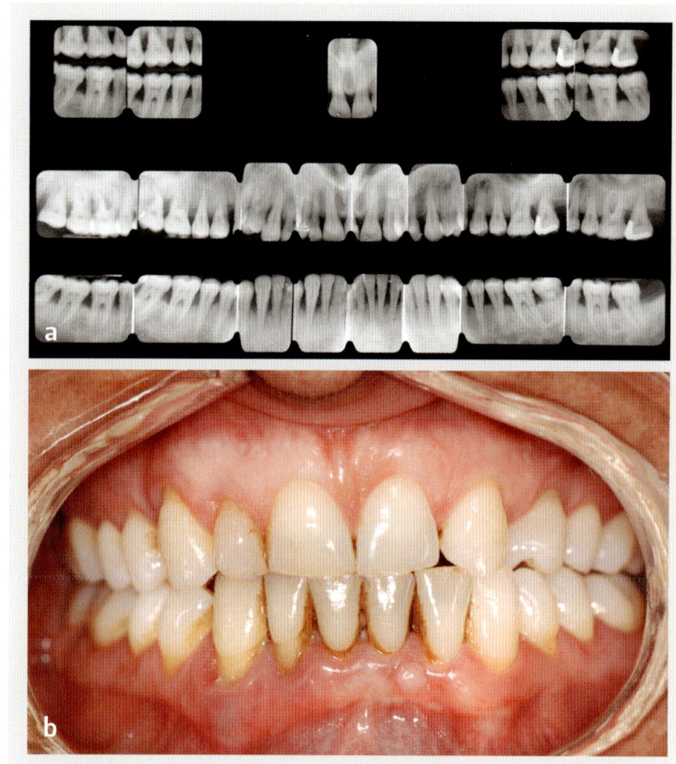

4.2 Clinical and radiographic exam of a case of periodontitis Stage III.

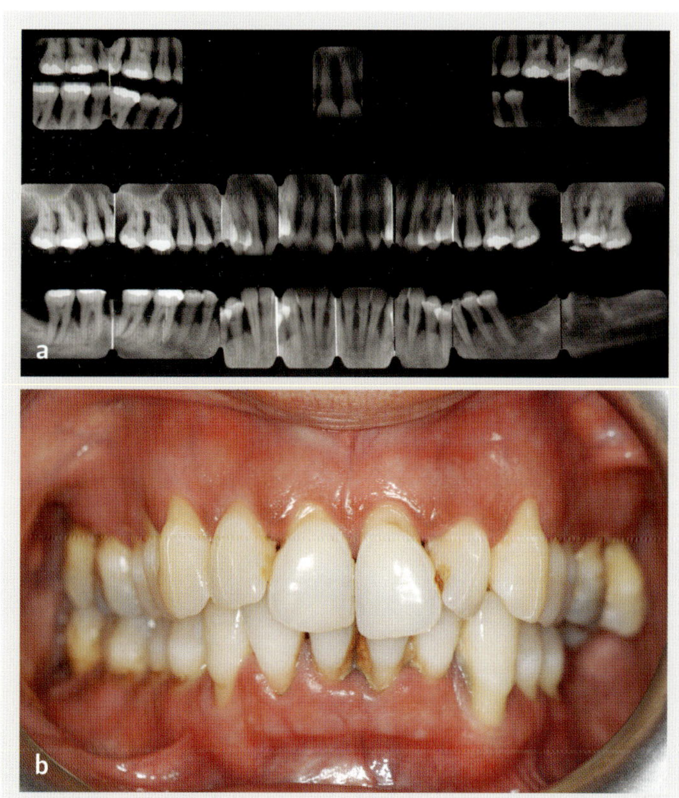

4.3 Clinical and radiographic exam of a case of periodontitis Stage IV.

Periodontal diagnostics

In orthodontic periodontal patients, periodontal situation and plaque control must be constantly monitored, not only during supportive periodontal therapy but also during treatment, orthodontic check-ups and periodic follow-ups[9]. We will not describe in detail how a complete periodontal examination is performed, but we will analyse the most important points to be taken into consideration in order to be able to intercept and refer the patient to the periodontist before starting treatment.

General history

In particular in younger patients, it is important to ask for family history regarding periodontal disease and for the presence of other conditions that could worsen the periodontal situation, such as uncontrolled diabetes. Smoking, stress and lifestyle habits can negatively affect the progression of the disease. It is essential to know the possible use of drugs (for example NSAIDs, antidepressants, bisphosphonates, chemotherapeutic drugs), taking into account the influence they can have on bone metabolism.

Radiographic exam

In addition to cephalometric and panoramic Rx, the periodontal patient also needs the execution of the full (16 or 21) radiographic status, including periodontal bite-wings (4.4).

The radiographic examination is important, as it allows to distinguish the bone loss pattern[10] based on:

1. Extension (localized or generalized).
2. Severity (mild, moderate, advanced).
3. Trend (horizontal, vertical).

If a previous radiographic examination is obtained, the evolution of bone loss over time can also be estimated. This data is important for studying the degree of progression of periodontal disease according to the new classification. However, it must be remembered that the 30-50% of bone destruction occurs before it can be radiologically detected and that some incipient defects can appear radiologically even years later. This reaffirms the importance of carrying out the complete diagnostic protocol and not just the radiographic one.

Periodontal probing

Periodontal probing is the main diagnostic tool for collecting periodontal biometric parameters and for evaluating the inflammation of periodontal tissues. These values are reported in a paper or digital chart (periodontal charting), (4.5). In this text we will use a digital chart, the Online periodontal charting tool, available on the website www.perio-tools.com (Ramseier CA, Wolf CA, The Online Periodontal Charting Tool, www.periodontalchart-online.com, copyright © 2011, University of Bern, Unitectra Technology Transfer reference number UB-12/297). The data are collected with a periodontal probe in order to measure the pocket depth and a "Nabers" probe for furcations probing (4.6), creating a synoptic diagram of the patient's periodontal situation.

Periodontal 6 sites per tooth probing (4.7) and furcations probing (paying attention to the first upper premolars) is recommended, since the complete periodontal examination is of primary importance for a complete description of the periodontal situation[11-13]. It is essential to perform an accurate periodontal probing,

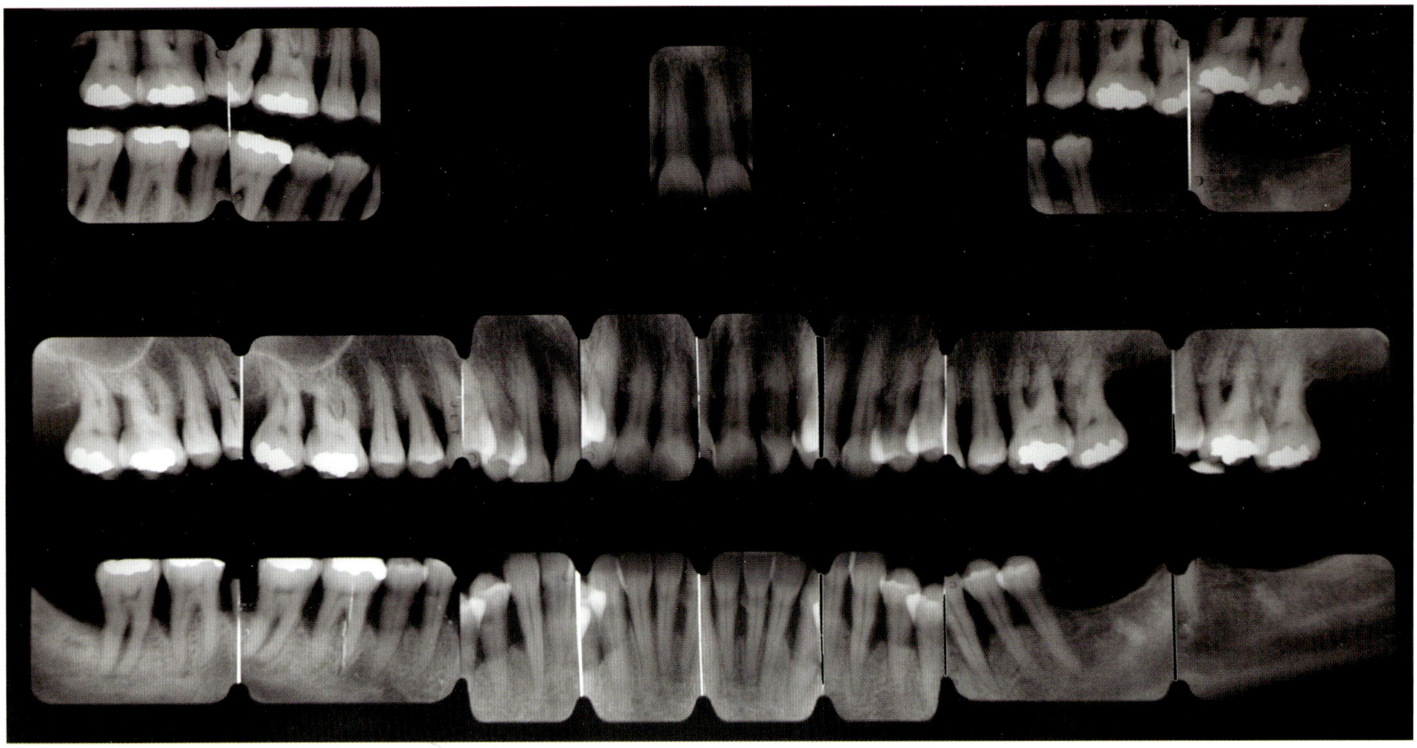

4.4 Complete radiographic status with 21 X-rays where the vertical trend of bone loss, generalized extension of the disease and gravity can be observed.

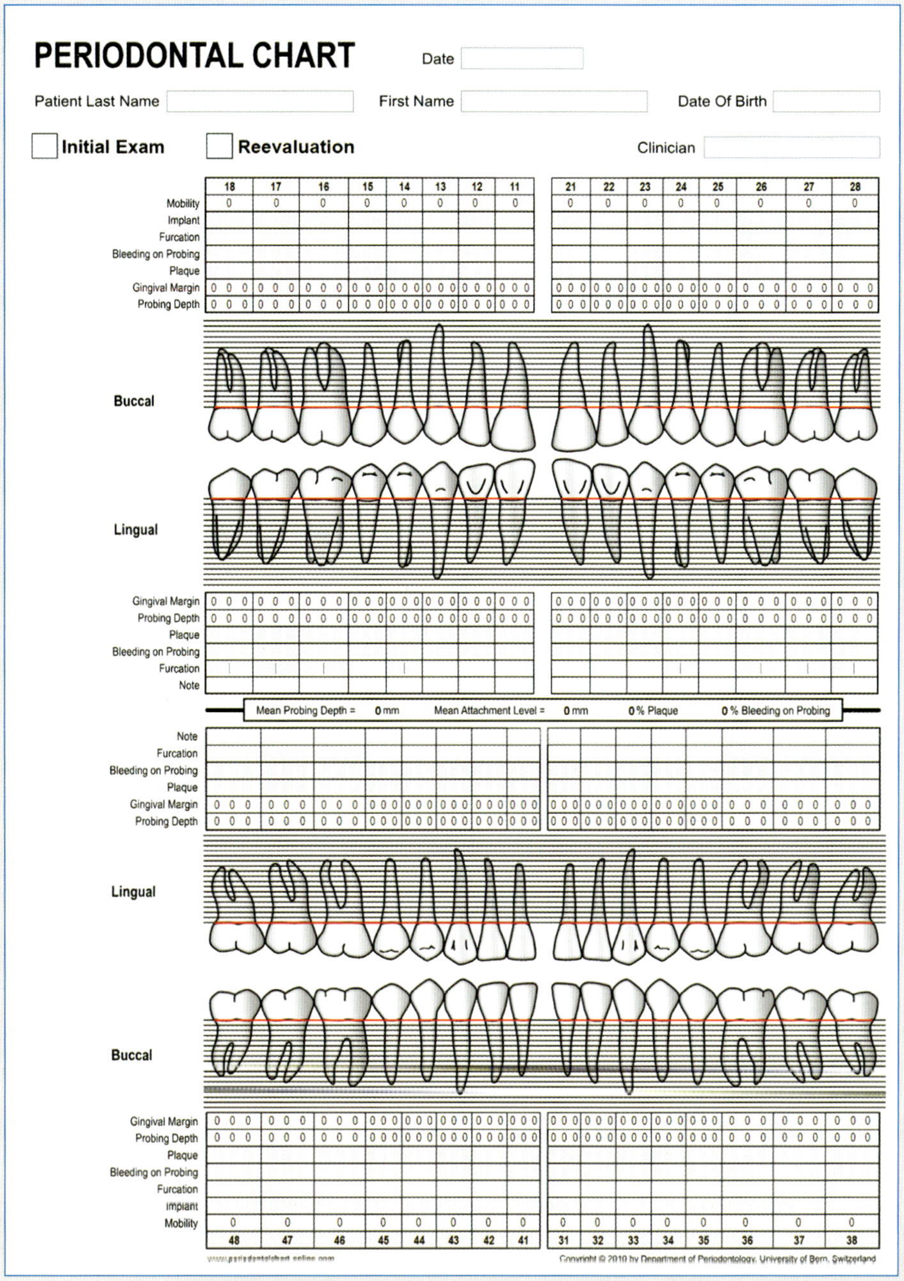

4.5 Example of periodontal charting (Ramseier CA, Wolf CA, The Online Periodontal Charting Tool, www.periodontalchart-online.com, copyright © 2011, University of Bern, Unitectra Technology Transfer reference number UB-12/297).

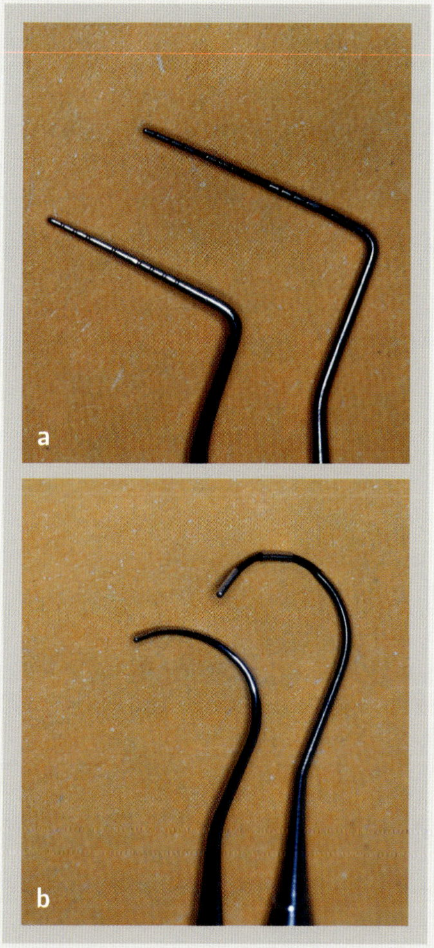

4.6 (**a**) Periodontal probe (Williams 10 mm and UNC 15 mm); (**b**) Nabers probe for furcations (simple and colour-coded).

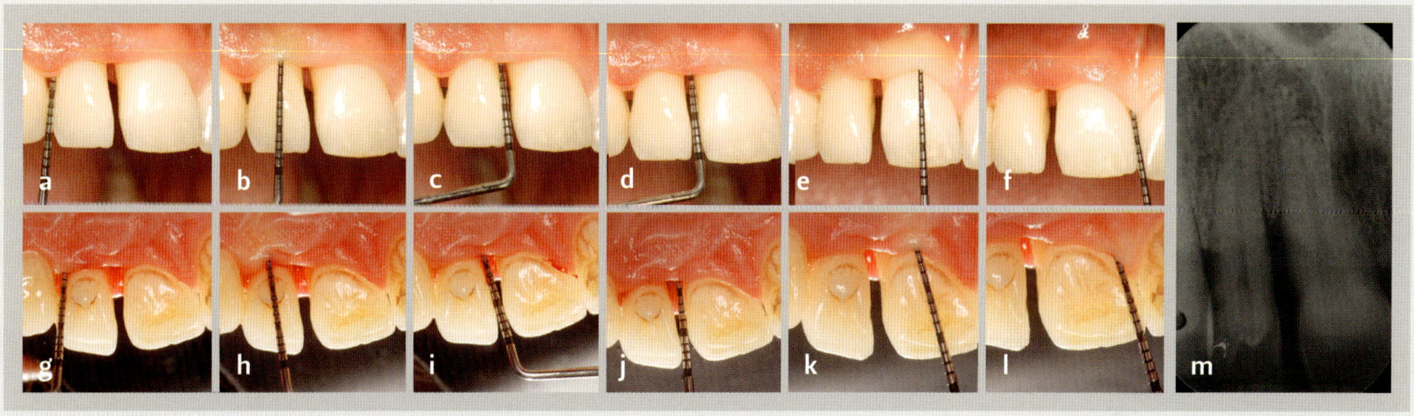

4.7 6-point periodontal probing (mesial/central/distal) on the vestibular and palatal aspect where, “browsing” the gingival sulcus, the 3D anatomy of the bone defect can be visualized, confirmed by X-ray and soft tissue observation.

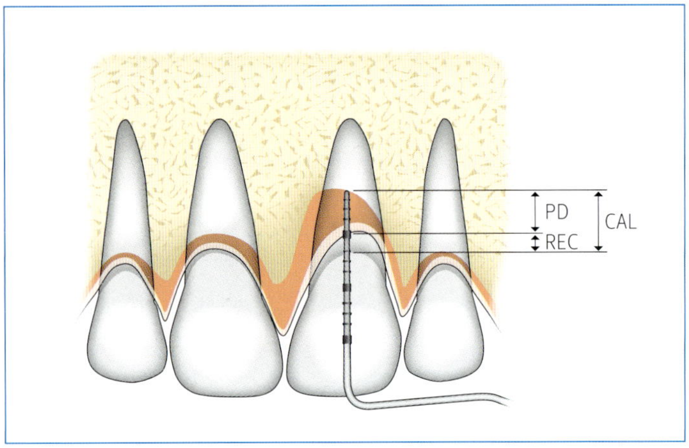

4.8 CAL: Clinical Attachment Loss; PD: Probing Depth; REC: Recession.

and not just a screening test as the Periodontal Screening and Recording (PSR), because even during the active orthodontic treatment a defect can be located on some sites of certain teeth that can be difficult to diagnose and can result unnoticed. Therefore, it is always necessary to pay attention to the patient's entire periodontal condition throughout the duration of the treatment in order to avoid worsening of the periodontal situation[14].

The complete periodontal charting should be used as a baseline to monitor the condition of the tissues during and after orthodontic treatment, as a comparison in the re-evaluation of the periodontal status and during the follow-ups over time. In charting different data are recorded (4.8): PD (Probing Depth; distance between the gingival margin and the bottom of the periodontal pocket), which together with the recession (REC, Recession) determines the CAL (Clinical Attachment Loss); BOP (Bleeding On Probe); furcations involvement; dental mobility; PI (Plaque Index). From these data various periodontal indexes are obtained: FMBS (Full Mouth Bleeding Score), FMPS (Full Mouth Plaque Score) and the number of sites in millimetres of periodontal attachment loss (normally divided into ≤4 mm, 5-6 mm, ≥7 mm).

In order to safely perform orthodontic treatment in an adult patient, to diagnose periodontal problems and to avoid the recurrence and/or worsening of a previous periodontal disease, periodontal charting is fundamental and mandatory: it is an examination that cannot be avoided at all.

The periodontal probing provides five points that must be always taken into account[15]:

1. Sulcus depth around the tooth: this data allows us to determine the periodontal attachment, its morphology and the three-dimensional nature of the bone defect. In a combined treatment plan, this information is very important, because tooth movements can modify the anatomy of the defect increasing the predictability of surgical treatment, where necessary, and probing helps to determine if and what type of surgical treatment should be performed.
2. Bleeding on probing (BOP): index of site inflammation and activity of the periodontal disease. It is important to remember that BOP has a high negative predictive value for disease progression, as the absence of BOP is a good indicator for maintaining periodontal stability, while the positive predictive value of BOP for attachment loss and progression of disease is low or moderate[16]. On a practical level, the absence of BOP is one of the gingival tissue health prediction parameters regardless of pocket depth, while its presence is one of the many risk factors associated with progressive bone loss due to periodontitis[3]. Orthodontic patients with persistent BOP should be considered at risk and should be referred to a strict regimen of periodontal control[3]. Bleeding from a pocket, therefore, is a prognostic indicator that is correlated to disease progression[17,18].
3. Degree of furcations involvement, important in uprighting movements.
4. Gingival recessions. The staging of recessions is outlined for the evolution over time of mechanical and inflammatory stresses[9].
5. Tooth mobility.

Bone defects anatomy

The data collected allow the mapping of the patient's periodontal situation, required to plan the treatment plan. According to the classification of Papapanou and Tonetti[19], the bone defects are classified into:

1. Suprabony defect (defect in which the base of the pocket is positioned coronally to the alveolar crest) (4.9a and 4.10).
2. Infrabony defect (defect in which the base of the

pocket is positioned apically to the alveolar ridge) (📷 4.9b and 4.11), which can be divided into:

   a. Intrabony (3-2-1 walls and combined) (📷 4.12-4.14).
   b. Crater (📷 4.15).

3. Interradicular defect:
   a. Horizontal (Class I, II, III) (📷 4.16).
   b. Vertical (Subclass A, B, C) (📷 4.17).

The knowledge of the three-dimensional anatomy of the defect is important from an orthodontic point of view, since it allows to understand if and how the movement can modify, reduce or eliminate the defect or if the defect complicates the orthodontic movement. This modification can increase the predictability of subsequent surgical treatment to the point of completely avoiding surgery. Missing diagnosis of these defects can lead to orthodontic movements that can be unsupported by a healthy and, therefore, not physiological periodontium.

Periodontal probing, therefore, is fundamental in the routine and in the early diagnosis of periodontal defects that could otherwise remain unmanifest and that could lead to complications that could have been avoided with a diagnosis and therapy of periodontal relevance, offering a real contribution to the patient's health.

📷 **4.9** Schematic diagram showing the difference between suprabony (**a**) and infrabony (**b**) defect.

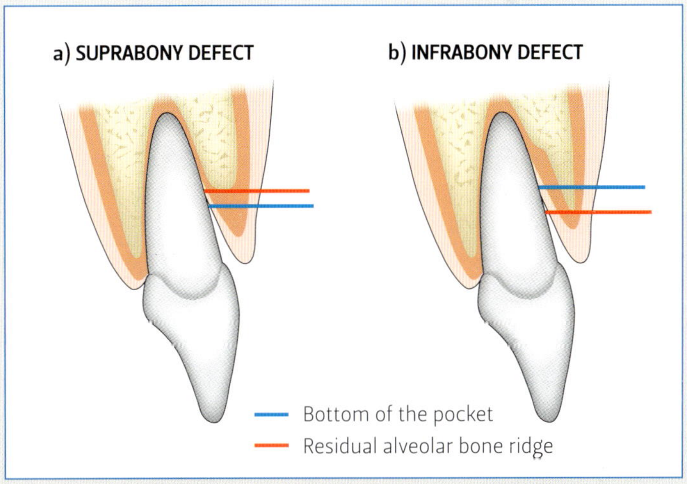

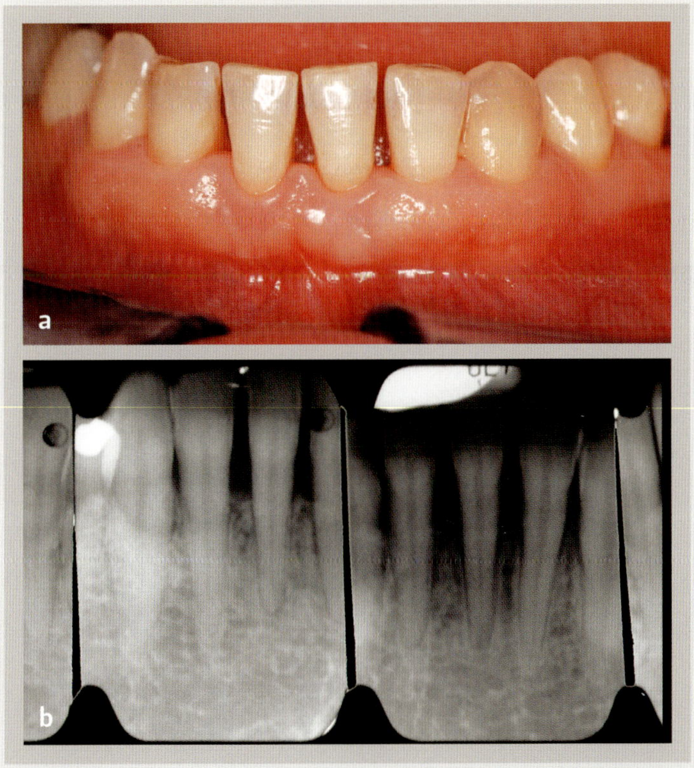

📷 **4.10** Clinical example of suprabony defect: soft tissue morphology and radiographic aspect.

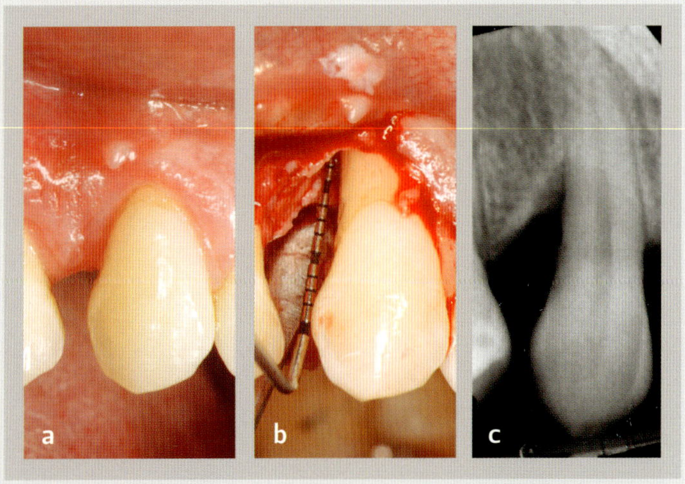

📷 **4.11** Clinical example of infrabony defect (2-wall intrabony defect): soft tissue morphology, periodontal probing and radiographic aspect.

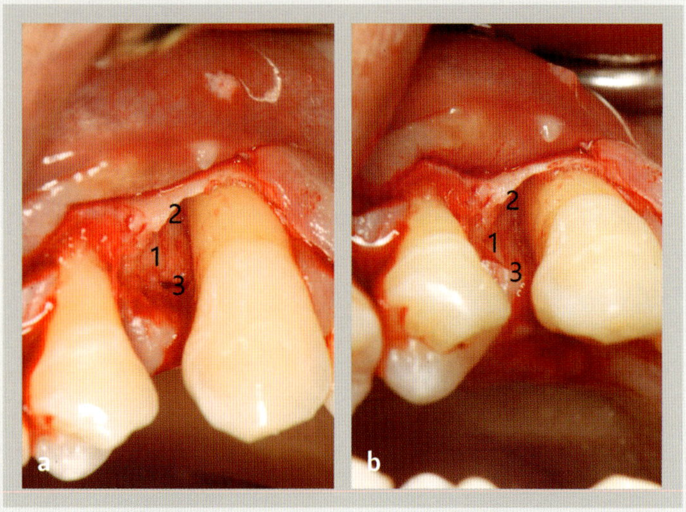

4.12 3-wall Intrabony defect where the three walls (1, 2, 3) can be seen.

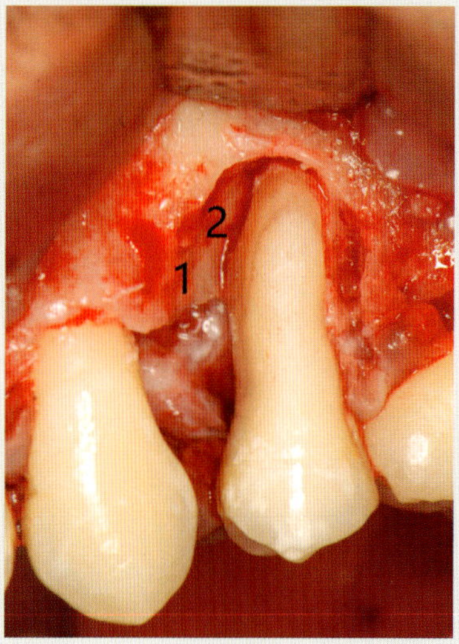

4.13 2-wall Intrabony defect where the two walls (1, 2) can be seen.

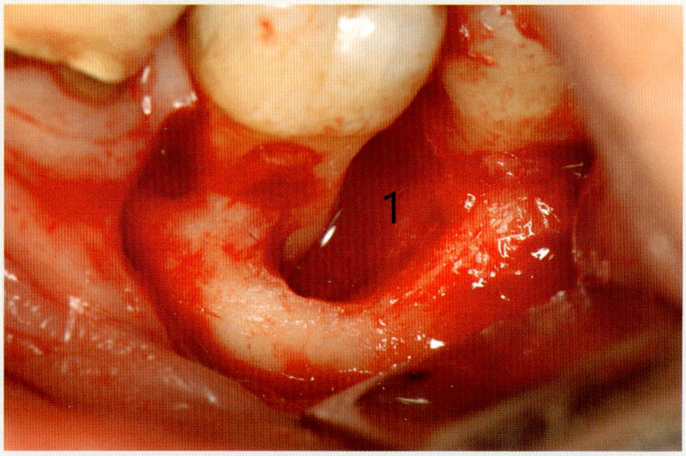

4.14 1-wall Intrabony defect where the residual bone wall (1) can be seen.

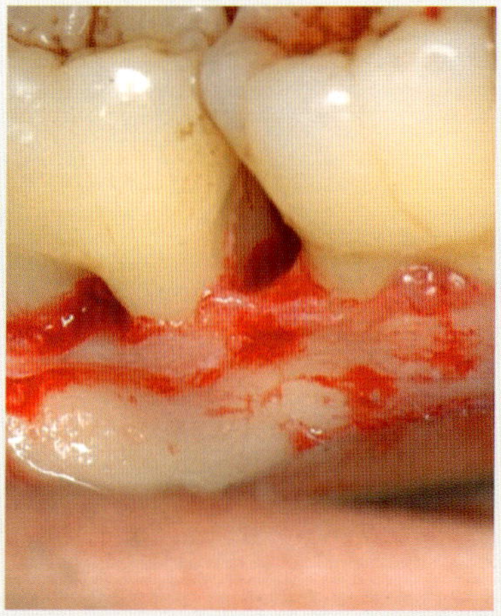

4.15 Bone crater. Clinical view where the remaining vestibular wall and the lack of the root interproximal bone peaks can be seen.

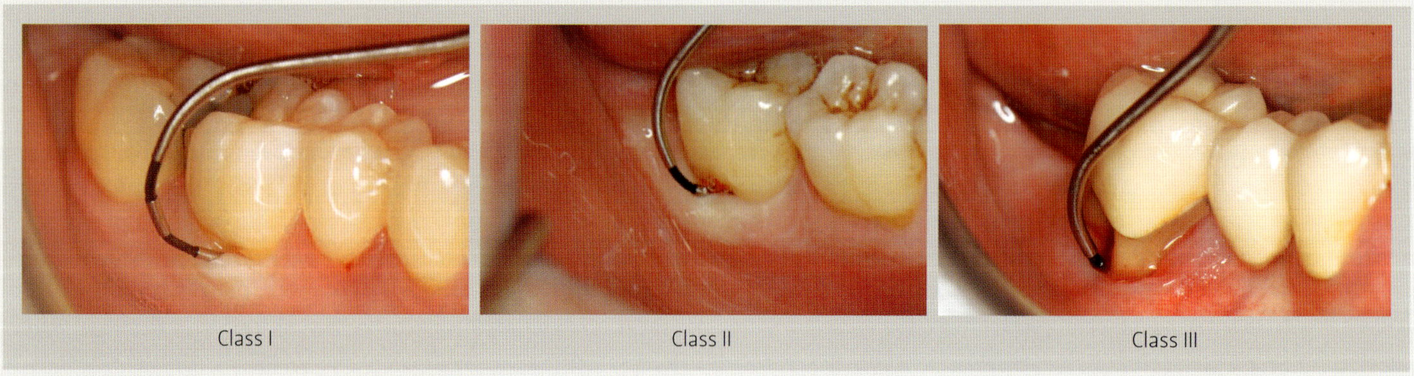

4.16 Furcations probing. Horizontal measurement (Class I, II, III).

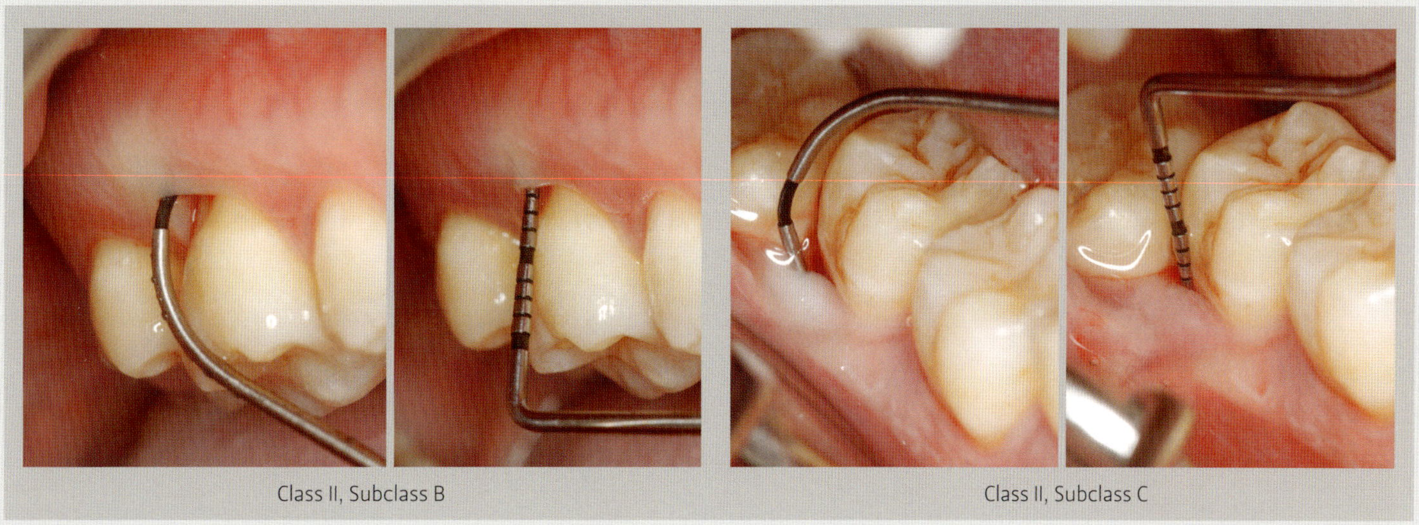

4.17 Furcations probing. Vertical measurement (Subclass B and C).

Orthodontic signs in the periodontal patient

Now we will see the orthodontic signs mainly shown in the periodontal patients, focusing not only on the periodontal aspect, but also pointing out how an orthodontic request can lead the patient to become aware of an unknown periodontal problem during the first orthodontic visit.

In the periodontal patient (4.18) can be observed[1,10,20,21]:

- proclination of the maxillary anterior teeth (PTM) with extrusion and deflection of teeth (4.19);
- irregular interdental spaces, diastema;
- overeruption;
- loss of teeth;
- rotation;
- migration;
- mobility;
- recessions.

Considerations on Pathologic Tooth Migration

PTM is the modification of the dental position that occurs when there is an imbalance in the forces that keep teeth in their normal relationship[10,22]. Flaring and drifting of the incisors is a common sign of advanced periodontal destruction. In literature, its prevalence varies from 11.4%[23] to 30.03%[22], up to 55.8%, and it is related to the amount of bone loss, tooth loss and gingival inflammation[24]. The possibility of having PTM is three times higher for teeth that are affected by bone loss[24]. In fact, in patients with aggressive periodontitis PTM is more frequent (72%) than in those with chronic periodontitis (46%)[25]. Several pathogenetic factors are reported as the cause of dental migration: proprioceptive disorders between the soft tissues (lips, tongue) and the periodontal attachment apparatus, pressure of the inflammatory granulation tissue in the intrabony defect, tension of the contralateral healthy periodontal fibres, bad habits, collapse of the posterior vertical dimension due to loss and inclination of teeth[26-28]. Periodontal complications and loss of posterior teeth can lead to posterior occlusion collapse and reduction in the vertical dimension which causes most of the reported signs (proclination, spaces and overeruption of the anterior teeth). Changes in dental position cause difficulties in oral hygiene care, traumatize the periodontium and lead to esthetic and functional discomfort[22,26]. There is probably no single etiopathogenetic factor, but periodontal bone loss is the primary factor, followed by tooth loss and gingival inflammation[24]. Migrated teeth have a greater clinical attachment loss (4.79 ± 0.28 mm) than non-migrated contralateral ones (3.21 ± 0.18 mm)[22]. Migration occurs when the pressure of the inflamma-

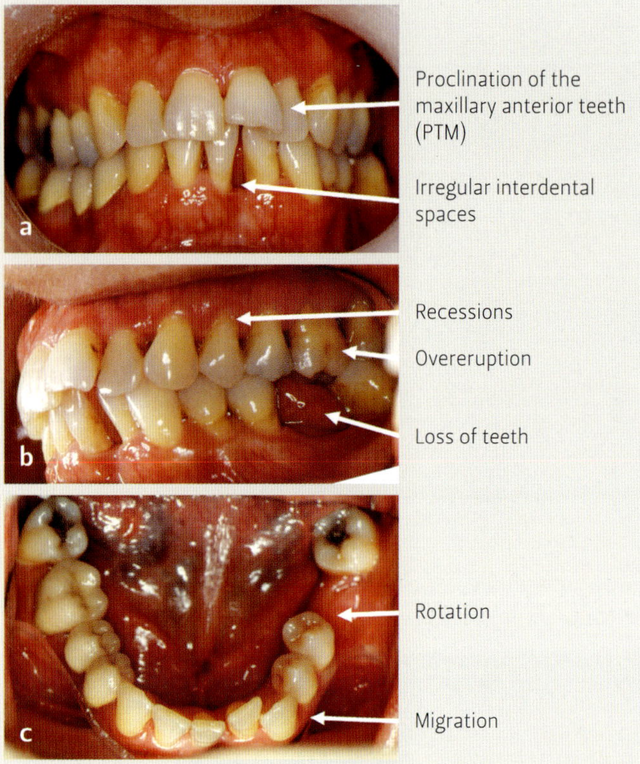

4.18 Clinical view of the orthodontic signs in the periodontal patient.

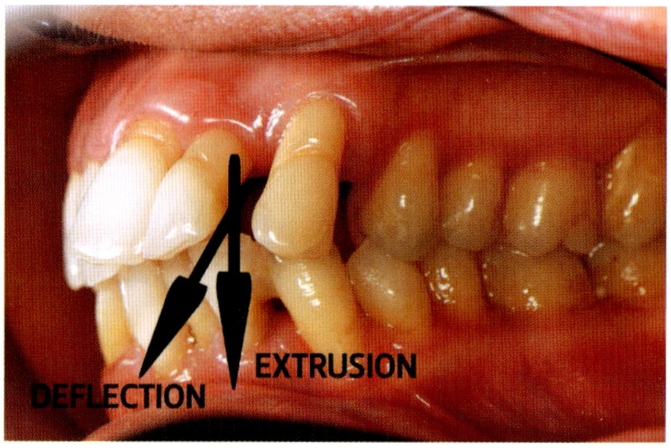

4.19 Dental deflection and extrusion in the PTM.

tory tissue of the defect (increased capillary filtration and pressure of the interstitial fluid) creates a tension in the periodontal ligament and the tooth moves away from the defect[10] (see 4.19). Often the esthetic problems of PTM are the triggering event that leads patients to look for the help of the orthodontist and periodontist[10], discovering for the first time that they are affected by periodontal disease. A typical example is the diagnosis of periodontitis when the patient asks for an orthodontic consultation for an anterior vestibular displacement of the incisors[24] complaining not only about an esthetic but also about an occlusal change with the formation of premature contacts that can accelerate the loss of periodontal support structures due to inflammation and negatively affect dental esthetics. PTM, therefore, can increase insidiously as periodontal destruction progresses and precipitates in proclination, extrusion and rotation of these teeth. Probably, the treatment of periodontal disease offers the best and most effective method to prevent PTM[26], in some cases through the spontaneous correction of the diastema ($\leq$1 mm)[29-33]. Today orthodontic treatment can be considered the first choice for the therapy of teeth that have undergone migration in adult periodontal patients[34], especially in cases in which spontaneous closure of the diastema does not occur and also in those in which esthetic deformities are disabling for the patient.

Clinical case 1

The patient's request is an aesthetic rehabilitation of anterior teeth and the resolution of the lower tooth loss. She shows facial symmetry and sagittal harmony, labial competence (4.20), canine and molar class I, increased overjet (OVJ) and overbite (OVB) (4.21), absence of 1.8, 2.8, 3.1, 3.6, 3.7, 3.8, 4.5, 4.8, normodivergent skeletal class I (4.22) (4.3). The patient is diagnosed as periodontitis stage III generalized grade C[7,8] with medium-high periodontal risk (Perio Risk: 14)[35-37] (4.23), She was provided with the initial periodontal therapy controlling the biofilm and improving the oral hygiene care. Once reduced the probing depth and FMBS-FMPS less than 20%, orthodontic treatment begins. Orthodontics is performed with a vestibular orthodontic mechanics in Tweed© technique, brackets slot .022×.028 (4.24), aimed at the correction of the PTM, the maintenance of the dental class and the control of OVJ and OVB taking into account the presence of only three lower incisors, in presence of a favourable Bolton. After stabilizing the dental situation, the implants (Frialit-2® Dentsply) are placed with a customized template (4.25 and 4.26) and, after their osteointegration, during the second surgical phase, a vestibular connective tissue graft is performed (4.27) and the prosthetic phase is realized with a cement-retained fixed denture (see 4.27; 4.28 and 4.29). At the end of the therapy the patient shows a skeletal balance (4.30) (see 4.3). After 3 years there is stability in facial balance (4.31), dental class I (4.32), in periodontal indexes (4.33) and the implant osteointegration (4.34). The patient at a long-term check (10 year follow-up) shows stability concerning orthodontic results (4.35 and 4.36), osteointegration (4.37) and periodontal (4.38) indexes. The combined treatment and supportive therapy lead the patient to a medium-low periodontal risk (Perio Risk: 5)[35-37] that she kept stable throughout the long-term period (10 years).

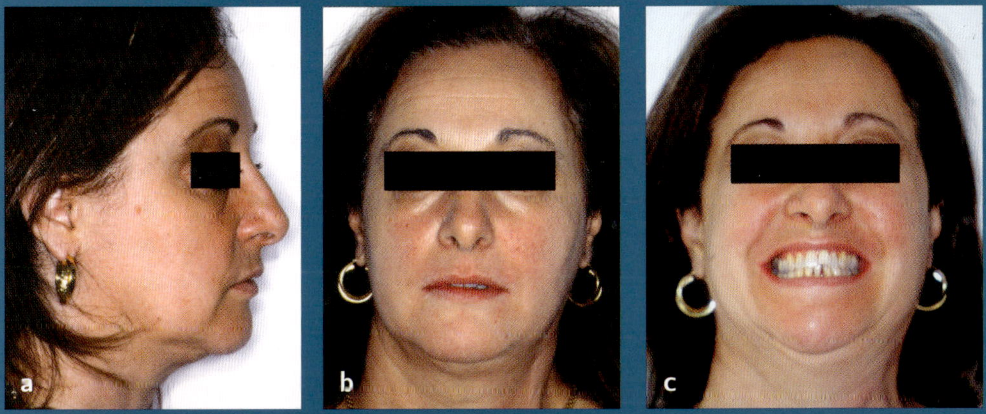

4.20 Extraoral pre-treatment photos.

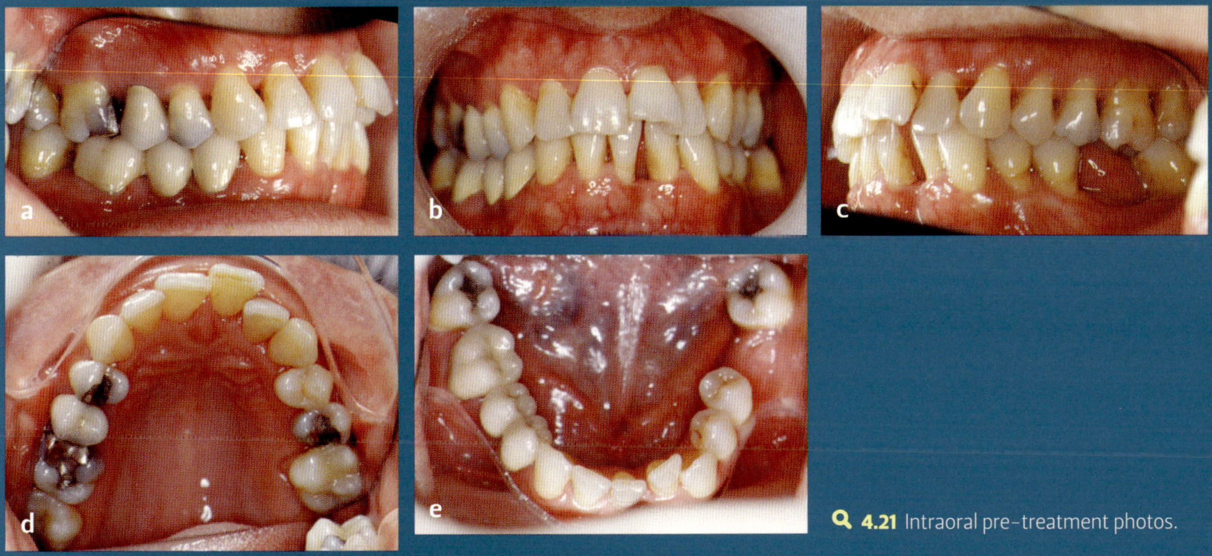

4.21 Intraoral pre-treatment photos.

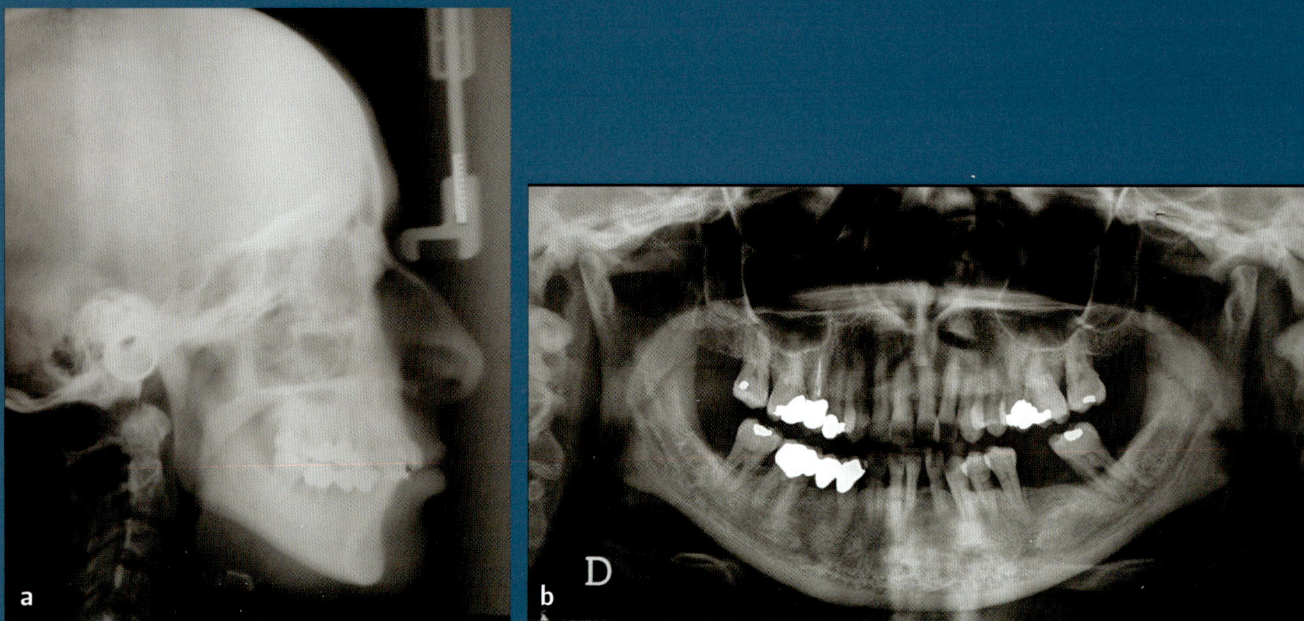

4.22 Pre-treatment cephalometric Rx (**a**) and panoramic Rx (**b**).

Tab. 4.3 Cephalometric values

Sagittal skeletal relationships	Pre-treatment	Post-treatment	Mean	DS
Maxillary sagittal relationship SNA	79°	78°	82°	3.5°
Mandibular sagittal relationship SNPg	76°	77°	80°	3.5°
Intermaxillary sagittal relationship ANPg	3°	1°	2°	2.5°
Vertical skeletal relationships				
Maxillary vertical relationship SN / ANS-PNS	10°	8°	8°	3.0°
Mandibular vertical relationship SN / Go-Gn	41°	40°	33°	2.5°
Intermaxillary vertical relationship ANS-PNS / Go-Gn	31°	32°	25°	6.0°
Dento-basal relationships				
Upper incisor inclination $\underline{1}$ - ANS-PNS	120°	116°	110°	6.0°
Lower incisor inclination $\overline{1}$ - Go-Gn	92°	93°	94°	7.0°
Lower incisor compensation $\overline{1}$ - A-Pg (mm)	+3	+3	2	2.0
Dental relationships				
Overjet (OVJ, mm)	4	3	3,5	2.5
Overbite (OVB, mm)	3	3	2	2.5
Interincisal angle $\underline{1}$ / $\overline{1}$	116°	118°	132°	6.0°

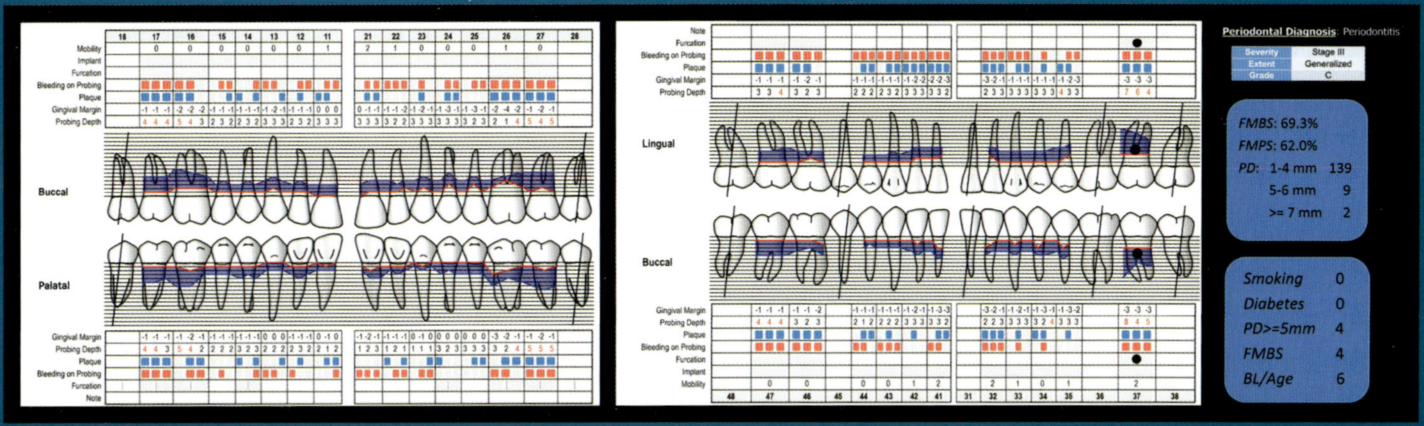

4.23 Initial periodontal probing, periodontal indexes, periodontal diagnosis, risk assessment (Online periodontal charting tool from www.perio-tools.com).

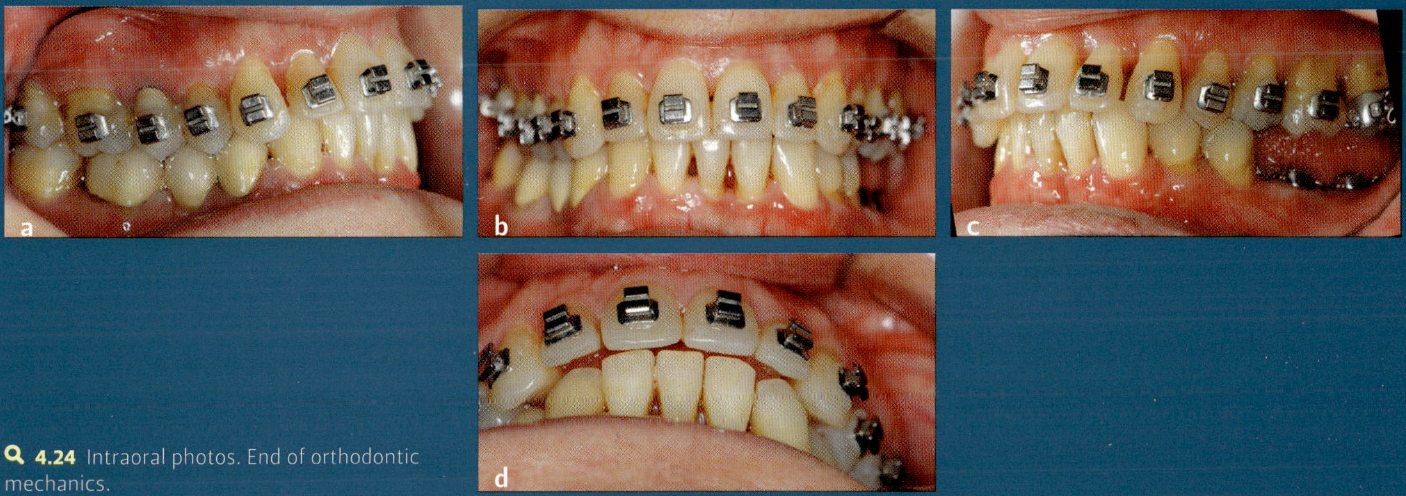

4.24 Intraoral photos. End of orthodontic mechanics.

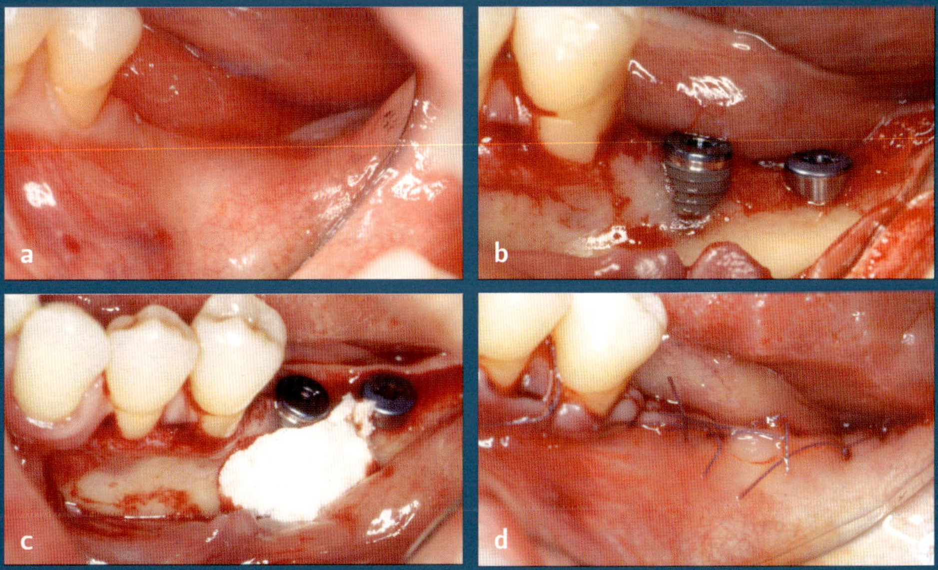

4.25 Tissue aspect at the implant placement time (**a**), implants inserted (**b**), graft material on the mesial implant (**c**), flap suture with a double line of suture (internal mattress and interrupted suture) (**d**).

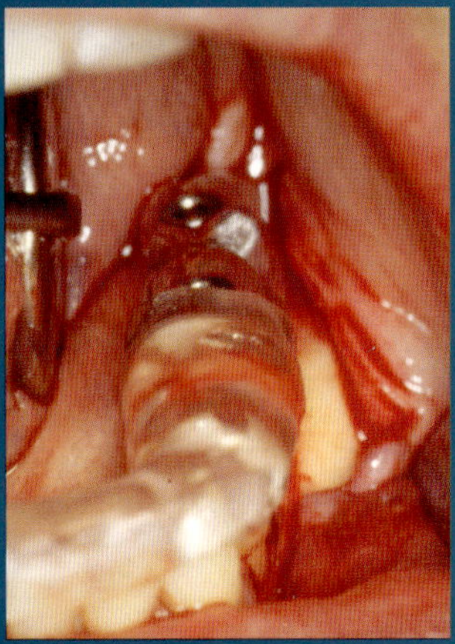

4.26 Customized template for implant placement.

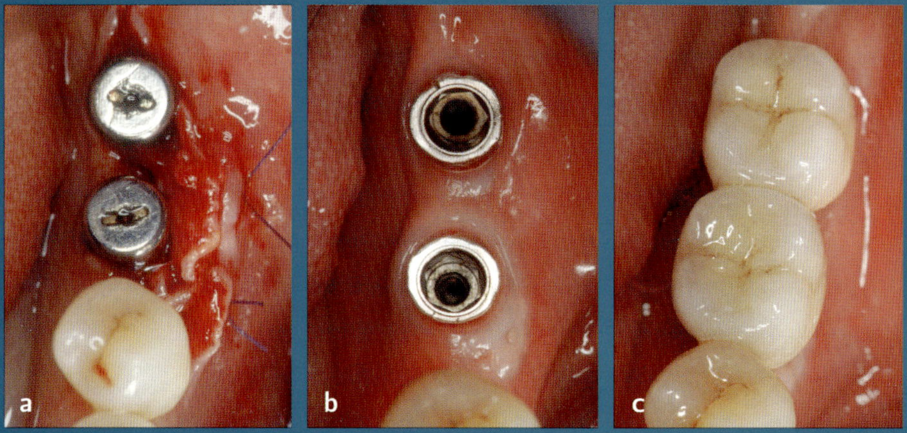

4.27 Vestibular connective tissue graft (**a**), occlusal view of the soft tissues at cementation time (**b**), fixed partial denture (**c**).

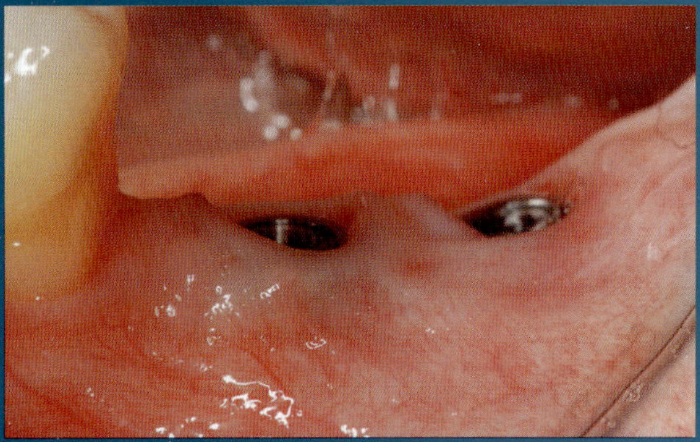

4.28 Vestibular view of the soft tissues at cementation time.

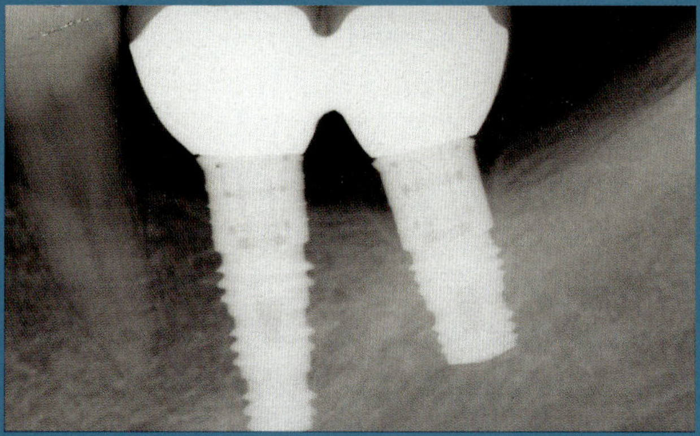

4.29 X-ray check of the osteointegration at cementation time.

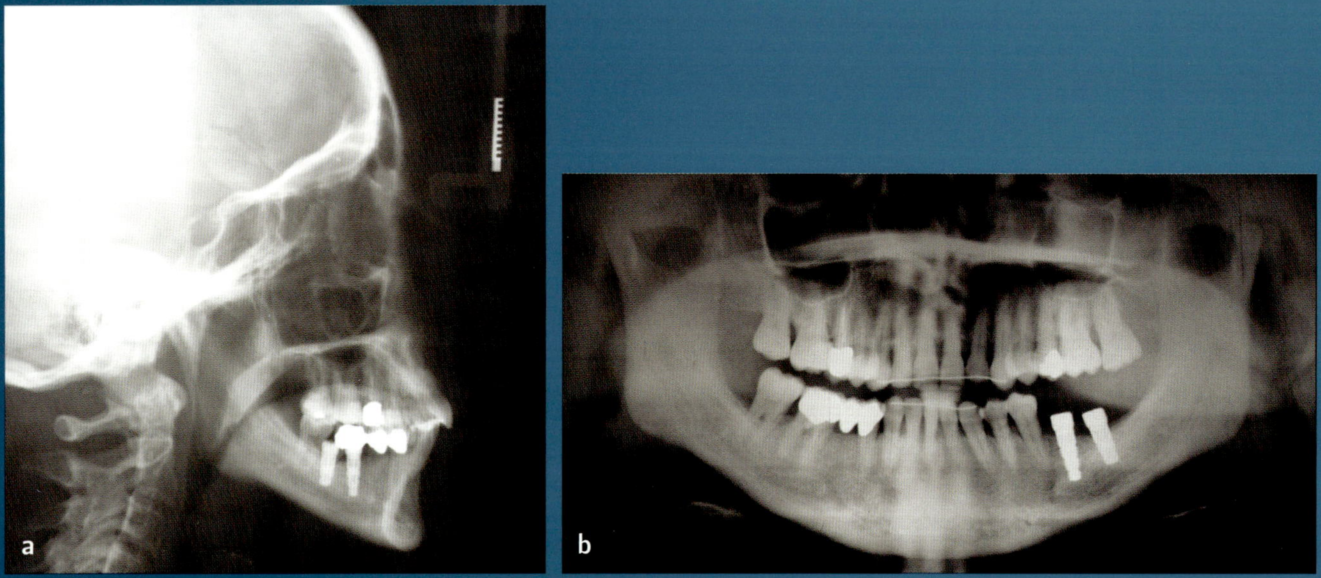

4.30 Post-treatment cephalometric Rx (**a**) and panoramic Rx (**b**).

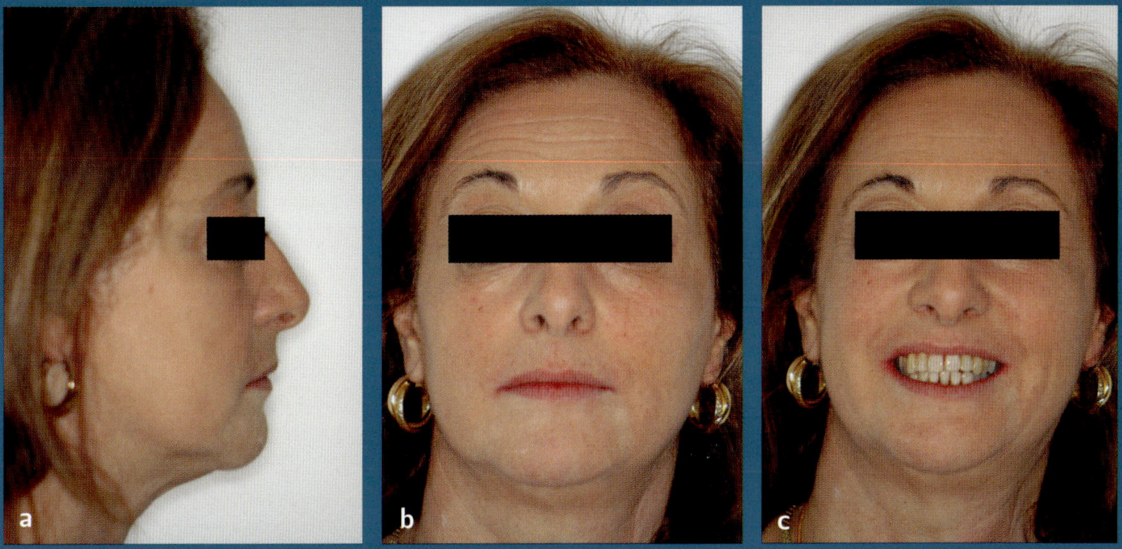

4.31 Extra-oral photos at 3-year follow-up.

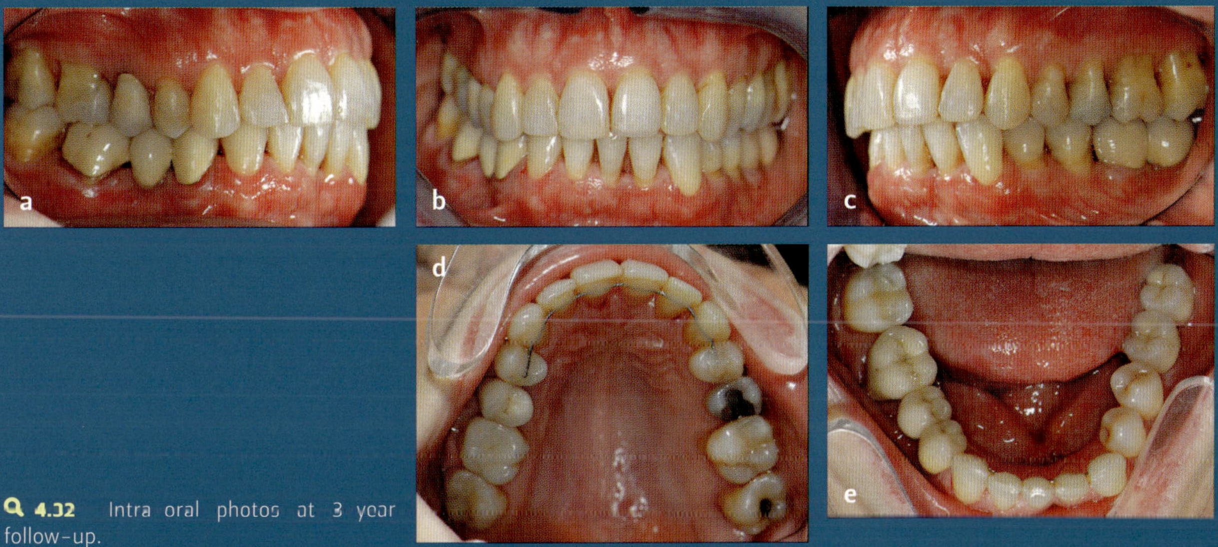

4.32 Intra oral photos at 3 year follow-up.

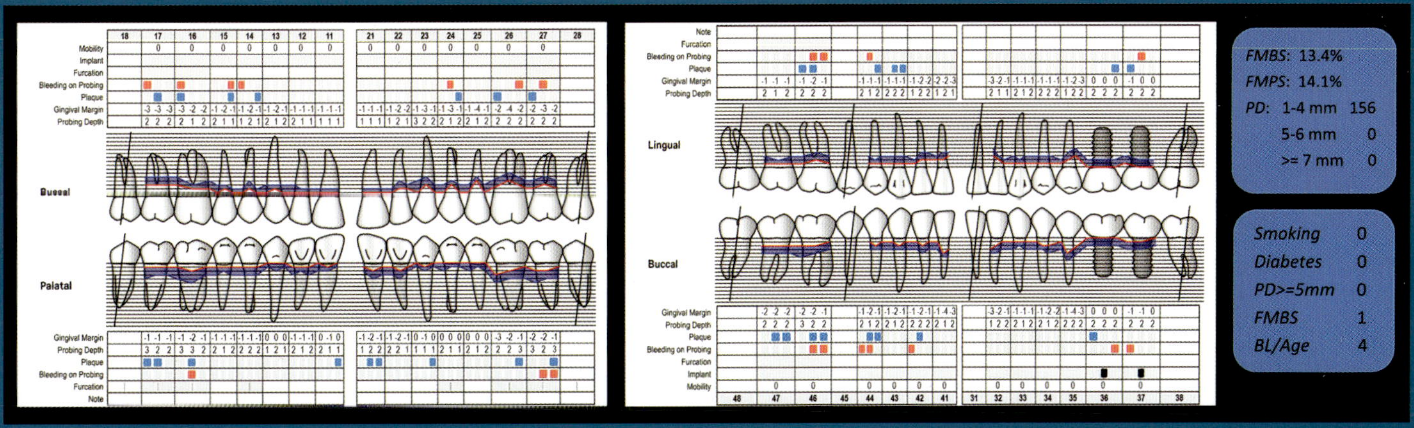

4.33 Periodontal probing, periodontal indexes, risk assessment at 3-year follow-up (Online periodontal charting tool from www.perio-tools.com).

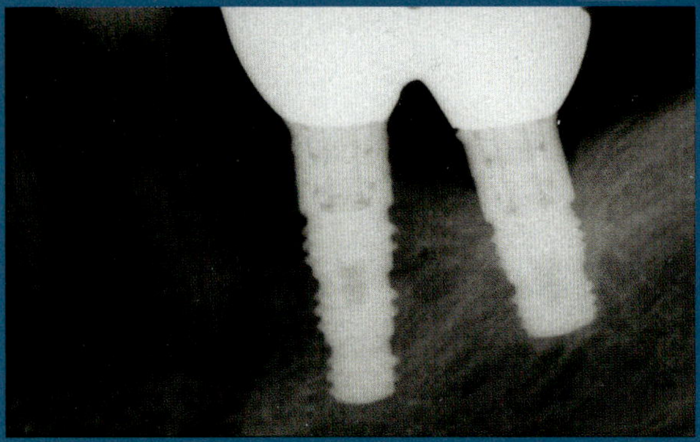

4.34 Implants X-ray check at 3-year follow-up.

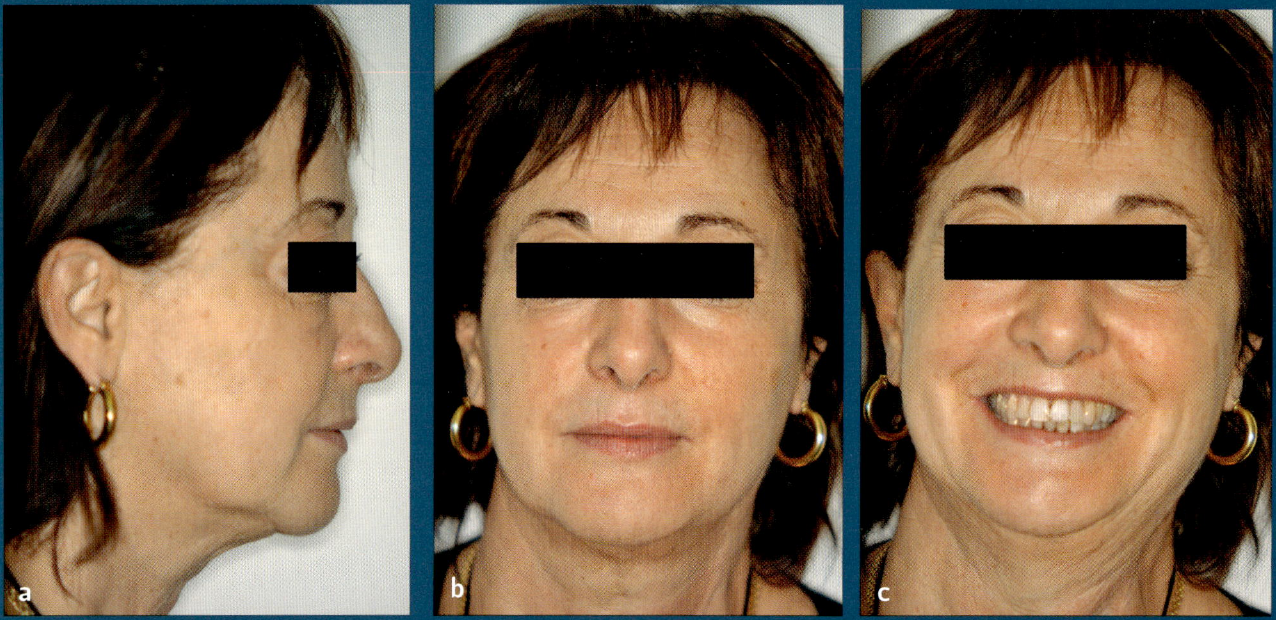

4.35 Extra-oral photos at 10-year follow-up.

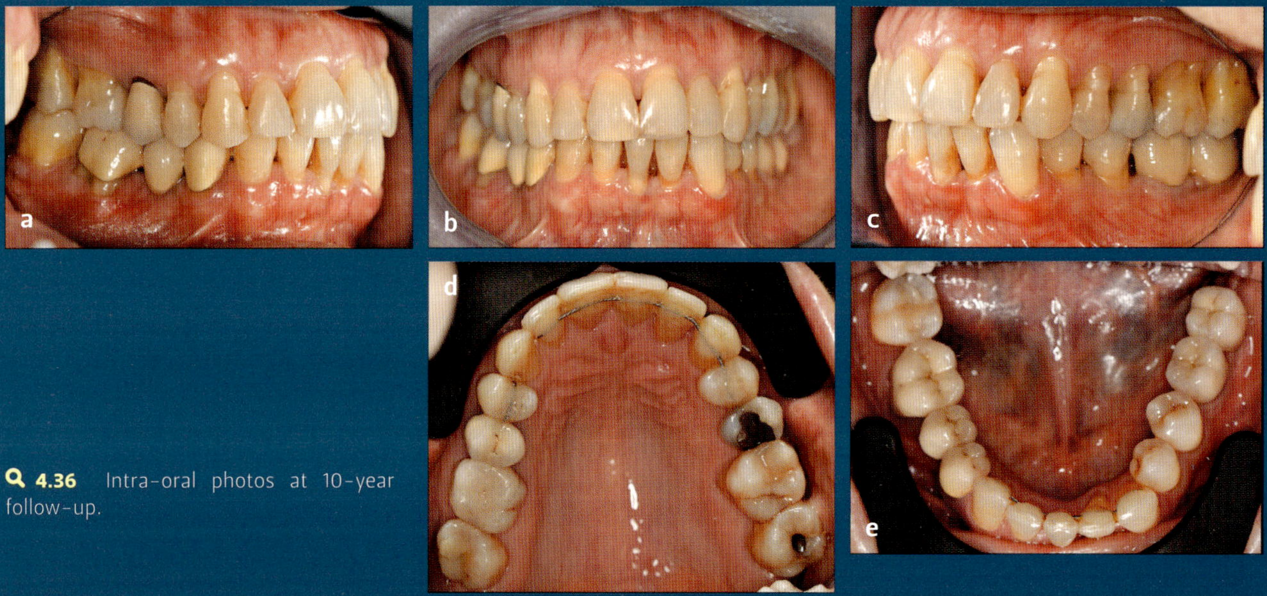

4.36 Intra-oral photos at 10-year follow-up.

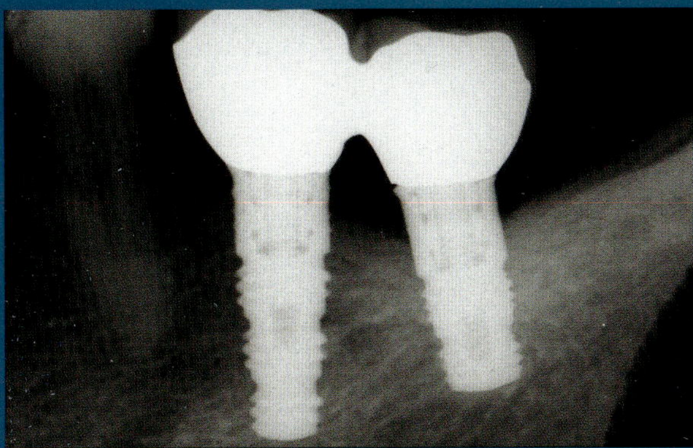

4.37 Implants X-ray check at 10-year follow-up.

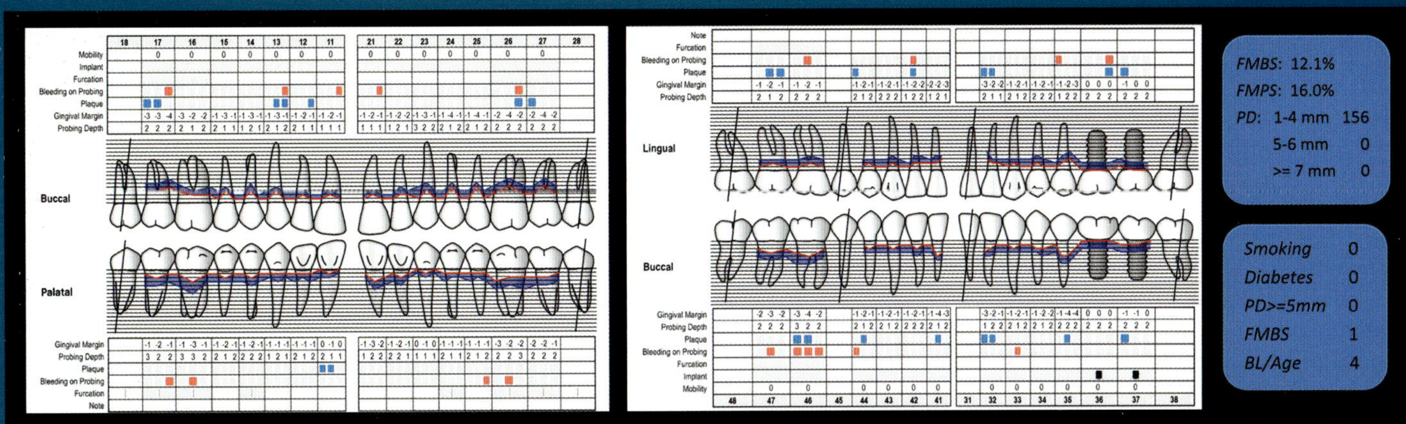

4.38 Periodontal probing, periodontal indexes, risk assessment at 10-year follow-up (Online periodontal charting tool from www.perio-tools.com).

REFERENCES

1. GKANTIDIS N, CHRISTOU P, TOPOUZELIS N. The orthodontic-periodontic interrelationship in integrated treatment challenges: a systematic review. *J Oral Rehabil.* 2010;37(5):377-390.

2. ELKORDY SA, PAOLOMO L, PALOMO JM, MOSTAFA YA. Do Fixed Orthodontic appliances adversly affect the periodontium? A systematic review of systematic reviews. *Semin Orthod.* 2019;25(2):130-157.

3. PALOMO L, PAOLOMO JM, BISSADA NF. Salient periodontal issues for the modern biologic Orthodontist. *Semin Orthod.* 2008;14(4):229-245.

4. HAZAN-MOLINA H, LEVIN L, EINY S, AIZENBUD D. Aggressive periodontitis diagnosed during or before orthodontic treatment. *Acta Odontol Scand.* 2013;71(5):1023-1031.

5. CHACKARTCHI T, CHAUSHU S, STABHOLZ A. Orthodontic treatment in patients with severe periodontal disease. In: Eliades T, Katsaros C. *The ortho-perio patient: clinical evidence & therapeutic guidelines.* Batavia, IL. Quintessence Publishing Co; 2019:189-210.

6. TONETTI MS, SANZ M. Implementation of the new classification of periodontal diseases: decision-making algorithms for clinical practice and education. *J Clin Periodontol.* 2019;46(4):398-405.

7. KORNMAN KS, TONETTI MS. Proceedings of the World Workshop on the Classification of Periodontal and Peri-Implant Diseases and Conditions. *J Periodontol.* 2018;89 Suppl 1:S1-S291.

8. KORNMAN KS, TONETTI MS. Proceedings of the World Workshop on the Classification of Periodontal and Peri-Implant Diseases and Conditions. *J Clin Periodontol.* 2018;45(Suppl 20):S1-S291.

9. GORBUNKOVA A, PAGNI G, BRIZHAK A ET AL. Impact of orthodontic treatment on periodontal tissues: a narrative review of multidisciplinary literature. *Int J Dent.* 2016;2016:4723589.

10. CARDAROPOLI D, GAVEGLIO L, ABOU-ARRAJ RV. Orthodontic movement and periodontal bone defects: rationale, timing, and clinical implications. *Semin Orthod.* 2014;20(3):177-187.

11. SUSIN C, KINGMAN A, ALBANDAR JM. Effect of partial recording protocols on estimates of prevalence of periodontal disease. *J Periodontol.* 2005;76(2):262-267.

12. KINGMAN A, ALBANDAR JM. Methodological aspects of epidemiological

studies of periodontal diseases. *Periodontol 2000.* 2002;29(1):11-30.

13. **Boyd RL, Baumrind S.** Periodontal considerations in the use of bonds or bands on molars in adolescents and adults. *Angle Orthod.* 1992;62(2):117-126.
14. **Zoizner R, Arbel Y, Yavnai N et al.** Effect of orthodontic treatment and comorbidity risk factors on interdental alveolar crest level: a radiographic evaluation. *Am J Orthod Dentofacial Orthop.* 2018;154(3):375-381.
15. **Kokich VG.** Don't start without the charting. *Am J Orthod Dentofacial Orthop.* 2011;139(4 Suppl):S14.
16. **Lang NP, Adler R, Joss A, Nyman S.** Absence of bleeding on probing. An indicator of periodontal stability. *J Clin Periodontol.* 1990;17(10):714-721.
17. **Trombelli L, Simonelli A, Franceschetti G et al.** What periodontal recall interval is supported by evidence? *Periodontol 2000.* 2020;84(1):124-133.
18. **Farina R, Tomasi C, Trombelli L.** The bleeding site: a multi-level analysis of associated factors. *J Clin Periodontol.* 2013;40(8):735-742.
19. **Papapanou PN, Tonetti MS.** Diagnosis and epidemiology of periodontal osseous lesions. *Periodontol 2000.* 2000;22(1):8-21.
20. **Antoun JS, Mei L, Gibbs K, Farella M.** Effect of orthodontic treatment on the periodontal tissues. *Periodontol 2000.* 2017;74(1):140-157.
21. **Feng X, Oba T, Oba Y, Moriyama K.** An interdisciplinary approach for improved functional and esthetic results in a periodontally compromised adult patient. *Angle Orthod.* 2005;75(6):1061-1070.
22. **Towfighi PP, Brunsvold MA, Storey AT et al.** Pathologic migration of anterior teeth in patients with moderate to severe periodontitis. *J Periodontol.* 1997;68(10):967-972.
23. **Khorshidi H, Moaddeli MR, Golkari A et al.** The prevalence of pathologic tooth migration with respect to the severity of periodontitis. *J Int Soc Prev Community Dent.* 2016;6(Suppl 2):S122-S125.
24. **Martinez-Canut P, Carrasquer A, Magán R, Lorca A.** A study on factors associated with pathologic tooth migration. *J Clin Periodontol.* 1997;24(7):492-497.
25. **Czochrowska EM, Rosa M.** The orthodontic/periodontal interface. *Semin Orthod* 2015;21(1):3-14.
26. **Brunsvold MA.** Pathologic tooth migration. *J Periodontol.* 2005;76(6):859-866.
27. **Diedrich P, Fritz U, Kizinger G.** Interrelationship between periodontics and adult orthodontics. *Perio.* 2004;1(3):143-149.
28. **Proffit WR.** Equilibrium theory revisited: factors influencing position of the teeth. *Angle Orthod.* 1978;48(3):175-186.
29. **Livada R, Shiloah J, Hottel TL.** Non-orthodontic, non-restorative closure of acquired diastemata. *J Tenn Dent Assoc.* 2015;95(2):34-38.
30. **Thakur AM, Baburaj MD.** Analysis of spontaneous repositioning of pathologically migrated teeth: a clinical and radiographic study. *Quintessence Int.* 2014;45(9):733-741.
31. **Sato S, Ujiie H, Ito K.** Spontaneous correction of pathologic tooth migration and reduced infrabony pockets following nonsurgical periodontal therapy: a case report. *Int J Periodontics Restorative Dent.* 2004;24(5):456-461.
32. **Singh J, Deshpande RN.** Pathologic migration - spontaneous correction following periodontal therapy: a case report. *Quintessence Int.* 2002;33(1):65-68.
33. **Gaumet PE, Brunsvold MI, McMahan CA.** Spontaneous repositioning of pathologically migrated teeth. *J Periodontol.* 1999;70(10):1177-1184.
34. **Cardaropoli D.** Orthodontics for the adult periodontal patient: first or second choice treatment? *Prog Orthod.* 2009;10(2):88-96.
35. **Trombelli L, Minenna L, Toselli L et al.** Prognostic value of a simplified method for periodontal risk assessment during supportive periodontal therapy. *J Clin Periodontol.* 2017;44(1):51-57.
36. **Trombelli L, Farina R, Ferrari S et al.** Comparison between two methods for periodontal risk assessment. *Minerva Stomatol.* 2009;58(6):277-287.
37. **Farina R, Ferrari S, Pasetti P et al.** Comparison between two methods for periodontal risk assessment. Abstracts of the 6th International Congress of the European Federation of Periodontology (Europerio 6), Stockholm, June 4-6 2009. *J. Clin Periodontol.* 2009;36(S9):82(abstr. #157).

Dental movement in the periodontal patient. Concepts of biomechanics

Introduction

Literature agrees on the possibility of moving teeth with reduced, but healthy periodontal tissue, without detrimental effects on the attachment level[1,2]. During the orthodontic movement, the whole attachment system, including the bone structures, the periodontal ligament and the soft tissues, moves together with the tooth. The same phenomenon also occurs in patients with a reduced healthy periodontium[3]. Periodontal inflammation must be eliminated before starting orthodontic movement and excellent oral hygiene must be maintained, otherwise, subgingival plaque, before and during orthodontic treatment, can lead to severe attachment loss[4]. It is the presence of plaque in the bone defect that causes the exacerbation and progression of periodontal disease[2,4,5]. As a consequence, the orthodontic movement, in presence of periodontal inflammation, can induce a rapid increase in pocket depth and a greater bone loss than in chronic inflammation alone[6]. Hence, cooperation between clinicians and patients in maintaining oral hygiene is essential to minimize subsequent loss of periodontal bone support during orthodontic movement[7].

Bodily movement does not cause connective attachment loss if the periodontal tissue is free from inflammation, regardless of the height of the periodontium[2,7,8-11]. A failure in the control of plaque on periodontal tissues during orthodontic treatment starts an inflammatory process that accelerates the progression of periodontal destruction, with loss of clinical attachment, increased probing and conversion from gingivitis to periodontitis[7,12,13]. In addition to the inflammatory process, the formation of a hyalinization zone due to the application of excessive force to a periodontally compromised tooth could be very serious, because in the presence of bacterial infection the regeneration of the periodontal ligament does not occur, resulting in severe destruction of the alveolar bone[14,15].

Tooth movement in the presence of periodontal disease has already been analysed by Ericsson and Lindhe[16,17], who have shown on Beagle dogs that there is a worsening effect on the progression of periodontal disease when trauma due to *jiggling* forces[18] is added to angular defects without proper periodontal treatment, increasing the risk of progression of periodontal disease. These jiggling forces, under certain conditions, can act as a co-destructive factor and can increase the worsening effect of plaque[16], where the combination of inflammation/tooth movement/occlusal trauma can produce a more rapid destruction of periodontal tissue[19].

Stating that orthodontics does not appear to be a contraindication when marginal bone has been lost due to periodontal disease under conditions of inflammation control [14,15,20-22], we will analyse the movements that can be performed in the periodontal patient.

Movements in the periodontal patient

Most of the studies on orthodontic movements have been carried out on animal models with induced and unnatural periodontal disease[23], where bone metabolism is different from the one in humans[20]. Hence, we must face the difficulty of extrapolating data and adapting them to the human model where the loss of attachment and the result of a chronic pathology are very slow and occur over a long-term period; moreover, in the human model, the host response is very variable and there are differences in the regeneration capability of the periodontal tissues that follow the movement of the teeth in bone defects[24]. Therefore, the presence of a "real" and not experimentally induced disease can influence and modify the data[25]. Such researches are ideal for histological studies, a field in which they find their main indication[24].

Even knowing that the real orthodontic movement is a combination of several movements, we will divide the

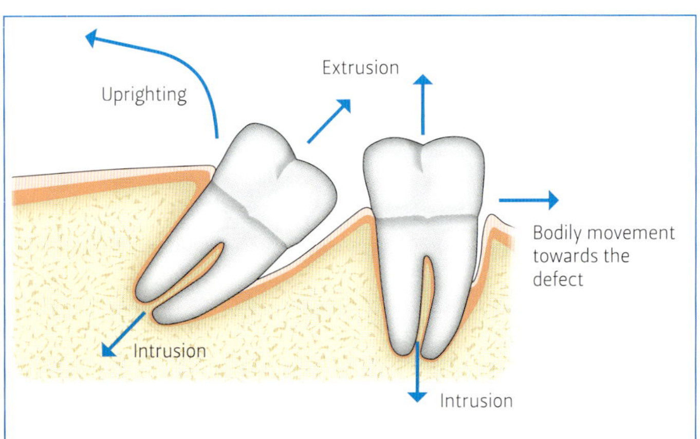

5.1 Schematic diagram of the orthodontic movements in relation to periodontal defect.

various dental movements, with respect to the periodontal defect (5.1), into:

1. Movements towards the defect: bodily and non-bodily movements and intrusion movements.
2. Movements away from the defect: extrusion and uprighting movements.

Movements towards the bone defect

BODILY AND NON-BODILY MOVEMENTS

The idea underneath the use of bodily movement in the periodontal patient is to move the tooth towards the bone defect, with the hypothetical aim of obtaining its reduction or elimination (5.2).Polson et al.[1] investigated the effect of bodily movement of a tooth towards an intraosseous defect in monkeys after plaque removal. In the control specimens not subjected to orthodontic movement there were bony angular defects with epithelium on the root surface; in the tested teeth, the angular defect was eliminated by the orthodontic movement, but with no gain in the residual attachment level. There was only a very thin epithelial layer covering the root surface, with an increase of cement on the side of tension, and the alveolar bone adjacent to the orthodontically moved tooth had no longer an angular morphology. In conclusion, there was no effect on the connective attachment level and no regeneration of the support apparatus was observed, but there was also no further attachment loss; while performing a containment action on the apical growth of the epithelium, the orthodontic movement did not completely avoid the formation of long junctional epithelium[26].

It is therefore possible to move the teeth with a reduced, but healthy, periodontal support without detrimental effects on the level of periodontal attachment. These observations by Polson et al.[1] were also confirmed by Diedrich et al.[21], who demonstrated that conventional periodontal therapy (with a reparative, not regenerative, approach), in combination with the orthodontic movement, has no effect on the level of connective tissue attachment. However, in the presence of inflammation, bodily movement towards an intraosseous defect can increase attachment loss. This situation is particularly evident when the tooth is moved within intrabony pockets, when it is necessary to align teeth that are tipped, elongated and vestibularly displaced as

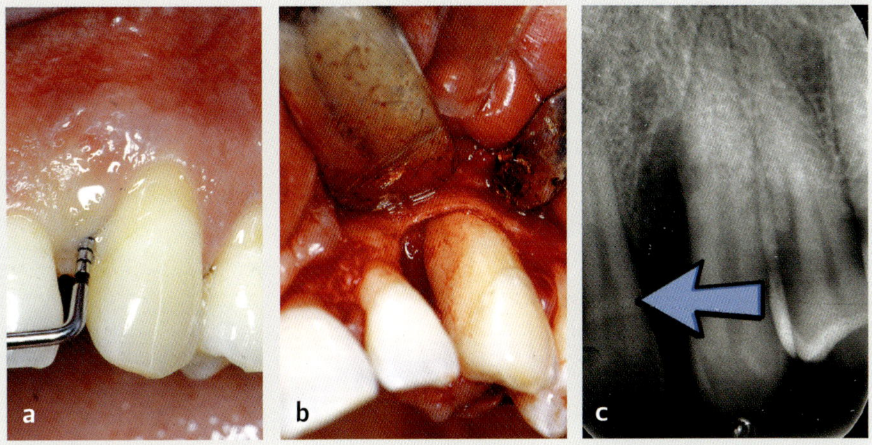

5.2 Bodily movement towards the defect.

a consequence of periodontal disease[12]. Movements towards the intraosseous defect, with a healthy periodontium and a good oral hygiene can be performed without additional loss of periodontal support[20,21].

Orthodontic movement in the bone defect is also given by a combination of various movements. Diedrich et al.[27] histologically studied the intrusive movement associated with a bodily movement towards the defect and away from the defect started 1 month after surgical regenerative treatment (open flap debridement with EMD and Vicryl® membrane) in dogs. At the end of the experiment, after 6 months of orthodontic movement in the sites associated with the intrusion, the Authors detected a slight epithelial growth towards the bottom of the pockets and an orthodontically induced remodeling with extensive cementoneogenesis and osteonegenesis; these situations are also present on the tension site in the group with a movement of translation; the experimentally created bone pockets were no longer observable after orthodontics and there was a substantial formation of cement and bone. This osteoinduction by the orthodontic movement has also been confirmed by Nemcovsky et al.[28] and Vardimon et al.[29] on Wistar rats, reiterating that orthodontic movement appears to be a stimulating factor for bone apposition.

For what concerns literature in humans, there are some case reports. A study by Corrente et al.[30] demonstrated a gain in clinical attachment and a radiographic filling of the bone defect by movement in the bone defect (not pure but combined with an intrusion and associated with periodontal surgery). Ahn et al[31] confirmed that the movement of the teeth in an intraosseous defect can modify its morphology, solve it radiologically and reduce the PPD.

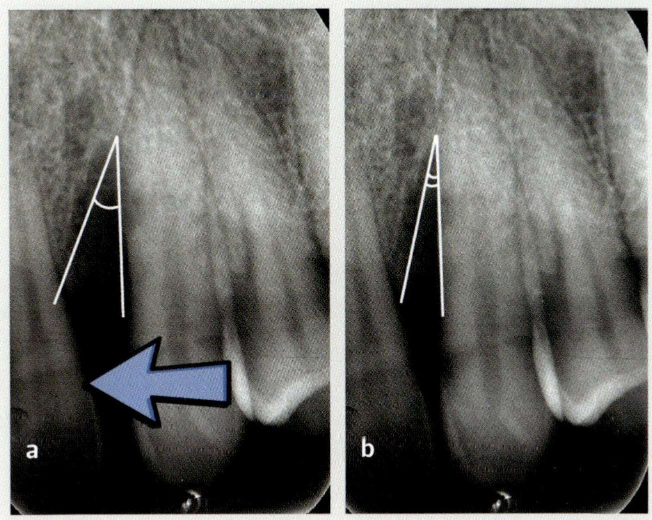

5.3 Closing of the intrabony defect angle after the bodily movement.

So, we can move teeth bodily inside infraosseous defects, without further loss of connective attachment but also without any regeneration too[32], filling the contact area through long junctional epithelium. This type of movement, as suggested by some Authors[32], could only be useful to close the angle at the base of the defect in the presence of a large intrabony defect, increasing the surgical regenerative predictability and therefore, the healing ability[33] (5.3). The movement must always take place in the absence of plaque and tissue inflammation[12].

INTRUSIVE MOVEMENTS

In theory, intrusion could find multiple applications in the correction of pathological results in the periodontal and rehabilitative patient, such as diastemas correction in anterior teeth, therapy of PTM, treatment of deep-bites with impingement of the anterior group, pre-restorative mechanics, high verticality cases with open-bite, discrepancies in the occlusal plane[24,34]. In intrusive movement a thin epithelial layer is formed which covers the root to the deepest point of the root planing with junctional epithelium which can also proliferate under the alveolar ridge[21]. Erkan et al.[35] and Murakami et al.[36] quantified the displacement of tissues in relation to the extent of the intrusive movement (5.4). Melsen et al.[37,38] demonstrated in histological studies in monkeys new cement formation and new collagen attachment following the surgical procedures if the oral hygiene was maintained, and that the intrusion improved the quantity of new attachment if carried out under healthy conditions. Intrusion was performed under a control of a light biomechanics force system (5-15 g). These forces realised an apical bodily movement with the action line passing from 0 to 1 mm the center of resistance[37]. In the group treated with periodontal flap surgery with curettage, the new attachment ranged from 0.7 to 2.3 mm. In the group without oral hygiene care there was an aggravation of periodontal bone loss, with pockets of 3-4 mm and no new attachment could be detected. Intrusion appeared possible even in the case of loss of periodontal support and could lead to a gain of connective attachment, but a regular curettage was crucial for the outcome of the treatment[38]. During this intrusive movement, the orthodontic displacement would cause a stretching of the collagen fibres in gingivo-apical direction, so that the periodontal ligament cells close to the alveolar bone, known to be the most active ones, would find themselves more gingival during the intrusion movement. This shift might favourably contribute to the competition of the turnover rate between the junctional epithelial cells and the more coronal periodontal ligament cells. Bodily apical displacement with light forces would reduce the stress in the most marginal part of the periodontal ligament, with a limitation of the hyalinization, which, instead, could have favoured an epithelial downgrowth[38]. With light forces, therefore, no compression of the marginal part of the alveolous would occour but a stretching of the fibers and an increased cellular activity is observed[39]. The intrusion, therefore, could be perceived as a bend of the alveolar walls produced by the pull from the Sharpey fibers; this event would cause the formation of new bone at the level of the middle and coronal third of the root[24,38]. At the apex the load would be minimal and the fibers would not appear to be subjected to traction, therefore the resorption of the apical bone can be read as a remodeling. Furthermore, the effect of a load that could be so big to generate hyalinization and to increase in bone density in the direction of movement, might increase the risk of apical root resorption, since the dense bone with high extension of osteoid would be absorbed less easily than the trabecular bone, initially, during the removal of the hyalinization tissue, and subsequently when woven bone must be replaced[38-40] (5.1). Some Authors report that, at the cell's level, the intrusion movement reduces

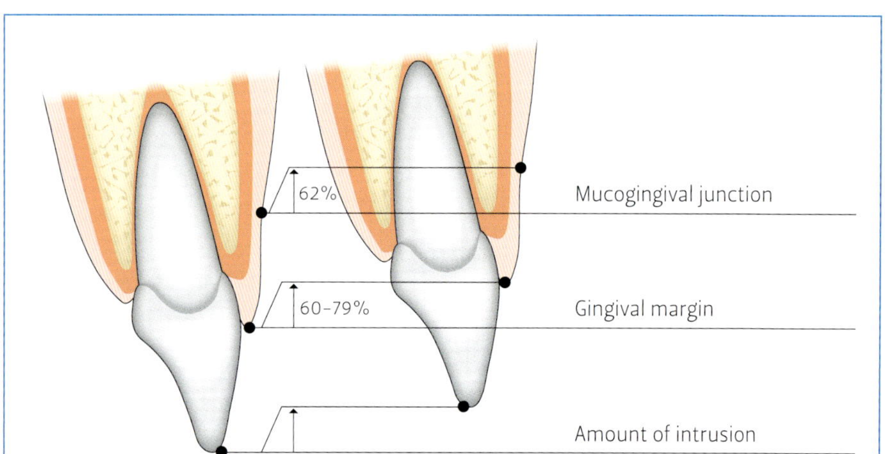

5.4 Amount of the displacement of the gingival margin and of the mucogingival junction after intrusion.

Tab. 5.1 Forces effect on intrusion movement

Light forces → Fibers stretching → Bone apposition	
Heavy forces → Hyalinization → Bone and root resorption	

the thickness of the periodontal ligament, increases the cell density, the number of mitoses and the periradicular cells and stimulates the formation of the cellular cement[19]. According to some Authors, in order to obtain the regeneration of the deep tissues with intrusive movements it is necessary to perform GTR (Guided Tissue Regeneration) surgery in which are observed collagen fibers of the periodontal ligament that are functionally oriented and inserted into the new cement[41]; otherwise there would just be a repair of the periodontal attachment. Intrusive movement, however, can displace supragingival plaque into a subgingival location[13], with the possibility of creating infrabony defects and loss of periodontal attachment with its apical displacement. This is confirmed in studies in dogs through a tipping and intrusive movement (tilting) with continuous and not jiggling forces, in teeth out of occlusion in the presence of plaque.

Melsen et al.[37] and Melsen[39] analysed other data: when relating the change in the distance between the marginal gengiva and the cemento-enamel junction to the amount of intrusion and the change in marginal bone level, major infrabony pockets had developed during treatment. Since failure to measure the pockets' depth did not imply that new attachment had taken place but the reduction in probing measurement could be a sign of the resolution of the inflammatory process, with an increase in tissue resistance to probing[37]. Gingival remodeling during intrusion and retrusion occurs mostly on the lingual aspect[25]. In a recent review[25] a significant reduction of PPD has been demonstrated where the intrusion has been used to correct the position of the extruded maxillary incisors, with radiological presence of infrabony defect and PD ≥6 mm, while associating retrusion to the intrusion. Even in the presence of furcations, a clinical attachment gain after intrusive movements is reported in the literature[42]. Papageorgiou et al.[43], in a recent meta-analysis, showed that the anterior teeth intrusion appears to be associated with a slight, although minimal, gain in periodontal clinical attachment of the treated incisors, with an average of 0.63 mm (0.54- 0.71 mm).

In human clinical studies, according to some Authors, sufficient clinical and radiographic data[20,22,30,37,44-46], such as PPD, clinical crown length, marginal bone level, radiological dimension of the defect and root length, suggest that the intrusion of central incisors with pathological migration and angular defects in patients with advanced periodontal disease, after proper surgical periodontal treatment, can be a reliable treatment in the maintenance of these teeth, thanks to a positive modification of both the alveolar bone and the soft tissues, with an improvement in clinical and radiographic parameters (realignment of treated incisors, radiological bone filling, attachment level gain, reduction of probing depth and gingival recession) and an average increase of 2.05 mm in marginal bone level (distance between the root apex and the marginal bone level without a radicular length reduction). A 50% reduction in gingival recession was also observed after intrusion, regardless of gingival thickness[45]. Intrusion can also be associated with regenerative procedures before moving teeth, with new bone formation and attachment gain[41,47]. These clinical findings were confirmed as stable in long-term period[22], but there is no histological confirmation describing whether such healing occurred by long junctional epithelium or deep tissue regeneration. The orthodontic mechanics had been applied 7-10 days after periodontal therapy with intrusive mechanics (cantilever or utility arches) in segmented technique, .017×.025 in β-titanium, with forces of 10-15 g with a palatal arch as anchorage; they were of variable duration of 4, 6, 9 months and stabilized with lingual fixed retainer[15]. It is possible to carry out the intrusion movement in bone defects even in the presence of bone grafts[30,44]; in this case the bone degradation is enhanced by the orthodontic movement[48,49], and it is also confirmed in surgical re-entries[47]. All the studies demonstrate the efficacy of a combined orthodontic-periodontal approach in the clinical treatment of extruded teeth with periodontal disease and intrabony defects[19,50,51]. Vanarsdall[32], however, reports that the intrusion alters the position of the cemento-enamel junction and creates a clinical attachment with the root formed just by epithelial tissue. For this reason, susceptible patients are at risk of breakdown or triggering of periodontal disease[32].

Some Authors have observed that dental intrusion, because the forces are concentrated at the apical level, can cause apical root resorption, pulpal disturbances and incomplete root formation in young patients[24,32,52], and reduction of alveolar bone[53]. Using light force (5-15 g per tooth)[37,54-56] the risk of apical root resorption is reduced, since this risk is more correlated, in addition to the genetic predisposition, also to the intensity of the intrusive force, to the extent of the displacement of tooth[24] and to the periodontal condition of the tooth itself[53]. Minch et al.[53], by a finite elements study, have shown that in the intrusive movement the concentration of stress occurs on a small surface at the level of the upper part of the alveolus and at the root apex. These concepts must be kept in mind and are of great importance in teeth with a reduced periodontium, in order to safeguard the residual periodontal support and not to further reduce the crown/root ratio[20]. The individualization on a periodontal, mechanical and genetic basis of this force, which must not exceed the patient's adaptation degree, always together with a strict control of inflammation, are the crucial factor for the success of the intrusion of teeth with reduced periodontal support.

Regarding the flared and elongated incisors that have horizontal bone defects, whose bone morphology is not a candidate for periodontal regenerative procedures[57], some authors[58] suggest that, by intrusion, this morphology can be modified, converting the bone defect from horizontal to angular vertical (5.5); this modification should make regenerative procedures feasible and capable of improving periodontal tissues and long-term stability, promoting bone circulation and creating better conditions for surgical GTR procedures[58,59]. In this perspective, other Authors have carried out an intrusion with supracrestal fibrotomy, an effective treatment for the intrusion of the anterior group, with the aim of changing the shape of the bone defect from horizontal to angular, obtaining a *cone-shaped* defect[60 61], with significantly greater crestal bone augmentation in cases of fibrotomy[62].

Clinically, what it is important to diagnose when planning an intrusion movement (5.6) is the location of the bone peak in relation to the cemento-enamel junction. As it can be seen in the 5.7, the mesial bone peak of 2.6, where no attachment loss occurred, is in a correct relationship with the cemento-enamel junction. This involves its levelling with the intrusive movement of the tooth (see 5.7). If, on the other hand, the interproximal level is horizontal, the intrusive movement, as we have seen in the 5.5, would create an intraosseous defect.

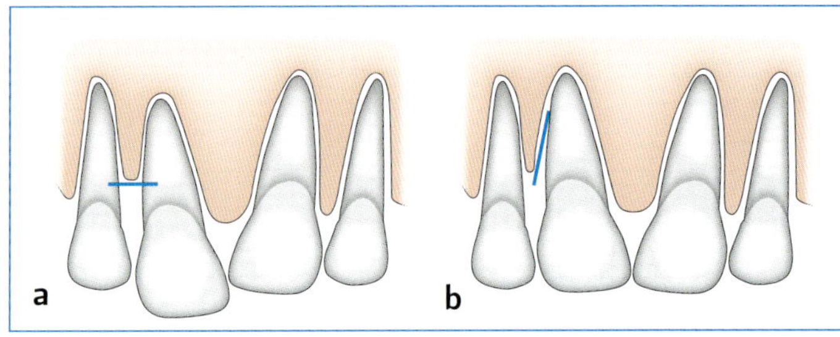

5.5 Intrabony defect creation from a suprabony defect after intrusion.

If the treatment plan, in the presence of a vertical defect, requires an intrusion in some patients, it is important to perform a surgical-periodontal therapy before the orthodontic movement in order to reduce the depth of the existing periodontal pocket[24] and to modify the bone morphology by programming it in relation to the orthodontic movement.

Movements away from the bone defect

EXTRUSION

Extrusion, as orthodontic movement, is the most predictable technique to solve single morphological defects caused by periodontal disease or by supracrestal tissue invasion. Extrusion of individual teeth can reduce pocket depth, provide physiological gingival and bone topography and preserve the maximum amount of periodontal attachment available. Therefore, the movement of choice to improve bone architecture is the extrusion which can eliminate or reduce the defect, by moving the tooth away from the defect itself[27,32,63]. The idea of using extrusion as a tool to manage one- and two-wall defects has created a new orthodontic opportunity for the periodontal patient[24,64]. Berglundh et al.[65] reported that, during extrusion, the relationship between the bone margin and the cemento-enamel junction remains unchanged and that the bone follows the extrusive movement.

The same unchanged relationship is found between

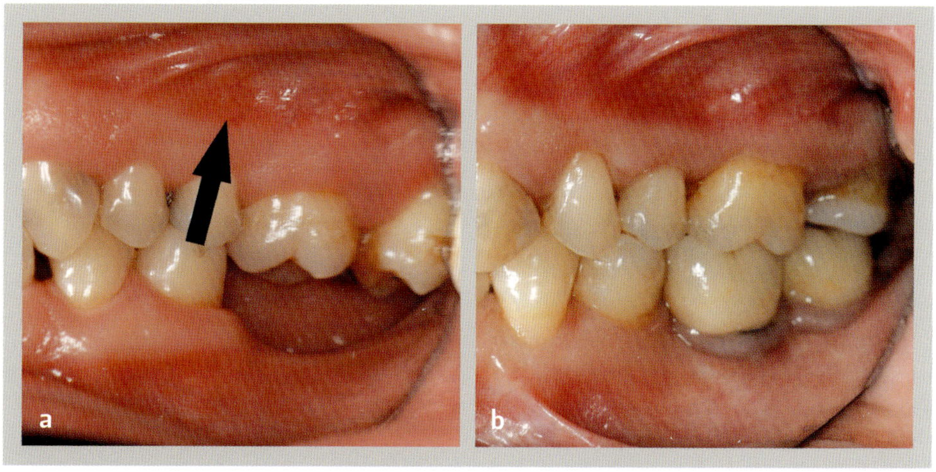

5.6 Intrusion of upper posterior teeth where the mucogingival juction stability can be seen.

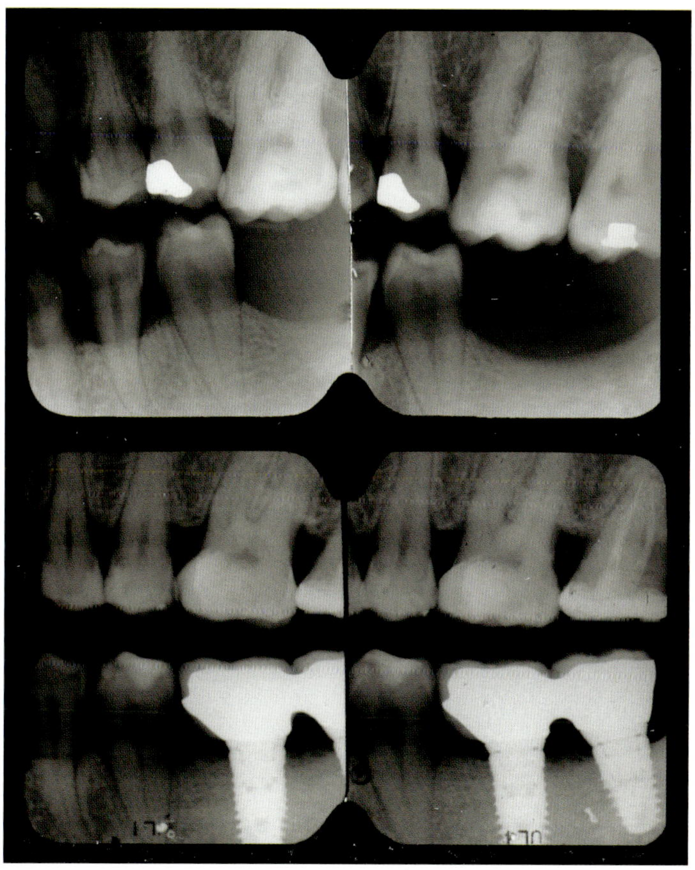

5.7 Radiographic exam of the intrusive movement of the case in 5.6 where the mesial bone peak over 2.6 joined to cemento-enamel juction can relocate the bone level without bone defect creation after the intrusive movement.

the periodontium and the cemento-enamel junction[66]. Movement occurs in the coronal direction where gingiva and bone migrate in the same direction, leading to a coronal displacement of the bone[67]; the gingival margin, therefore, migrates in the coronal direction, while the position of the mucogingival junction remains stable[68]. In fact, orthodontic extrusion does not create a new attachment but only relocates the pre-existing periodontal one[69]. The amount of the displacement was quantified by Kajiyama et al.[70] and Pikdoken et al.[71], who demonstrated that by extrusive movement the soft tissues move in the same direction as the tooth movement does, as it can be observed in 5.8.

By the extrusive movement, the stresses applied to the alveolar bone lead to the stimulation of angiogenic growth factors that contribute to the formation of gingival tissue and periodontal fibers and to the deposition of new bone through osteoblastic activity[67].

The improvements in periodontal conditions resulting from extrusive movement are due to physiological and microbiological changes in the local environment of the teeth. This movement could lead to a change in the plaque formation from subgingival to a supragingival one, with subsequent reduction of its pathogenicity and its effect on gingival tissue[72]. The clinical application of extrusion will be discussed in more detail in Chapter 8.

UPRIGHTING

Mesial tooth tipping, especially at the molars, often causes premature occlusal contact and, consequently, trauma. This trauma alone does not lead to attachment loss, but, in the presence of soft tissue inflammation, it can lead to a worsening of the defect. The plaque maintenance is extremely difficult due to the inclination of the tooth, which makes the hygiene of the mesial side difficult, inducing a con-

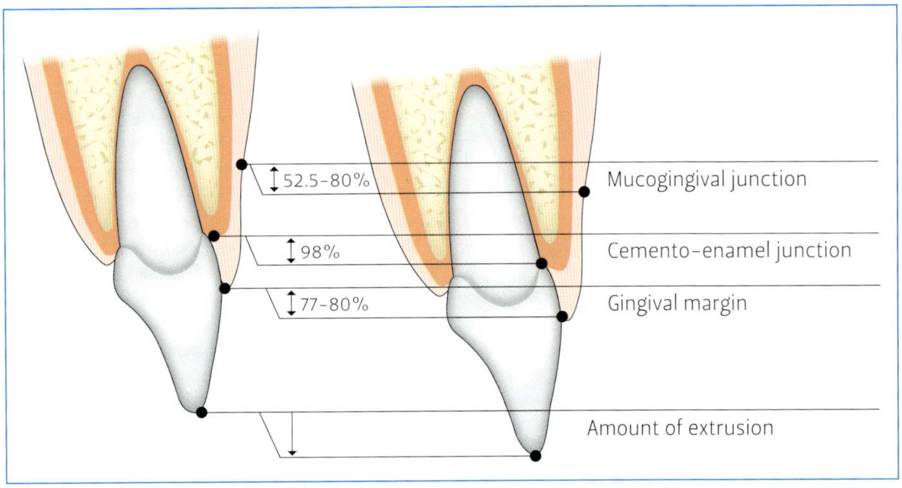

5.8 Amount of displacement of the gingival margin, cemento-enamel junction and mucogingival junction after extrusion.

tinuous worsening of the periodontal situation if the problem is not treated. The tipped molar starts a periodontal problem: its inclination leads to the formation of a pseudopocket on the mesial aspect due to the tendency of the bone to follow the cemento-enamel junction[24]. The mesial alveolar bone ridge moves apically, creating an acute-angled bone contour. In severe inclination, the marginal gingiva on the mesial side is often compressed and shows hypertrophy due to plaque-induced inflammation[21]. This microenvironment creates plaque retention which tends to induce a loss of attachment and subsequently deepens the pocket, predisposing the area to rapid periodontal worsening.

Some bacterial samples were taken from mesial pockets of the mesially tipped molars then subjected to an uprighting movement using the same mesially inclined site of the contralateral tooth as a case control. The sites were not subjected to plaque control, without scaling and root planing. At the end of the treatment, all the uprighted sites exhibiting at the start of the treatment *Bacteroides forsythus*, *Porphyromonas gingivalis*, *Prevotella intermedia* and *Actinobacillus actinomycetemcomitans* showed a significant decrease in these bacterial species[73]. The same pathogen reduction occurred in another study with DNA probe at the same sites for the *Bacteroides*[32]. On the mesial surface of the crestal bone margin of these teeth there are often signs of mesial bone resorption not related to periodontal inflammation but, probably, to a non-physiological occlusal stresses (5.9). Orthodontics can improve these problems by correcting the inclination of the tooth, removing non-physiological contacts and creating a maintainable periodontal environment, thus leading to a marked improvement (reduction of PPD, bleeding and plaque accumulation)[21]. It can be observed how the orthodontic resolution of the molar inclination can solve this problem, increase the mineralization of the *lamina dura*, reaching its full corticalization (5.10). The uprighting movement of mesially tipped molars reduces pocket depth and improves bone morphology; this happens because the connective attachment on the mesial aspect of the molar and on the bone ridge creates tension allowing bone remodeling[74,75] (5.11). This facilitates the oral care maintenance by the patient and improves the self-maintaining of soft tissue health[32] and access to the margins of the restoration (where necessary)[24]. At the end of the movement, corrective surgery can be performed to solve residual periodontal defects, if they are still present[76]. If the surgery is performed before

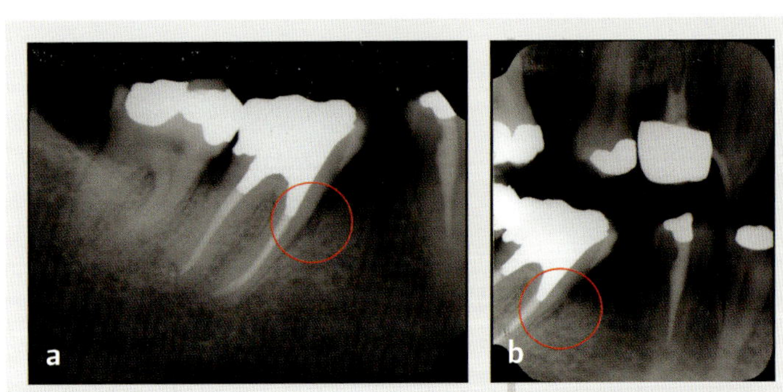

5.9 Radiographic mesial bone resorption on the mesial tipped teeth.

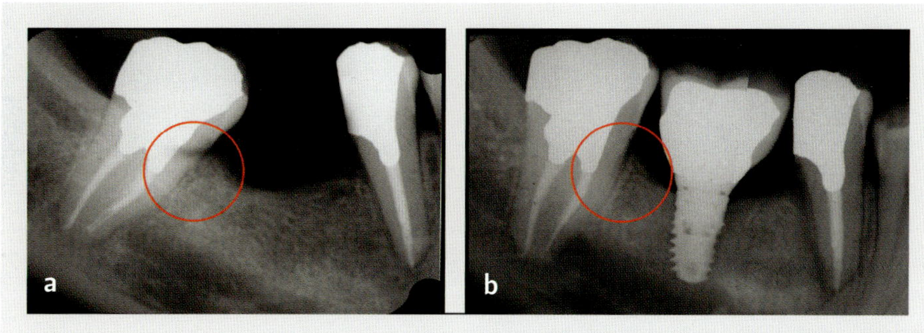

5.10 Cortical bone remineralization of the mesial resorption due to the molar uprighting.

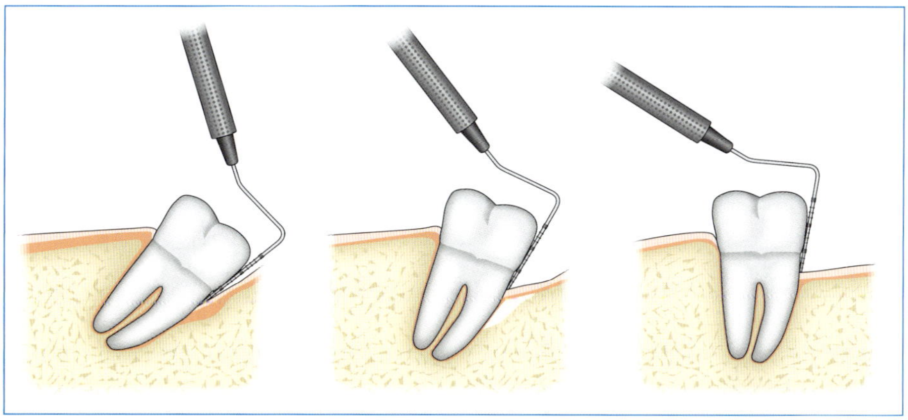

5.11 Periodontal improvement of the mesial crestal bone after uprighting with probing depth reduction and mesial bone remineralization.

the movement, as in the case of regenerative therapy, the orthodontic movement will not interfere with the healing of the defects[77].

Along with the periodontal problems, the tipped molar also presents other problems that must be solved and which we summarize below (5.12):

1. Mechanical: extra-axial stresses and occlusal interferences.
2. Rehabilitative: divergence of the prosthetic abutments and narrow spaces for pontics.
3. Periodontal: marginal gingival compression, plaque retention and acute tooth/bone angle topography.

During the procedures of molars uprighting with furcation involvement there is an increased risk of worsening of periodontal problems in about half of the population with moderate periodontitis that should be taken into account very seriously, because the simultaneous extrusion can increase the severity of the furcation defect, especially if the area is not maintainable by the patient[78]. An alternative or an integration to the orthodontic movement, is the root separation (5.13) of the tooth affected by the movement[20], the root resection[79] (5.14) or GTR[80] (5.15), according to the chosen treatment plan.

The uprighting movement, as well as the intrusive movement, can be performed in conjunction with other movements. The extrusive component of the uprighting movement is a key factor in tipped molars with angular mesial lesion, because moving the tooth away from the bone defect coronalizes the tilted bone

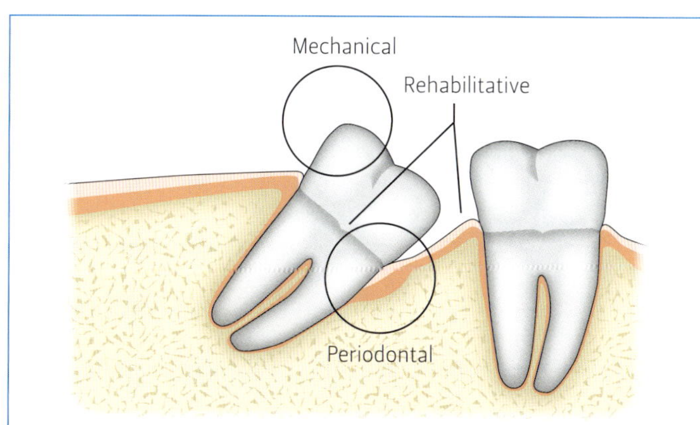

5.12 Schematic diagram of the tipped molar related problems.

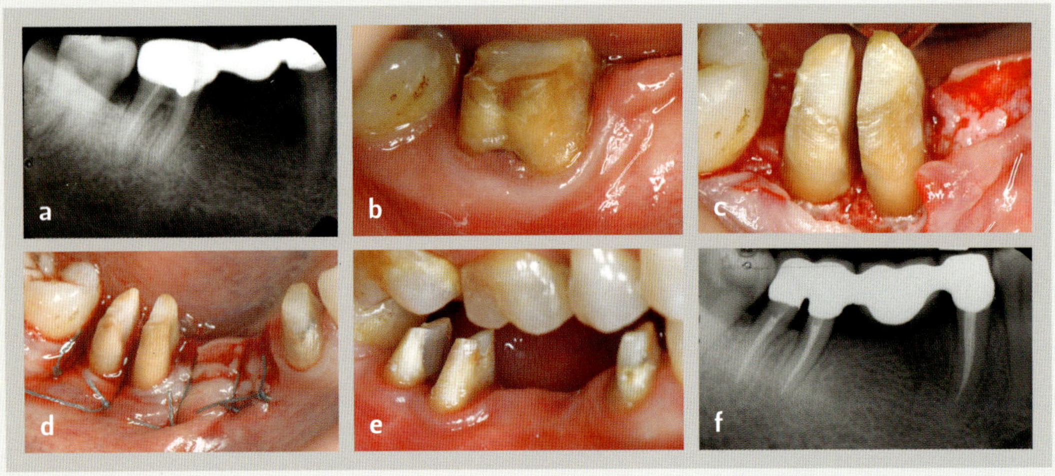

5.13 Clinical example of root separation with osseous resective surgery and prosthetic rehabilitation.

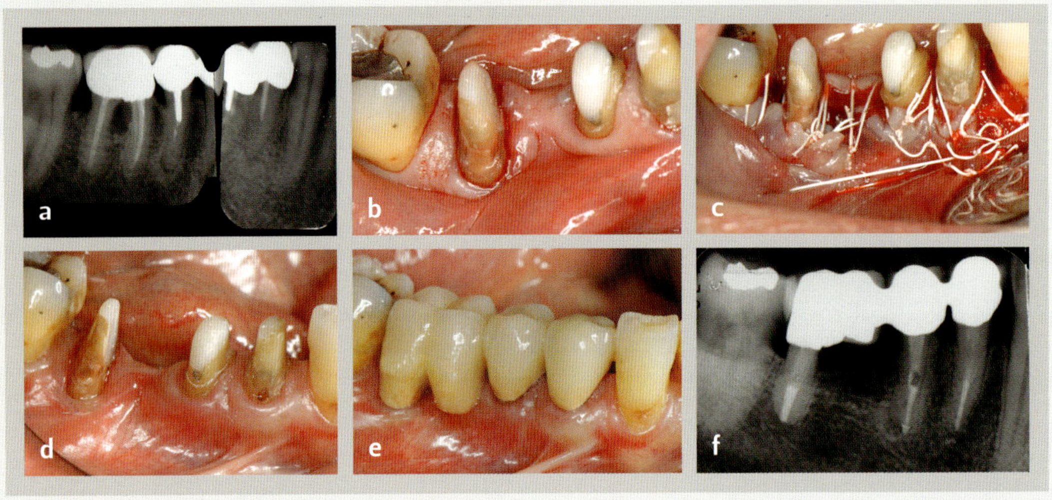

5.14 Clinical example of root resection with osseous resective surgery and prosthetic rehabilitation.

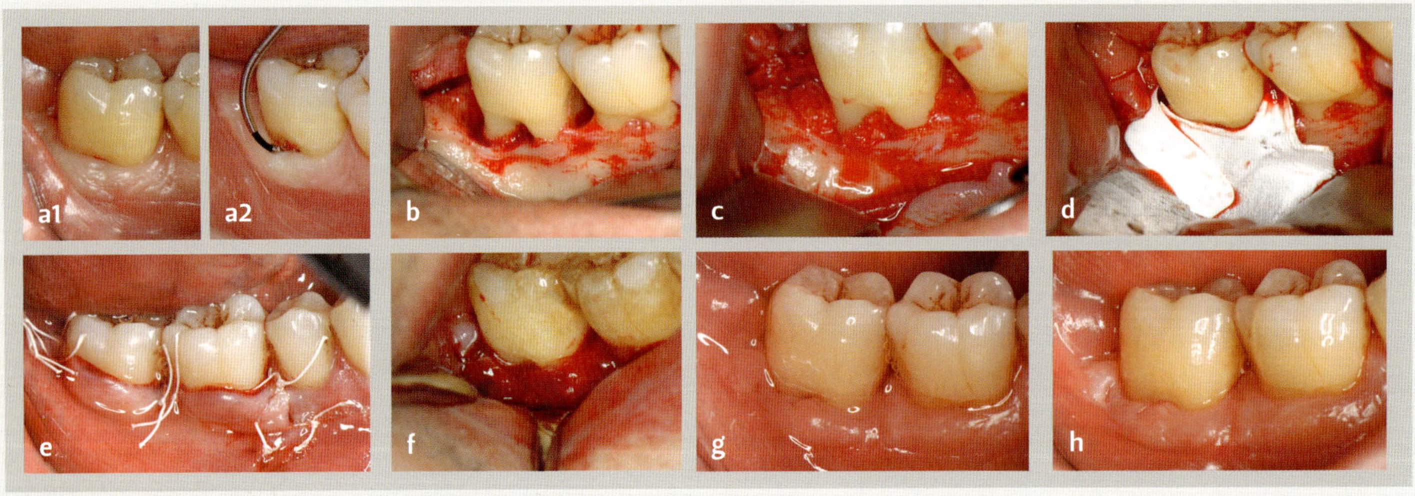

5.15 Clinical example of class II furcation regenerative treatment with non-resorbable membrane with (**g**) 2- and (**h**) 4-year follow-up.

contour. Due to the tensions on the collagen fibers of the periodontal ligament, the alveolar bone follows the movement of the tooth, leaving the level of the connective attachment unchanged on the mesial side[41], thus allowing to combine the advantages of the extrusive movement with those of uprighting; however, very often an endodontic treatment and a prosthetic restoration are necessary to realign the occlusal plane[81], always taking into account the evaluation of any furcation defect[78]. If an intrusive movement is associated, with the aim of obtaining a physiological "occlusal-functional" repositioning of the tooth, an intrabony defect could be created which must then be regenerated[58].

Biomechanics in the periodontal patient

Knowledge and control of orthodontic forces are essential for optimizing tooth movement even in the patient with loss of periodontal support[32]. The pre-existing attachment loss has three effects on orthodontic biomechanics due to the modification of the action area on the periodontal ligament[21]:

1. The reduced surface area of the root/alveolar bone interface requires an adaptation of the intensity of the forces (5.16a).
2. The apical displacement of the center of resistance involves a different system of forces according to the type of movement to be obtained (5.16b);the tooth is more prone to tipping rather than to bodily movement.
3. Periodontally compromised teeth may offer reduced anchorage quality.

Orthodontic biomechanics considerations

Dental movement is not a pure movement of a free body, but it is affected by the periodontal support structures surrounding the tooth. The application of an orthodontic force on a tooth is therefore not part of the mechanics of free bodies, which can be assimilated to a point, but in the one of constrained bodies. The tooth is a body bound to a peculiar external constraint: first of all, it is a triple constraint, interlocking, mobile as it varies over time, peculiar because the bone is a constraint that changes with the bone resorption itself. Furthermore, the tooth is not a simple cantilever, as it is immersed for the whole root or for part of it in the bone through the periodontal ligament which, with its typical viscoelastic characteristics, becomes a particular biological constraint, moreover in continuous evolution[82].

For a free solid body a hypothetical point can be identified, inside or outside the body itself, that can be called "center of mass" or "center of gravity", which the force of gravity appears to act. When the body is constrained the effect of a force is to put the body in motion in relation to the constraint and/or to produce a deformation of the constraints that prevent the body from moving.

In orthodontics, for what concerns the "tooth-bone" constrained system, we do not speak of a center of gravity or center of mass, but of a "center of resistance" defined as the point along which the line of action of force, passing through it, produces a transla-

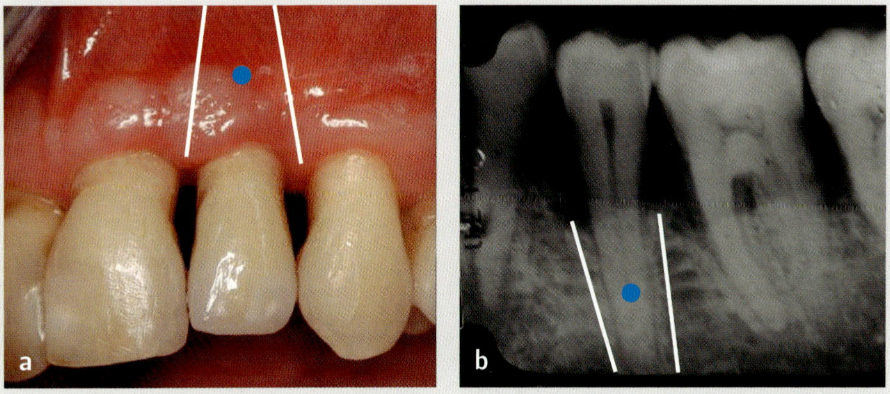

5.16 Biomechanical modification in teeth with reduced periodontal tissues: reduction of the root/bone surface (*white lines*); apical shifting of the center of resistance (*blu spot*).

tion movement[83]. In physics, when all the points of a rigid body have the same speed, the motion is called translatory. The center of resistance of a tooth depends on the morphology, size and root surface, but also on the periodontal bone surrounding the tooth itself, on its morphology, on its level and density and on asymmetry and anisotropy of the periodontal ligament[84-86]. Furthermore, the center of resistance is not a simple point on a two-dimensional plane, but three-dimensionally[87] it is a resistance volume in which the center of resistance should be built on the projection of the force vector in the three planes of space[85]. In relation to the ligament and bone areas subjected to tension and compression, we know from the literature that in bone the tension areas are more predominant than the compression ones even in the conventionally defined "compression" areas, so that bone resorption directed on the front of the roots subjected to "compression" movement would begin as a consequence of a hypophysiological tension load below the minimum effective[39,88]. The change in shape of the alveolar circumference would result from the stretching of the periodontal ligament fibers which, reducing the radius of the alveolar wall and flexing the bone in the tension zone, would produce bony apposition on the alveolar wall as a reaction to the bending that can be comparable to bony apposition load on long bones reported by orthopedists[39]. In the same way, the RAP (Regional Acceleratory Phenomenon) would occur, which would lead to an increased bone turnover in case of trauma; a continuous mechanical stimulus can also lead to an increase in density called SATMU (Structural Adaptation To Mechanical Usage)[39,40,89]. Furthermore, it must always be kept in mind that the tensions and tractions on the alveolar bone are mediated by the periodontal ligament and that the alveolar process is considered an "envelope" that contains the tooth, unlike the long bones which have a completely different function.

The center of resistance of a single-rooted tooth with healthy periodontal support is located on the long axis of the tooth itself between the middle 1/3 and 1/2 of the root length apical to the alveolar ridge. In a multi-rooted tooth the center of resistance is probably between the roots, 1-2 mm apical to the furcation; this happens in conditions of ideal bone support[83]. The position of the center of resistance depends on the length of the root; for example, since the maxillary canines have a longer root than the lateral incisors, they will have a center of resistance further away from the brackets[83]. Furthermore, the center of resistance varies with the height of the bone, therefore the initial assessment of the root situation, such as the presence of apical root resorption or periodontal bone loss, is important[83,90]. If the vector of the resulting force passes through the center of resistance of the tooth, a translation will occur[83]; otherwise, there will be a resultant moment, a couple of forces with a rotational component and consequent tipping if the resultant has a mesiodistal component, or torque if the resultant has a vestibulolingual component. During the incisors retraction, the moment of the retraction force (M_{ret}) will be given by the product of the retraction force (F_{ret}) and the horizontal component of the distance (d_x) from the point of application of the force to the center of resistance[83]. The control of the center of rotation during tooth movement is based on two components: the use of a couple of forces with direction and amplitude that creates a retraction moment M_{ret} and the counter-torque forces F_{tor} with a predominantly apical action opposite moment (F_{tor})[91]. If we relate the resulting moments of the couple of counter-torque forces acting on the tooth (M_{tor}) and the moment of the retraction force M_{ret}, we know that[83,92-96]:

- when the M_{tor}/M_{ret} ratio is equal to 1, it means that the M_{tor}/F_{ret} ratio is equal to the distance d_x of the center of resistance from the brackets, the movement is bodily and the center of rotation is at infinity;
- when the M_{tor}/M_{ret} ratio is less than 1, i.e. the M_{tor}/F_{ret} ratio is less than the distance d_x of the center of resistance from the brackets, the center of rotation is at the apex and the movement is a controlled tipping;
- when the M_{tor}/M_{ret} ratio is greater than 1, i.e. the M_{tor}/F_{ret} ratio is greater than the distance d_x of the center of resistance from the brackets, the center of rotation is at the incisor margin and there is a root movement.

$$\frac{M_{tor}}{M_{ret}} = 1 \text{ (with } M = F \cdot d\text{)}; \frac{F_{tor} \cdot d_y}{F_{ret} \cdot d_x} = 1; \frac{F_{tor} \cdot d_y}{F_{ret}} = d_x; \frac{M_{tor}}{F_{ret}} = d_x$$

We can write M_{tor} as $F_{tor} \times d_y$, where d_y indicates the distance of the force d_y from the center of resistance and F_{tor} is the sum of the total counter-torque forces , and F as F_{ret}, i.e. the resultant of the retraction forces. To simplify we will write M/F meaning $F_{tor} \times d_y/F_{ret}$: the bodily movement occurs for a M/F ratio that coincides with d_x in which the ratio between the two moments is equal to 1. This consideration is very important for teeth that have lost periodontal bone support where the distance from the center of resistance is increased.

Center of resistance and periodontal bone loss

The loss of alveolar bone in the periodontal patient causes an apical displacement of the tooth center of resistance compared to a tooth with healthy periodontium (5.17)and increases the distance *d* between the point of application of the force and the center of resistance, resulting in increasing of the moment (*M*)[95,96]. The ratio *M*/*F* increases of 0.65% for each millimeter of bone loss[95,97]. So in a tooth that has lost periodontal bone support, *d* increases, and the greater the *d*, the greater the resulting *M*/*F* ratio (5.18); therefore, in the case of periodontal bone loss, minor forces will be enough to have an identical resulting moment, i.e. a tipping, but to have a translation movement the counter-torque force at the apical level would result huge, beyond the physiological limits. Teeth with periodontal bone loss are, therefore, more prone to tipping than to bodily movement[14,85,90,92,95,98,99].

STRATEGIES TO BE IMPLEMENTED IN THE PERIODONTAL PATIENT TO CHECK THE M/F RATIO

In the previous paragraph we saw that, in order to have a translation movement, the *M*/*F* ratio must be equal to the distance between the point of application of the force (brackets) and the center of resistance of the tooth. To obtain a root movement, however, this ratio must be greater; if, therefore, as in the periodontal patient the distance increases, a huge *F*, that most likely would result harmful for root health, should be used, to achieve a ratio $M/F \geq d$ and this is unacceptable. To solve this difficulty and to reduce the *M*/*F* ratio, two strategies can be implemented:

1. Change the apico-coronal positioning of the brackets. The distance between the point of application of the force and the center of resistance of the tooth, apart from depending on the periodontium anatomy, which is invariable for the clinician when they begin to apply the mechanics, can be modified by changing the position of the brackets, which is the point of application of the force; brackets can be positioned more or less apically and thus the *M* component of the *M*/*F*[93] ratio vary.

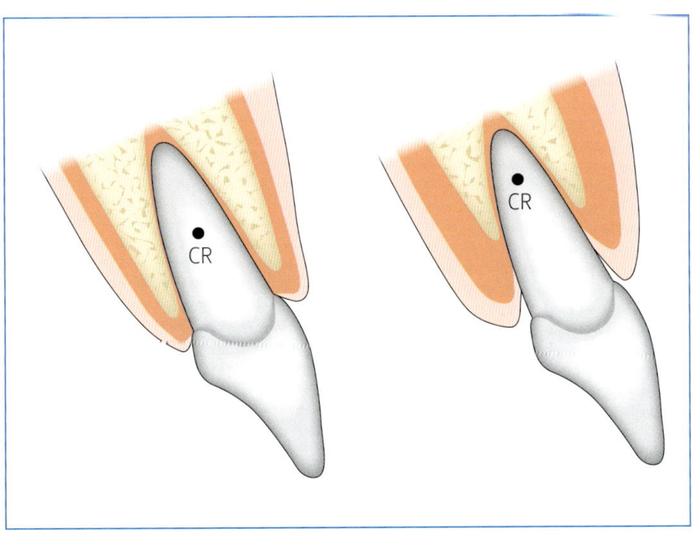

5.17 Schematic diagram showing the apical shifting of the center of resistance in healthy and reduced periodontal tissues.

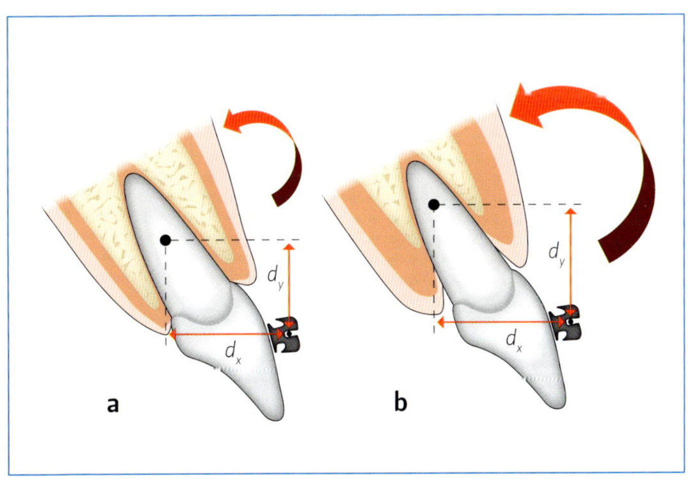

5.18 Schematic diagram showing the increase in distance (*d*: d_x x-axis distance; d_y y-axis distance) from the force application point to the center of resistance in the tooth with reduced periodontium, with resulting increase of moment (*M*) and therefore of *M*/*F* ratio. (**a**) Healthy periodontium; (**b**) reduced periodontium.

❷ Incorporate loops. As far as loops are concerned, the loops that must be chosen are not the ones with coils, as we know from the literature that coils do not influence the *M/F* ratio but only the load/deflection trend[94], but *T*- loops with horizontal wire components[92, 94].

Considerations on lingual mechanics

The position of the center of resistance does not vary with the orthodontic technique. What can be varied, with orthodontic mechanics, is the center of resistance-brackets distance (point of application of the force) (5.19a), i.e. the resulting moment with outcomes on the *M/F* ratio[100]. The moments created in lingual mechanics with the same *F* are smaller than in vestibular one, because the distance *d* brackets-center of resistance on the sagittal plane is less[9] (5.20a) and therefore, the forces required to obtain a translational movement are less. This is also applied in the periodontal patient, where the increase in the distance *d* of resistance center-point of force application is relatively lower in lingual compared to vestibular mechanics (5.19b), for these reasons, the forces that are necessary in lingual mechanics (lingual orthodontics remains a self-anchoring mechanics) and the moments are smaller (5.20b). Therefore, since in lingual orthodontics the brackets are close to the center of resistance in the sagittal plane, a pure intrusive movement[100] will be appropriate to have a bodily movement. Since, on the other hand, the distance on the vertical plane is greater, there will be a greater moment with a greater tendency to torque loss; this trend must be planned in lingual mechanics[100] and in particular in patients with periodontal bone loss.

CONSIDERATIONS ON THE UPPER ANTERIOR GROUP IN PERIODONTAL PATIENTS

For the upper anterior group the position of the center of resistance of the 6 anterior teeth is 14.5 mm apical and 9.5 mm distal from the incisal margin of the central incisors[101]. The distance between the point of application of the intrusive force and the center of resistance at the start of the intrusion and the variation at the end of the intrusion are not statistically significant[102]. The position of the brackets and the lingual coronal morphology require special consideration. We have seen how torque control in lingual mechanics, is more demanding than in vestibular ones, because the distance between the point of application of the force and the center of resistance is less; this is also due to the morphology of the lingual surface, where even a minimal variation of position creates large variations in the torque[95,103,104]. Reading Geron et al.[95] we know that the application of an intrusive force in vestibular mechanics brings to a counterclockwise moment and a coronovestibular torque for an initial inclination of the upper incisor from -20° up to +45°,

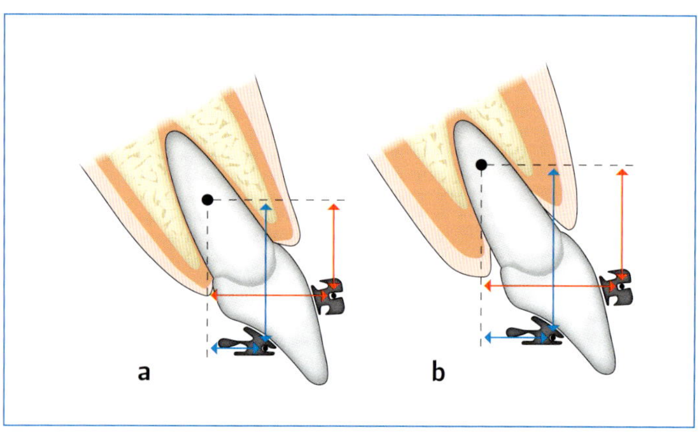

5.19 (**a**) Schematic diagram in lingual technique of the less distance *d* of the force application point (lingual bracket) from the center of resistance of tooth; healthy parodontium. (**b**) Schematic diagram showing how, in reduced periodontium, the distance *d* of the force application point (lingual brackets) from the center of resistance is proportionally increased, but to a lesser extent than in the vestibular technique.

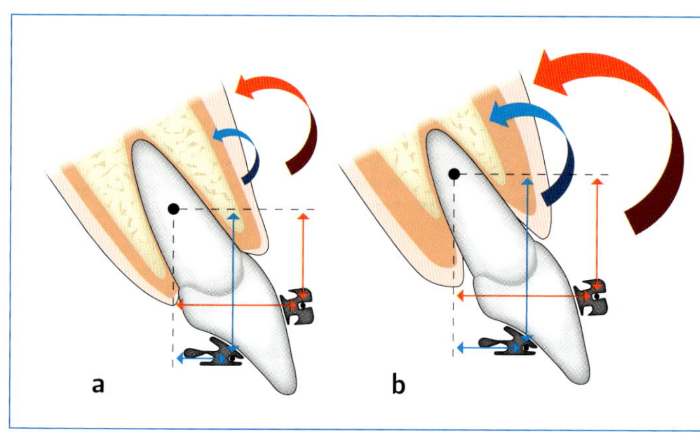

5.20 (**a**) Schematic diagram of the force moments (*M*) created in lingual mechanics that, with the same *F*, are less, because the variation of the distance *d* brackets-center of resistance is smaller. (**b**) Since in the periodontal patient the increase in the distance *d* between the center of resistance and the point of application of the force is less in the lingual technique than in the vestibular technique, the increase of the moment *M* and, therefore, of the resulting *M/F* ratio will be smaller.

while in lingual mechanics the counterclockwise moment occurs only for an inclination of the upper incisor greater than +20°. Only when the incisors start from an inclination of +20°, defined by the Authors as the transition point between the clockwise and counterclockwise moments, a pure intrusion occurs[95]. In lingual mechanics, therefore, it becomes important to control the *M/F* ratio by reducing the retraction force, increasing the torque[105] also with the aid of TADs (see Chapter 6, *Clinical case 1*) or by splitting the mechanics of the anterior group with a retraction first of the lateral sectors of the arch including the canines and only in a second time retracting the four upper incisors (see Chapter 6, *Clinical case 2*). In fact, in vestibular mechanics the incorporation of a root-lingual torque together with retraction creates a translation with a center of rotation at infinity, while in lingual mechanics it causes an uncontrolled tipping with a center of rotation 4.2 mm above the apex[105]. In lingual mechanics, in the periodontal patient, since the brackets-center of resistance distance is increased, if an intrusive and retracting force is applied, the rotational components take over; however, since the increase in this distance is smaller than in the vestibular mechanics, because of the position of the lingual attachment, the increase in moment will be proportionately less and the control of the retraction mechanics will be less complex. In teeth with periodontal bone loss the transition point is smaller than in healthy periodontal teeth and depends on the bone level, the initial tooth inclination and the width of the brackets[95]. Furthermore, lingual mechanics offers a valid anchorage in the retraction mechanics[106], since in the lingual technique the component of the reactions on the molars during retraction mechanics of the anterior group is self-anchoring; if this is not sufficient, an additional anchorage such as a palatal bar or TADs can be applied. It will be the integration of the periodontal clinical evaluation of the residual bone support and of the "en masse" retraction mechanics of the six anterior teeth or, rather, of only the four incisors that will ask for these auxiliary anchorage systems[107-109] (see Chapter 6, *Clinical Cases 1* and *2*; Chapter 7, *Clinical case 1*).

REFERENCES

1. **Polson A, Caton J, Polson AP et al.** Periodontal response after tooth movement into intrabony defects. *J Periodontol.* 1984;55(4):197-202.
2. **Ericsson I, Thilander B.** Orthodontic forces and recurrence of periodontal disease. An experimental study in the dog. *Am J Orthod.* 1978;74(1):41-50.
3. **Gorbunkova A, Pagni G, Brizhak A et al.** Impact of orthodontic treatment on periodontal tissues: a narrative review of multidisciplinary liter ature. *Int J Dent.* 2016;2016:4723589.
4. **Sanders NL.** Evidence-based care in orthodontics and periodontics: a review of the literature. *J Am Dent Assoc.* 1999;130(4):521-527.
5. **Boyd RL, Leggott PJ, Quinn RS et al.** Periodontal implications of orthodontic treatment in adults with reduced or normal periodontal tissues versus those of adolescents. *Am J Orthod Dentofacial Orthop.* 1989;96(3):191-198.
6. **Kessler M.** Interrelationships between orthodontics and periodontics. *Am J Orthod.* 1976;70(2):154-172.
7. **Artun J, Urbye KS.** The effect of orthodontic treatment on periodontal bone support in patients with advanced loss of marginal periodontium. *Am J Orthod Dentofacial Orthop.* 1988;93(2):143-148.
8. **Zoizner R, Arbel Y, Yavnai N et al.** Effect of orthodontic treatment and comorbidity risk factors on interdental alveolar crest level: a radiographic evaluation. *Am J Orthod Dentofacial Orthop.* 2018;154(3):375-381.
9. **Zachrisson BU.** Clinical implications of recent orthodontic-periodontic research findings. *Semin Orthod.* 1996;2(1):4-12.
10. **Boyd RL, Baumrind S.** Periodontal considerations in the use of bonds or bands on molars in adolescents and adults. *Angle Orthod.* 1992;62(2):117-126.
11. **Ericsson I, Thilander B, Lindhe J.** Periodontal conditions after orthodontic tooth movements in the dog. *Angle Orthod.* 1978;48(3):210-218.
12. **Wennström JL, Stokland BL, Nyman S, Thilander B.** Periodontal tissue response to orthodontic movement of teeth with infrabony pockets. *Am J Orthod Dentofacial Orthop.* 1993;103(4):313-319.
13. **Ericsson I, Thilander B, Lindhe J, Okamoto H.** The effect of orthodontic tilting movements on the periodontal tissues of infected and non-infected dentitions in dogs. *J Clin Periodontol.* 1977;4(4):278-293.

14. Cardaropoli D, Gaveglio L. The influence of orthodontic movement on periodontal tissues level. *Semin Orthod.* 2007;13(4):234-245.

15. Cardaropoli D, Re S, Manuzzi W et al. Bio-Oss collagen and orthodontic movement for the treatment of infrabony defects in the esthetic zone. *Int J Periodontics Restorative Dent.* 2006;26(6):553-559.

16. Ericsson I, Lindhe J. Effect of longstanding jiggling on experimental marginal periodontitis in the beagle dog. *J Clin Periodontol.* 1982;9(6):497-503.

17. Lindhe J, Ericsson I. The effect of elimination of jiggling forces on periodontally exposed teeth in the dog. *J Periodontol.* 1982;53(9):562-567.

18. Lindhe J, Svanberg G. Influence of trauma from occlusion on progression of experimental periodontitis in the beagle dog. *J Clin Periodontol.* 1974;1(1):3-14.

19. Cardaropoli D, Gaveglio L, Abou-Arraj RV. Orthodontic movement and bone defects: rationale, timing, and clinical implications. *Semin Orthod* 2014;20(3):177-187.

20. Gkantidis N, Christou P, Topouzelis N. The orthodontic-periodontic interrelationship in integrated treatment challenges: a systematic review. *J Oral Rehabil.* 2010;37(5):377-390.

21. Diedrich P, Fritz U, Kizinger G. Interrelationship between periodontics and adult orthodontics. *Perio.* 2004;1(3):143-149.

22. Re S, Corrente G, Abundo R, Cardaropoli D. Orthodontic treatment in periodontally compromised patients: 12-year report. *Int J Periodontics Restorative Dent.* 2000;20(1):31-39.

23. Elkordy SA, Palomo L, Palomo JM, Mostafa YA. Do fixed orthodontic appliances adversly affect the periodontium? A systematic review of systematic reviews. *Semin Orthod.* 2019;25(2):130-157.

24. Antoun JS, Mei L, Gibbs K, Farella M. Effect of orthodontic treatment on the periodontal tissues. *Periodontol 2000.* 2017;74(1):140-157.

25. Zasciurinskiene E, Lindsten R, Slotte C, Bjerklin K. Orthodontic treatment in periodontitis-susceptible subjects: a systematic literature review. *Clin Exp Dent Res.* 2016;2(2):162-173.

26. Nemcovsky CE, Sasson M, Beny L et al. Periodontal healing following orthodontic movement of rat molars with intact versus damaged periodontia towards a bony defect. *Eur J Orthod.* 2007;29(4):338-344.

27. Diedrich P, Fritz U, Kinzinger G, Angelakis J. Movement of periodontally affected teeth after guided tissue regeneration (GTR)-an experimental pilot study in animals. *J Orofac Orthop.* 2003;64(3):214-227.

28. Nemcovsky CE, Beny L, Shanberger S et al. Bone apposition in surgical bony defects following orthodontic movement: a comparative histomorphometric study between root- and periodontal ligament-damaged and periodontally intact rat molars. *J Periodontol.* 2004;75(7):1013-1019.

29. Vardimon AD, Nemcovsky CE, Dre E. Orthodontic tooth movement enhances bone healing of surgical bony defects in rats. *J Periodontol.* 2001;72(7):858-864.

30. Corrente G, Abundo R, Re S et al. Orthodontic movement into infrabony defects in patients with advanced periodontal disease: a clinical and radiological study. *J Periodontol.* 2003;74(8):1104-1109.

31. Ahn JC, Lee JH, Yoon JH et al. Interdisciplinary treatment of a patient with multiple missing teeth and periodontitis. *Am J Orthod Dentofacial Orthop.* 2018;153(2):278-289.

32. Vanarsdall RL. Orthodontics and periodontal therapy. *Periodontol 2000.* 1995;9(1):132-149.

33. Cortellini P, Tonetti MS. Clinical concepts for regenerative therapy in intrabony defects. *Periodontol 2000.* 2015;68(1):282-307.

34. Melsen B, Agerbaek N. Orthodontics as an adjunct to rehabilitation. *Periodontol 2000.* 1994;4(1):148-159.

35. Erkan M, Pikdoken L, Usumez S. Gingival response to mandibular incisor intrusion. *Am J Orthod Dentofacial Orthop.* 2007;132(2):143.e9-143.e1.43E13.

36. Murakami T, Yokota S, Takahama Y. Periodontal changes after experimentally induced intrusion of the upper incisors in Macaca fuscata monkeys. *Am J Orthod Dentofacial Orthop.* 1989;95(2):115-126.

37. Melsen B, Agerbaek N, Markenstam G. Intrusion of incisors in adult patients with marginal bone loss. *Am J Orthod Dentofacial Orthop.* 1989;96(3):232-241.

38. Melsen B, Agerbaek N, Eriksen J, Terp S. New attachment through periodontal treatment and orthodontic intrusion. *Am J Orthod Dentofacial Orthop.* 1988;94(2):104-116.

39. Melsen B. Tissue reaction to orthodontic tooth movement - a new paradigm. *Eur J Orthod.* 2001;23(6):671-681.

40. Melsen B. Biological reaction of alveolar bone to orthodontic tooth movement. *Angle Orthod.* 1999;69(2):151-158.

41. Diedrich PR. Guided tissue regeneration associated with orthodontic therapy. *Semin Orthod.* 1996;2(1):39-45.

42. da Silva VC, Cirelli CC, Ribeiro FS et al. Intrusion of teeth with class III furcation: a clinical, histologic and histometric study in dogs. *J Clin Periodontol.* 2008;35(9):807-816.

43. Papageorgiou SN, Papadelli AA, Eliades T. Effect of orthodontic treatment on periodontal clinical attachment: a systematic review and meta-analysis. *Eur J Orthod.* 2018;40(2):176-194.

44. Cardaropoli D, Re S, Corrente G, Abundo R. Intrusion of migrated incisors with infrabony defects in adult periodontal patients. *Am J Orthod Dentofacial Orthop.* 2001;120(6):671-677.

45. Re S, Cardaropoli D, Abundo R, Corrente G. Reduction of gingival recession following orthodontic intrusion in periodontally compromised patients. *Orthod Craniofac Res.* 2004;7(1):35-39.

46. Re S, Corrente G, Abundo R, Cardaropoli D. The use of orthodontic intrusive movement to reduce infrabony pockets in adult periodontal patients: a case report. *Int J Periodontics Restorative Dent.* 2002;22(4):365-371.

47. Re S, Corrente G, Abundo R, Cardaropoli D. Orthodontic move-

ment into bone defects augmented with bovine bone mineral and fibrin sealer: a reentry case report. *Int J Periodontics Restorative Dent.* 2002;22(2):138-145.

48. Araújo MG, Carmagnola D, Berglundh T et al. Orthodontic movement in bone defects augmented with Bio-Oss. An experimental study in dogs. *J Clin Periodontol.* 2001;28(1):73-80.

49. Hossain MZ, Kyomen S, Tanne K. Biologic responses of autogenous bone and beta-tricalcium phosphate ceramics transplanted into bone defects to orthodontic forces. *Cleft Palate Craniofac J.* 1996;33(4):277-283.

50. Hong SY, Shin JW, Hong C et al. Alveolar bone remodeling during maxillary incisor intrusion and retraction. *Prog Orthod.* 2019;20(1):47. Published 2019 Dec 23.

51. Jepsen K, Jaeger A, Jepsen S. Esthetic and functional rehabilitation of a severely compromised central incisor: an interdisciplinary approach. *Int J Periodontics Restorative Dent.* 2015;35(3):e35-e43.

52. Al-Zubair NM. Orthodontic intrusion: a contemporary review. *J Orthod Res.* 2014;2(3):118-24.

53. Minch LE, Sarul M, Nowak R et al. Orthodontic intrusion of periodontally-compromised maxillary incisors: 3-dimensional finite element method analysis. *Adv Clin Exp Med.* 2017;26(5):829-833.

54. Nakamura Y, Gomi K, Oikawa T et al. Reconstruction of a collapsed dental arch in a patient with severe periodontitis. *Am J Orthod Dentofacial Orthop.* 2013;143(5):704-712.

55. Weltman B, Vig KW, Fields HW et al. Root resorption associated with orthodontic tooth movement: a systematic review. *Am J Orthod Dentofacial Orthop.* 2010;137(4):462-476.

56. Johal A, Ide M. Orthodontics in the adult patient, with special reference to the periodontally compromised patient. *Dent Update.* 1999;26(3):101-108.

57. Scantlebury T, Ambruster J. The development of guided regeneration: making the impossible possible and the unpredictable predictable. *J Evid Based Dent Pract.* 2012;12(3 Suppl):101-117.

58. Rabie ABM, Gildenhuys R, Boisson M. Management of patients with severe bone loss: bone induction and orthodontics. *World J Orthod.* 2001;2(2):142-153.

59. Passanezi E, Janson M, Janson G et al. Interdisciplinary treatment of localized juvenile periodontitis: a new perspective to an old problem. *Am J Orthod Dentofacial Orthop.* 2007;131(2):268-276.

60. Cao T, Xu L, Shi J, Zhou Y. Combined orthodontic-periodontal treatment in periodontal patients with anteriorly displaced incisors. *Am J Orthod Dentofacial Orthop.* 2015;148(5):805-813.

61. Liu XF, Pan XG, Shu R. A preliminary study of combined periodontal-orthodontic approach for treating labial displacement of incisors in patients with periodontal diseases. *Shanghai Kou Qiang Yi Xue.* 2008;17(3):264-266.

62. Shi J, Zhou Y, Fu M. Computer tomograghy study on periodontal patients with anterior displaced teeth before and after combined orthodontic-periodontal treatment. *Beijing Da Xue Xue Bao Yi Xue Ban.* 2003;35(6):659-662.

63. González-Martín O, Solano-Hernandez B, González-Martín A, Avila-Ortiz G. Orthodontic extrusion: guidelines for contemporary clinical practice. *Int J Periodontics Restorative Dent.* 2020;40(5):667-676.

64. Ingber JS. Forced eruption: part II. A method of treating nonrestorable teeth--Periodontal and restorative considerations. *J Periodontol.* 1976;47(4):203-216.

65. Berglundh T, Marinello CP, Lindhe J et al. Periodontal tissue reactions to orthodontic extrusion. An experimental study in the dog. *J Clin Periodontol.* 1991;18(5):330-336.

66. Watanabe T, Marchack BW, Takei HH. Creating labial bone for immediate implant placement: a minimally invasive approach by using orthodontic therapy in the esthetic zone. *J Prosthet Dent.* 2013;110(6):435-441.

67. da Silva VC, de Molon RS, Martins RP et al. Effects of orthodontic tooth extrusion produced by different techniques, on the periodontal tissues: a histological study in dogs. *Arch Oral Biol.* 2020;116:104768.

68. Batenhorst KF, Bowers GM, Williams JE Jr. Tissue changes resulting from facial tipping and extrusion of incisors in monkeys. *J Periodontol.* 1974;45(9):660-668.

69. Hayashi J, Shin K. Implant site development by orthodontic extrusion and buccal root torque at a site showing severe gingival recession with periodontitis: a case report. *Int J Periodontics Restorative Dent.* 2019;39(4):589-594.

70. Kajiyama K, Murakami T, Yokota S. Gingival reactions after experimentally induced extrusion of the upper incisors in monkeys. *Am J Orthod Dentofacial Orthop.* 1993;104(1):36-47.

71. Pikdoken L, Erkan M, Usumez S. Gingival response to mandibular incisor extrusion. *Am J Orthod Dentofacial Orthop.* 2009;135(4):432.e1-433.

72. Rotundo R, Bassarelli T, Pace E et al. Orthodontic treatment of periodontal defects. Part II: A systematic review on human and animal studies. *Prog Orthod.* 2011;12(1):45-52.

73. Mihram WL, Murphy NC. The orthodontist's role in 21st century periodontic-prosthodontic therapy. *Semin Orthod.* 2008;14(4):272-289.

74. Promchaiwattana P, Suzuki B, Krisanaprakornkit S, Suzuki EY. Periodontal ligament enhancement in mesio-angulated impaction of third molars after orthodontic tooth movement: A prospective cohort study. *Am J Orthod Dentofacial Orthop.* 2020;158(4):495-504.

75. Wise RJ, Kramer GM. Predetermination of osseous changes associated with uprighting tipped molars by probing. *Int J Periodontics Restorative Dent.* 1983;3(1):68-81.

76. Harshita N, Kamath DG, Kadakampally D. Perio-ortho interactions. A review. *J Pharm Sci & Res.* 2018;10(5):1053-1056.

77. Cirelli CC, Cirelli JA, da Rosa Martins JC et al. Orthodontic movement of teeth with intraosseous defects: histologic and histometric study in dogs. *Am J Orthod Dentofacial Orthop.* 2003;123(6):666-675.

78. Burch JG, Bagci B, Sabulski D, Landrum C. Periodontal changes in fur-

cations resulting from orthodontic uprighting of mandibular molars. *Quintessence Int.* 1992;23(7):509-513.

79. Mokbel N, Kassir AR, Naaman N, Megarbane JM. Root resection and hemisection revisited. Part I: A systematic review. *Int J Periodontics Restorative Dent.* 2019;39(1):e11-e31.

80. Jepsen S, Gennai S, Hirschfeld J et al. Regenerative surgical treatment of furcation defects: a systematic review and Bayesian network meta-analysis of randomized clinical trials. *J Clin Periodontol.* 2020;47 (Suppl 22):352-374.

81. Maeda S, Ono Y, Nakamura K, Kuwahara T. Molar uprighting with extrusion for implant site bone regeneration and improvement of the periodontal environment [published correction appears in *Int J Periodontics Restorative Dent.* 2008 Oct;28(5):451]. *Int J Periodontics Restorative Dent.* 2008;28(4):375-381.

82. Saffar JL, Lasfargues JJ, Cherruau M. Alveolar bone and the alveolar process: the socket that is never stable. *Periodontol 2000.* 1997;13(1):76-90.

83. Smith RJ, Burstone CJ. Mechanics of tooth movement. *Am J Orthod.* 1984;85(4):294-307.

84. McCormack SW, Witzel U, Watson PJ et al. The biomechanical function of periodontal ligament fibres in orthodontic tooth movement. *PLoS One.* 2014;9(7):e102387.

85. Viecilli RF, Budiman A, Burstone CJ. Axes of resistance for tooth movement: does the center of resistance exist in 3-dimensional space? *Am J Orthod Dentofacial Orthop.* 2013;143(2):163-172.

86. Halazonetis DJ. Computer experiments using a two-dimensional model of tooth support. *Am J Orthod Dentofacial Orthop.* 1996;109(6):598-606.

87. Nägerl H, Burstone CJ, Becker B, Kubein-Messenburg D. Centers of rotation with transverse forces: an experimental study. *Am J Orthod Dentofacial Orthop.* 1991;99(4):337-345.

88. Cattaneo PM, Dalstra M, Melsen B. The finite element method: a tool to study orthodontic tooth movement. *J Dent Res.* 2005;84(5):428-433.

89. Epker BN, Frost HM. Correlation of bone resorption and formation with the physical behavior of loaded bone. *J Dent Res.* 1965;44:33-41.

90. Tanne K, Nagataki T, Inoue Y et al. Patterns of initial tooth displacements associated with various root lengths and alveolar bone heights. *Am J Orthod Dentofacial Orthop.* 1991;100(1):66-71.

91. Burnstone JC. *Application of bioengineering to clinical orthodontics.* In: Graber LW, Vanarsdall RL Jr, Vig KWL, Huang GJ. *Orthodontics. Current principles and techniques.* 6th ed. St. Louis: Elsevier; 2017:154-186.

92. Manhartsberger C, Morton JY, Burstone CJ. Space closure in adult patients using the segmented arch technique. *Angle Orthod.* 1989;59(3):205-210.

93. Burstone CJ, Pryputniewicz RJ. Holographic determination of centers of rotation produced by orthodontic forces. *Am J Orthod.* 1980;77(4):396-409.

94. Burstone CJ, Koenig HA. Optimizing anterior and canine retraction. *Am J Orthod.* 1976;70(1):1-19.

95. Geron S, Romano R, Brosh T. Vertical forces in labial and lingual orthodontics applied on maxillary incisors - a theoretical approach. *Angle Orthod.* 2004;74(2):195-201.

96. Proffit W. *Special considerations in comprehensive treatment for adults.* In: Proffit W, Fields HW, eds. *Contemporary orthodontics.* 3rd ed. St. Louis: Mosby; 2000:644-674.

97. Siatkowski RE. Optimal orthodontic space closure in adult patients. *Dent Clin North Am.* 1996;40(4):837-873.

98. Geisinger ML, Abou-Arraj RV, Souccar NM et al. Decision making in the treatment of patients with malocclusion and chronic periodontitis: scientific evidence and clinical experience. *Semin Orthod.* 2014;20(3):170-176.

99. Williams S, Melsen B, Agerbaek N, Asboe V. The orthodontic treatment of malocclusion in patients with previous periodontal disease. *Br J Orthod.* 1982;9(4):178-184.

100. Romano R. Concepts on control of the anterior teeth using the lingual appliance. *Semin Orthod.* 2006;12(3):178-185.

101. Choy K, Kim KH, Burstone CJ. Initial changes of centres of rotation of the anterior segment in response to horizontal forces. *Eur J Orthod.* 2006;28(5):471-474.

102. van Steenbergen E, Burstone CJ, Prahl-Andersen B, Aartman IH. The relation between the point of force application and flaring of the anterior segment. *Angle Orthod.* 2005;75(5):730-735.

103. Riolo C, Finkleman SA, Kaltschmidt C. Lingual orthodontics: understanding the issues is the key to success with lingual mechanics. *Semin Orthod.* 2018;24(3):271-285.

104. Geron S. Finishing with lingual appliances, problems, and solutions. *Semin Orthod.* 2006;12(3):191-202.

105. Liang W, Rong Q, Lin J, Xu B. Torque control of the maxillary incisors in lingual and labial orthodontics: a 3-dimensional finite element analysis. *Am J Orthod Dentofacial Orthop.* 2009;135(3):316-322.

106. Geron S. Anchorage considerations in lingual orthodontics. *Semin Orthod.* 2006;12(3):167-177.

107. Riolo C. Lingual orthodontics: adding value to the care we offer our patients. *Semin Orthod.* 2018;24(3):269-270.

108. Kim JS, Kim SH, Kook YA et al. Analysis of lingual en masse retraction combining a C-lingual retractor and a palatal plate. *Angle Orthod.* 2011;81(4):662-669.

109. Kyung HM. The use of microimplants in lingual orthodontic treatment. *Semin Orthod.* 2006;12(3):186-190.

Orthodontics as a periodontal treatment

Introduction

Orthodontic movement can help the periodontal treatment plan not only for what concerns the movement of a single tooth nearby a defect with the aim of changing its three-dimensional morphology, but also working on the entire dentition, at several levels:

1. Changing the bone levels.
2. Redistributing spaces and planning the position of dental abutments to reduce or eliminate the implant rehabilitation.
3. Resolving dental crowding.

Change in bone levels

The orthodontic movement achieves bone levelling and corrects defects and, consequently, reduces or eliminates compromised local topographies, modifies surgery or even allows to avoid more invasive surgery, creates a physiological bone and gingival topography and preserves the greatest quantity of the available attachment apparatus preparing the patient for long-term maintenance[1].

Specially in the anterior area, as we saw in Chapter 4 for PTM (Pathologic Tooth Migration), dental malposition creates esthetic and psychological discomfort[2] in the patient and dental repositioning must be precisely planned. From this point of view, the evaluation of the trend in the bone levels is very important, because it allows to understand how to deal with dental movement, in particular when it is necessary to associate movements in the presence of vertical defects, or how to take advantage from the movement by levelling the bone defects in the presence of a predominantly horizontal bone pattern.

The apical displacement of the center of resistance due to the progressive loss of periodontal support has as consequence an easier vestibular displacement of the crowns, in particular at the incisors' level, which, being subject to both masticatory forces and to anterolaterally directed parafunctional activities, are no longer protected from occlusal forces; we are accustomed to observe this situation every day in increased overjet in class II[3]. This unesthetic displacement induces the patient to ask for correction and it is very often accompanied by bone lesions; these lesions make the intrusive movement difficult, which could be more easily achieved in conditions of a homogeneous and flat periodontal level[4]. When there are vertical defects and the anterior teeth must be retracted and intruded, there are two possibilities: to intrude in conditions of infection control and absence of inflammation, after having performed regenerative periodontal treatment where it is necessary, or to modify angular defects bringing to a horizontal homogeneity with extrusive sectorial micro-movements, carrying out the intrusion later on. This approach is best indicated when the bone level trend is slightly horizontal or if there are minimal intrabony defects, which can be eliminated with the aforementioned micro-movements. When the angular defects are deep, it is necessary to perform regenerative techniques before the orthodontic movement, as we will see in detail in Chapter 9. When such minimal angular defects are present, just a part of the periodontal tissues must follow the tooth by extrusion, keeping in mind that, often, further surgical therapy, such as a localized clinical crown lengthening, may be indispensable and necessary after the end of orthodontic therapy to obtain normally scalloped soft and hard tissues[5].

If an extrusion is performed to reconstruct the alveolar bone, and then the extrusion is followed by an intrusion, part of the bone apposition obtained by the extrusion remains stable and is maintained during the subsequent intrusion, provided that gingival health is preserved during treatment[1,6]. These sectorial extrusions of anterior teeth to level the interproximal bone, are preparatory to the retraction of the upper anterior group and may require balancing and remodeling of the incisal margins or more extensive restorative or prosthetic approaches[6]. The bone level, therefore, has the absolute priority of diagnosis and mechanics, leading to a subsequent necessity of modification of the anatomy of the dental crowns which will require occlusal equilibration or reconstructive-prosthetic modifications[7], in order to level marginal ridges and allow occlusion. Overcorrection in the positioning of the brackets is a strategy to always be kept in mind from the very beginning to obtain a control of dental movement, correcting bone leveling and root positioning. This is important in the closure of orthodontic spaces and in the correction of periodontal interproximal defects, which will be described in the orthodontic extrusions and in sectoral extrusions in Chapter 8[8]. This approach determines that some periodontal defects, whose correction might have been initially surgical, become non-surgical after orthodontic treatment[7] and that bone development improves through orthodontic movements[9].

Clinical case 1

The patient's request is a complete rehabilitation aimed at restoring a functional and esthetic balance. After having been proposed elsewhere a prosthetic-rehabilitative treatment plan that she considered to be too demolishing, she asked for a different solution. She shows facial symmetry, reduced nasolabial angle, reduced neck-chin length, increased chin-labial sulcus and incompetent lips with lingual interposition, symmetrical movements, without dysfunctions (🔍 6.1). Several teeth are absent: 1.8, 2.6, 3.1, 4.6; 3.6 and 3.5 require an endodontic-restorative treatment, 3.8 has unrestorable decay and will be extracted. At the intraoral and cast examination the patient shows a molar and canine class II on the right; on the left, the molar and canine classes are not fully assessable, as several teeth are missing; OVJ (15 mm) and OVB (7 mm) are increased (🔍 6.2).The cephalometric values confirm a normal prognathism of the maxilla, with a slight reduction of the mandibular prognathism and resulting in an increased sagittal discrepancy. At the vertical evaluation, the maxilla is normoinclined, with an increase in mandibular verticality. The upper incisors are in great vestibuloversion, the lower ones are in slight linguoversion with a resulting decreased interincisal angle and an OVJ of 15 mm, mainly of dental origin, partly of skeletal origin; the OVB is increased and, despite the increased verticality, it is of dental origin (🔍 6.3) (📁 6.1).

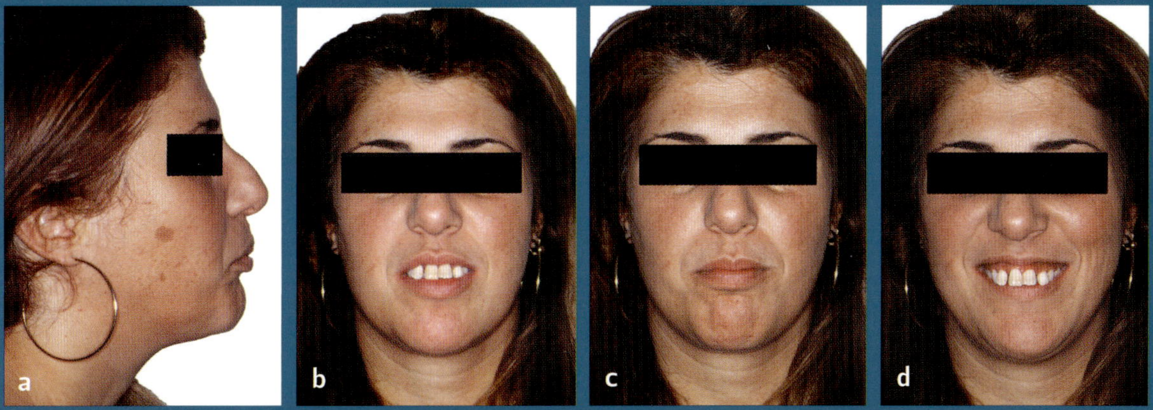

6.1 Extraoral pre-treatment photos. (Reproduced from "Paolone MG, Kaitsas R, Kaitsas F. Lingual orthodontics in an adult patient with upper premolar extraction: case report. *Int Orthod.* 2020;18(1):165-177". ©CEO. Published by Elsevier Masson SAS. All rights reserved. With permission.)

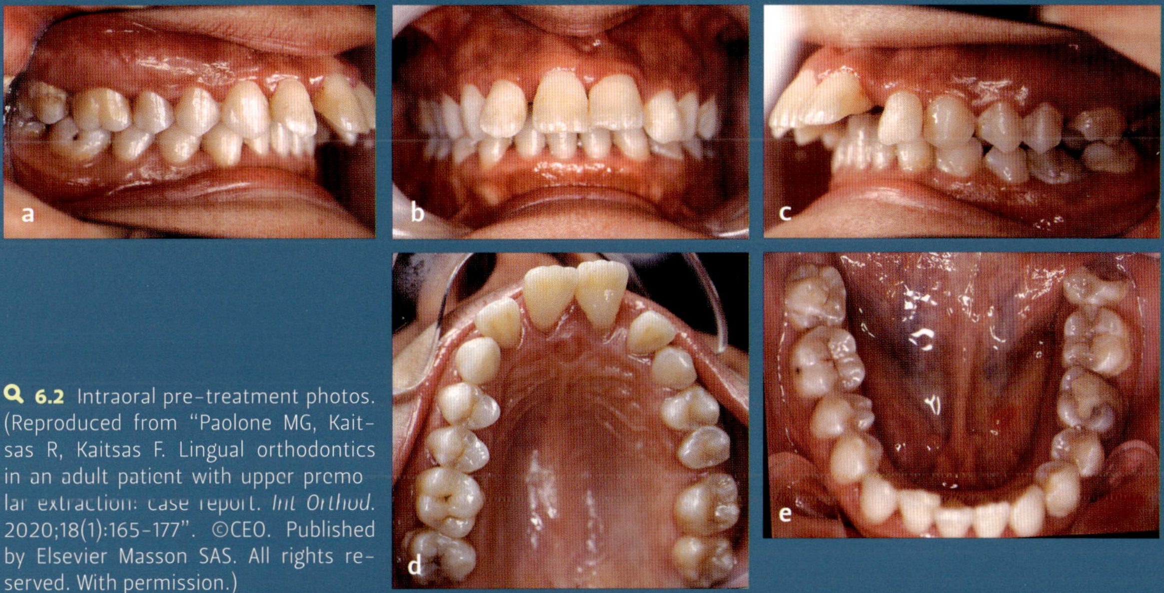

6.2 Intraoral pre-treatment photos. (Reproduced from "Paolone MG, Kaitsas R, Kaitsas F. Lingual orthodontics in an adult patient with upper premolar extraction: case report. *Int Orthod.* 2020;18(1):165-177". ©CEO. Published by Elsevier Masson SAS. All rights reserved. With permission.)

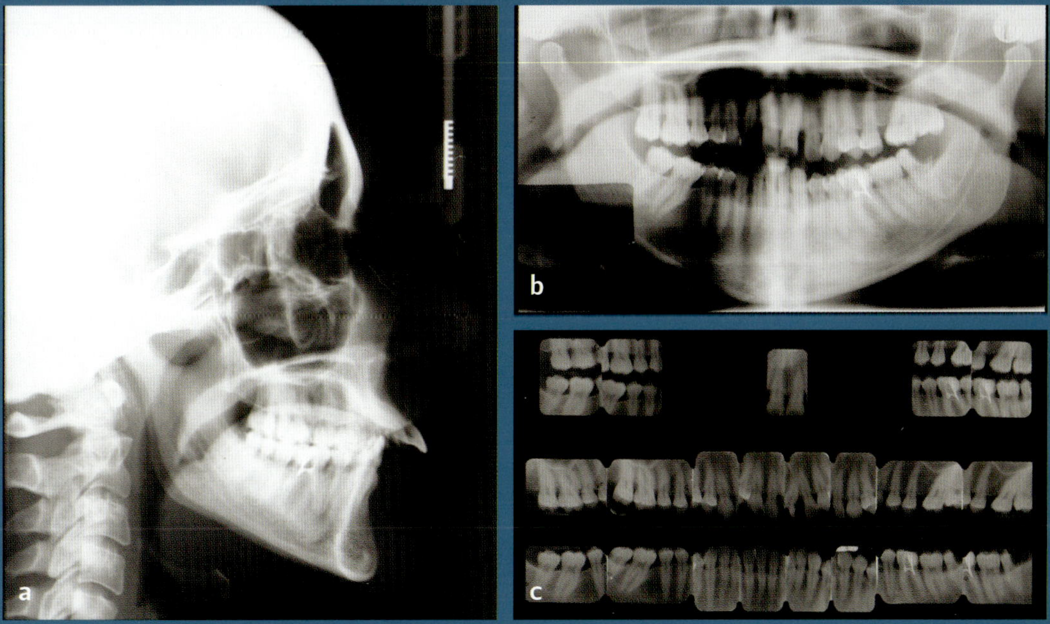

6.3 Pre-treatment cephalometric Rx (**a**), panoramic Rx (**b**), full radiographic periodontal status (**c**). (Reproduced from "Paolone MG, Kaitsas R, Kaitsas F. Lingual orthodontics in an adult patient with upper premolar extraction: case report. *Int Orthod.* 2020;18(1):165-177". ©CEO. Published by Elsevier Masson SAS. All rights reserved. With permission.)

Tab. 6.1 Cephalometric values

Sagittal skeletal relationships	Pre-treatment	Post-treatment	Retention	Mean	DS
Maxillary sagittal relationship SNA	80°	79°	79°	82°	3.5°
Mandibular sagittal relationship SNPg	76°	78°	78°	80°	3.5°
Intermaxillary sagittal relationship ANPg	4°	1°	1°	2°	2.5°
Vertical skeletal relationships					
Maxillary vertical relationship SN / ANS-PNS	9°	8°	8°	8°	3.0°
Mandibular vertical relationship SN / Go-Gn	40°	40°	40°	33°	2.5°
Intermaxillary vertical relationship ANS-PNS / Go-Gn	31°	32°	32°	25°	6.0°
Dento-basal relationships					
Upper incisor inclination $\underline{1}$ – ANS-PNS	125°	108°	107°	110°	6.0°
Lower incisor inclination $\overline{1}$ – Go-Gn	85°	87°	90°	94°	7.0°
Lower incisor compensation $\overline{1}$ – A-Pg (mm)	0	2	2	2	2.0
Dental relationships					
Overjet (OVJ, mm)	15	3	3	3.5	2.5
Overbite (OVB, mm)	7	1	1	2	2.5
Interincisal angle $\underline{1}$ / $\overline{1}$	115°	131°	132°	132°	6.0°

The patient has a class II/1 with an increased OVJ of dentoalveolar and skeletal origin, molar class II, deep dental OVB. After periodontal probing examination and complete radiographic status (6.4), the diagnosis is periodontitis Stage II localized Grade B[10,11] with medium-high risk assessment (Perio Risk: 12)[12-14]. Initial periodontal therapy and periodontal re-evaluation (6.5), are performed followed by an open flap debridement, although the patient mainly shows suprabony defects with a horizontal trend (absence of pockets >4 mm); these defects are maintainable with supportive therapy but a conservative surgical therapy (open flap debridement) limited to the anterior teeth was performed to stabilize the periodontal situation according to the subsequent orthodontic treatment. Initially, the patient's compliance is only partial (as it can be seen from the high values of FMBS and FMPS, but always below 20%), since she is resigned and disappointed by the conditions of her oral health and by the esthetic aspect; oral hygiene motivation will become increasingly improved during treatment for esthetic and dental improvement and rehabilitation.

The therapy involves the extraction of the two upper first premolars with lingual orthodontics in maximum anchorage in order to obtain a molar class II on the right and a class I molar on the left, a repositioning of the upper incisors and a normal lip function (6.6). The self-anchoring possibilities inherent in lingual mechanics, the application of miniscrews and the cooperation with class II elastics allow to obtain an occlusion in which the 3.3 is set in the 3.2 position and the 3.4 in the 3.3 one. Great attention is paid to the control of the verticality and to the correction of the position of the incisors. Lingual mechanics (Kurz 7th Generation®, Ormco) is made with indirect bonding that incorporates sectorial extrusive set-ups led by the morphology of periodontal defects. First it is applied a .016 CuNiTi archwire during the first month, then a .016 β-titanium archwire with loops and elastic chains for canine retraction. A rectangular .017×.017 β-titanium archwire is then applied with extrusive steps, and then a .017×.025 β-titanium archwire for torque control before retraction of the anterior group. The same archwire with T, helix and teardrop retraction loops, together with miniscrews, allows retraction, torque and pre - restorative intrusion of the anterior group. Finishing and stabilization are realized with a .017×.017 β-titanium archwire. The intrusion, retraction and torque control of the upper anterior group involve a first phase of sectoral extrusions aimed at bone levelling (see 6.6) and a subsequent intrusion with great torque control is carried out in a second moment with an extra-anchorage by

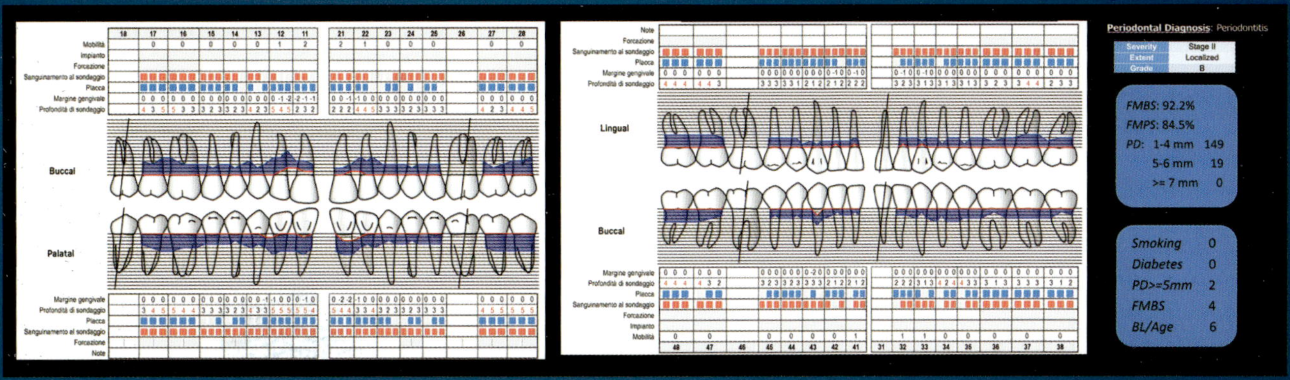

6.4 Initial periodontal probing, periodontal indexes, periodontal diagnosis, risk assessment. (Online periodontal charting tool from www.perio-tools.com) (Reproduced from "Paolone MG, Kaitsas R, Kaitsas F. Lingual orthodontics in an adult patient with upper premolar extraction: case report. *Int Orthod*. 2020;18(1):165-177". ©CEO. Published by Elsevier Masson SAS. All rights reserved. With permission.)

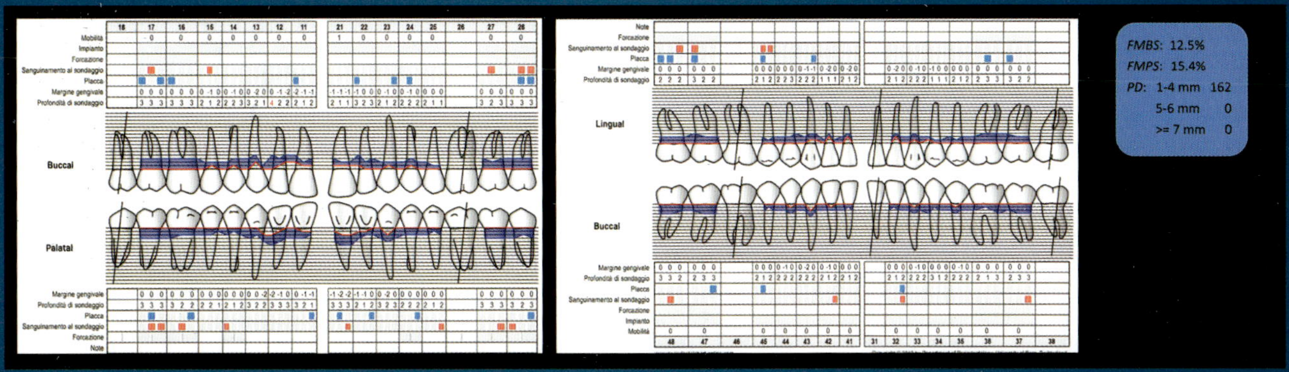

6.5 Re-evaluation periodontal probing and periodontal indexes (Online periodontal charting tool from www.perio-tools.com).

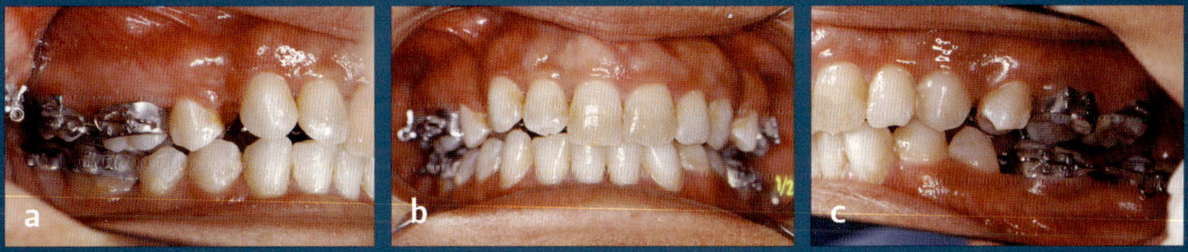

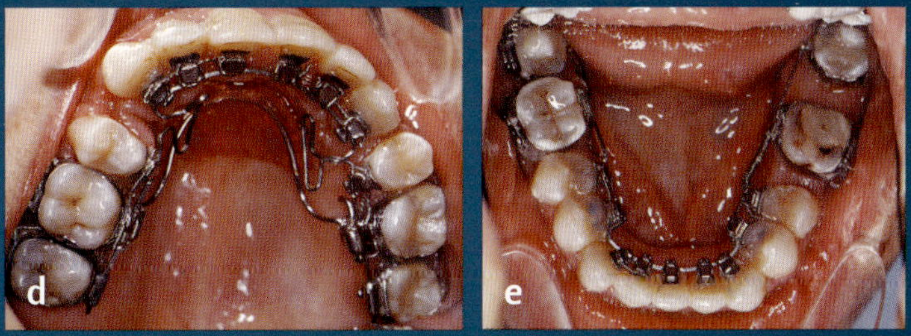

6.6 Lingual mechanics, .017×.025 β-titanium retraction archwire, with T-loops after sectorial extrusions lower.017×.025 β-titanium archwire.

miniscrews (6.7-6.9). At the end of the therapy the patient shows facial balance (6.10), a class II molar occlusion on the right and a class I molar occlusion on the left; at the canine level, on the right she shows a class I, on the left a class I where the upper canine is in occlusion with the 3.4 in 3.3 position (6.11) and normalization of the cephalometric values, levelling of the marginal bone (6.12) (see 6.1). These esthetic, dental and skeletal results are stable after 7 years (6.13-6.15) (see 6.1). Despite the absence and the atypical morphology of multiple dental elements, a prosthetic contribution was not necessary but only a restorative one of the anterior group. The patient will decide for a further definitive restorative approach. The apical root resorption is compatible with the amount of incisive retraction and intrusive movement. The movements took place without increasing the verticality. As it can be observed from the periodontal charting, at the end of the therapy the patient no longer presents pockets >4 mm and she is able to maintain a good oral hygiene, with FMBS at 10% and FMPS at 16% (6.16). The risk value is now reduced to medium-low (Perio Risk: 5)[12-14]. This reduction was obtained not only by the reduction of inflammatory indexes and pathological probing depths, but also by influencing the BL/Age ratio (Bone Level loss/Age), since residual bone levels were modified through orthodontics with sectorial movements on the teeth, which otherwise would have required resective periodontal surgery (see 3.14).

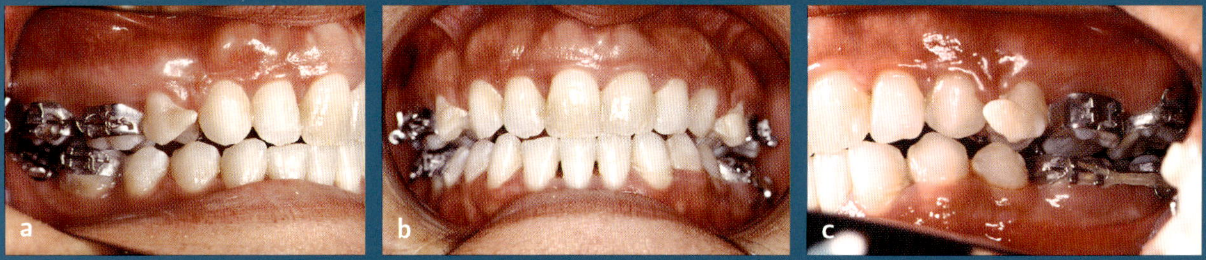

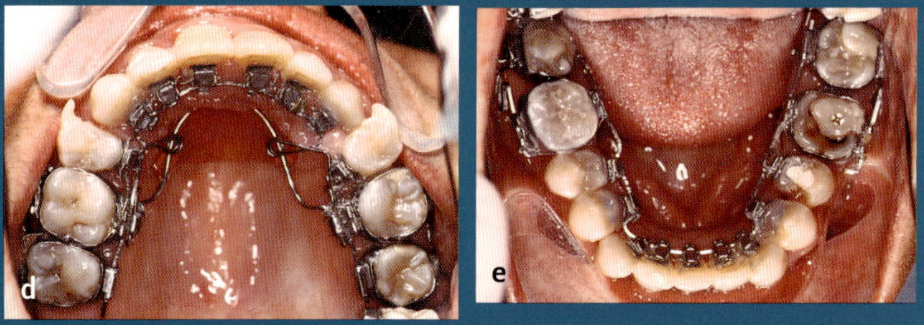

6.7 Lingual mechanics, .017×.017 β-titanium retraction archwire, with helix-loops after sectorial extrusions 1.2, 1.3. (Reproduced from "Paolone MG, Kaitsas R, Kaitsas F. Lingual orthodontics in an adult patient with upper premolar extraction: case report. *Int Orthod*. 2020;18(1):165-177". ©CEO. Published by Elsevier Masson SAS. All rights reserved. With permission.)

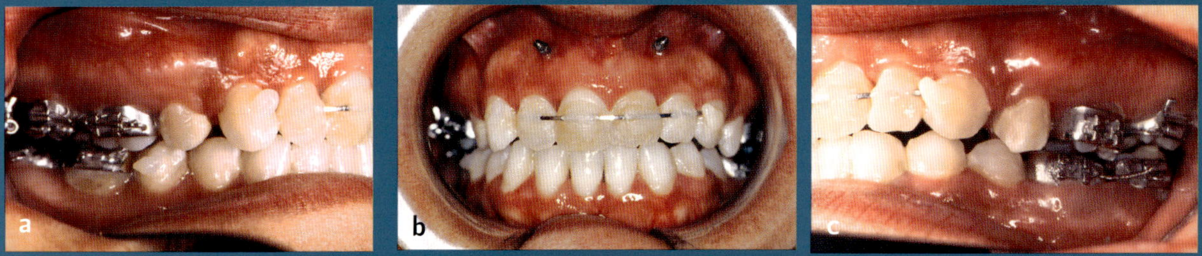

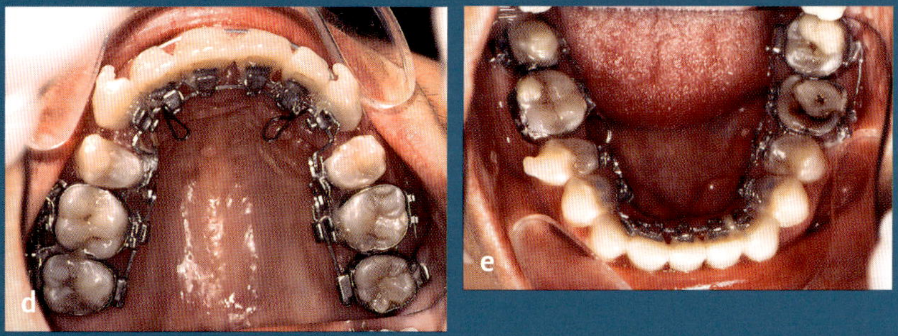

6.8 Lingual mechanics, .017×.025 β-titanium retraction archwire, with tear-drops-loops, TADs anchorage, antibowing loops, anterior group intrusion after sectorial extrusions. (Reproduced from "Paolone MG, Kaitsas R, Kaitsas F. Lingual orthodontics in an adult patient with upper premolar extraction: case report. Int Orthod. 2020;18(1):165-177". ©CEO. Published by Elsevier Masson SAS. All rights reserved. With permission.)

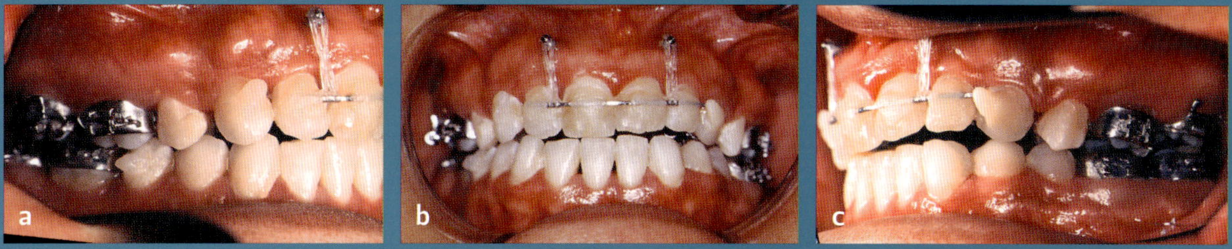

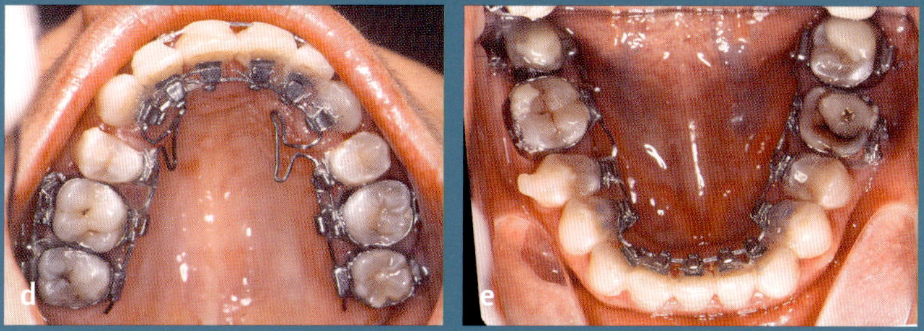

6.9 Lingual mechanics, .017×.025 β-titanium retraction archwire, with T-loops, TADs anchorage, extrusive step 1.1. (Reproduced from "Paolone MG, Kaitsas R, Kaitsas F. Lingual orthodontics in an adult patient with upper premolar extraction: case report. *Int Orthod.* 2020;18(1):165-177". ©CEO. Published by Elsevier Masson SAS. All rights reserved. With permission.)

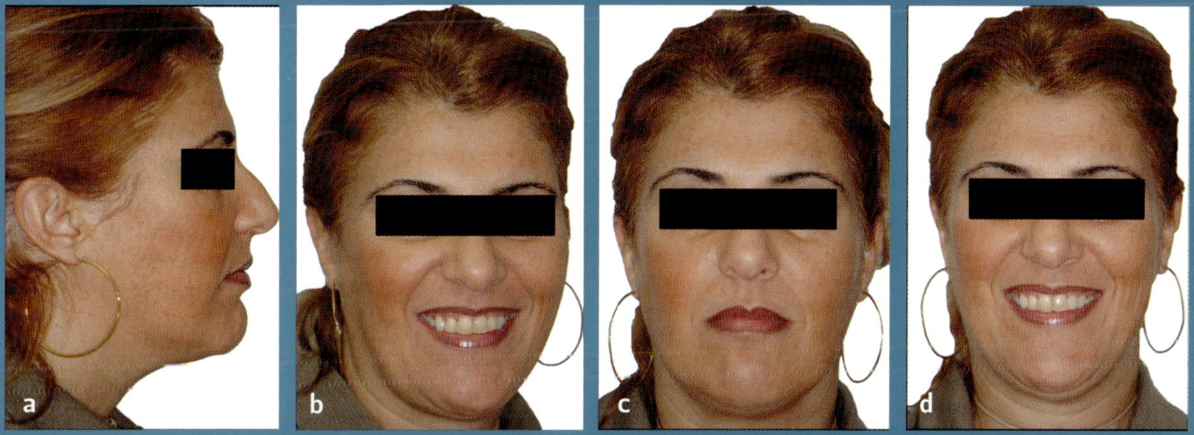

6.10 Extraoral post-treatment photos. (Reproduced from "Paolone MG, Kaitsas R, Kaitsas F. Lingual orthodontics in an adult patient with upper premolar extraction: case report. *Int Orthod.* 2020;18(1):165-177". ©CEO. Published by Elsevier Masson SAS. All rights reserved. With permission.)

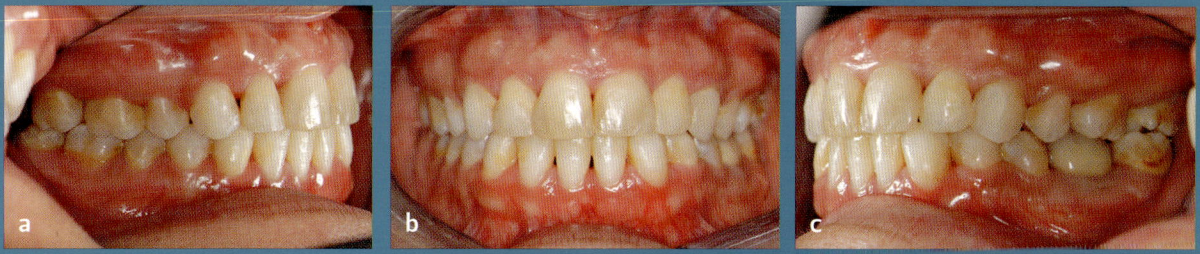

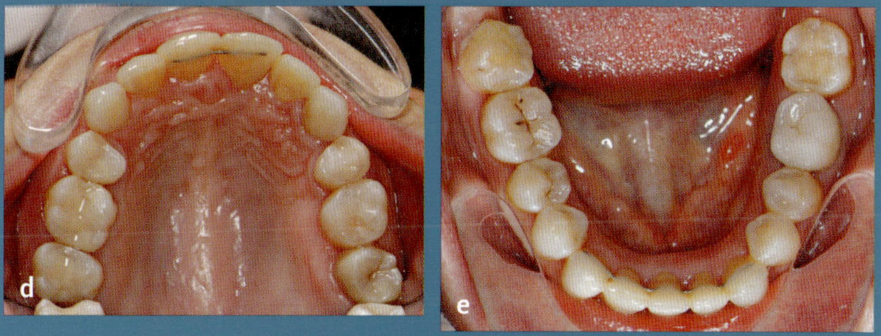

6.11 Intraoral post-treatment photos. (Reproduced from "Paolone MG, Kaitsas R, Kaitsas F. Lingual orthodontics in an adult patient with upper premolar extraction: case report. *Int Orthod.* 2020;18(1):165-177". ©CEO. Published by Elsevier Masson SAS. All rights reserved. With permission.)

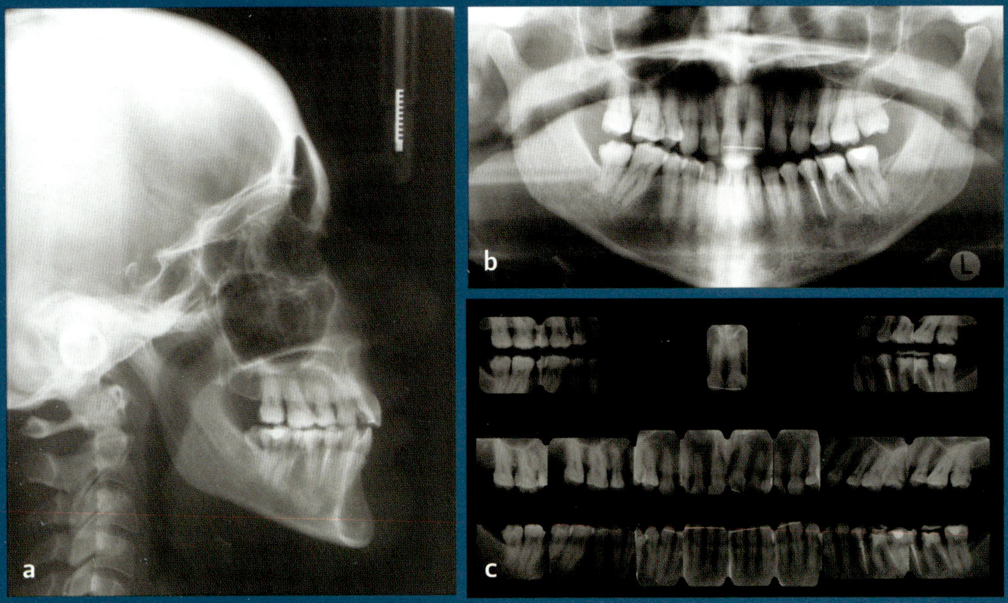

6.12 Post-treatment cephalometric Rx (**a**), panoramic Rx (**b**), full radiographic periodontal status (**c**). (Reproduced from "Paolone MG, Kaitsas R, Kaitsas F. Lingual orthodontics in an adult patient with upper premolar extraction: case report. *Int Orthod.* 2020;18(1):165-177". ©CEO. Published by Elsevier Masson SAS. All rights reserved. With permission.)

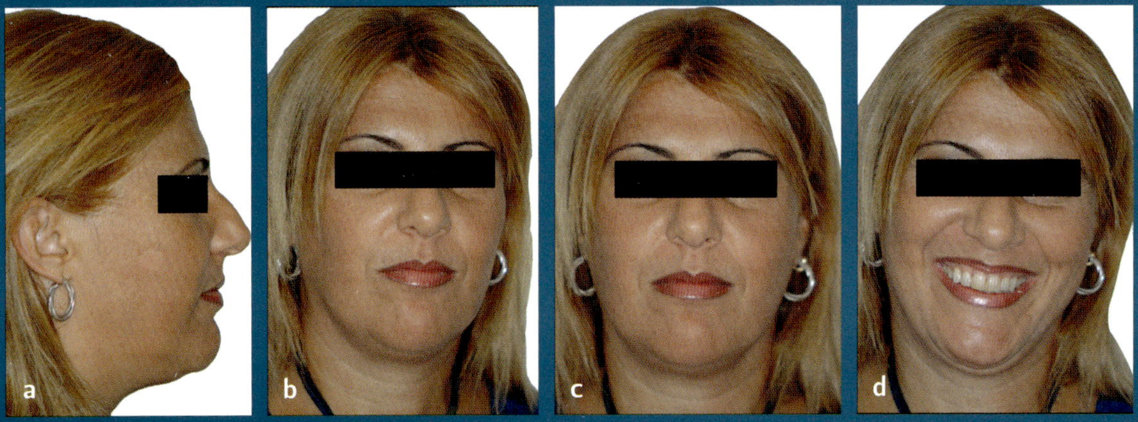

6.13 Extraoral 7-year post-retention photos. (Reproduced from "Paolone MG, Kaitsas R, Kaitsas F. Lingual orthodontics in an adult patient with upper premolar extraction: case report. *Int Orthod.* 2020;18(1):165-177". ©CEO. Published by Elsevier Masson SAS. All rights reserved. With permission.)

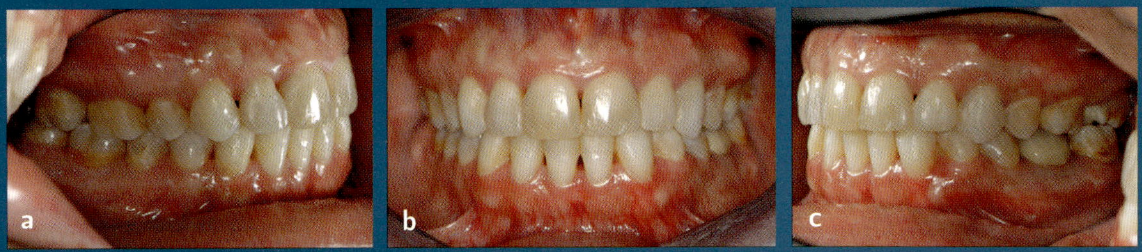

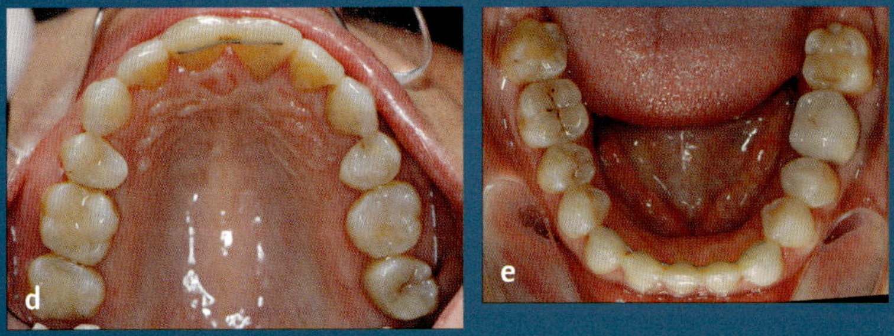

6.14 Intraoral 7-year post-retention photos. (Reproduced from "Paolone MG, Kaitsas R, Kaitsas F. Lingual orthodontics in an adult patient with upper premolar extraction: case report. *Int Orthod.* 2020;18(1):165-177". ©CEO. Published by Elsevier Masson SAS. All rights reserved. With permission.)

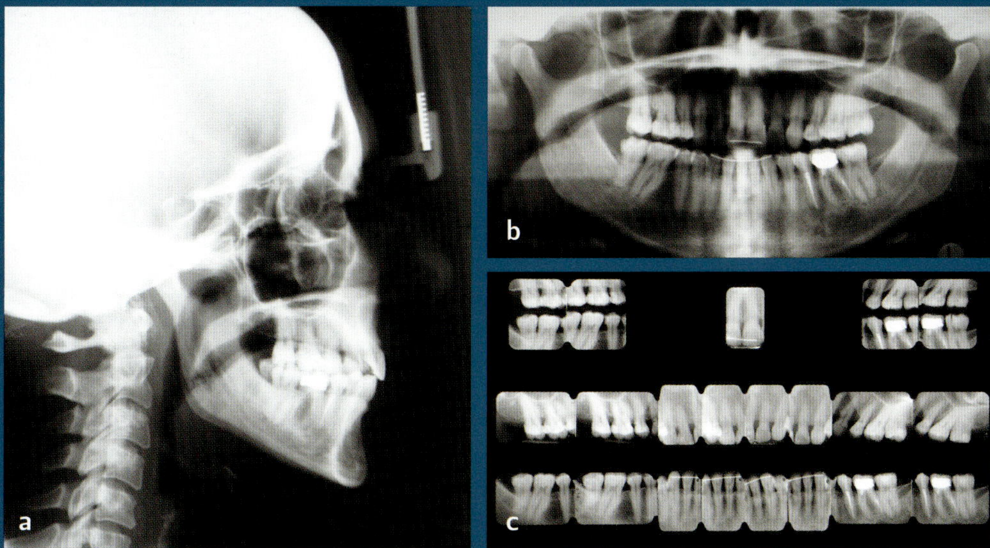

6.15 7-year post-retention cephalometric Rx (**a**), panoramic Rx (**b**), full radiographic periodontal status (**c**). (Reproduced from "Paolone MG, Kaitsas R, Kaitsas F. Lingual orthodontics in an adult patient with upper premolar extraction: case report. *Int Orthod.* 2020;18(1):165-177". ©CEO. Published by Elsevier Masson SAS. All rights reserved. With permission.)

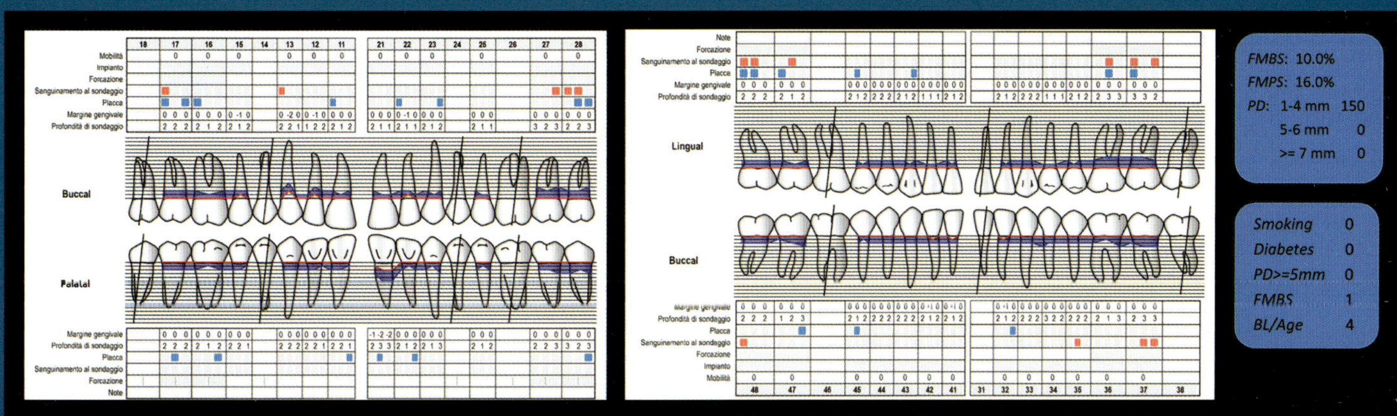

6.16 7-year post-retention periodontal probing, periodontal indexes, risk assessment (Online periodontal charting tool from www.perio-tools.com).

Orthodontics and space redistribution

Space redistribution within an interdisciplinary orthodontic-periodontal treatment can be developed in two ways, with two distinct indications:

1. Movement of the dental abutments in order to parallelize them for prosthetic purposes or for a correct implant placement, together with movements to bring abutment closer to modify spaces and reduce or avoid the number of implants.
2. Moving the teeth in edentulous areas to regenerate bone between the shifted elements by recreating adequate bone volumes to reduce the complexity of any GBR surgery or implant rehabilitation, eventually performing them in more posterior areas of the arch.

Prosthetic spaces redistribution

Prosthetic conventional and implant rehabilitation can offer some difficulties in the presence of reduced bone volumes, which require complex GBR (Guided Bone Regeneration) surgical techniques, and in the case in which the abutments that need to be prepared are healthy teeth that require, in conventional prosthesis, a root canal treatment. The orthodontic closure of the spaces reduces the costs that are necessary for rehabilitation with implant therapy, such as GBR and grafts[15] (6.17 and 6.18; see *Clinical case 2*). Although this type of choice brings multiple benefits to the treatment plan, it is not always accepted by clinicians because of mucogingival and periodontal risks, imperfect root parallelism, incomplete space closure, increased treatment time and possible relapse[15,16].

On the other hand, it must always be taken into account that, using natural abutments, the possibility of a future exacerbation and progression of the periodontal disease could lead to the failure of prosthetic denture on natural abutments[17]. One of the advantages of the redistribution of spaces and the use of natural dentition is to reduce the number of implants, and this data assume an important meaning when we consider that periodontal patients are more susceptible to develop peri-implant diseases[18,19].

Several case reports have reported techniques for orthodontic space closure, and extrapolating the data we can conclude that there is a slight loss of height of the mesial crestal bone of the tooth that is moved into the edentulous area, probably because of the initial tipping movement which would cause a compression of the marginal tissues, and a consequent stress at the marginal level of the alveolar bone, where the periodontal ligament is inserted. This large stress normally occurs on the marginal tissue and likely it causes a negative remodeling and thus bone loss[20,21].

It is therefore important, taking into account these considerations, to carry out the closure of the edentulous spaces by carrying out a bodily movement from the very beginning to try to reduce these side effects[16]. For this reason we prefer, when possible, to make a movement towards the edentulous ridge which is first a radicular movement and then a coronal uprighting, with or without TADs.

Factors that can improve, rather than worsen, the patient's periodontal situation must always be taken into account, including the use of light forces, bodily movements, absence of marginal inflammation, excellent oral hygiene care and the patient's age. It is important to always prevent the risk of mucogingival defects and attachment loss in adjacent sites before the closure of the spaces[16].

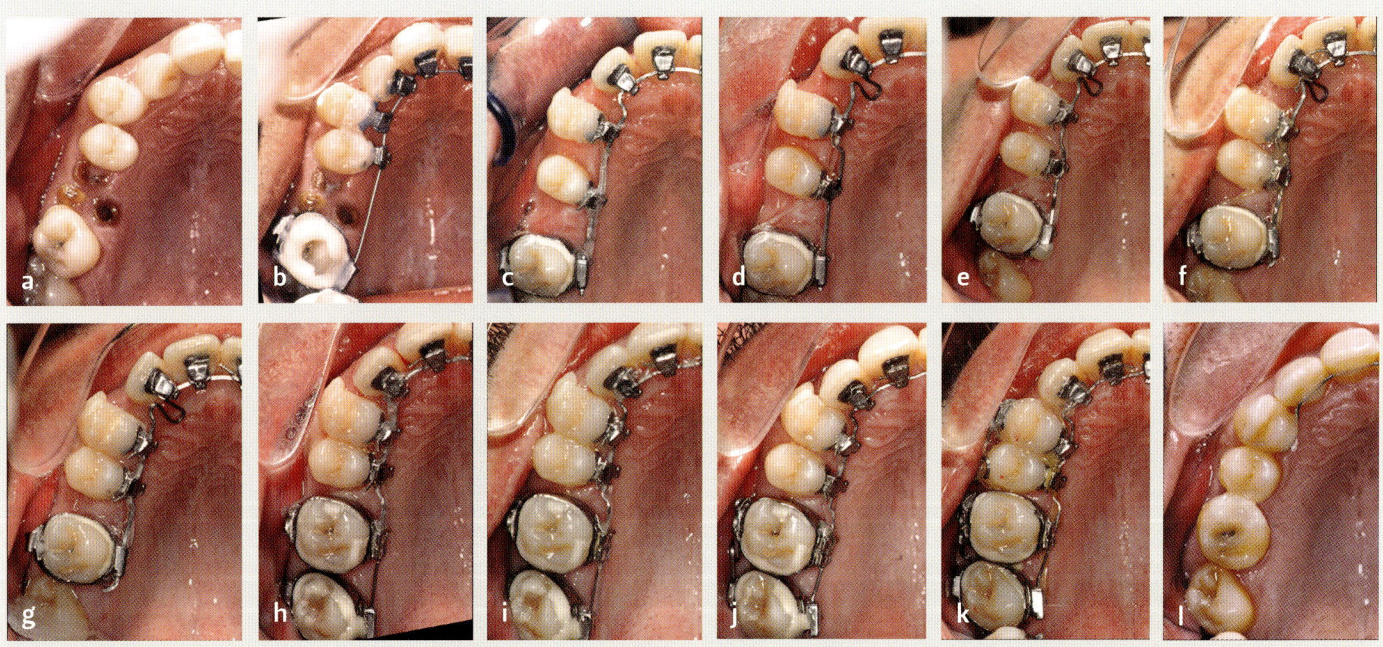

6.17 Orthodontic space closure, solution without implant-prosthetic rehabilitation. Upper Right sector (see *Clinical case 2*).

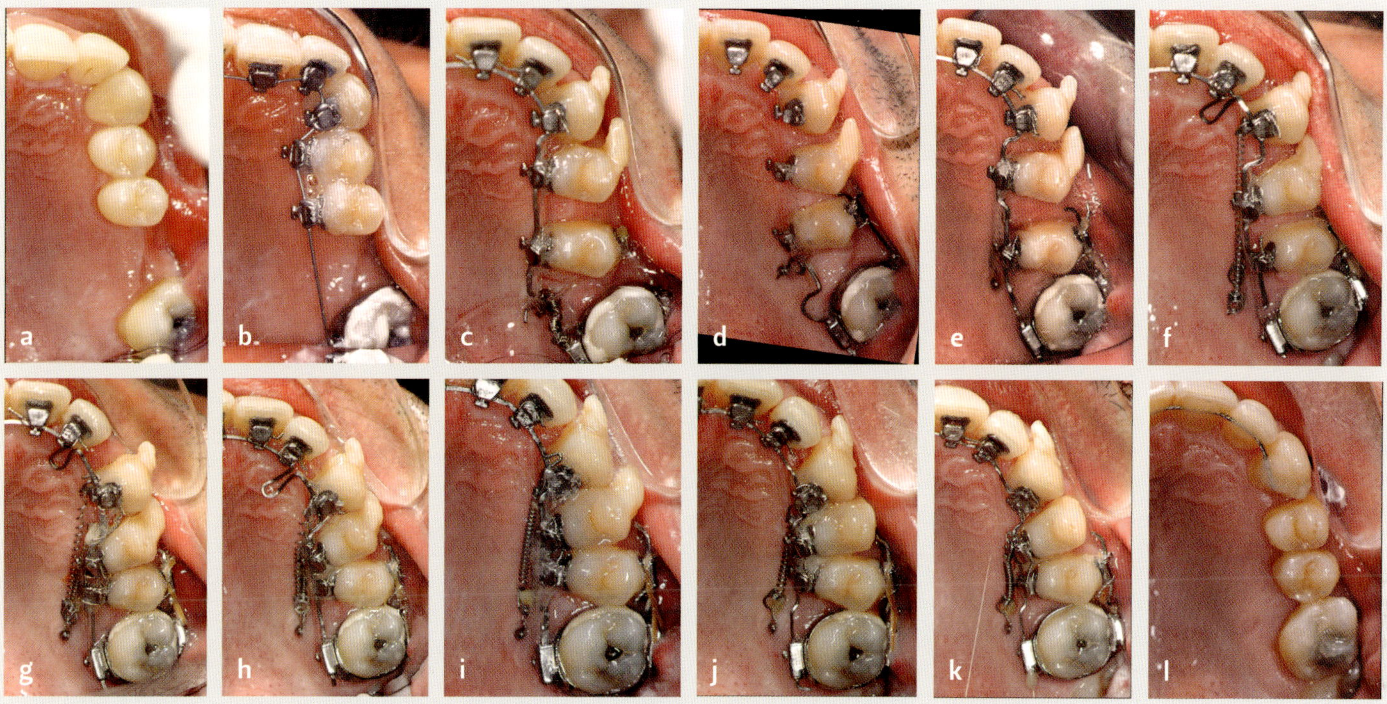

6.18 Orthodontic space closure, solution without implant-prosthetic rehabilitation. Upper Left sector (see *Clinical case 2*).

Clinical case 2

The patient's request consists in a complete and esthetic rehabilitation of the mouth and in a resolution of crowding and edentulousness. The presence of several dental overeruptions and extrusions of teeth in the absence of the antagonists and the need for correction of the bone level suggests for an orthodontic-periodontal treatment with restorative solution. The patient shows facial symmetry, normal nasolabial angle, reduced neck-chin length and competent lips (6.19), absence of 1.3, 1.6, 2.6, 3.6, 3.7, 4.6 and 4.7, class II/2, molar and canine class not completely evaluable on the right due to the absence of different teeth and a left canine class II, non-evaluable left molar class, normal OVJ, increased OVB (6.20), normodivergent skeletal class I and linguoversion of the upper and lower incisors (6.21) (6.2). The patient is diagnosed as periodontitis Stage II localized Grade B[10,11], which is confirmed by the fact that the tooth loss is due to decays and not to periodontal disease (6.22 and 6.23) with medium-high risk assessment (Perio Risk: 10)12-14.

The set-up and the indirect lingual bonding (Kurz 7th Generation®, Ormco) are applied to the two arches, first with a .016 archwire CuNiTi , then with a 0.016 β-titanium archwire and subsequently with a .017× .017 β-titanium with retraction loops for a sectorial torque of 1.2 with a palatal miniscrew between 2.5 and 2.7 (6.24). The retraction is achieved by implementing a variation of the classical lingual mechanics, finalizing it to the correction of the torque and to the final retraction of the upper incisors sector only. Therefore, at a first phase, the retraction concerns only the left premolar and canine segments with NiTi springs with TADs anchorage, together with 2.7 mesialization and retraction of the left upper premolars and 1.7 mesialization. Only in a second time the torque of the upper incisors is over-corrected, then retraction is carried out with a .017×.025 β-titanium archwire with retraction loops (6.25), class II elastics; at the same time an uprighting of the third molars is performed at the lower arch with NiTi springs. During the last 6 months of orthodontic detailing (6.26), the implants (Frialit-2®, Dentsply) (6.27) with conventional osteotomy are placed in the lower edentulous ridges and then detailing is realised with a .017×.017 β-titanium archwire (6.28).

At the end of the treatment the patient presents facial balance, canine class I, in which the 1.4 is in 1.3 position, class II molar on the right and class I molar and canine on the left, normalization of the OVB and cephalometric values of the incisive inclination (6.29-6.32; see 6.2); after 5 years he shows stability in retention (6.33-6.34).

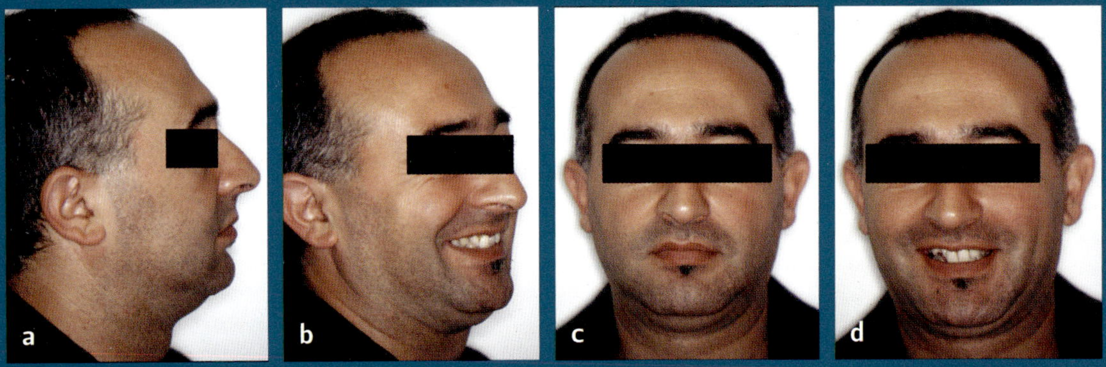

6.19 Extraoral pre-treatment photos.

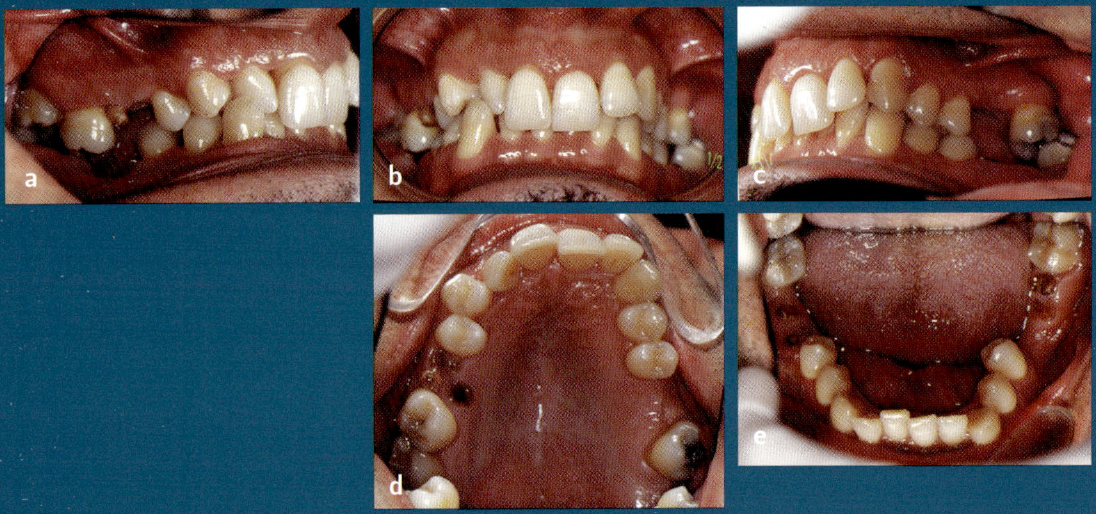

6.20 Intraoral pre-treatment photos.

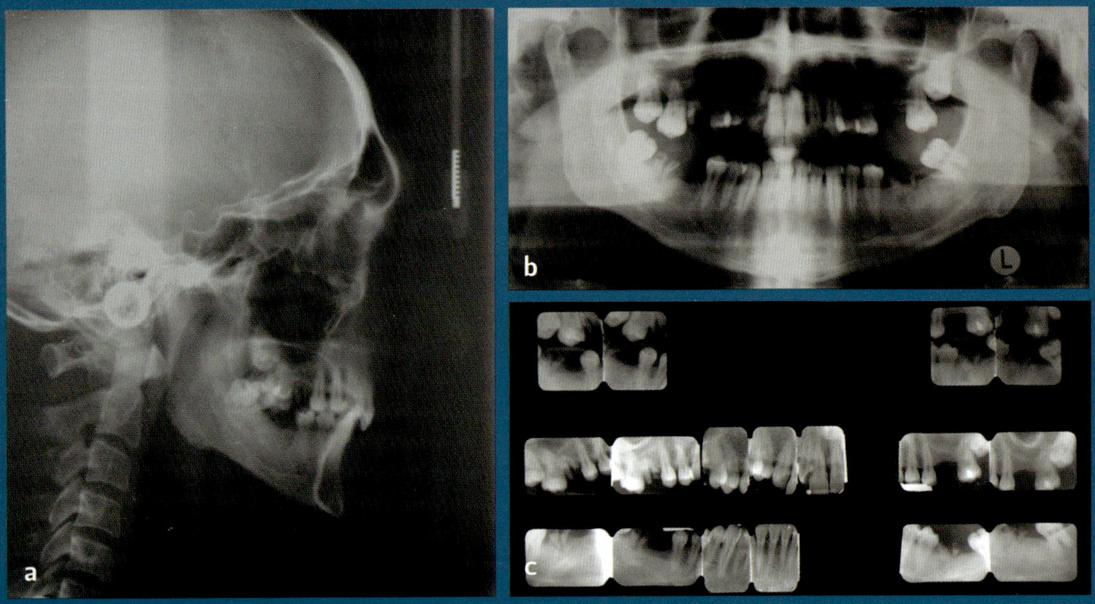

6.21 Pre-treatment cephalometric Rx (**a**), panoramic Rx (**b**), full radiographic periodontal status (**c**).

Tab. 6.2 Cephalometric values

Sagittal skeletal relationships	Pre-treatment	Post-treatment	Mean	DS
Maxillary sagittal relationship SNA	81°	81°	82°	3.5°
Mandibular sagittal relationship SNPg	79°	79°	80°	3.5°
Intermaxillary sagittal relationship ANPg	2°	2°	2°	2.5°
Vertical skeletal relationships				
Maxillary vertical relationship SN / ANS-PNS	10°	10°	8°	3.0°
Mandibular vertical relationship SN / Go-Gn	31°	32°	33°	2.5°
Intermaxillary vertical relationship ANS-PNS / Go-Gn	21°	22°	25°	6.0°
Dento-basal relationships				
Upper incisor inclination 1 – ANS-PNS	95°	108°	110°	6.0°
Lower incisor inclination 1 – Go-Gn	90°	94°	94°	7.0°
Lower incisor compensation 1 – A-Pg (mm)	-5	-1	2	2.0
Dental relationships				
Overjet (OVJ, mm)	4	2	3,5	2.5
Overbite (OVB, mm)	8	2	2	2.5
Interincisal angle 1 / 1	150°	139°	132°	6.0°

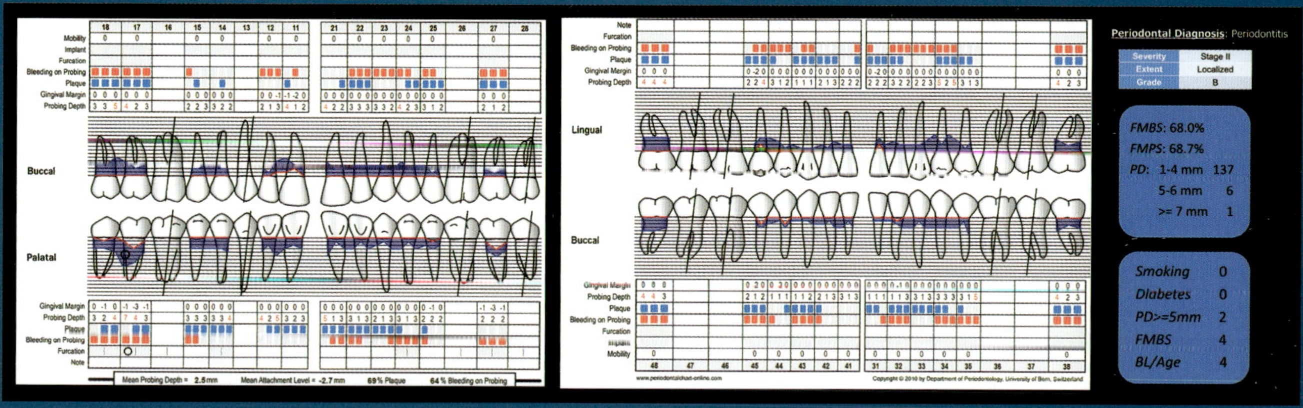

6.22 Initial periodontal probing, periodontal indexes, periodontal diagnosis, risk assessment (Online periodontal charting tool from www.perio-tools.com).

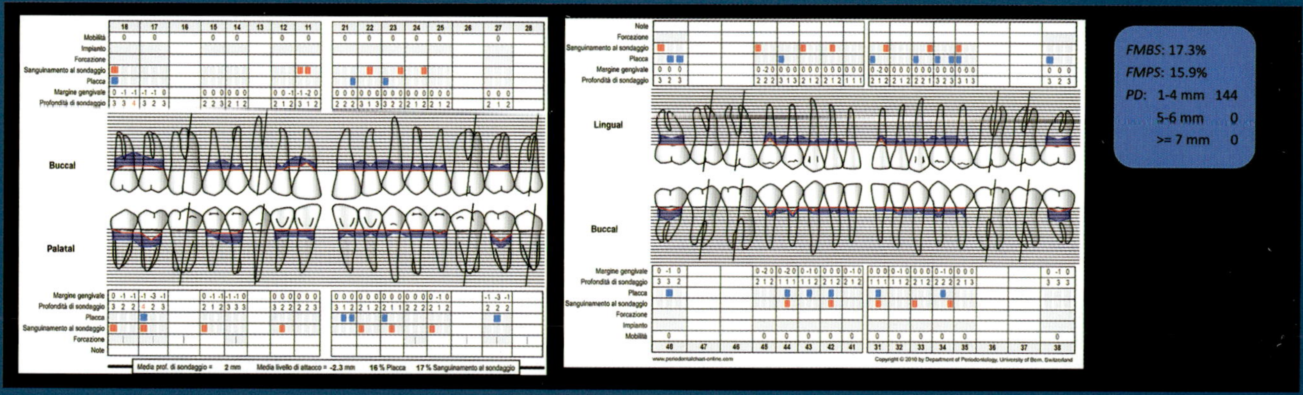

6.23 Re-evaluation periodontal probing and periodontal indexes (Online periodontal charting tool from www.perio-tools.com).

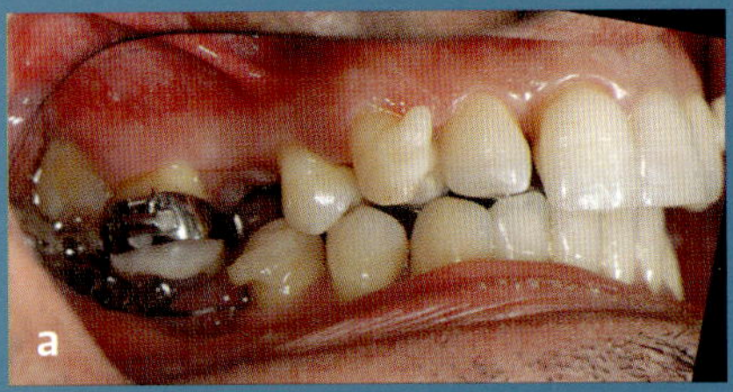

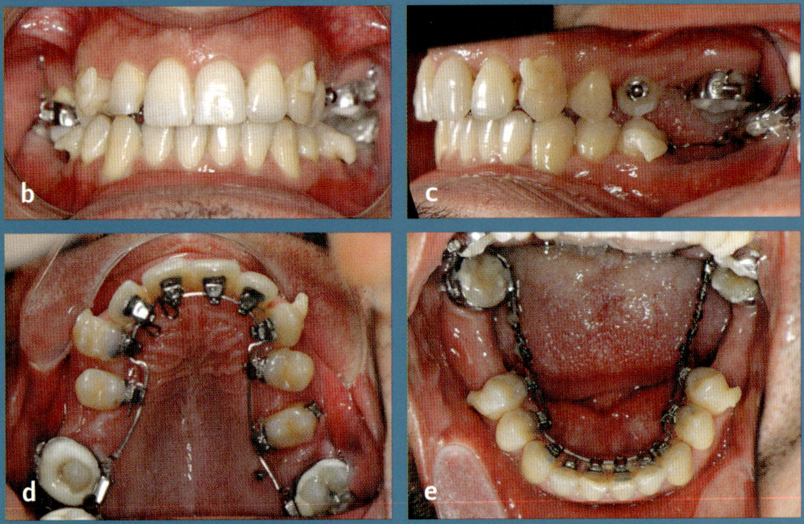

6.24 Lingual mechanics, .017×.017 β-titanium archwires, with teardrop-loops with a sectorial torque 1.2, with a palatal anchorage TADs between 2.5 and 2.7.

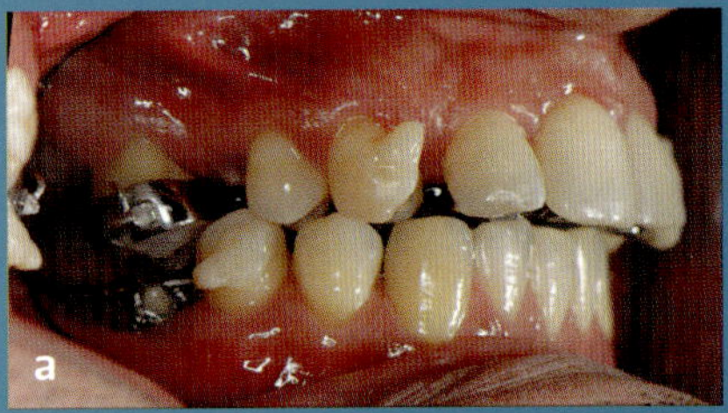

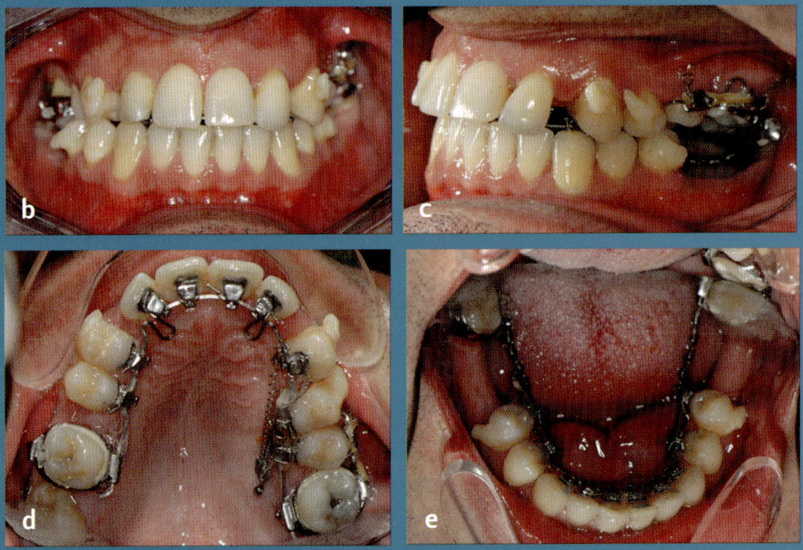

6.25 Lingual mechanics, .017×.025 β-titanium archwires, with teardrop retraction loops with a palatal anchorage TADs between 2.5 and 2.7.

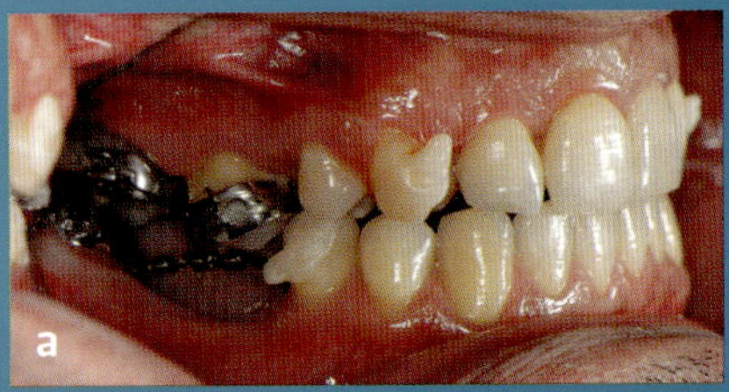

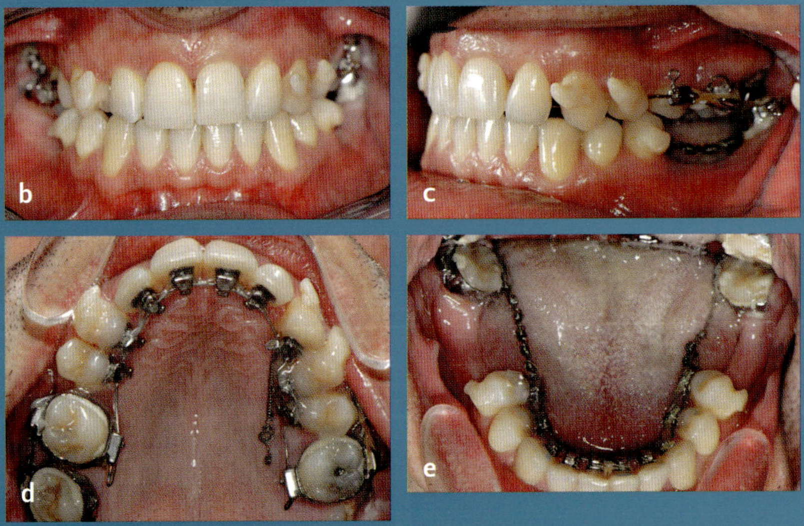

6.26 Detailing, .017×.017 β-titanium archwires.

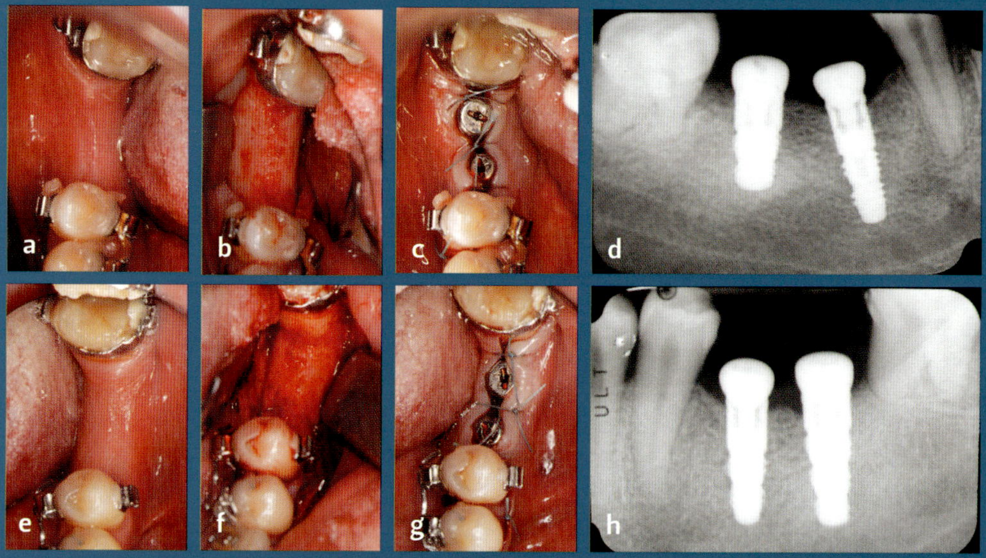

6.27 Implant surgery in the lower arch in 3.6, 3.7, 4.6, 4.7 sites and healing abutments placement in the same surgical procedure.

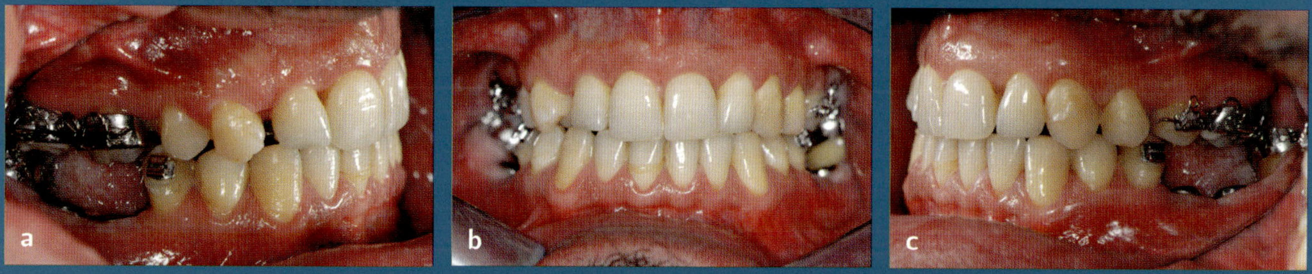

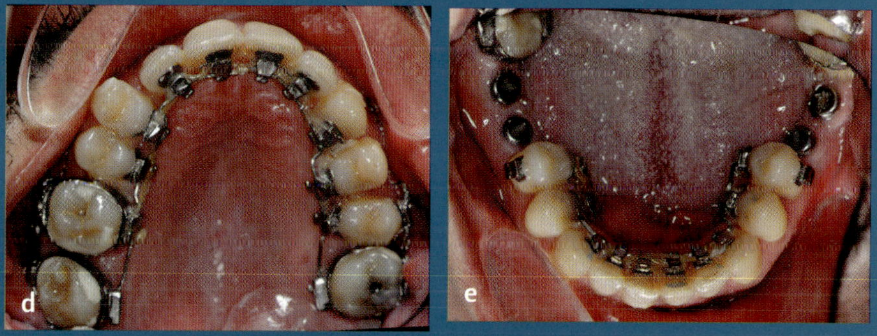

6.28 Detailing, .017×.017 β-titanium archwires.

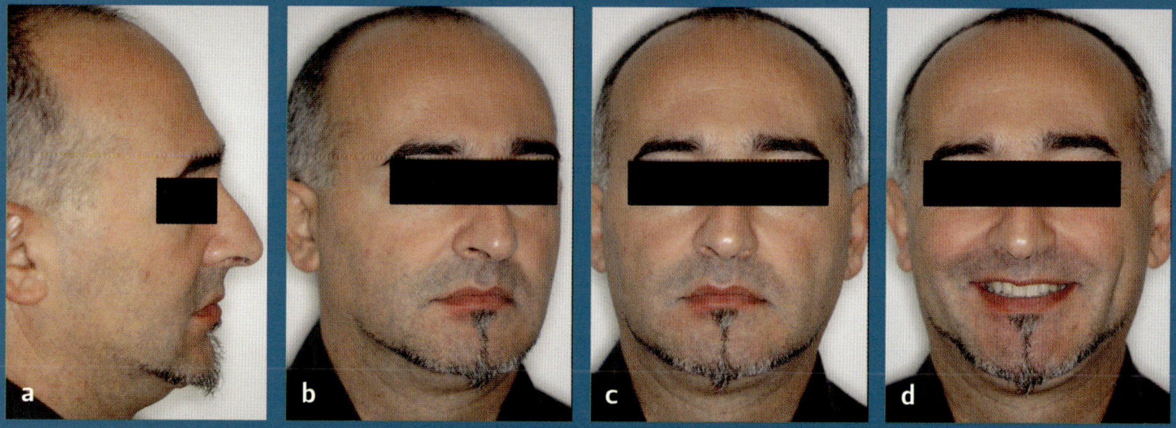

6.29 Post-treatment extraoral photos.

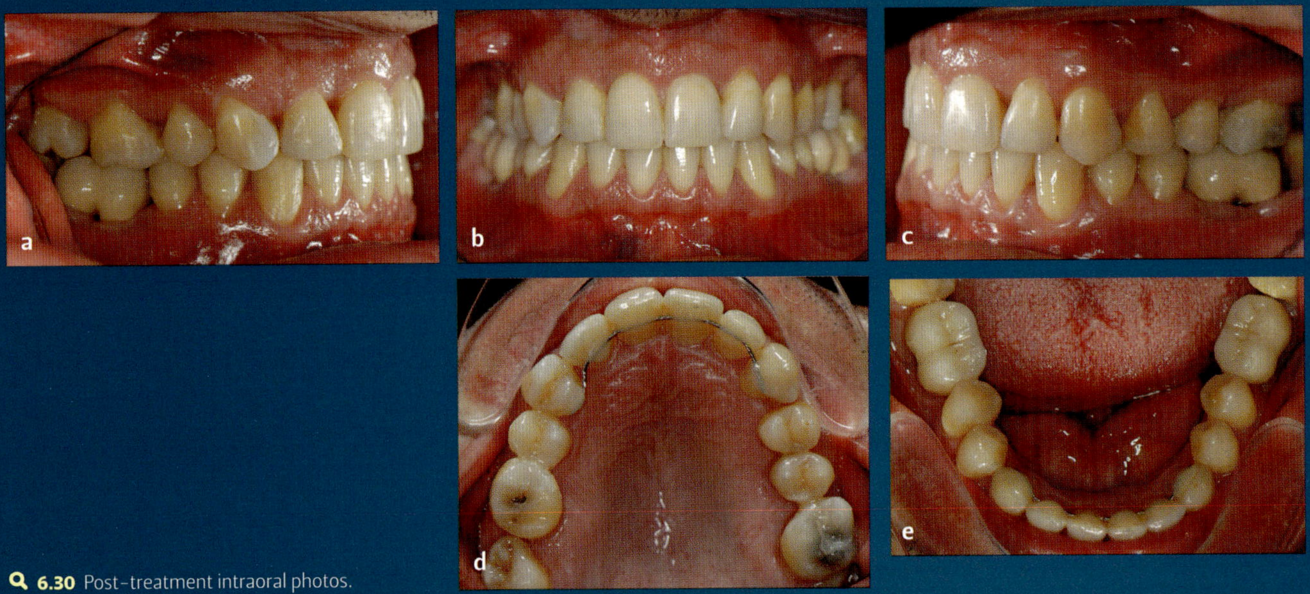

6.30 Post-treatment intraoral photos.

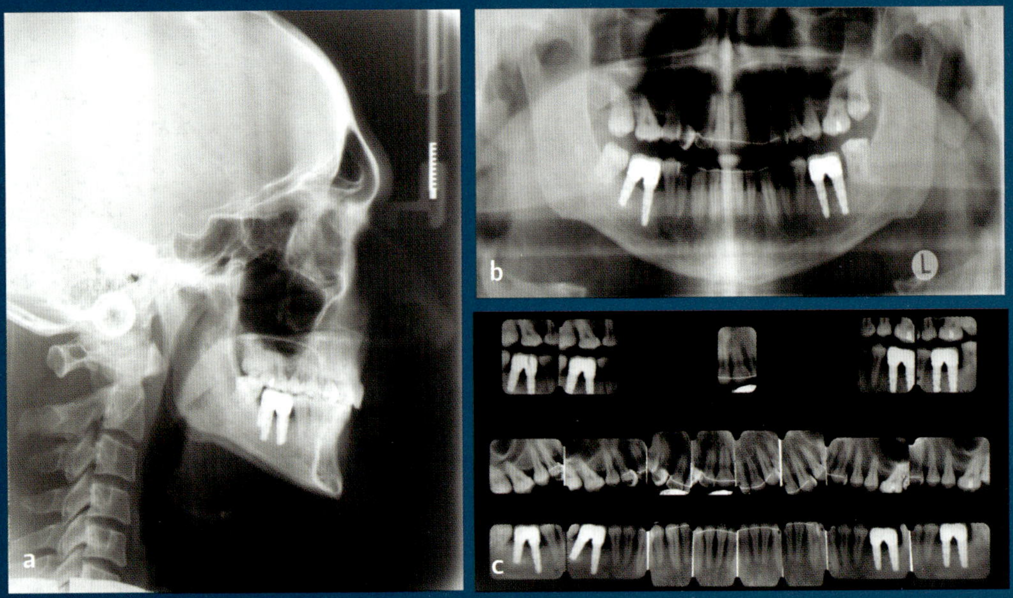

6.31 Post-treatment cephalometric Rx (**a**), panoramic Rx (**b**) and full radiographic periodontal status (**c**).

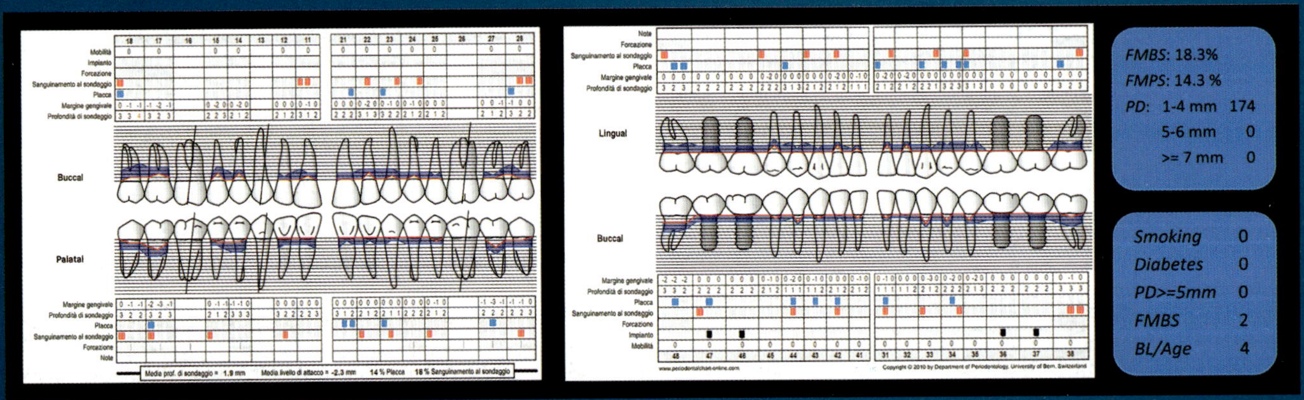

6.32 Post-treatment periodontal probing, periodontal indexes, risk assessment (Online periodontal charting tool from www.perio-tools.com).

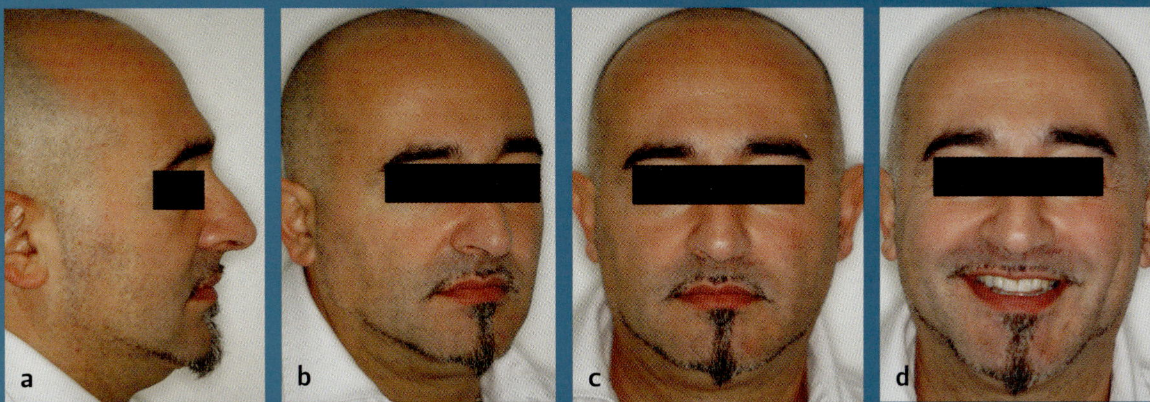

6.33 Extraoral 5-year post-retention photos.

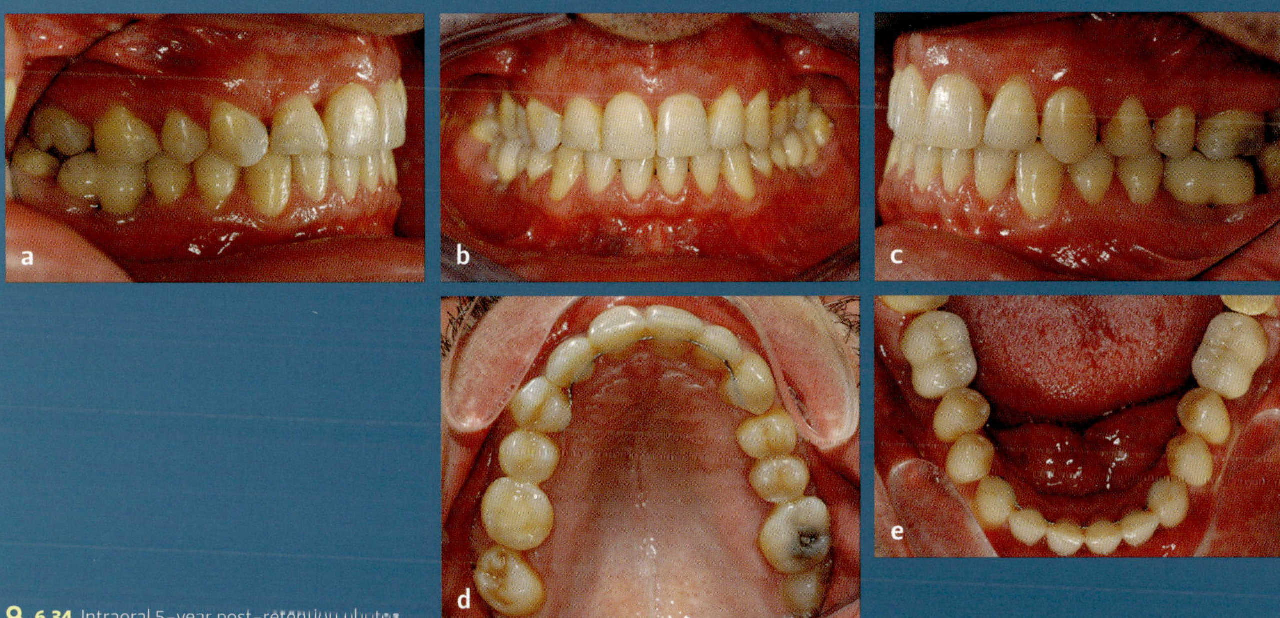

6.34 Intraoral 5-year post-retention photos.

Movement in edentulous areas

Orthodontic tooth movement in edentulous areas is a viable option to improve crestal anatomy by recreating a new regularized "regenerated" bone crest between the moved teeth. The orthodontic movement of the teeth towards atrophic ridges is followed by the movement of the alveolar bone associated with the tooth and orthodontics has been proposed as an alternative to the surgical augmentation of atrophic ridges in sites adjacent to natural teeth.

Developed by Fontenelle[22,23] and Kokich[24], and also called Orthodontic Implant Site Switching (OISS)[25], it is a technique for implant site development that allows the creation of a suitable edentulous ridge without complex regenerative surgical techniques, associated with minimal changes in the periodontal support of the transposed tooth. This leads to the expansion of the alveolar bone in the tension side of the orthodontic movement. This technique can be used in tooth agenesis to generate sufficient bone volume for implant placement, for example in the area of the lateral incisors and premolars[25]. A clinical case is reported in which the second upper right premolar after GTR of the distal bone defect is moved towards the mesial edentulous ridge with a contextual movement of extrusion with anchorage on TADs to recreate a ridge as regular as possible in order to place implants (see Chapter 11, *Clinical case 1*) (6.35-6.37; see 9.2-9.10).

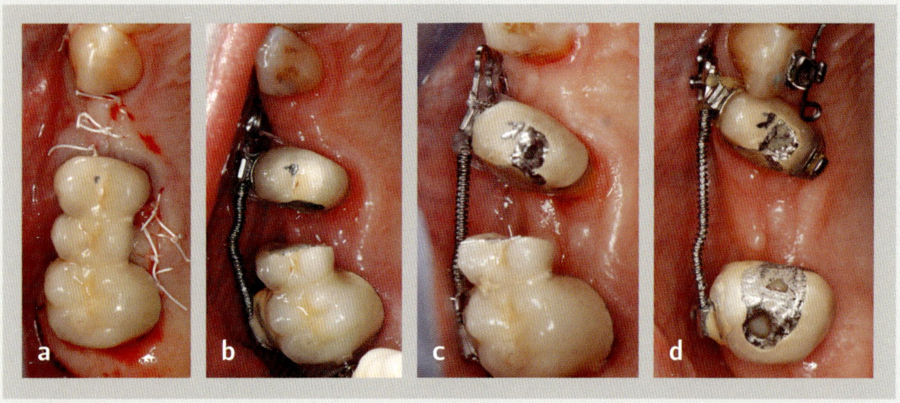

6.35 Mesial movement of the 1.5 to regenerate a distal regular edentulous ridge (occlusal view).

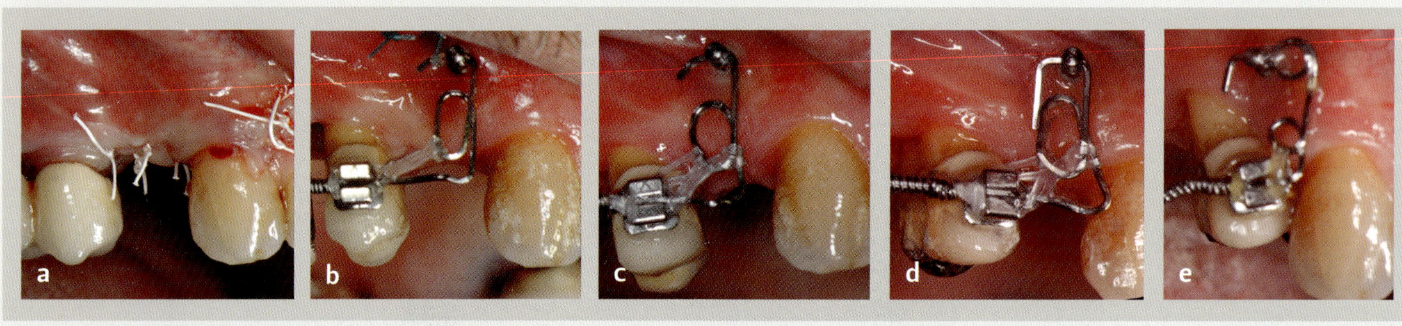

6.36 Mesial movement of the 1.5 to regenerate a distal regular edentulous ridge (vestibular view).

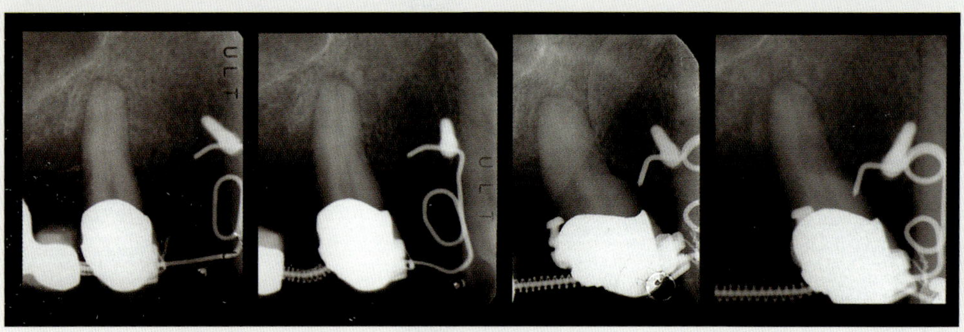

6.37 X-ray check of the mesial movement of the tooth in Fig. 6.35-6.36.

The closure and the management of edentulous spaces in very resorbed and thin long alveolar ridges (that are almost always present in the case of long-standing extractions and rehabilitation of edentulous patients), such as in the cases of loss of a deciduous tooth with permanent agenesis or after the extraction of a tooth with a very compromised and non-restorable root is a biomechanical and anatomical challenge for orthodontics and a key for a surgical-prosthetic rehabilitative solution[16]. Experimentally, it has been shown that a tooth with a normal height of the periodontal support can be moved orthodontically with very light forces in an area where the bone height is markedly reduced, while maintaining the height of the periodontal attachment of the tooth itself. In partially edentulous patients with a normal periodontal support, movements towards an edentulous area with a reduced bone volume have led to encouraging results, as long as the tooth movements are bodily and performed with light orthodontic forces[26,27]. Although a greater distance was found between the cemento-enamel junction and the bone crest on the pressure side of the orthodontically moved teeth in relation to the non-moved contralateral ones, the bone level of all the sample teeth was positioned more coronally than the original bone level that was reduced in the area towards which the test tooth was moved[28].

Movement in the mandible is particularly hard due to the presence of dense cortical bone and a greater susceptibility to the bone crest resorption[16]. Radiological evaluation often detects slight root resorption on the compression side of the tooth moving within thin ridge; this resorption appears independent from the periodontal parameters but seems directly correlated with the orthodontic force[29]. The presence of thin bone ridges with cortical predominance produces most of the pressure stress[29]. The prevalence of this root resorption is 40.6%, and it is on average 2.3 mm[30]. After tooth movement these resorption areas are repaired with the deposition of new cement, a time-dependent process that is less reactive after the application of strong orthodontic forces[31]. In cases of reduced buccolingual thickness of the edentulous ridge, movement along the cortex may be delayed and vestibular or lingual dehiscences may occur. In these cases, alveolar bone augmentation procedures are recommended prior to movement[32,33]. An age-dependent effect on the amount of increase in alveolar bone thickness, where newly formed bone would follow the tooth moving into the edentulous space has been reported in young growing patients, but not necessarily in older patients[34].

Clinical case 3

The patient comes to rehabilitate the lower left sector (6.38). Elsewhere, an extraction of the remaining root of 3.4 and the placement of an implant in the edentulous area between 3.5 and 3.7 had been proposed.

By carefully observing that the amount of remaining dental tissue is enough for the maintenance of the root as abutment, it is decided to rehabilitate the sector using the teeth as prosthetic abutments without inserting any implant, to recover the parallelism of the abutments and to create an adequate prosthetic space between the elements 3.4 and 3.5, moving the future prosthetic abutments in the edentulous crest. Therefore, through the use of a small orthodontic sectional .019×.025 ss on the Tweed® slot .022×.028 (6.39), 3.4, 3.5 and 3.6 (6.40a-d) are repositioned in the arch, allowing a prosthetic recovery after surgical crown lengthening (6.40e-f, 6.41 and 6.42) and reconstruction of the abutments. The obtained parallelism allowed the application of a conventional fixed partial denture saving a root that had been intended for extraction, without use of any implant (6.43 and 6.44).

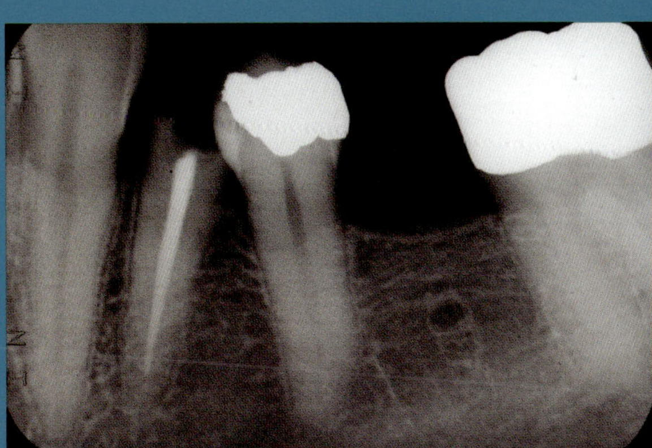

6.38 Initial X-ray showing the absence of parallellism of the dental abutments and the prosthetic space reduction for the 3.4.

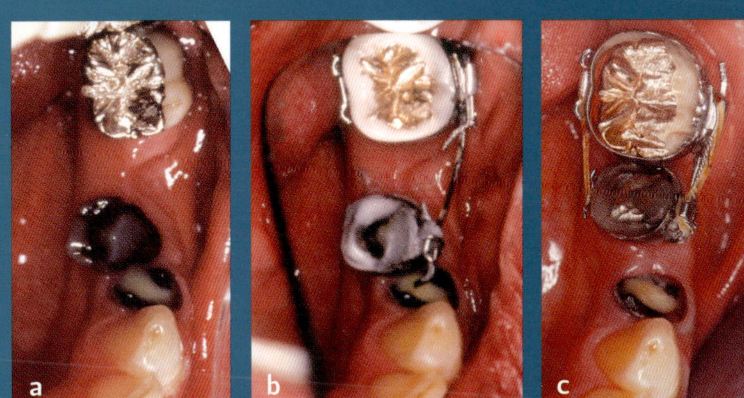

6.39 Occlusal view.

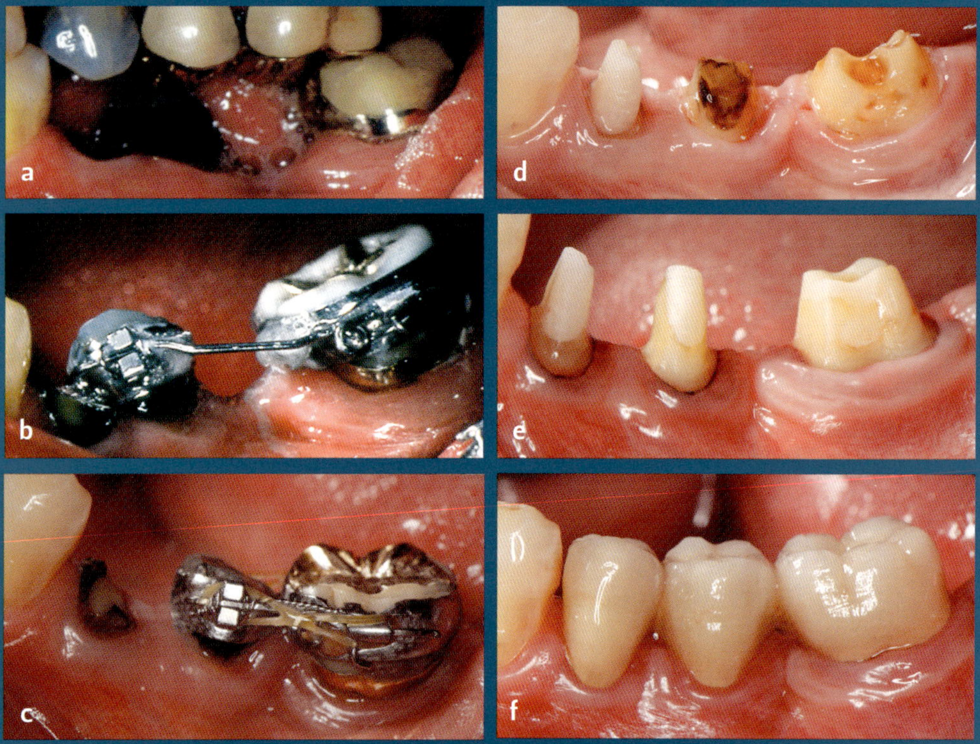

6.40 Lateral view.

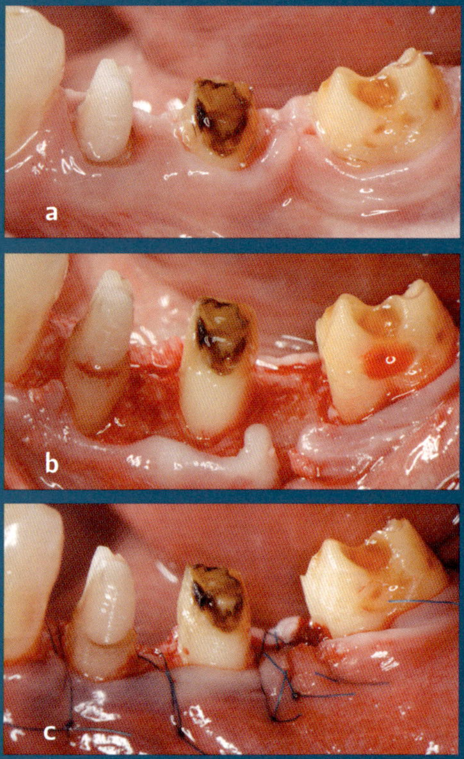

6.41 The three dental abutments after alignment and the recovery of the healthy dental hard tissue after surgical crown lengthening.

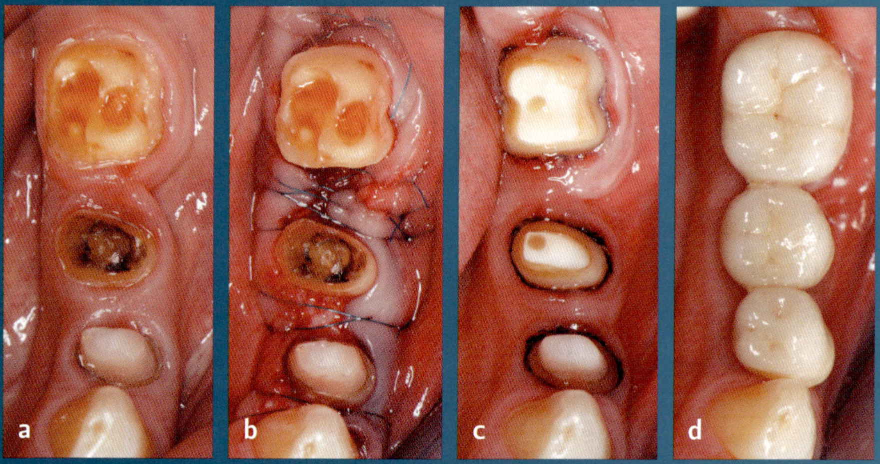

6.42 Dental alignment of the abutments, suture, definitive impression and the fixed partial denture.

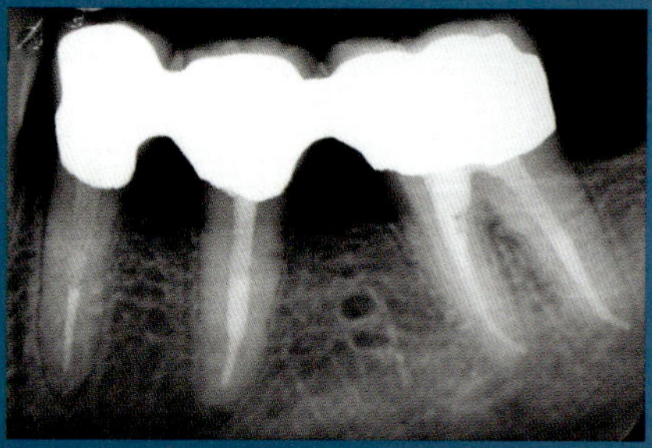

6.43 X-ray check of the fixed partial denture.

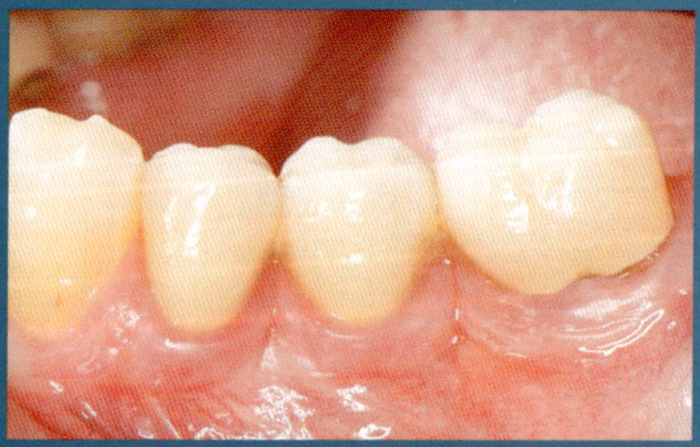

6.44 Vestibular view of the fixed partial denture.

Crowding

Dental crowding makes it difficult to control the plaque of the proximal surfaces of the teeth and the orthodontic correction of this problem allows to have a more advantageous access for oral hygiene and improves the morphology of marginal soft and hard tissues. The combination of periodontal and orthodontic treatment improves periodontal health and restores physiologically right dentition[35]. In fact, an acceptable level of plaque control requires an oral environment that allows the patient to perform these maneuvers[1]. A higher plaque index was statistically found in the mandible than in the maxilla, probably due to the fact that dental crowding is more frequent in the mandible[35]. Plaque and gingival indexes of crowded teeth are also significantly higher than those of uncrowded teeth[36,37]. The number and composition of periodontal pathogenic bacterial species on crowded teeth are higher than in non-crowded ones and the uprighting of tipped teeth can eliminate plaque retentive areas, with modification of the bacterial flora, and reduce the pocket depth on the mesial surfaces[38], as described in Chapters 3 and 5. Once the teeth are aligned, the tissue shows less tendency to bleed on probing and requires less rate of supportive care[1]. Approximately 3 months after the resolution of the crowding, the periodontal indexes are reduced, as the conditions of maintenance of hygiene have improved and the patient has been motivated already from the first months of treatment[39].

Clinical case 4

The patient requires a resolution of crowding and esthetic compromise of the smile. He has a symmetrical face, competent lips (6.45), dental class I on the right, dental class II on the left, normal OVJ and OVB, absence of 4.6 and several teeth show extensive restorative and endodontic treatments (6.46), skeletal class I, normodivergence, slight linguoversion of the upper and lower incisors (6.47) (6.3). Taking into account that the lower arch has a slight crowding in the presence of a reduced lower incisor angle/mandibular plane, we choose to extract only the first upper left premolar to solve the crowding in the 2.3 area. From a periodontal point of view the periodontal indexes, FMBS and FMPS, are higher than 90% (6.48 and 6.49) and it is hard for the patient to maintain home hygiene due to crowding; for these reasons orthodontics appears to be the ideal therapy for the resolution of the crowding, becoming a periodontal treatment, and sublimating and legitimizing the initial esthetic request proposed by the patient. The resolution of the lower edentulism with the uprighting of the 4.7 molar allows the placement of the implant in 4.6 position, recreating an ideal site[40], in an environment that is more favourable to maintain the oral hygiene.

An indirect (Hiro System®[41]) lingual (Kurz 7th Generation®, Ormco) bonding is performed, first with a .016 CuNiTi archwire (6.50 and 6.51), then with a .016 β-titanium archwire and subsequently with a .017×.017 β-titanium, with torque control of 2.3 (6.52 and 6.53) and, then, with a .017×.025 β-titanium for stabilization and correction of the torque of the upper left canine. An implant (Xive®, Dentsply) is placed in the 4.6 edentulous area, after 4.7 uprighting to correct the tooth parallelism (6.54; see 3.5). At the end of the therapy the patient shows facial symmetry and labial competence (6.55), a class II molar occlusion on the left and class I molar on the right, canine class I (6.56) and normalization of the cephalometric values (6.57) (see 6.3). The periodontal indexes (FMBS and FMPS) (6.58) at the end of the therapy are reduced below 15%, confirming the periodontal contribution by orthodontic treatment.

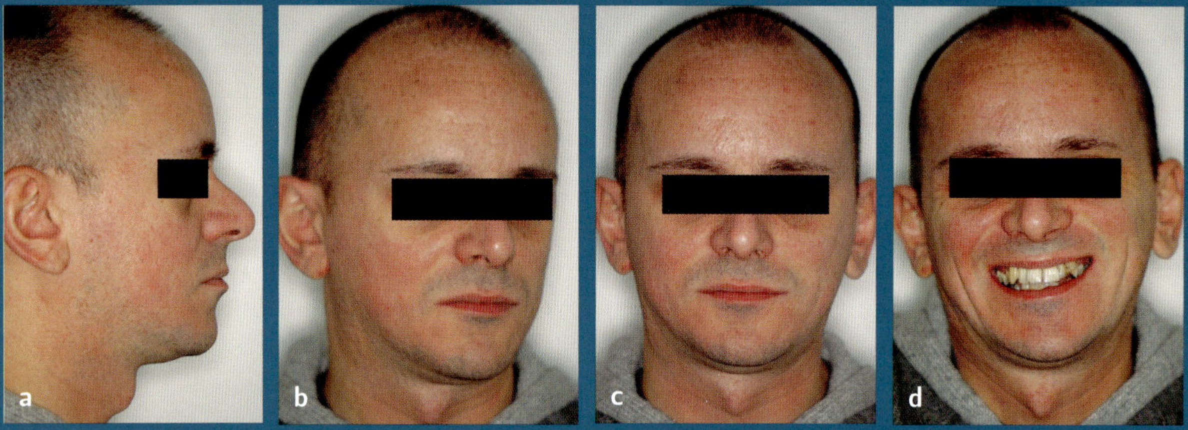

6.45 Extraoral pre-treatment photos.

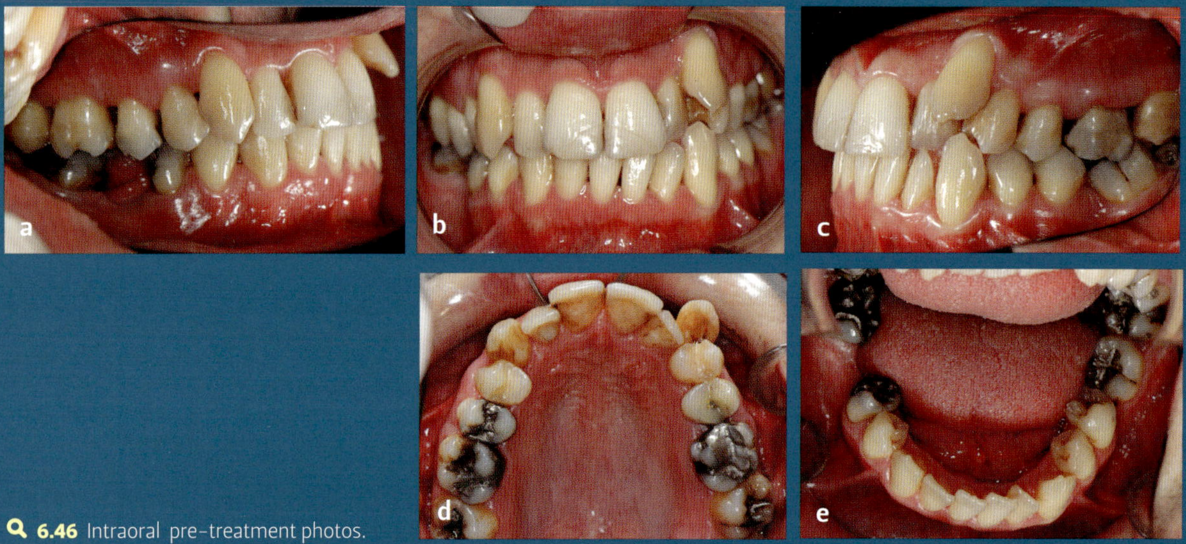

6.46 Intraoral pre-treatment photos.

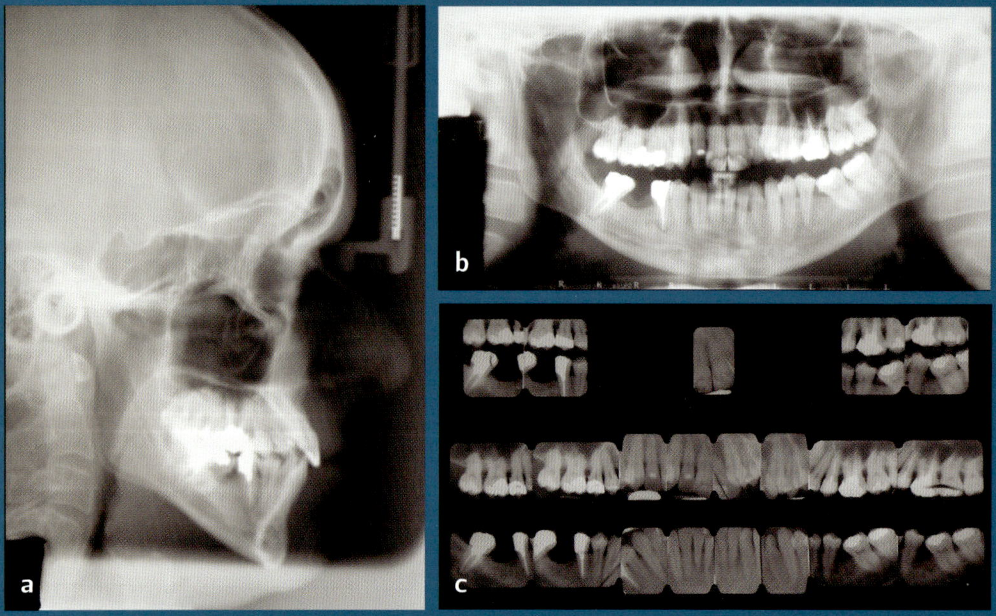

6.47 Pre-treatment cephalometric Rx (**a**), panoramic Rx (**b**), full radiographic periodontal status (**c**).

Tab. 6.3 Cephalometric values

Sagittal skeletal relationships	Pre-treatment	Post-treatment	Mean	DS
Maxillary sagittal relationship SNA	84°	85°	82°	3.5°
Mandibular sagittal relationship SNPg	83°	84°	80°	3.5°
Intermaxillary sagittal relationship ANPg	1°	1°	2°	2.5°
Vertical skeletal relationships				
Maxillary vertical relationship SN / ANS-PNS	6°	3°	8°	3.0°
Mandibular vertical relationship SN / Go-Gn	32°	30°	33°	2.5°
Intermaxillary vertical relationship ANS-PNS / Go-Gn	26°	27°	25°	6.0°
Dento-basal relationships				
Upper incisor inclination 1 - ANS-PNS	114°	108°	110°	6.0°
Lower incisor inclination 1 - Go-Gn	84°	85°	94°	7.0°
Lower incisor compensation 1 - A-Pg (mm)	+2	+2	2	2.0
Dental relationships				
Overjet (OVJ, mm)	3	2	3,5	2.5
Overbite (OVB, mm)	3	2	2	2.5
Interincisal Angle 1 / 1	137°	137°	132°	6.0°

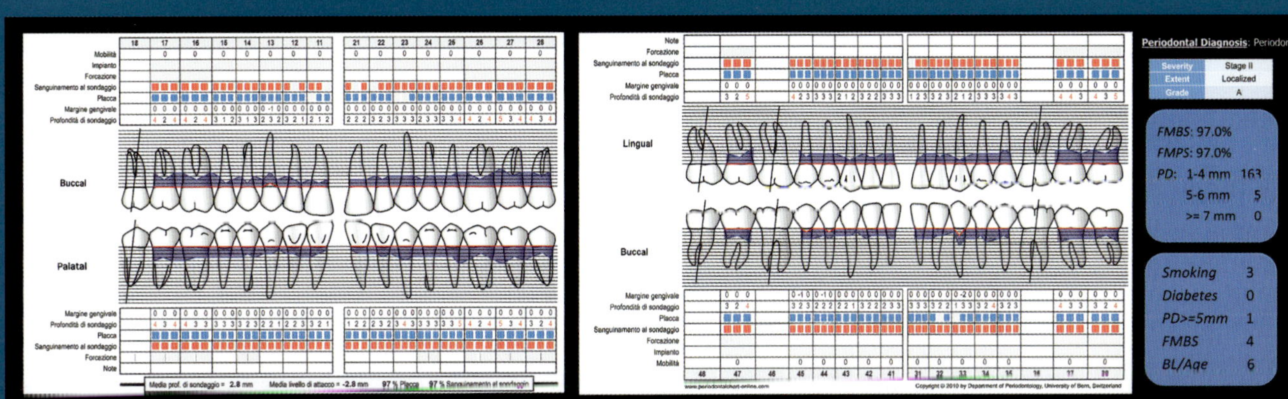

6.48 Initial periodontal probing, periodontal indexes, risk assessment (Online periodontal charting tool from www.perio-tools.com).

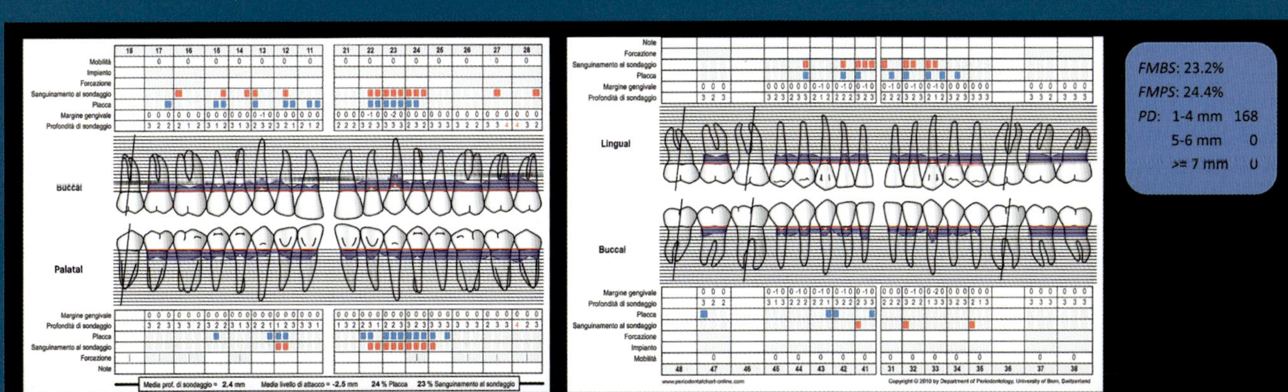

6.49 Re-evaluation periodontal probing and periodontal indexes (Online periodontal charting tool from www.perio-tools.com).

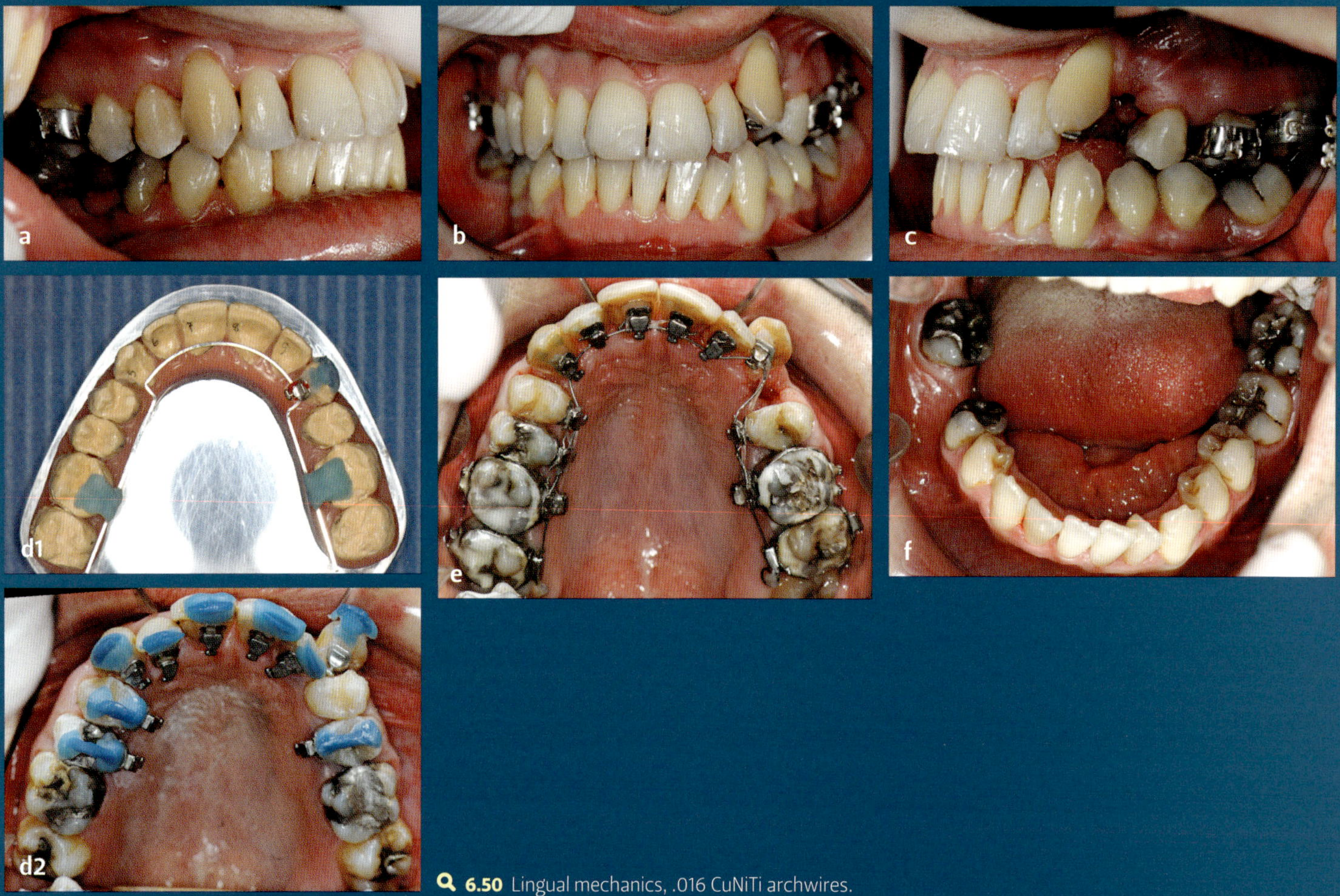

6.50 Lingual mechanics, .016 CuNiTi archwires.

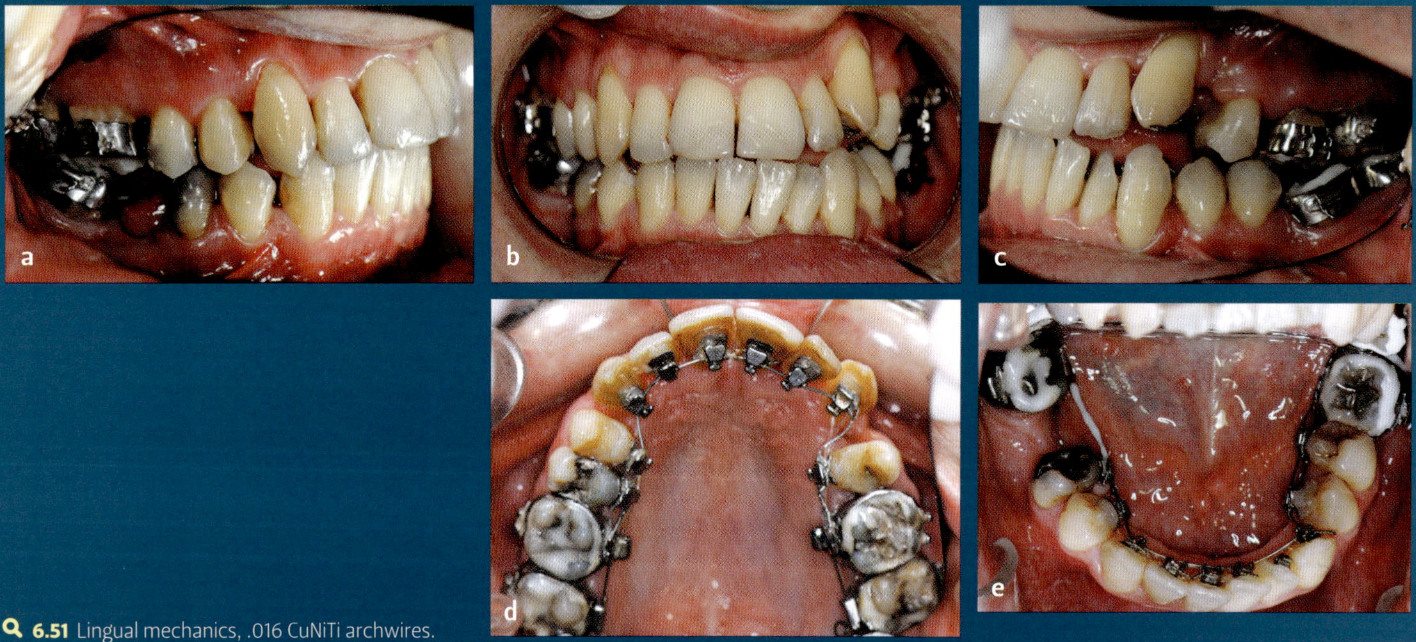

6.51 Lingual mechanics, .016 CuNiTi archwires.

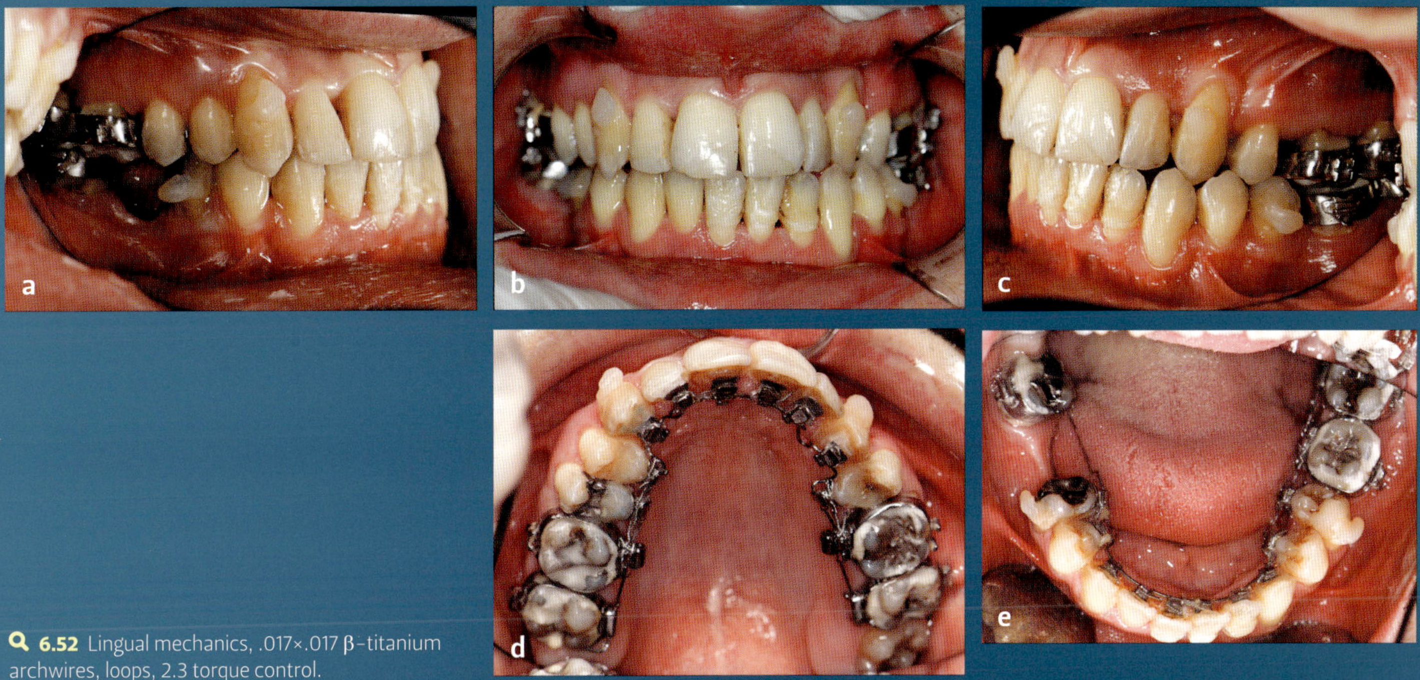

6.52 Lingual mechanics, .017×.017 β-titanium archwires, loops, 2.3 torque control.

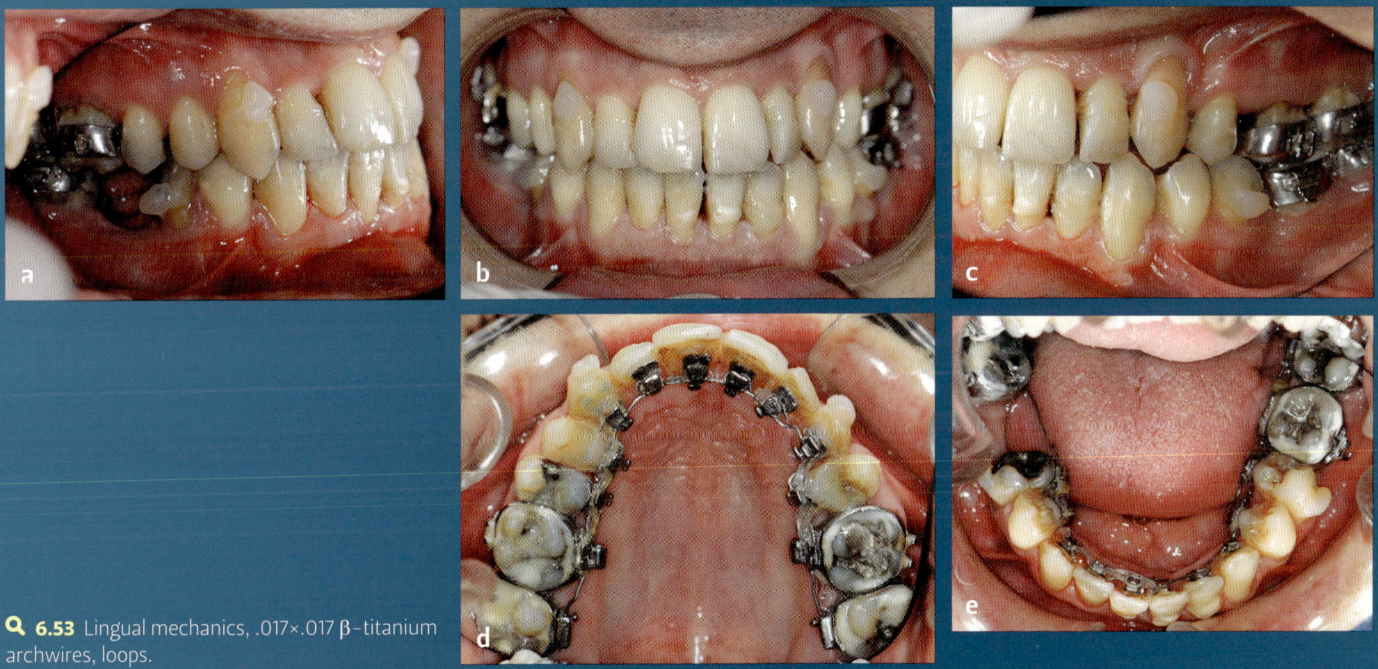

6.53 Lingual mechanics, .017×.017 β-titanium archwires, loops.

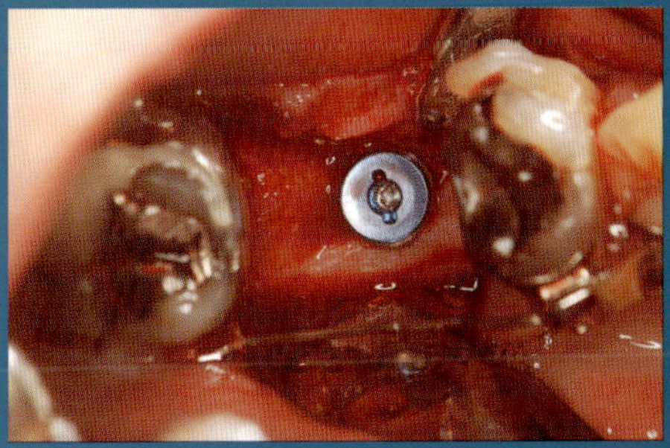

6.54 Clinical view of the implant placement.

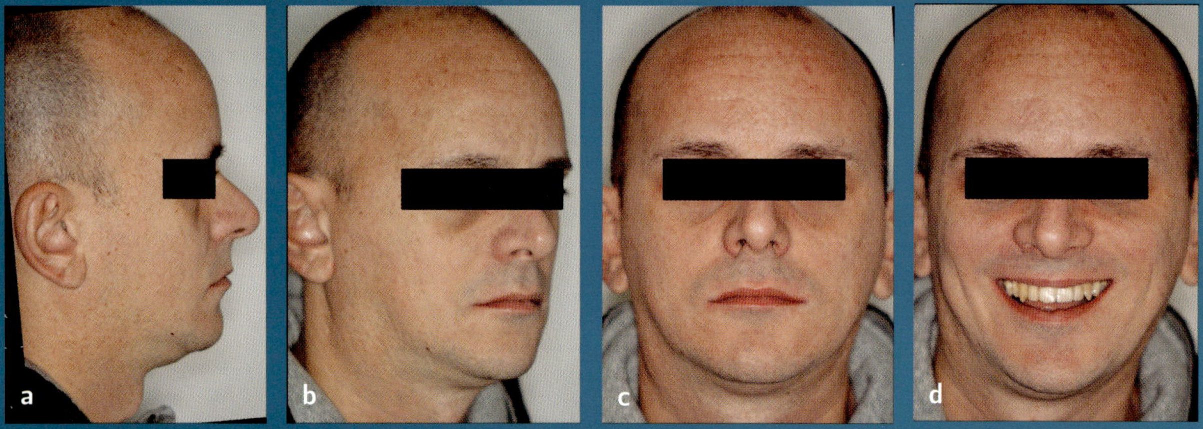

6.55 Extraoral post-treatment photos.

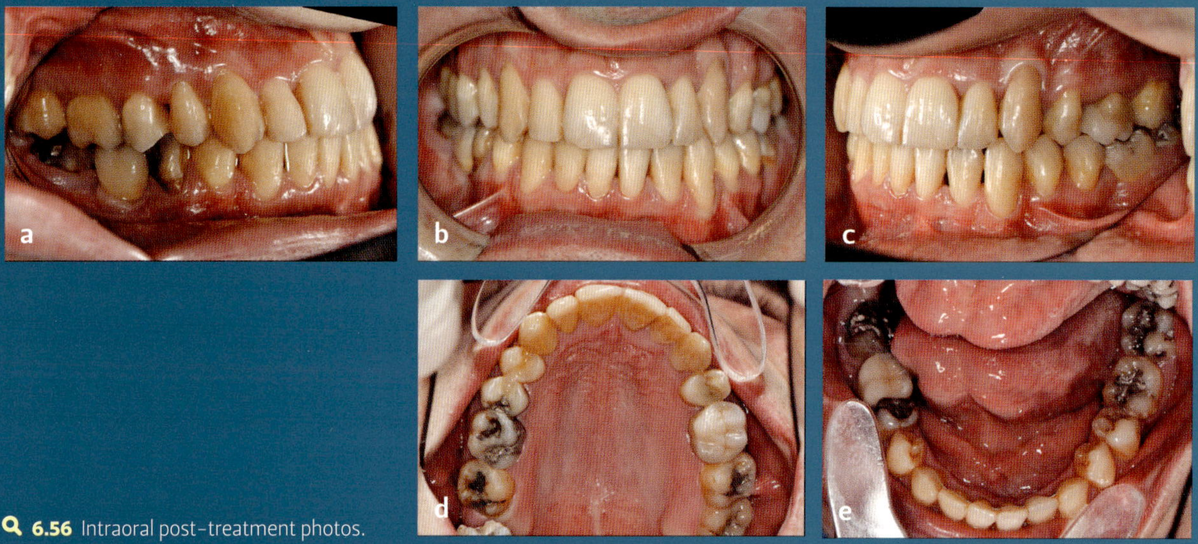

6.56 Intraoral post-treatment photos.

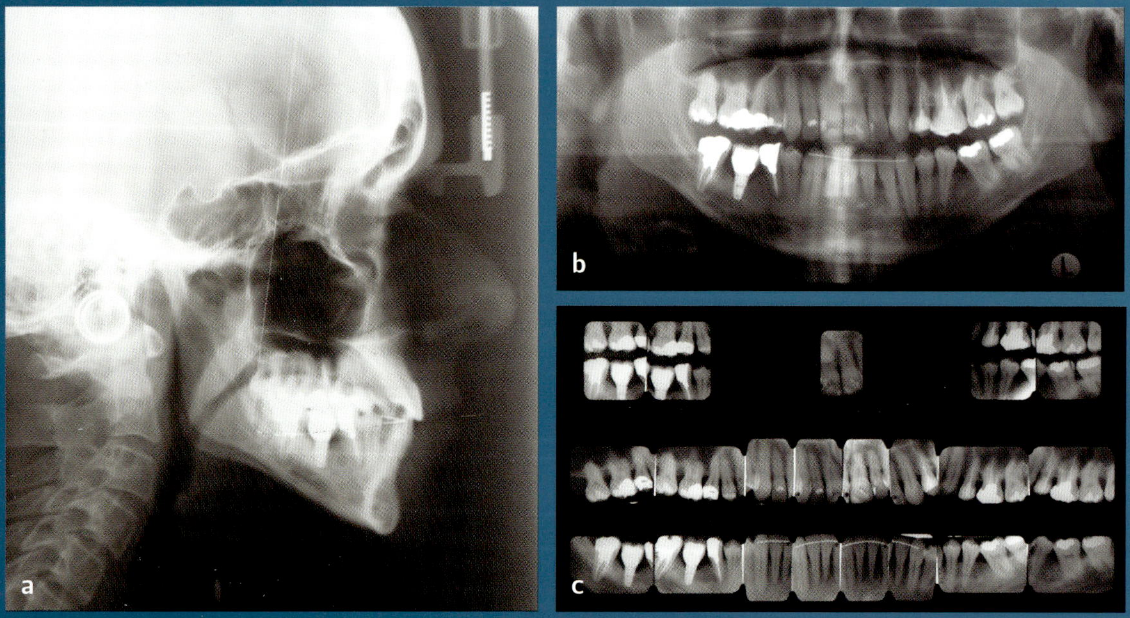

6.57 Post-treatment cephalometric Rx (**a**), panoramic Rx (**b**), full radiographic periodontal status (**c**).

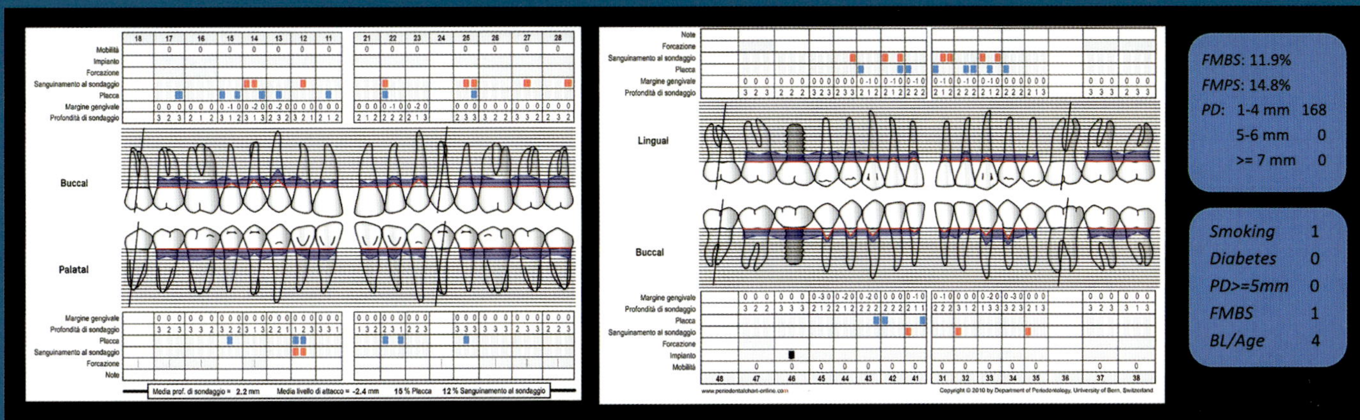

6.58 Post-treatment periodontal probing, periodontal indexes, risk assessment (Online periodontal charting tool from www.perio-tools.com).

REFERENCES

1. VANARSDALL RL. Orthodontics and periodontal therapy. *Periodontol 2000*. 1995;9(1):132-149.
2. MELSEN B, AGERBAEK N. Orthodontics as an adjunct to rehabilitation. *Periodontol 2000*. 1994;4(1):148-159.
3. CARDAROPOLI D, GAVEGLIO L. The influence of orthodontic movement on periodontal tissues level. *Semin Orthod*. 2007;13(4):234-245.
4. PAOLONE MG, KAITSAS R, KAITSAS F. Lingual orthodontics in an adult patient with upper premolar extraction: case report. *Int Orthod*. 2020;18(1):165-177.
5. BRAGA G, BOCCHIERI A. A new flapless technique for crown lengthening after orthodontic extrusion. *Int J Periodontics Restorative Dent*. 2012;32(1):81-90.
6. JANSON M, JANSON G, MURILLO-GOIZUETA OE. A modified orthodontic protocol for advanced periodontal disease in Class II division 1 malocclusion. *Am J Orthod Dentofacial Orthop*. 2011;139(4 Suppl):S133-S144.
7. MATHEWS DP, KOKICH VG. Managing treatment for the orthodontic patient with periodontal problems. *Semin Orthod*. 1997;3(1):21-38.
8. KOKICH VG. *Adjunctive role of orthodontic therapy*. In: Newman MG, Takei HH, Klokkevold PR, Carranza FA. *Clinical periodontology*, 13th Ed. Philadelphia, Elsevier; 2019:582-583e1-e13.
9. PALOMO L, PAOLOMO JM, BISSADA NF. Salient periodontal issues for the modern biologic orthodontist. *Semin Orthod*. 2008;14(4):229-245.
10. KORNMAN KS, TONETTI MS. Proceedings of the World Workshop on the Classification of Periodontal and Peri-Implant Diseases and Conditions. *J Periodontol*. 2018;89(Suppl 1):S1-S291.
11. KORNMAN KS, TONETTI MS. Proceedings of the World Workshop on the Classification of Periodontal and Peri-Implant Diseases and Conditions. *J Clin Periodontol*. 2018;45(Suppl 20):S1-S291.
12. TROMBELLI L, MINENNA L, TOSELLI L ET AL. Prognostic value of a simplified method for periodontal risk assessment during supportive periodontal therapy. *J Clin Periodontol*. 2017;44(1):51-57.
13. TROMBELLI L, FARINA R, FERRARI S ET AL. Comparison between two methods for periodontal risk assessment. *Minerva Stomatol*. 2009;58(6):277-287.
14. FARINA R, FERRARI S, PASETTI P ET AL. Comparison between two methods for periodontal risk assessment. Abstracts of the 6th International, Congress of the European Federation of Periodontology (Europerio 6), Stockholm, June 4-6 2009. *J. Clin Periodontol*. 2009;36(S9):82(abstr. #157).
15. SAGA AY, MARUO IT, MARUO H ET AL. Treatment of an adult with several missing teeth and atrophic old mandibular first molar extraction sites. *Am J Orthod Dentofacial Orthop*. 2011;140(6):869-878.
16. ANTOUN JS, MEI L, GIBBS K, FARELLA M. Effect of orthodontic treatment on the periodontal tissues. *Periodontol 2000*. 2017;74(1):140-157.
17. CZOCHROWSKA EM, ROSA M. The orthodontic/periodontal interface. *Semin Orthod* 2015;21(1):3-14.
18. DREYER H, GRISCHKE J, TIEDE C ET AL. Epidemiology and risk factors of peri-implantitis: a systematic review. *J Periodontal Res*. 2018;53(5):657-681.
19. PAPAPANOU PN, SANZ M, BUDUNELI N ET AL. Periodontitis: consensus report of workgroup 2 of the 2017 World Workshop on the Classification of Periodontal and Peri-Implant Diseases and Conditions. *J Periodontol*. 2018;89(Suppl 1):S173-S182.
20. MELSEN B. Tissue reaction to orthodontic tooth movement - a new paradigm. *Eur J Orthod*. 2001;23(6):671-681.
21. REITAN K. Clinical and histologic observations on tooth movement during and after orthodontic treatment. *Am J Orthod*. 1967;53(10):721-745.

22. **Fontenelle A.** Concetti parodontali dello spostamento dentale guidato. *S.I.D.O. Syllabus*. 1992;2.

23. **Fontenelle A.** Une conception parodontale du mouvement dentaire provoqué: évidences cliniques [A periodontal concept of induced tooth movement: clinical evidence]. *Rev Orthop Dento Faciale*. 1982;16(1):37-53.

24. **Kokich VG.** Maxillary lateral incisor implants: planning with the aid of orthodontics. *J Oral Maxillofac Surg*. 2004;62(9 Suppl 2):48-56.

25. **Borzabadi-Farahani A, Zadeh HH.** Adjunctive orthodontic applications in dental implantology. *J Oral Implantol*. 2015;41(4):501-508.

26. **Gkantidis N, Christou P, Topouzelis N.** The orthodontic-periodontic interrelationship in integrated treatment challenges: a systematic review. *J Oral Rehabil*. 2010;37(5):377-390.

27. **Thilander B.** Infrabony pockets and reduced alveolar height in relation to orthodontic therapy. *Semin Orthod*. 1996;2(1): 55-61.

28. **Lindskog-Stokland B, Wennström JL, Nyman S, Thilander B.** Orthodontic tooth movement into edentulous areas with reduced bone height. An experimental study in the dog. *Eur J Orthod*. 1993;15(2):89-96.

29. **Chiu G, Chang C, Roberts WE.** Interdisciplinary treatment for a compensated Class II partially edentulous malocclusion: orthodontic creation of a posterior implant site. *Am J Orthod Dentofacial Orthop*. 2018;153(3):422-435.

30. **Diedrich PR, Fuhrmann RA, Wehrbein H, Erpenstein H.** Distal movement of premolars to provide posterior abutments for missing molars. *Am J Orthod Dentofacial Orthop*. 1996;109(4):355-360.

31. **Cheng LL, Türk T, Elekdağ-Türk S et al.** Repair of root resorption 4 and 8 weeks after application of continuous light and heavy forces on premolars for 4 weeks: a histology study. *Am J Orthod Dentofacial Orthop*. 2010;138(6):727-734.

32. **Amato F, Mirabella AD, Borlizzi D.** Rapid orthodontic treatment after the ridge-splitting technique - a combined surgical-orthodontic approach for implant site development: case report. *Int J Periodontics Restorative Dent*. 2012;32(4):395-402.

33. **Diedrich PR.** Guided tissue regeneration associated with orthodontic therapy. *Semin Orthod*. 1996;2(1):39-45.

34. **Stepovich ML.** A clinical study on closing edentulous spaces in the mandible. *Angle Orthod*. 1979;49(4):227-233.

35. **Han JY.** A comparative study of combined periodontal and orthodontic treatment with fixed appliances and clear aligners in patients with periodontitis. *J Periodontal Implant Sci*. 2015;45(6):193-204.

36. **El-Mangoury NH, Gaafar SM, Mostafa YA.** Mandibular anterior crowding and periodontal disease. *Angle Orthod*. 1987;57(1):33-38.

37. **Alexander AG, Tipnis AK.** The effect of irregularity of teeth and the degree of overbite and overjet on the gingival health. A study of 400 subjects. *Br Dent J*. 1970;128(11):539-544.

38. **Kraal JH, Digiancinto JJ, Dail RA et al.** Periodontal conditions in patients after molar uprighting. *J Prosthet Dent*. 1980;43(2):156-162.

39. **Glans R, Larsson E, Øgaard B.** Longitudinal changes in gingival condition in crowded and noncrowded dentitions subjected to fixed orthodontic treatment. *Am J Orthod Dentofacial Orthop*. 2003;124(6):679-682.

40. **Maeda S, Ono Y, Nakamura K, Kuwahara T.** Molar uprighting with extrusion for implant site bone regeneration and improvement of the periodontal environment [published correction appears in *Int J Periodontics Restorative Dent*. 2008;28(5):451]. *Int J Periodontics Restorative Dent*. 2008;28(4):375-381.

41. **Hiro T, Iglesia FD, Andreu P.** Indirect bonding technique in lingual orthodontics: the HIRO system. *Prog Orthod*. 2008;9(2):34-45.

Phenotypes and orthodontics

Notes on the new classification

Mucogingival conditions

The current classification of mucogingival conditions[1-3] takes into consideration the anatomy and it is therapy-oriented. It classifies recessions into:

- RT1: gingival recession without loss of interproximal attachment. The cemento-enamel junction is not clinically detectable on the mesial and distal aspects of the tooth (📷 7.1);
- RT2: gingival recession associated with a loss of interproximal attachment less than or equal to the loss of vestibular attachment (📷 7.2);
- RT3: gingival recession associated with a loss of interproximal attachment greater than the loss of vestibular attachment (📷 7.3).

The assessment of the exposed root surface was also included in the classification with the registration of the presence or absence of the cemento-enamel junction (class A/B) and the presence or absence of cervical abrasion >0.5 mm (+/–, present/absent) (📷 7.4).

Biotype and phenotype

From a tissutal point of view, three types of gingival biotype can be observed, with their own characteristics and different clinical behaviors[4]: thick, thin and mixed. In the 📷 7.5-7.7 the three types of biotype are represented and their clinical characteristics are shown in 📁 7.1.

After the introduction of the new classification it is preferred to use the term phenotype[1,2] instead of biotype, because this term combines genetic aspects with environmental factors. It must be noted that the gingival phenotype is site-specific, because it has gingival and bone components that can change over time in relation to environmental factors at the level of the single tooth itself and comparing them with the contralateral ones[5].

Anyhow, it is important to understand that gingival phenotypic expression always depends on a genetically predetermined biotype where external environmental factors can modify the locus, always acting on a genetic substrate. It is the knowledge of the clinical characteristics of these different phenotypes that allows to manage an orthodontic case in complete safety from a mucogingival point of view.

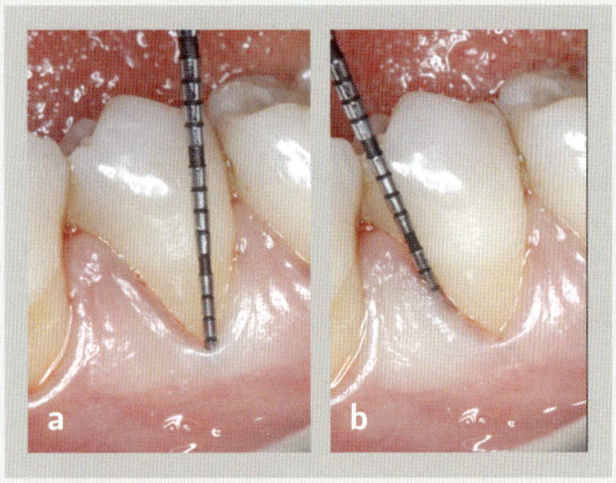

7.1 Recession RT1 type.

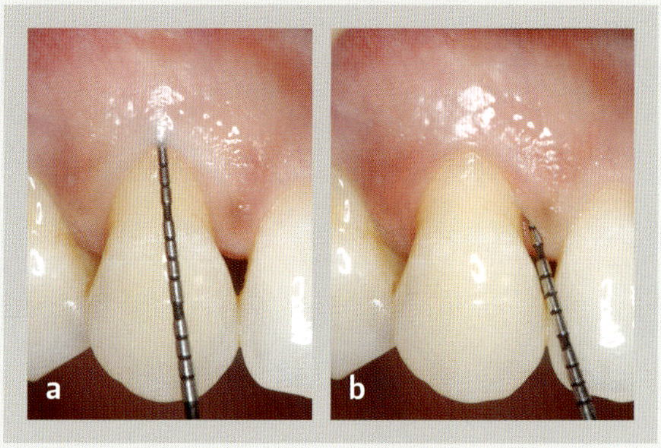

7.2 Recession RT2 type.

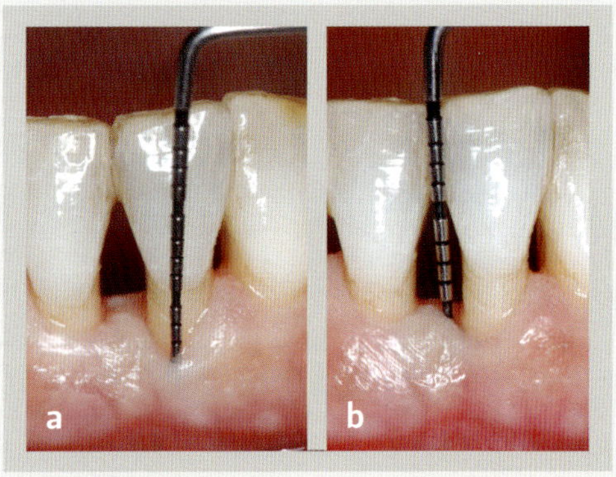

7.3 Recession RT3 type.

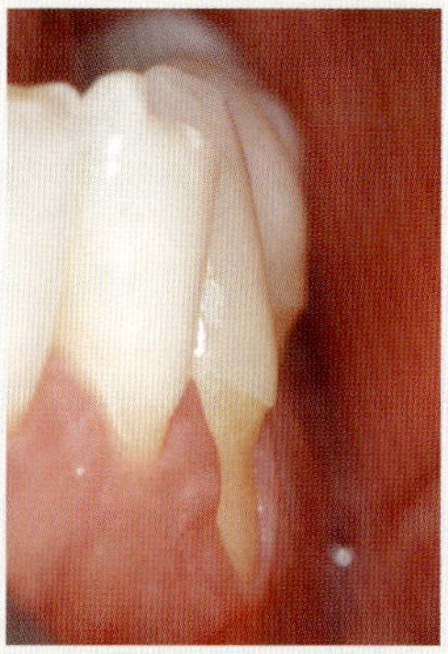

7.4 Lateral view of a recession with abrasion (Class B+).

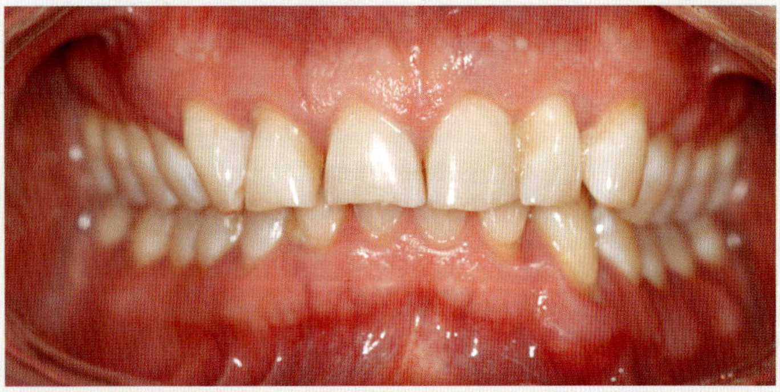

7.5 Clinical view of the thick biotype.

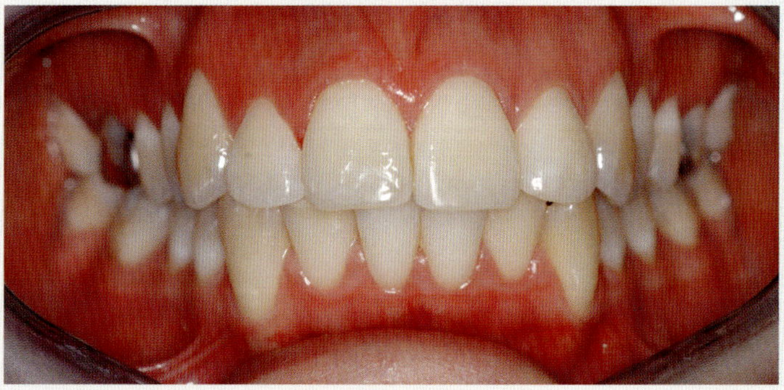

7.6 Clinical view of the thin biotype.

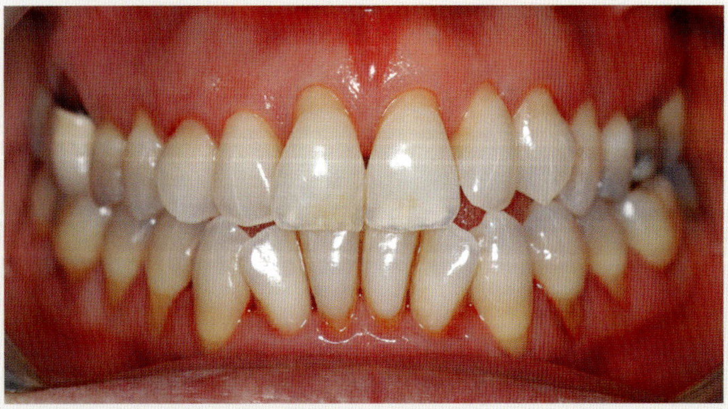

7.7 Clinical view of the thick scalloped biotype.

Tab. 7.1 Gingival biotype with related characteristic

Biotype	Clinical characteristic
Thick	Thick and voluminous gingiva with large area of KT (keratinized tissue)
	Slightly scalloped or flat margins
	Short and wide teeth
	Wide and more apical contact areas
	Short interdental papillae
Thin	Thin gingiva with narrow zone of KT (keratinized tissue)
	Scalloped gingival margins
	Long and slender teeth with conical shape
	Incisally positioned contact areas
Thick scalloped	Thick fibrotic gingiva
	Slender teeth
	Narrow area of KT
	Scalloped pronounced gingival margins

Substrate and irritative stimuli

In order to determine in which way the orthodontic movement is related to present and future mucogingival aspects, it is important to analyse the risk factors present in the patient before starting treatment and to be aware of the clinical characteristics that must alert the clinician about the future onset of mucogingival defects.

During tooth movement the periodontal tissues must hold a stable relationship around the cervical area of the tooth. An adequate amount of attached gingiva is needed to maintain gingival health and to allow orthodontic mechanics to provide controlled treatment[6]. As a consequence, it is important that the soft tissues maintain and/or increase their thickness and/or height in order to manage the keratinized gingiva during the orthodontic movement. It is not orthodontics that causes mucogingival problems, but it is the presence of irritative, traumatic or bacterial stimuli, with the increase of inflammation in a susceptible substrate, such as thin phenotypes. Therefore, as we have already previously stated, it is important to evaluate the risk factors that can determine a worsening of soft tissues situation, in particular not only the thickness of the tissue and the amount of keratinized gingiva, but also all the cofactors that determine the probability of developing gingival recessions.

Anatomical considerations and recessions

There is still a controversy about the relationship between orthodontic treatment and gingival recessions, since the scientific evidence regarding the role that orthodontic treatment plays in the development of the gingival recessions is insufficient. We must always keep in mind the signs that can evolve into recessions. Therefore, which factors need to be evaluated in particular in order to correlate – if there are any correlations – tooth movement with an increased risk of recession formation? Among many factors the literature in particular analyses the incisors inclination, the shape of the symphysis and the amount of keratinized tissue.

Incisors inclination

Renkema et al.[7], in 2013, limited to a study on plaster models, stated in the conclusions that orthodontic treatment and/or the retention phase may be risk factors for the development of labial gingival recessions, showing a greater vulnerability of the mandibular incisors, and that it is not possible to differentiate which element of orthodontic treatment among the position of the incisors, the appliance itself or retention, has a predominant effect on the occourence of recessions in the lower incisors. Their study was retrospective, with data collected from plaster models with no other periodontal parameters[7]. The same Authors[8], in the same year, reported that the prevalence of gingival recessions, always studied on plaster models, steadly increases after orthodontic treatment: the prevalence was higher in treated patients aged >16 years and there was a continuous increase of 7% at the end of the treatment, 20% at 2 years and 38% at 5 years, without association with the sex, extractions, or type of lingual fixed retainers[8]; this actually showed a trend which was similar to the one observed in epidemiological studies[8,9,10], with a higher risk on maxillary canines, first premolars and first molars and mandibular lower incisors and first premolars, and a higher prevalence in elderly patients compared to young patients[8].

Melsen and Allais[11] also demonstrated that in post-orthodontic patients the prevalence of recessions >0.1 mm increased from 21% pre-treatment to 35%; only 2.8% developed recessions >2 mm and 5% of pre-existing recessions improved. Some Authors, in various studies and systematic reviews[12-14], found no evidence on association between the proclination movement of incisors and gingival recessions, concluding that fixed orthodontic appliances cannot be considered a risk for gingival recession. Only slight inconsistent tissue recession (mean 0.03 mm [0.01-0.04 mm]) was found in patients with orthodontic appliances[15], and a recent meta-analysis[16] (0.06 mm; 0,01/0.13 mm) showed that this data is clinically irrelevant.

Gebistorf et al.[17] showed that, about 15 years after treatment, the prevalence of gingival recession (85.2%) in orthodontically treated patients was similar to the one of untreated patients; patients who experienced recession on single teeth during orthodontic treatment were at risk of developing recessions on other teeth after treatment[18,19]. These data indicate that the tendency to develop recessions is not correlated with the treatment but with the patient's own predisposition to develop recessions. Therefore, it can be said that there is no correlation between the incisors proclination and the development of gingival recessions, as also reported by Ruf et al.[20] in patients treated with Herbst with a proclination of the lower incisors up to a mean of 8.9°, and by Artun and Grobéty[21], Djeu et al.[22] and Tepedino et al.[13]. This movement does not increase the risk of developing a gingival recession[23], since it does not lead to a significant deterioration of the periodontium with an average recession value of 0.36 mm in treated patients and 0.22 mm in the controls[24].

Some Authors have related the development of recessions with the proclination movement of the lower incisors; these conclusions, reported in the systematic reviews by Joss-Vassalli et al.[25] and Bin Bahar et al.[26], because of the low level of evidence of the included studies and the contradictory results, should be interpreted with great caution. A slight correlation has also been reported in relation to the extent of proclination of the incisors by Antonarakis et al.[27], who state that an orthodontic-surgical proclination of the lower incisors beyond the limit of 10° increases the risk of inducing lingual gingival recessions, without reporting correlation with vestibular recessions. This value would seem to be the limit beyond which the orthodontic action on the lower incisors should not be pushed beyond; in these cases, the option to reduce this risk is represented by osteogenetic distraction[27].

The association between orthodontics and recession, therefore, is probably due to the fact that the positioning of the teeth in the alveolar process in the buccal-lingual direction shows an increased variability in relation to the gingival tissues. If orthodontic treatment is performed under conditions of biomechanical and periodontal control, the risk of developing periodontal damage due to protrusion of the incisors is minimal and the recessions of the lower incisors do not increase significantly during this movement[11,28].

Shape of the symphysis

Three types of symphysis (narrow, intermediate and wide) and the initial inclination of the lower incisors were compared on cephalometric X-rays; the initial inclination was initially greater in the broad symphysis group, but the change in incisor inclination (about 5°) was similar in all the three groups and remained stable 5 years after treatment with an anterior movement of the root at the alveolar level of 0.4 mm in uncontrolled tipping and 1.1 mm in controlled tipping[29]. It is important to keep in mind that the external dimensions of the symphysis are not *per se* equivalent to an increased or decreased thickness of the alveolar bone supporting the incisors[29]. There are no data that the general morphology of the symphysis is associated with the development of gingival recessions[29]. The relationship between the height of the symphysis and the width at the crestal level showed a statistically significant association with the presence of buccal and lingual recessions. A proclination of incisors >10° showed an association with the onset of recessions in 25%[30]. There is no association between the cephalometrically measured thickness of the alveolar process and the development of recessions, but it can be hypothesized that persons with a thin alveolar process are more susceptible to develop gingival recessions due to a possible gingival phenotype, that, providing a weaker support, is a predisposing factor to the progression of the recession caused by external etiological factors[30]. In a study with CBCT, Garlock et al.[31] analysed the relationship between the position of the incisors and the height of the alveolar marginal bone, evaluating the possible associations between the initial bone characteristics and the amount of changes in the vertical height of the alveolar bone. A pretreatment thinner mandibular symphysis and cortical bone at the dental apex were associated with an increased loss of buccal vertical bone, with thinning of the cortical bone on the surface that showed vertical bone loss. A change in the incisor inclination in the mandibular plane was not related to the loss of vertical vestibular bone, while movements of the apex of the mandibular incisors towards the cortical bone produced greater amounts of vertical bone loss. The greater was the movement of the root apex towards the vestibular cortical bone, the greater was the reduction of the vestibular bone; a cortical bone thinning occurred on the surface affected by vertical bone loss[31].

It is important to underline that the apex can move towards the cortical bone through different types of movement, such as uncontrolled tipping, translation or proclination with bodily movement, and that all these movements must be foreseen and constantly re-evaluated during the whole mechanics.

Soft tissue thickness and keratinized tissue

Two aspects have been analysed in relation to the effects of orthodontic movement on the mucogingival complex: the variation of the size of the gingival tissue and the request for a gingival width to maintain the integrity of the attachment apparatus in particular environmental stresses. Two considerations must be kept in mind in orthodontic movement: the first is the fact that the evolution and developmental of the dentition in the spontaneous change of the buccal-lingual dental position during eruption influences the gingival height[32,33], the second is the observation of the thickening of the vestibular tissue dimensions after a lingual movement in a more protected position in the alveolar process of a buccally positioned tooth[18,34].

Since the mucogingival line is genetically predetermined and, therefore, it is a non-modifiable anatomical landmark[35], and since the gingiva is anchored to the supracrestal portion of the root, we will have two effects: the gingiva will follow the tooth in its extrusive movements, increasing the mucogingival junction-gingival margin distance, and the bone tissue will follow the movement, increasing the height of the bone crest[36].

The experimental dental bodily movement on monkeys in areas with different thickness and soft tissue quality showed an apical displacement of the gingival margin and less resistance to probing, but not a histological loss of connective attachment level; furthermore, the size of the gingival unit was smaller in the buccally moved teeth at both the apico-coronal and the bucco-lingual level[37]. This lower resistance to probing can perhaps be explained, according to Wennström, with the reduction of the height and thickness of the soft tissues, which would enhance the destructive effect of the plaque and the associated inflammatory lesion on a reduced bucco-lingual dimension; this finding is validated by observations that, in the presence of plaque-induced gingivitis, a thin marginal tissue is more susceptible to destruction than a thick one[38,39], while an orthodontic bodily movement *per se* in the absence of plaque does not cause destruction of the connective tissue attachment[40]. Therefore, it was the plaque-induced inflammation and the thickness in terms of volume of the marginal soft tissues, rather than the quality (gingiva or alveolar mucosa) and the apico-coronal width of the keratinized attached gingiva, that were the determining factors for the development of gingival recessions during orthodontic movement[37]. It is important to remember that extensive tipping and intrusive orthodontic forces can promote attachment loss due to the subgingival displacement of plaque as reported by Ericsson et al.[41]

Thin tissues[5] and thin cortical bone are more prone to gingival recession than normal or thick tissues, with a range of 1.3-10%. It is reported that a minimum of 2 mm of keratinized gingiva should be present to counteract orthodontic forces and prevent recessions[42]. In the presence of a thin biotype, this value is considered the limit beyond which a site can evolve with the highest probability into a recession, a boundary beyond which a gingival augmentation could be indicated, knowing, however, that this data is based only on clinical observations with a low level of evidence[43]. When corrective surgery must be performed, sites with gingiva >1-2 mm are associated with more predictable positive surgical outcomes[5]. However, the elimination of the inflammatory infiltrate from the tissues through excellent oral hygiene[5] avoids the formation of gingival recessions regardless of the thickness of the present gingival tissue[44]. However, attached gingiva is important to maintain gingival health in patients with suboptimal plaque control[5,43]. In a recent meta-analysis[16] on gingival recessions in treated and untreated patients, orthodontic therapy appears to be associated with a higher risk of developing at least one recession, both at the patient level (a treated patient has a double risk of developing recession compared to the untreated ones) and at the tooth level (risk greater than 1.81 times). It is important to note that in this meta-analysis the assessment of the presence of recessions was performed in binary evaluation (present/not present) regardless of the extension. This resulted in a loss of information, because even small recessions were considered as a presence of recessions.

Yared et al.[45] evaluated the risk assessment putting into correlation the mucogingival tissues and the final inclination of the mandibular incisors concluding that the factors associated with the incidence and the severity of gingival recessions of the mandibular incisors are the thickness of the free gingival margin (<0,5 mm) and the incisors final inclination (>95°), where the tissue thickness is more important than the final inclination. Wennström[36] confirmed this observation, stating that the labial tooth movement or the dental proclination does not cause gingival recession *per se*, but that in some cases this proclination will result in a reduced bucco-lingual tissue thickness and thereby a reduced height of the free gingival portion and an increased clinical crown height which include regions of low resistance to the inflammation and trauma. In this regard, the 1993 Consensus of the European Workshop on Periodontology[46] had already established that a surgical increase in apico-coronal width cannot be justifiable to maintain periodontal health and prevent soft tissue recessions, since traumatic brushing is one of the main factors associated together with bacterial plaque even in orthodontic patients.

Although orthodontic treatment can be a contributing factor to the development of recessions, it does not necessarily lead to their formation. There is no single cause for the development of recessions[23]. A series of correlated risk factors have been proposed[11,16] which can be predisposing, because already present, or precipitating because leading to an acceleration of the defect[9,47,48] (Tab. 7.2). These factors are summarized by the same Authors with the acronym ABEF, where A (Anatomy) represents the anatomical data such as alveolar bone dehiscences and radicular proximity, where CBCT can be an aid to the pre-treatment diagnosis[49]; B (Biotype), the gingival biotype; E (Environment), hygiene, traumatic brushing, smoking, parafunctions, bad habits, piercing, fixed retainers, unsuitable mechanics, age, pregnancy and skeletal pattern; F (Functional Matrix), the small thickness of the symphysis and the ectopic eruption.

Tab. 7.2 Risk factors for gingival recessions

Predisposing factors	Precipitating factors
Anatomic and morphologic characteristic, like bone dehiscence	Traumatic tooth brushing
Gingival phenotype	Traumatic overbite
Skeletal pattern	Age
Ectopic eruption	Smoking habits
Symphysis	Parafunctional habits
	Pregnancy
	Piercing

To minimize the risk of recessions and maximize the benefits of orthodontic treatment, clinicians must take into account not only the dental crowns, but also the roots and their proximity to the cortical bone and the soft and hard tissues, through excellent oral hygiene throughout the treatment and during supportive therapy. Clinicians must help to eliminate the potential causes of recessions (piercing, smoking, traumatic brushing), avoid uncontrolled dentoalveolar movements, consider atypical extractions (for example compromised and non-restorable teeth), avoid jiggling and, above all, perform early treatment with orthopaedic-interceptive procedures and therapies in mixed dentition[47] (see *Clinical case 2*).

The clinical conclusions written by Wennström[36], published in 1996 but still current, are important: during the orthodontic movement there are alterations in the mucogingival complex, but these alterations are independent from the apico-coronal width of the gingiva. Lingual tooth displacement will result in an increased buccal soft tissue thickness with coronal migration of the soft tissue margin and decreased height of the clinical crown; so if this movement is planned there is no need either to perform pre-orthodontics gingival vestibular augmentation procedures in cases of thin gingiva, or to carry out a mucogingival surgical procedure to cover pre-orthodontic recession defects; in fact, after a lingual movement of the tooth towards the center of the alveolar process, the recession could decrease and a possible surgery could be more predictable. On the contrary, a vestibular movement will reduce the vestibulo-lingual and apico-coronal tissue thickness[36]. Recessions will not develop because of tooth movement within the alveolar process envelope, but in the case that the movement might result in a bone dehiscence. Furthermore, the thickness of the overlying soft tissues must be evaluated and cannot be considered a factor that influences the formation of recessions during and post orthodontic treatment; orthodontics, *per se*, does not cause recession, but an eventual resulting thin gingiva would be a *locus minoris resistentiae* in the presence of bacterial plaque and/or brushing trauma, which could encourage the development of soft tissue defects. That is why we prefer to talk about the gingival phenotype, and not just about the biotype. Also for this reason the interceptive orthodontic treatment must promote, as soon as possible, a physiological eruption in the alveolar process of the teeth that are at risk of retention or non-physiological eruptions.

Clinical behavior

We will distinguish the management of the gingival phenotype through three approaches:

1. *Orthodontic approach:* management of gingival phenotypes through orthodontic treatment both as maintenance and modification and as resolution of mucogingival defects with tooth movement.
2. *Surgical approach*: management of the gingival phenotype by surgical treatment before and after orthodontic treatment.
3. *Combined interceptive approach*: management of mucogingival problems during orthodontic treatment, combining periodontal surgical management of soft tissues with orthodontic therapy aimed at intercepting dental retentions and atypical eruptions.

Orthodontic approach

From an orthodontic point of view, treatments for recessions may involve just the repositioning of the teeth in the alveolar envelope where the correction of the position of the roots reduces the extent of gingival recessions (7.8-7.10), improving the prognosis for a total root coverage and creating a favourable surgical site for future mucogingival surgery[50]; moreover, but this is a pure clinical observation, there may be a maintenance of the tissues even in thin phenotypes and, possibly, their modification; an apparent "thickening" can be obtained with simple orthodontic treatment; this approach is a procedure that is not supported by the literature but it is clinically observable and there is a urgent need of high quality randomized controlled trials (RCTs). We will focus our attention on how orthodontic mechanics can control soft tissues without worsening them but, on the contrary, making them have a "thicker appearance".

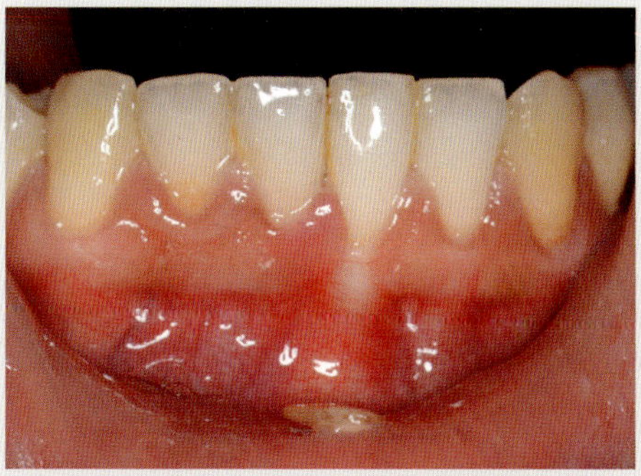

7.8 Recession on 3.1, labial piercing.

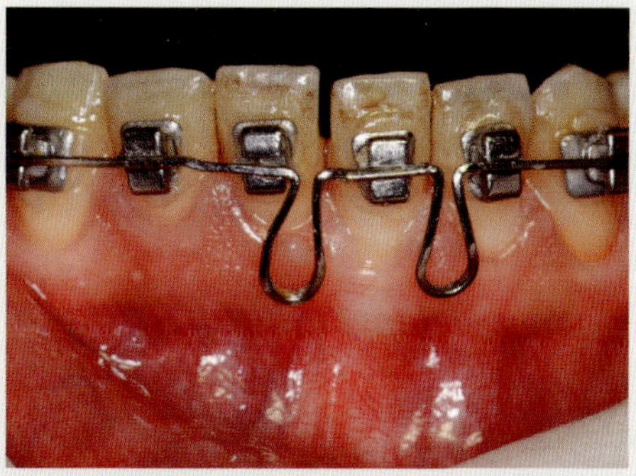

7.9 Vestibular mechanics, .019×.025ss archwire, with teardrops-loops, lingual root torque bending on 3.1, root tipping/uprighting bending on 4.1.

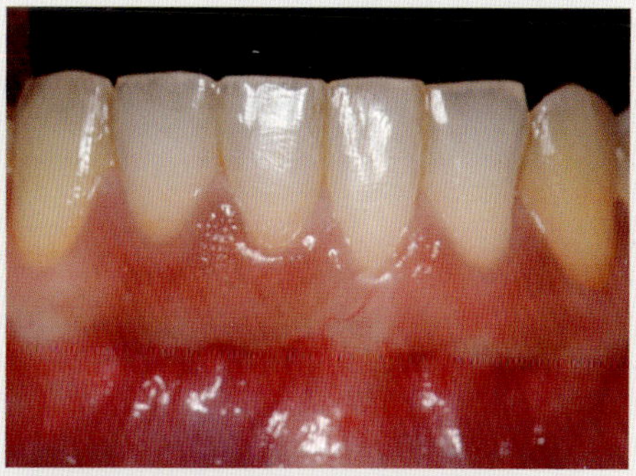

7.10 4-year follow-up.

Clinical case 1

The patient has facial symmetry, labial incompetence, gingival smile, reduced neck-chin length, biprotrusion (7.11), dental class I (7.12) and skeletal class II due to an increased maxillary prognatism with a slight increased vertical relationship, reduced interincisal angle due to an increased vestibular inclination of both upper and lower incisors (7.13 and 7.14) (7.3).

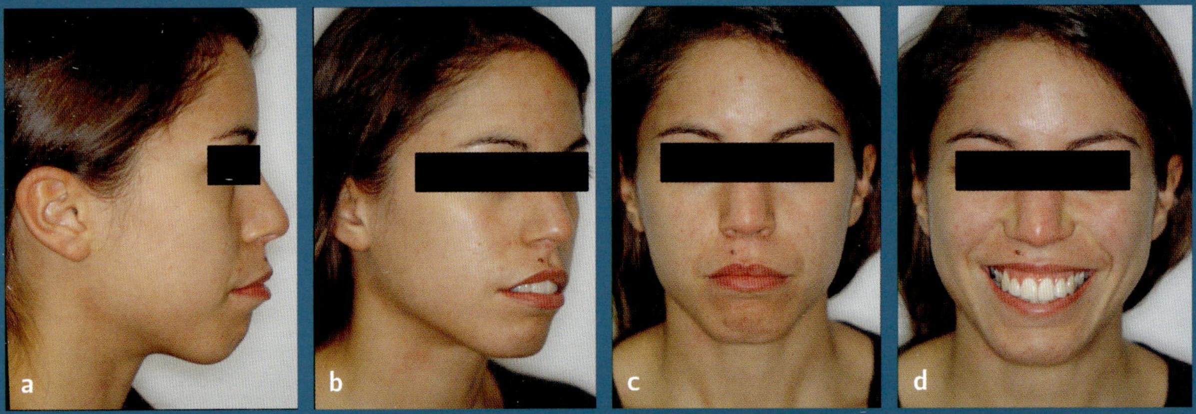

7.11 Extraoral pre-treatment photos.

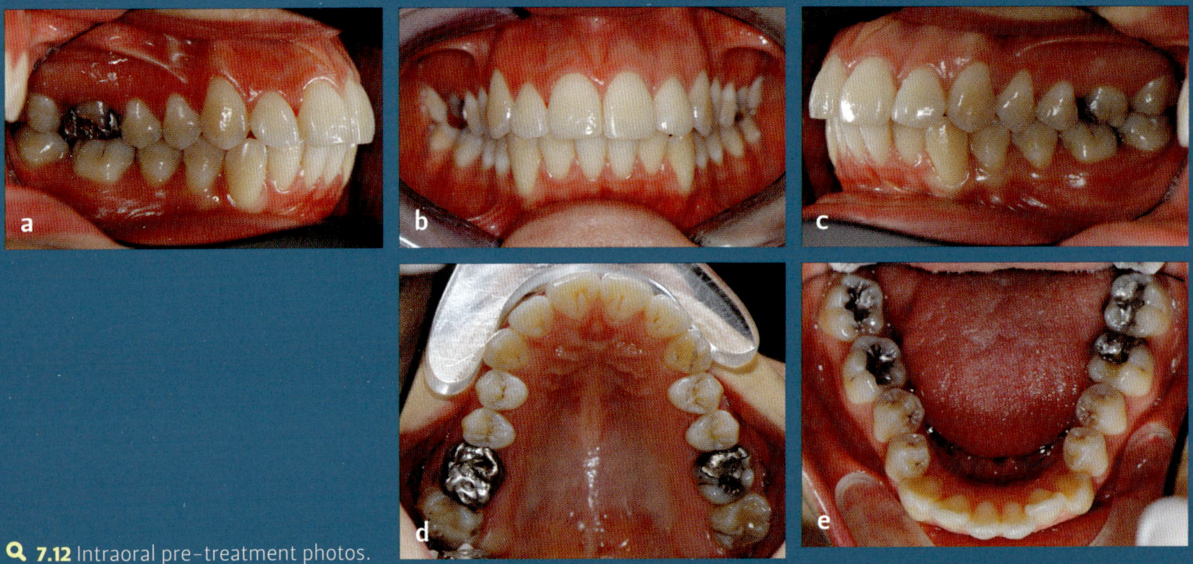

7.12 Intraoral pre-treatment photos.

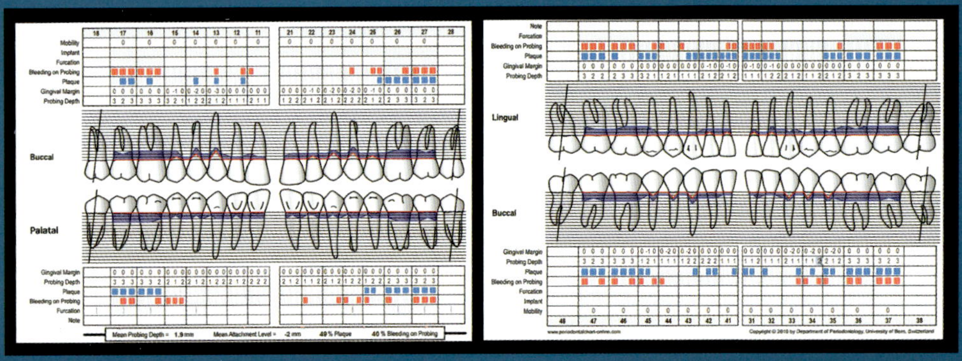

7.13 Initial periodontal probing where it can be seen the mucogingival problems (Online periodontal charting tool from www.perio-tools.com).

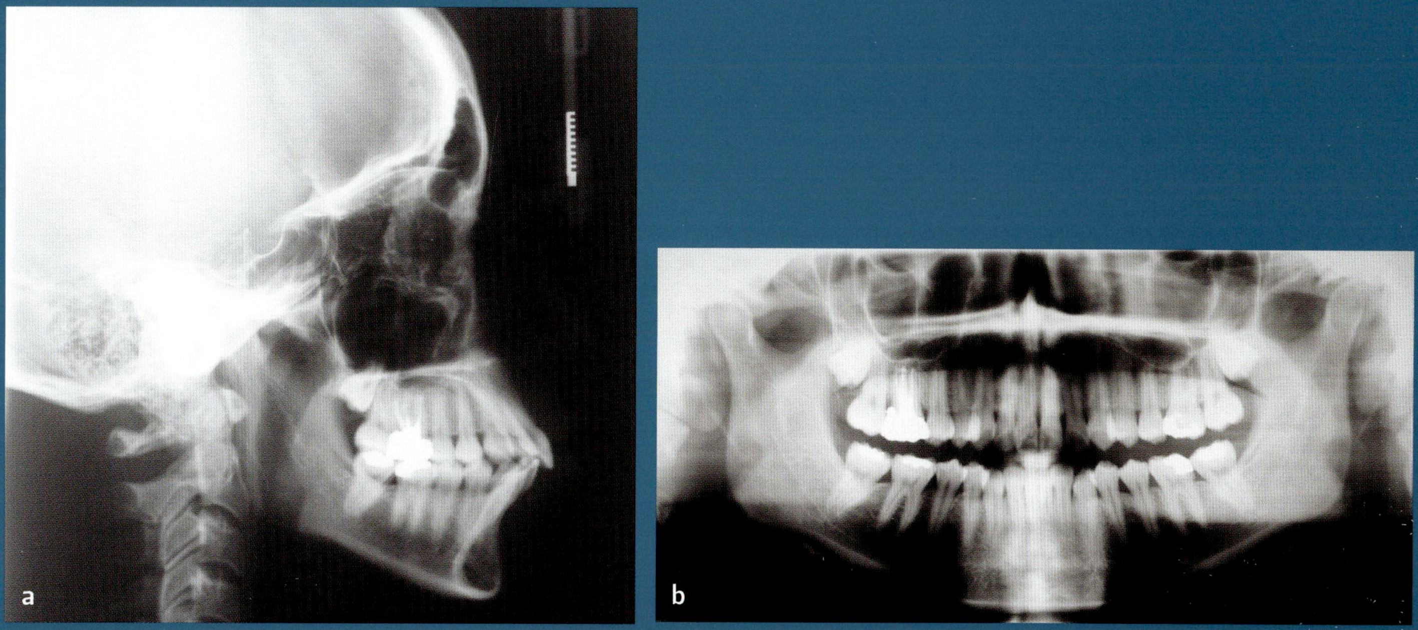

7.14 Pre-treatment cephalometric Rx (**a**) and panoramic Rx (**b**).

Tab. 7.3 Cephalometric values

Sagittal skeletal relationships	**Pre-treatment**	**Post-treatment**	**Mean**	**DS**
Maxillary sagittal relationship SNA	87°	85°	82°	3.5°
Mandibular sagittal relationship SNPg	80°	81°	80°	3.5°
Intermaxillary sagittal relationship ANPg	7°	4°	2°	2.5°
Vertical skeletal relationships				
Maxillary vertical relationship SN / ANS-PNS	6°	4°	8°	3.0°
Mandibular vertical relationship SN / Go-Gn	35°	32°	33°	2.5°
Intermaxillary vertical relationship ANS-PNS / Go-Gn	29°	28°	25°	6.0°
Dento-basal relationships				
Upper incisor inclination $\underline{1}$ - ANS-PNS	120°	100°	110°	6.0°
Lower incisor inclination $\overline{1}$ - Go-Gn	111°	90°	94°	7.0°
Lower incisor compensation $\overline{1}$ - A-Pg (mm)	+8	-1	2	2.0
Dental relationships				
Overjet (OVJ, mm)	5	3	3.5	2.5
Overbite (OVB, mm)	3	3	2	2.5
Interincisal angle $\underline{1}/\overline{1}$	102°	140°	132°	6.0°

The patient shows extensive restorative treatments of the first and lower second molars; she refused a combined orthodontic-surgical therapy and the extraction of the first molars, although compromised. A lingual orthodontic mechanics is applied (Kurz 7th Generation®, Ormco) with extraction of the first four premolars, indirect bonding and set-up (Hiro System®[51]), .016 CuNiTi archwire at first, then .016 β-titanium archwires, .017×.017 β-titanium archwires, mesial slicing of the first upper premolars to distalize the upper anterior group and mesial and distal slicing of the lower first premolars to mesialize the second premolars and retract the anterior group (7.15). The retraction of the upper canines is performed in sliding technique with a .017×.017 in β-titanium archwire (7.16), then with a .017×.025 in β-titanium archwire with TADs miniscrews anchorage and force translators to bring the force retraction point closer to the center of resistance (7.17). Then the incisive retraction is obtained with sliding mechanics and miniscrews for intrusion of the anterior group (7.18). The detailing is realized with a .017×.017 in β-titanium archwire (7.19).

At the end of therapy, the patient shows lip competence, reduction of the gingival smile with improvement of the profile (7.20), dental class I and normalization of OVJ and OVB, apparent different "expression" of the gingival phenotype (7.21 and 9.24 for comparision), reduction of verticality, normalization of cephalometric values and incisive inclination (7.22 and 7.23) (see 7.3).

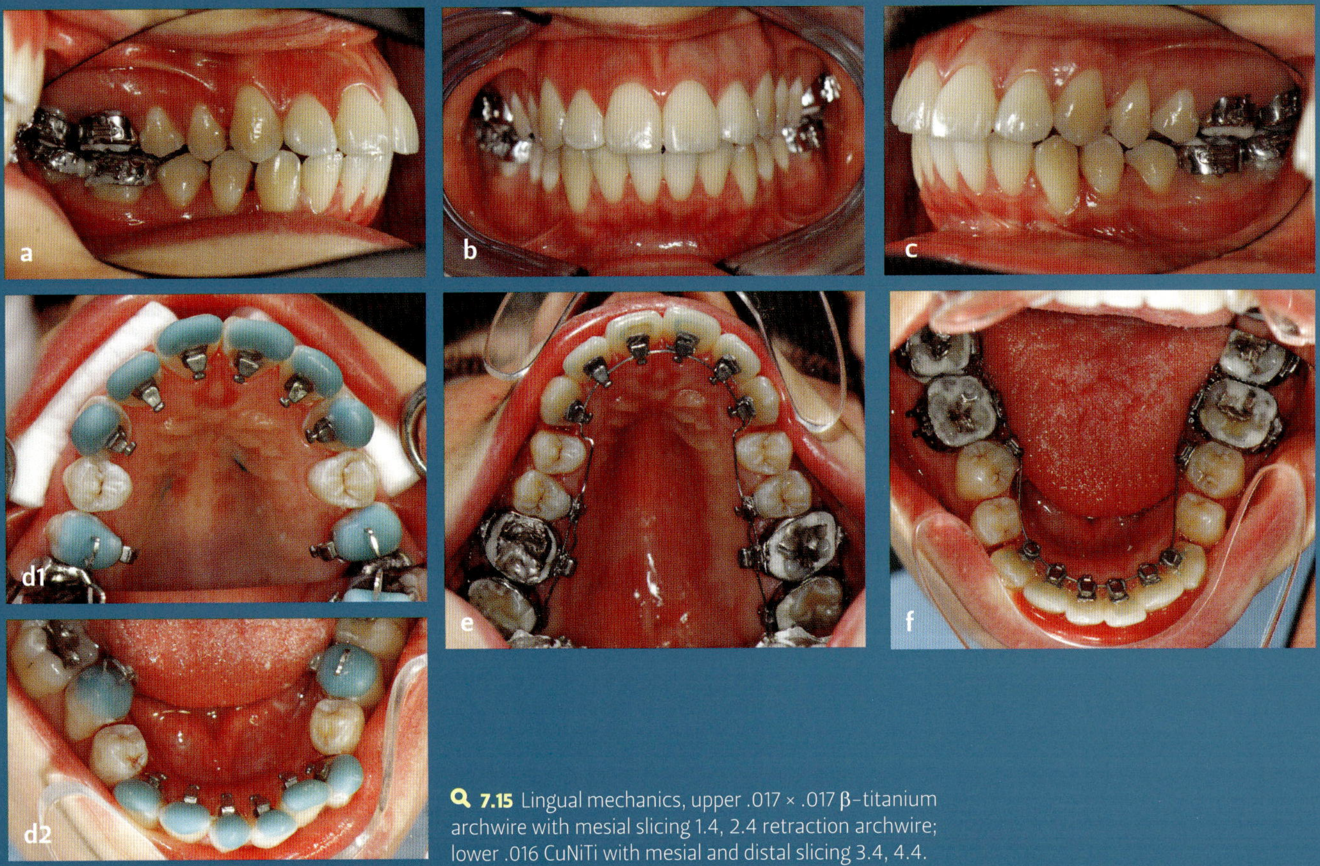

7.15 Lingual mechanics, upper .017 × .017 β-titanium archwire with mesial slicing 1.4, 2.4 retraction archwire; lower .016 CuNiTi with mesial and distal slicing 3.4, 4.4.

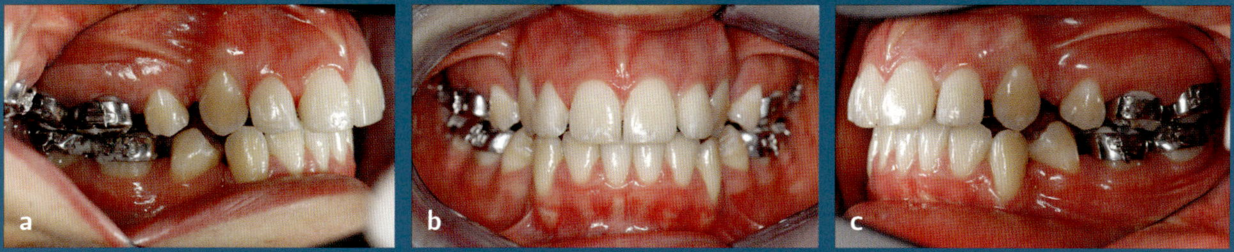
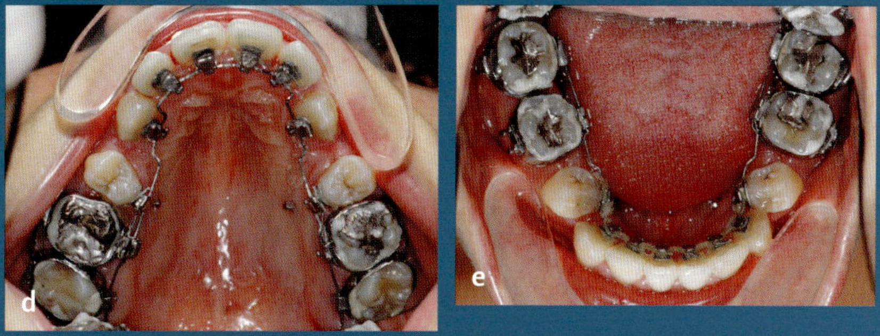

7.16 Lingual mechanics, upper canines retraction, .017×.017 β-titanium archwire, TADs anchorage.

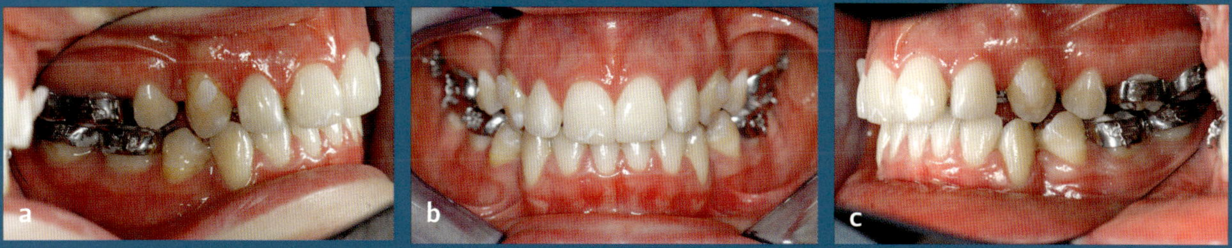
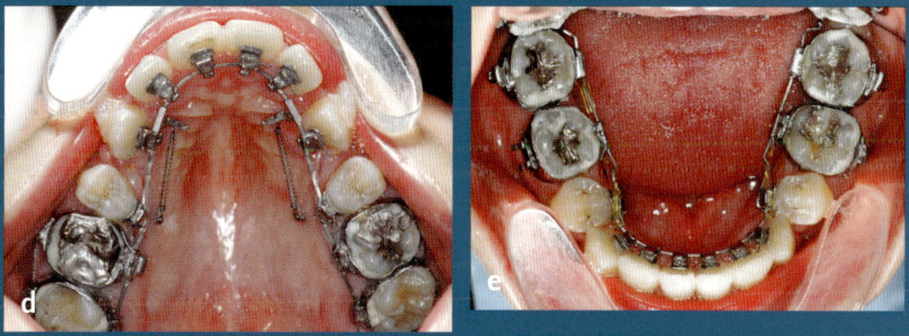

7.17 Lingual mechanics, .017×.017 β-titanium archwire with TADs anchorage, power arms to get closer the retraction force point to the center of resistance.

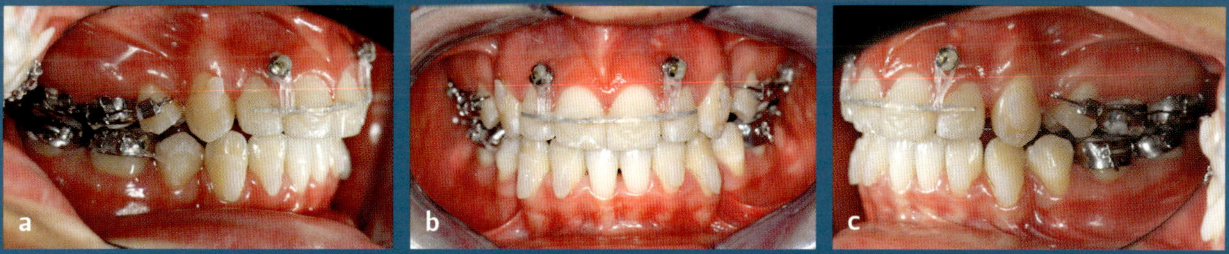
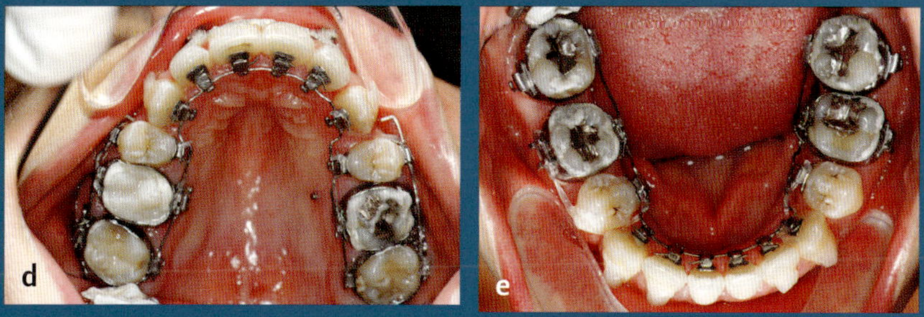

7.18 Lingual mechanics, incisors retraction archwire with sliding mechanics and TADs for anterior superior teeth intrusion.

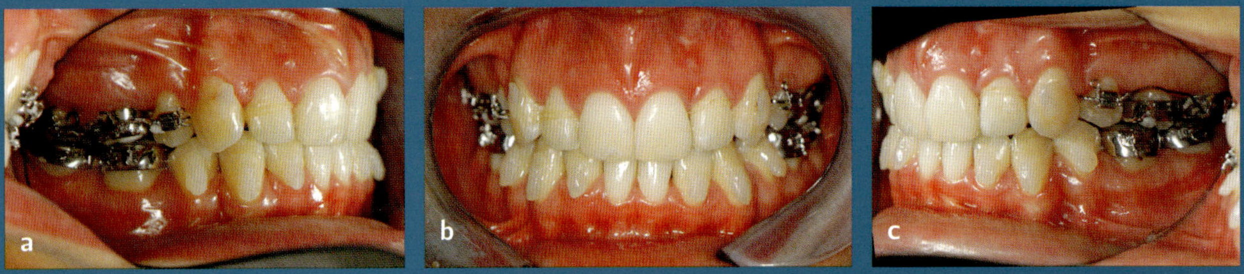
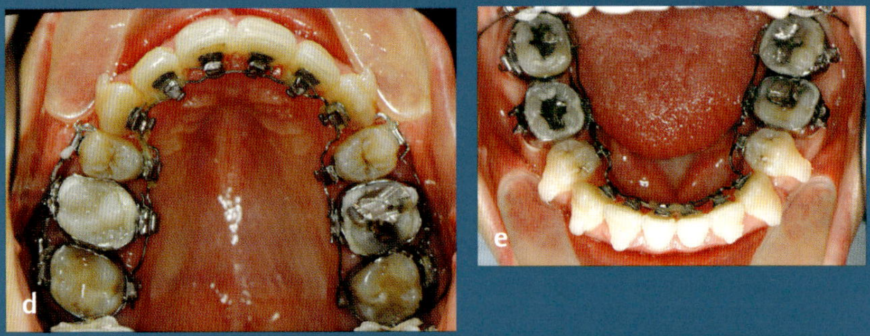

7.19 Lingual mechanics, detailing, .017× .017 β-titanium archwire.

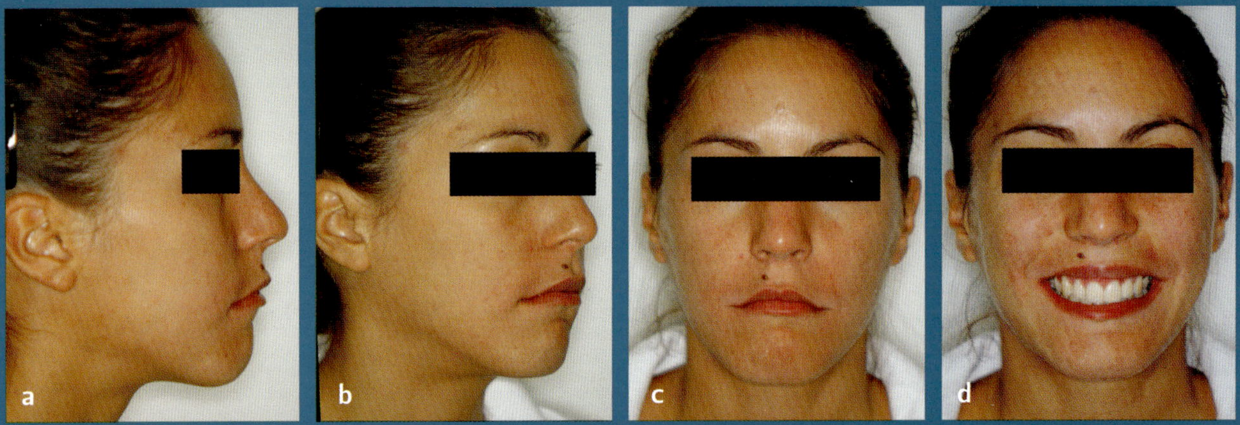

7.20 Extraoral post-treatment photos.

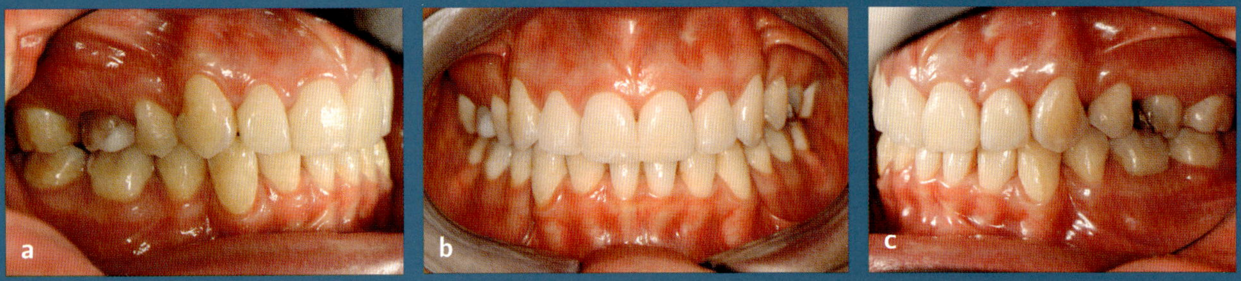
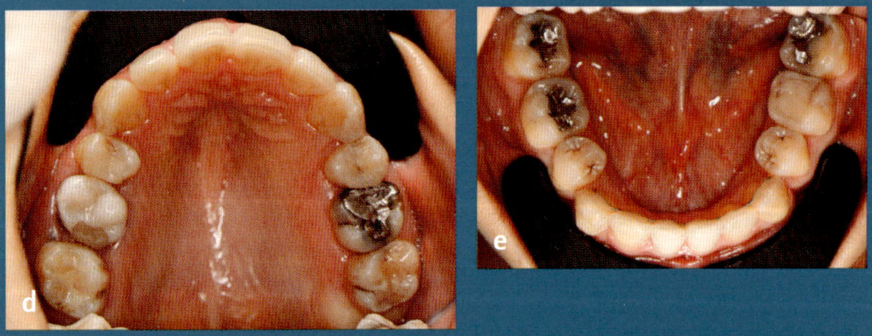

7.21 Intraoral post-treatment photos.

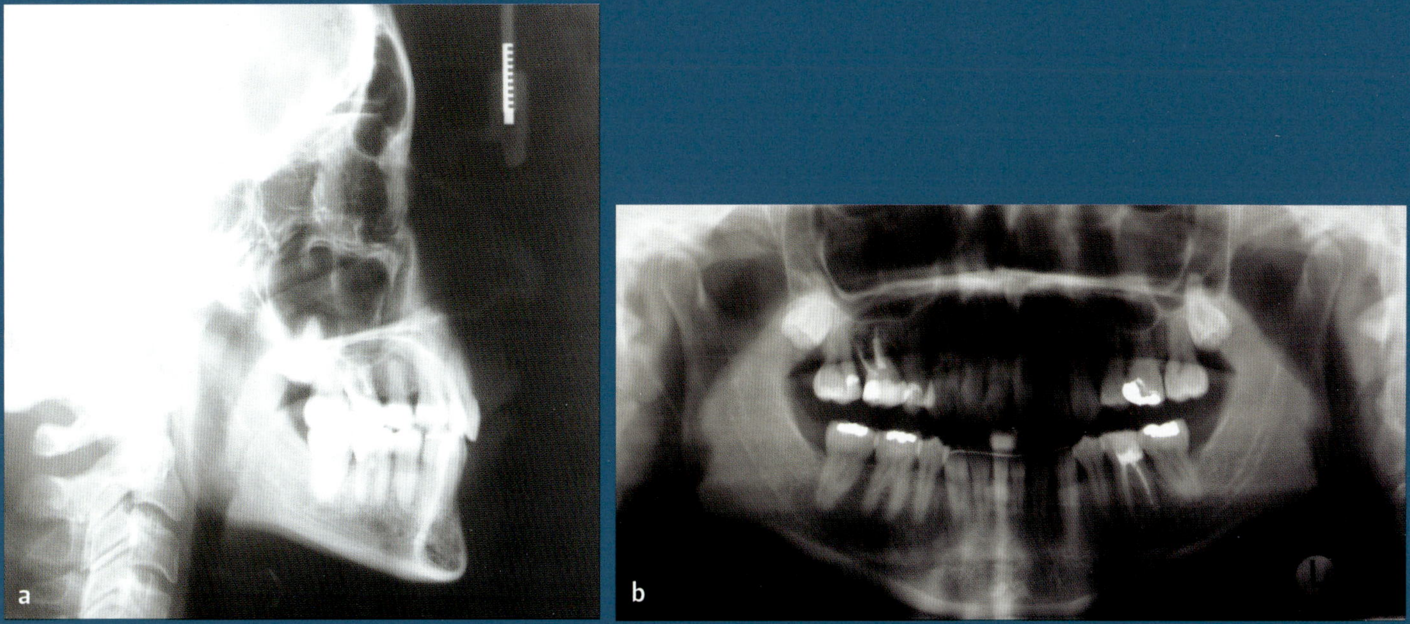

7.22 Post-treatment cephalometric Rx (**a**) and panoramic Rx (**b**).

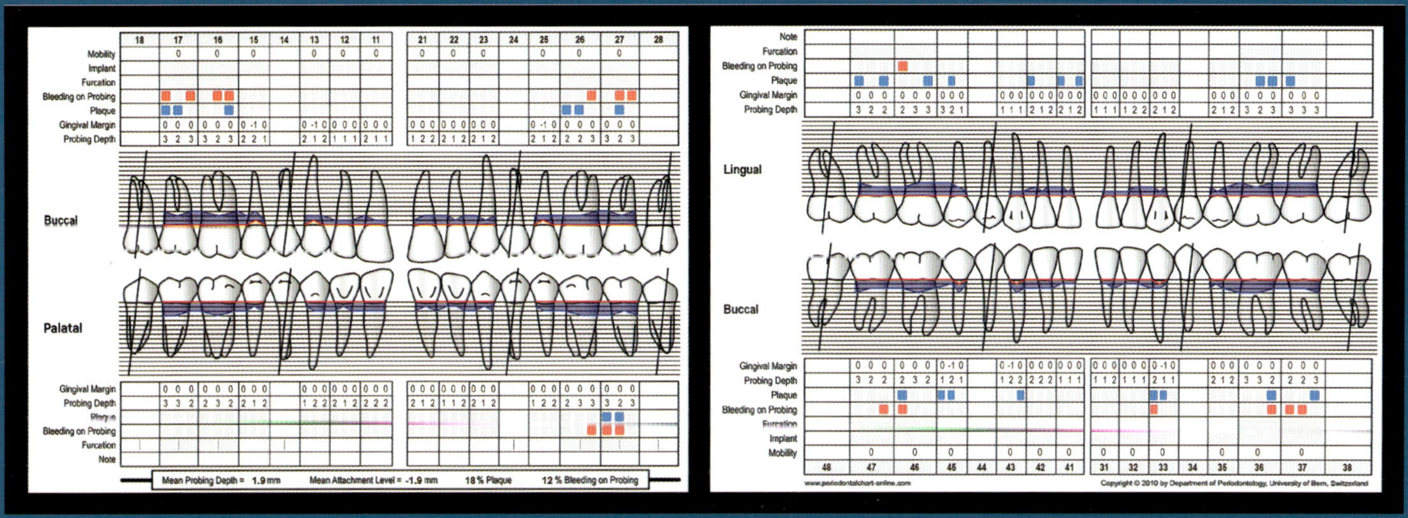

7.23 Post-treatment periodontal probing (Online periodontal charting tool from www.perio-tools.com).

Surgical approach

As we have seen in the literature, when it is necessary to increase the tissues before or after the orthodontic movement in order to modify the gingival phenotype, multiple surgical techniques are available. Among these, the most common are the coronally advanced flap[52] (7.24 to 7.27) and the coronally advanced flap with connective tissue graft[53] (7.28 and 7.29). These flaps, both with their own indications, can be used both before and after the end of orthodontic treatment.

Interceptive combined approach

When approaching soft tissues in orthodontic patients, particular attention must be paid to whatever concerns the treatment of teeth that risk to be retained or to erupt in an ectopic area. The same care that must be taken in the management of soft tissues in any mucogingival surgery e.g. covering recession or increasing keratinized gingiva, as we have seen in the previous paragraph, must also be observed in managing the soft tissues around a tooth at risk of retention; in this kind of teeth a sufficient keratinized tissue must be safeguarded for the future maintenance of teeth over time, including its eruption in the archwire mediated by orthodontics. If a tooth erupts buccally through the mucosa, no adjacent gingiva forms on the tooth surface[54].

Some Authors[36], in case of ectopic eruption, recommend a pre-eruptive surgical uncovering in the mucosa; others, however, prefer a "wait and see" attitude, because, under strict control of plaque, a spontaneous resolution of such defects during the growth may have place and surgery may be postponed to the end of the growth[55-57]. We prefer to manage soft tissue with a so-called "interceptive combined orthodontic" approach, choosing to early detect problems related to a non-physiological eruption in the arch of the retained tooth and to manage the position and the quantity of keratinized tissue present in the area where we are going to perform the uncovering surgery.

This interceptive treatment before the eruption and for ectopic eruptions before orthodontic treatment is also recommended by several authors[58,59]. This approach allows to maintain the thickness of the kerati-

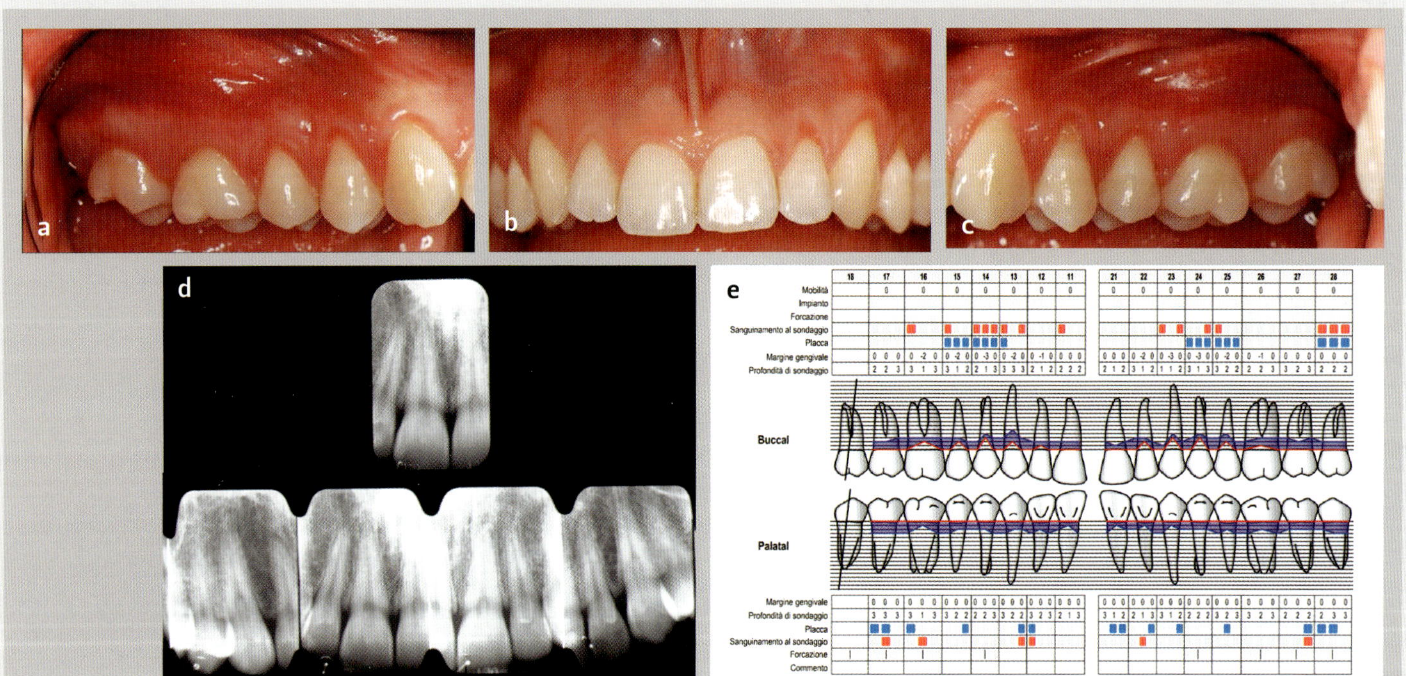

7.24 View of the upper arch where it can be seen the gingival recession from 1.6 up to 2.6 (RT1) with periodontal probing (Online periodontal charting tool from www.perio-tools.com).

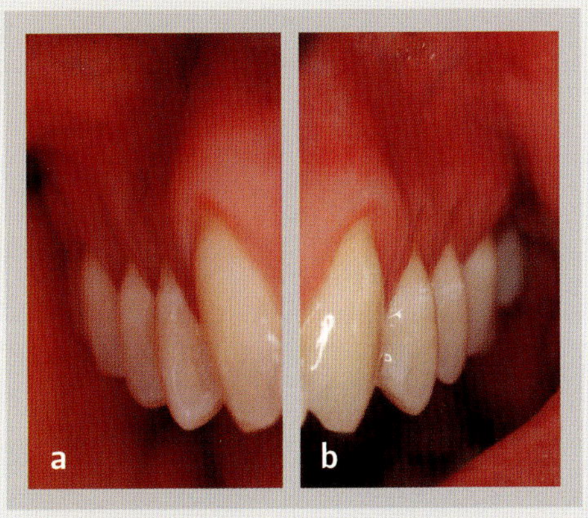

7.25 Recessions lateral view where it can be seen the cemento-enamel junction and the presence of cervical abrasion without step (Class A–).

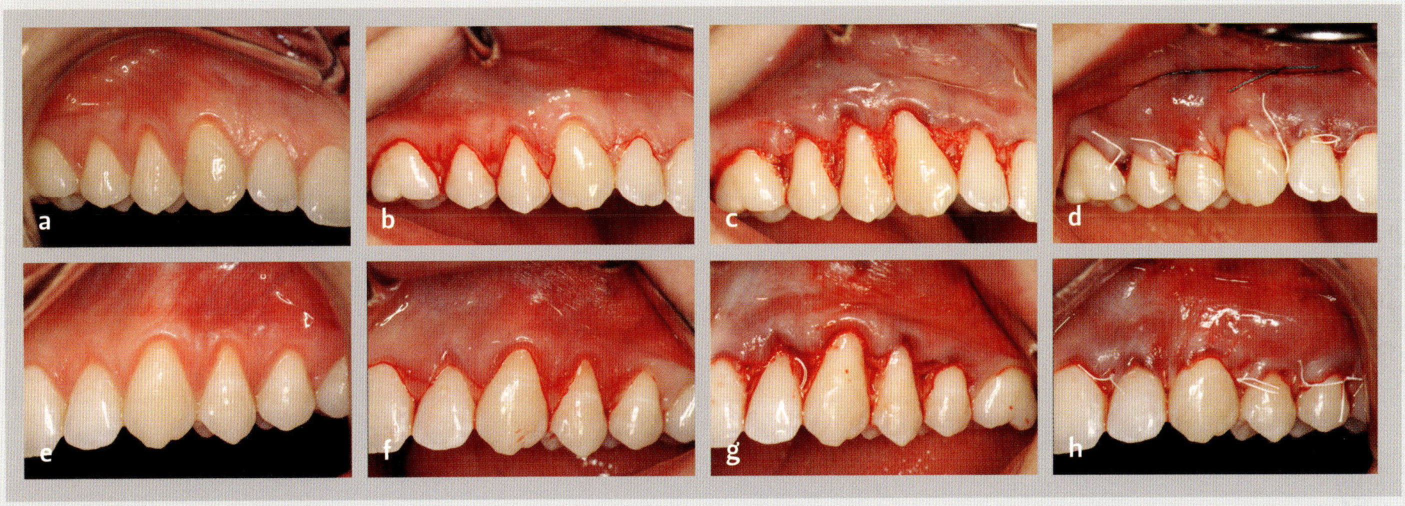

7.26 Surgical phase: flap design (**b, f**); papillae disepithelization (**c, g**); suture (**d, h**).

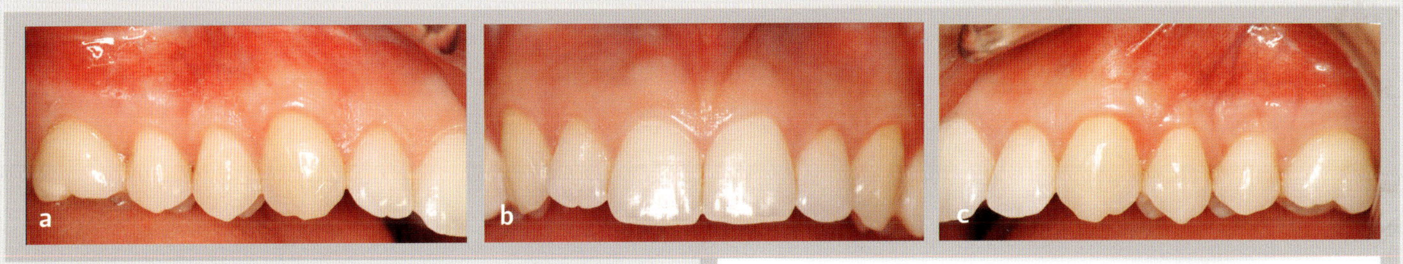

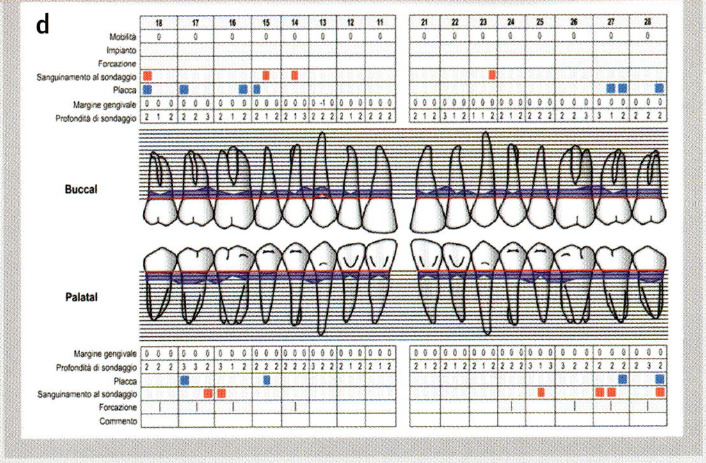

7.27 2-year follow-up (**a–c**) with periodontal probing (**d**) (Online periodontal charting tool from www.perio-tools.com).

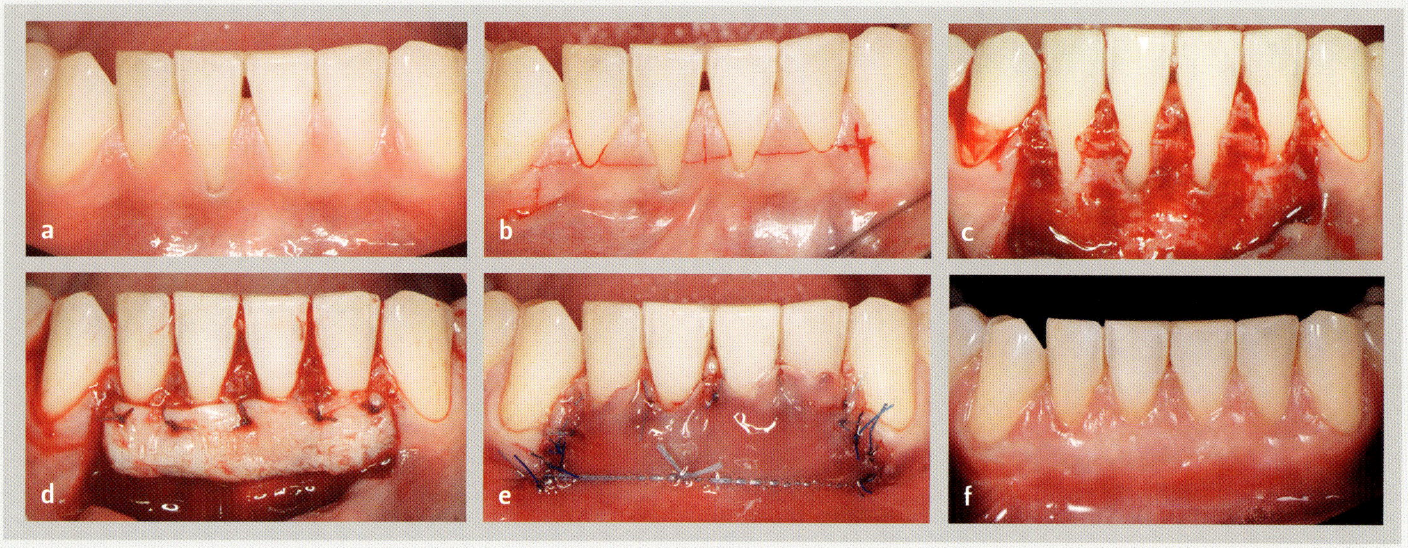

7.28 Vestibur view of the deep recessions on the lower incisors (**a**); flap design (**b**); papillae and periosteal recipient site preparation (**c**); suture of the connective tissue graft harvested from the palate (**d**); suture (**e**); 1-year follow-up (**f**).

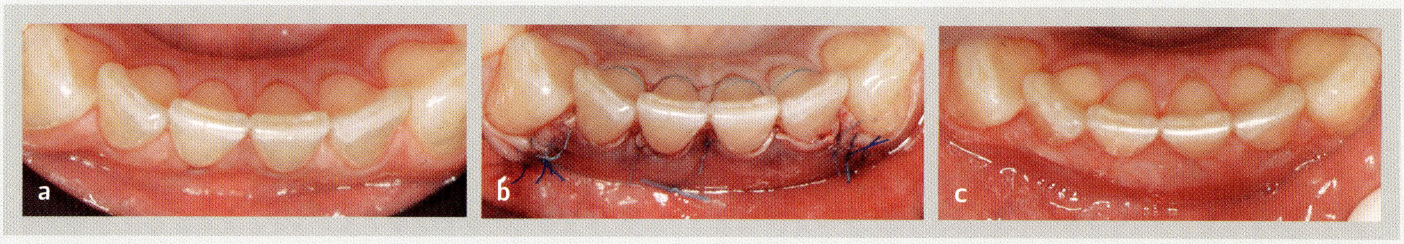

7.29 Clinical view of the tissue thickening obtained by the connective graft: after the suture (**b**) and after 1 year (**c**).

nized tissue in the long term. As it can be seen in the 7.30 and 7.31, great attention must be paid to two main factors: the position of the tooth and the surrounding tissues. The diagnostic factors that must be taken into account are the relationships between the retained tooth (position) and the overlying tissues (KT, Keratinized Tissue). This will determine the type of surgery to be performed for guaranteeing, during the orthodontically guided eruption phases, an adequate quantity of keratinized tissue to the tooth. For this reason it is important to manage the soft tissue in all the areas of the mouth, because all the teeth can have difficulties in eruption, from the anterior teeth (7.32 and 7.33), the non-erupted (7.34 and 7.35) and retained (see *Clinical case 2*) canines, up to correctly manage the flaps in the lower (7.36–7.39; see 9.22c,d for the 10-year X-ray check) and upper molars (7.40 and 7.41).

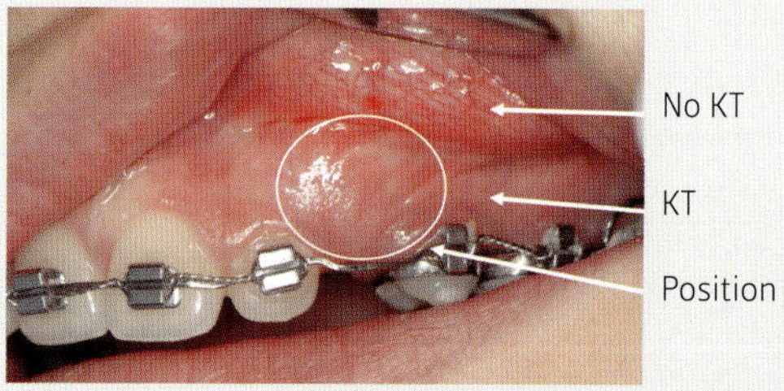

7.30 Favorable relationship between retained tooth and soft tissue. This relationship allows to perform more predictable mucogingival flaps.

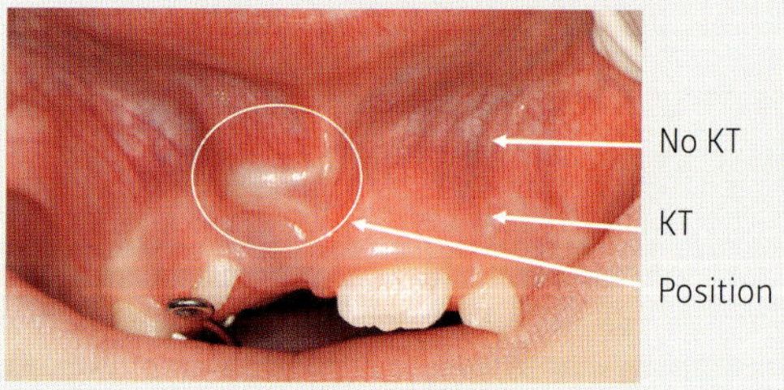

7.31 Unfavorable relationship between retained tooth and soft tissue. This relationship requires great attention about soft tissues management.

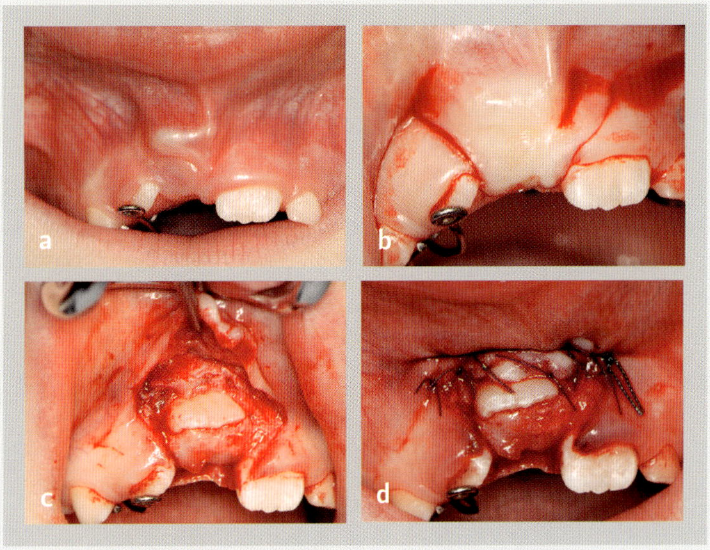

7.32 Apical repositioned flap to maintain the entire keratinized tissue that is present on site, allowing the orthodontic eruption with proper periodontal attachment.

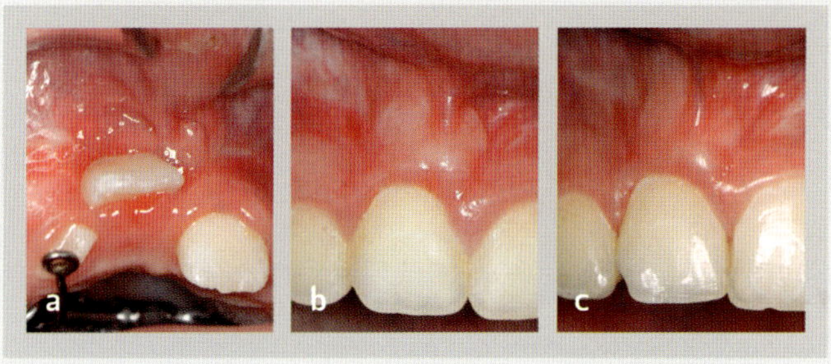

7.33 Soft tissue stability at a long-term follow-up (10 years) (**c**) of the case in 7.32.

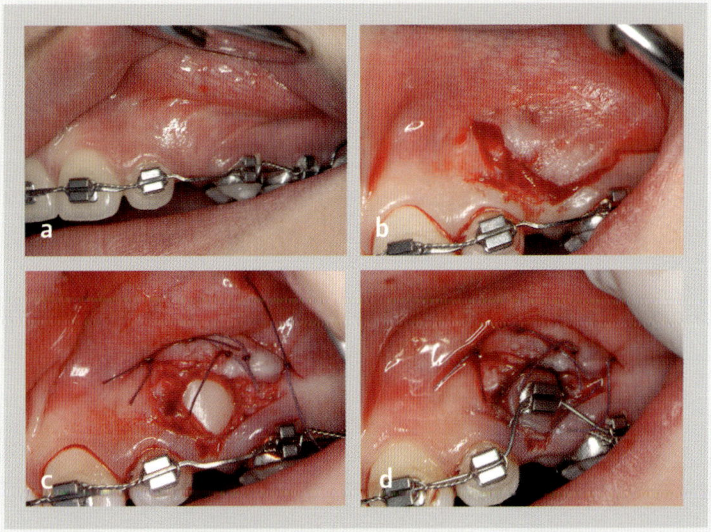

7.34 Apical repositioned flap to transpose the keratinized tissue along the canine cervical area.

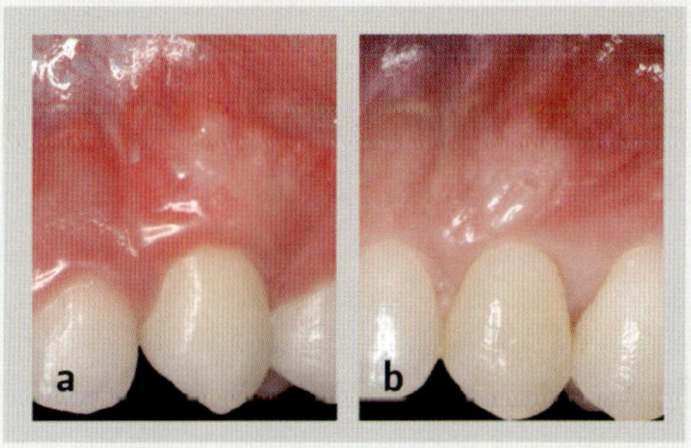

7.35 Long-term follow-up where can be seen the stability of the repositioned tissue after 14 years (**b**) of the case in 7.34.

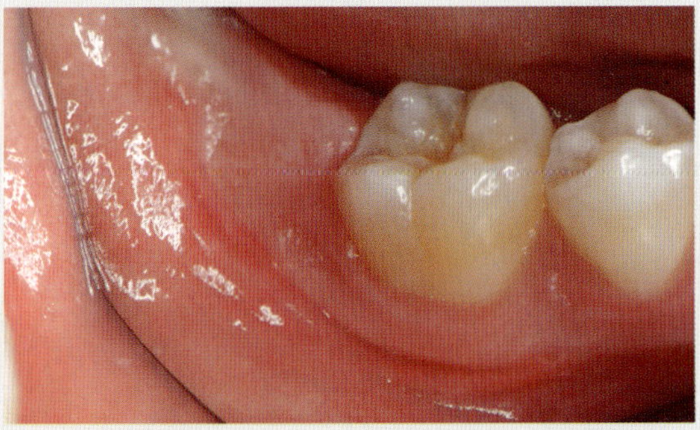

7.36 Horizontal impaction of the 4.7. Pre-surgical soft tissue aspect (pre-treatment X-ray in 9.18).

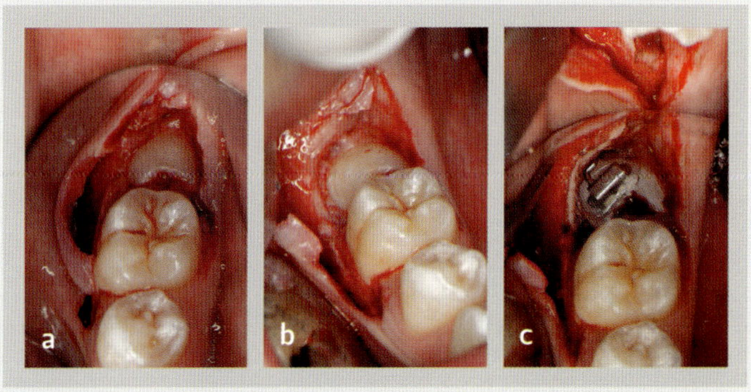

7.37 Uncovering surgical treatment with apical repositioned flap.

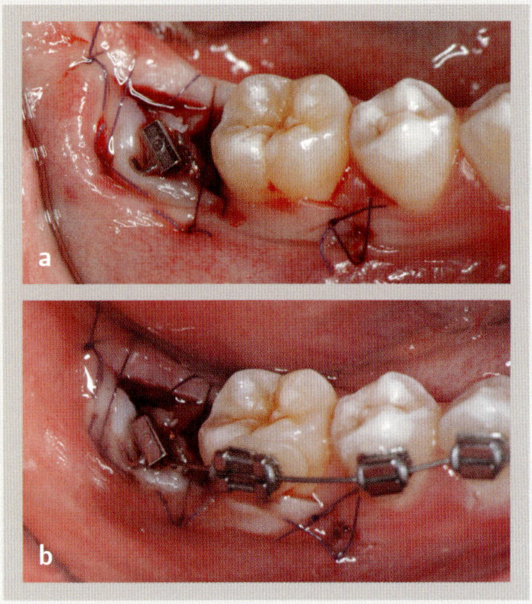

7.38 Brackets positioning, suture and orthodontic mechanics.

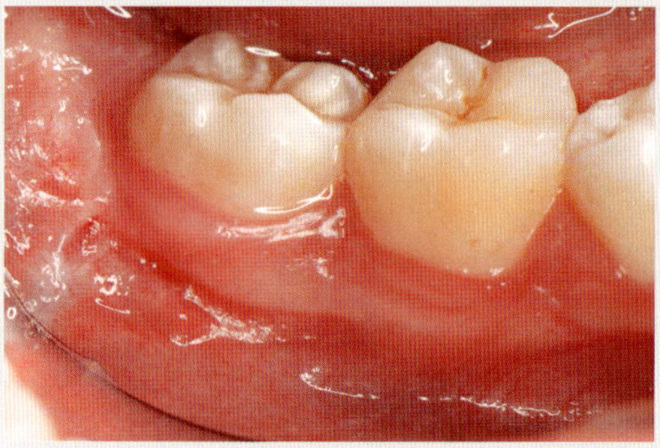

7.39 End-treatment soft tissue check.

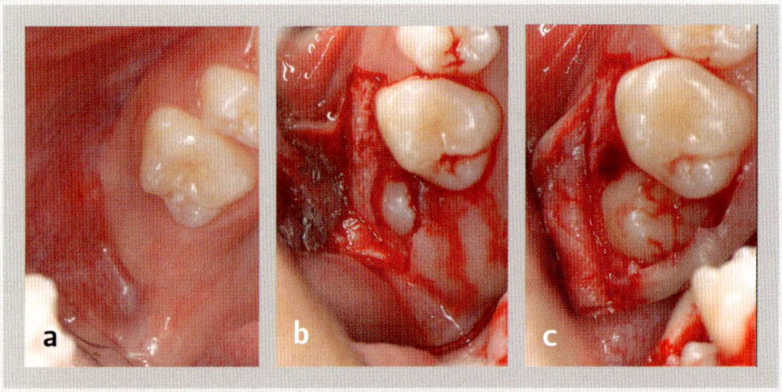

7.40 Uncovering surgical treatment of the second right upper molar (1.7).

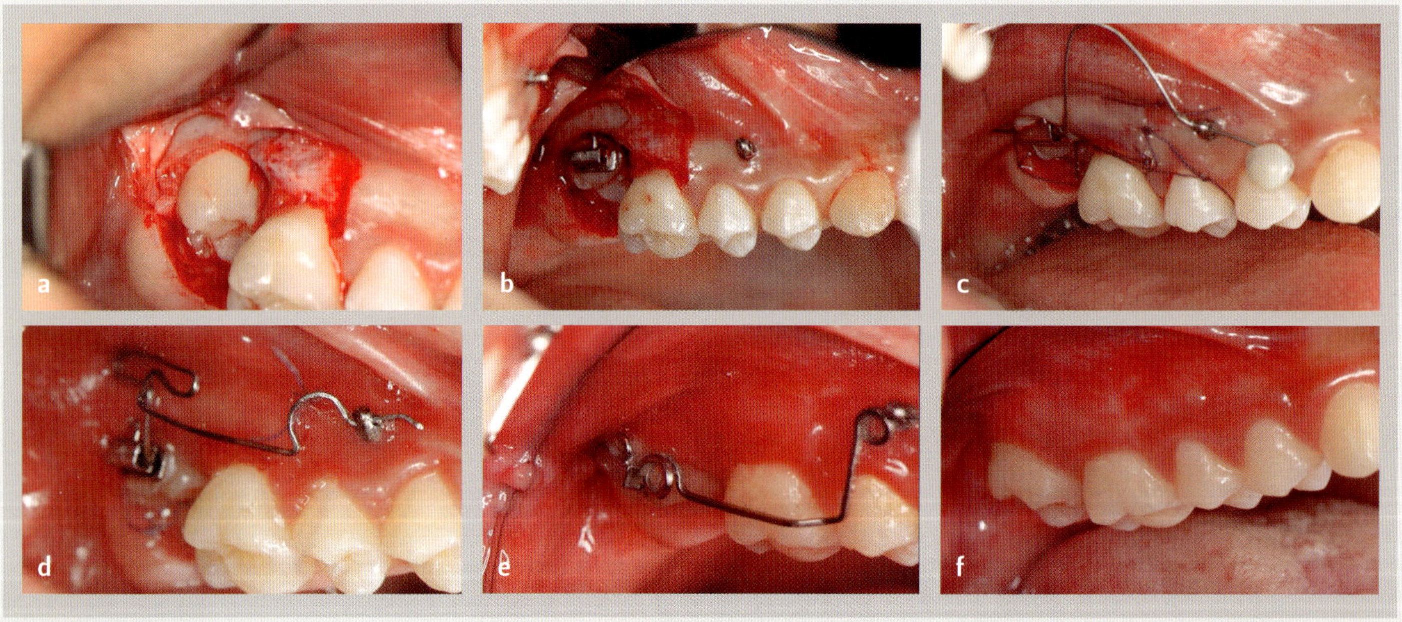

7.41 Flap design (**a**), orthodontic mechanics (**b**–**e**), post treatment soft tissue follow-up (**f**) of the case in 7.40.

Clinical case 2

The patient has a mild facial asymmetry, open nasolabial angle, biretrusion, competent and thin lips (7.42), maxillary contraction, dental and skeletal class I (7.43) hyperdivergence due to an increased mandibular verticality on a maxilla with a normal vertical inclination, biretrusion (7.44; 7.4).

The first phase of orthodontic therapy involves an expansion of the upper jaw, first with a rapid maxillary expansion[60,61], then with a fan-type rapid maxillary expansion (7.45), extraction of the deciduous canines[62-66], maintenance of the perimeter of the arch[67] with a modified palatal bar with a loop opened towards the incisors and springs welded with rests on the upper deciduous second molars (7.46), used with the bilateral uncovering surgery of 1.3 and 2.3 that are retained (7.47-7.49), creating a coronal eruptive tunnel by osteotomy connected to the post-extraction socket of the deciduous elements[68,69]. The orthodontic correction, alignment and intercuspidation are realised in a modified Tweed® mechanics, slot .022×.028, in particular with .018×.025ss archwire and retraction with tear retraction loops for the control of the root and crown position (tipping and torque) of 1.3 and 2.3 (7.50).

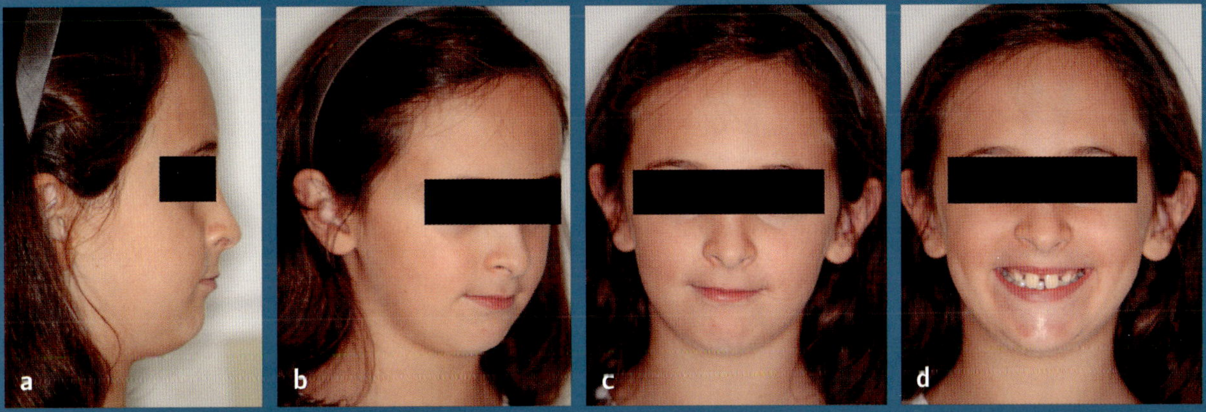

7.42 Extraoral pre-treatment photos.

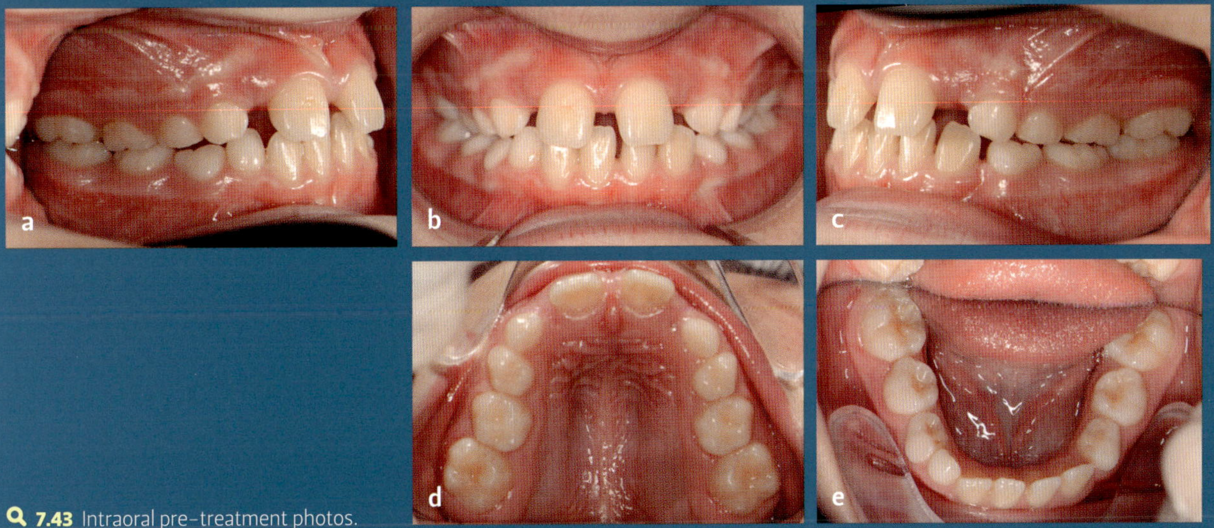

7.43 Intraoral pre-treatment photos.

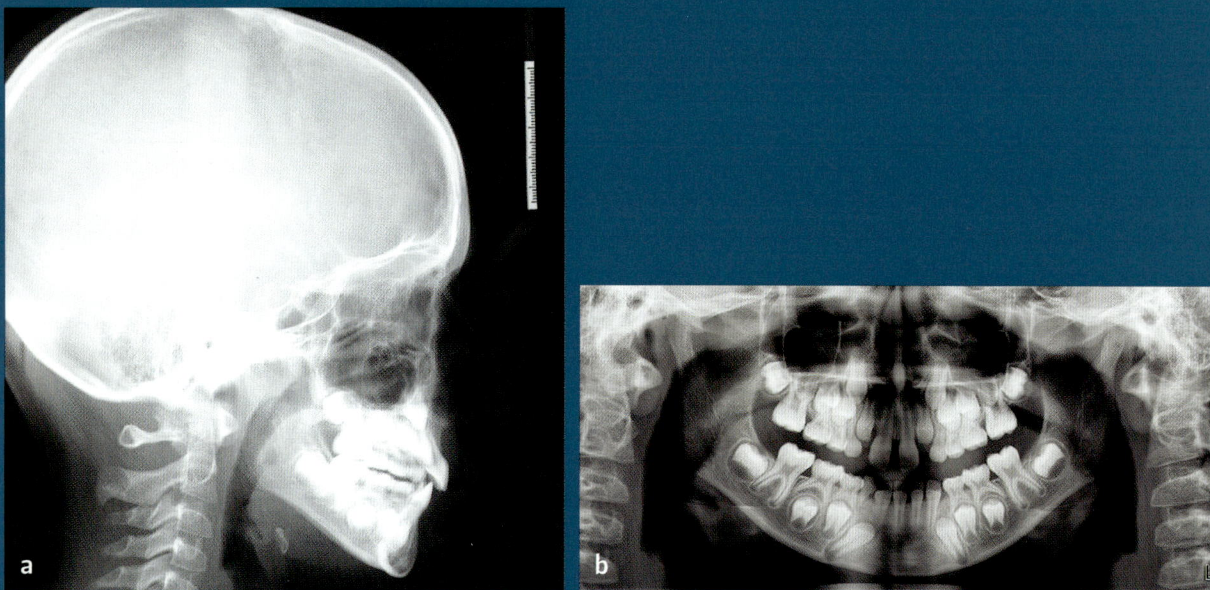

7.44 Pre-treatment cephalometric Rx (**a**) and panoramic Rx (**b**).

Tab. 7.4 Cephalometric values

Sagittal skeletal relationships	Pre-treatment	Post-treatment	Mean	DS
Maxillary sagittal relationship SNA	78°	77°	82°	3.5°
Mandibular sagittal relationship SNPg	76°	75°	80°	3.5°
Intermaxillary sagittal relationship ANPg	2°	2°	2°	2.5°
Vertical skeletal relationships				
Maxillary vertical relationship SN / ANS-PNS	6°	10°	8°	3.0°
Mandibular vertical relationship SN / Go-Gn	41°	43°	33°	2.5°
Intermaxillary vertical relationship ANS-PNS / Go-Gn	35°	33°	25°	6.0°
Dento-basal relationships				
Upper incisor inclination $\underline{1}$ - ANS-PNS	105°	115°	110°	6.0°
Lower incisor inclination $\overline{1}$ - Go-Gn	88°	92°	94°	7.0°
lower incisor compensation $\overline{1}$ - a-pg (mm)	0	+2	2	2.0
Dental relationships				
Overjet (OVJ, mm)	3	2	3,5	2.5
Overbite (OVB, mm)	2	2	2	2.5
Interincisal angle $\underline{1}$ / $\overline{1}$	128°	120°	132°	6.0°

At the end of the treatment, the patient has facial symmetry, normal nasolabial angle (7.51), dental class I, normal transverse relationships (7.52) and skeletal class I, vertical control and correction of the incisor inclinations (7.53) (see 7.4). Soft tissue stability is observed at the 2-year follow-up after surgical treatment in 7.54.

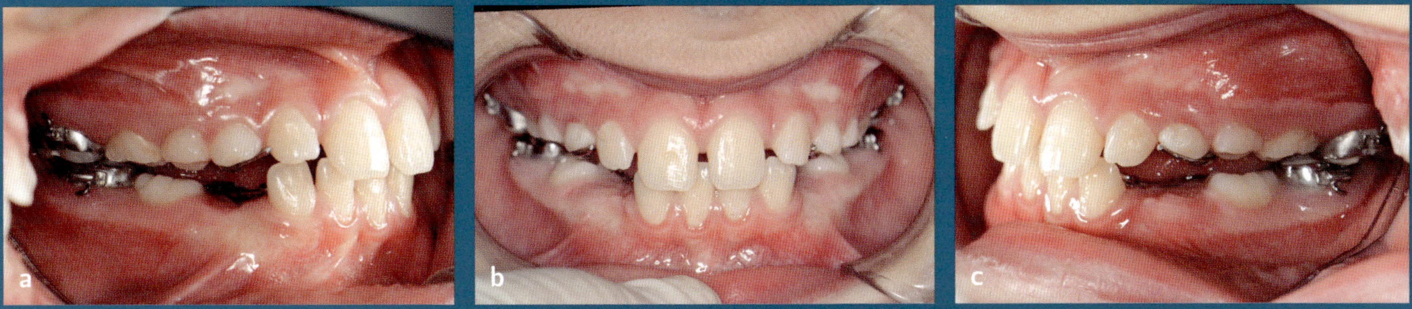

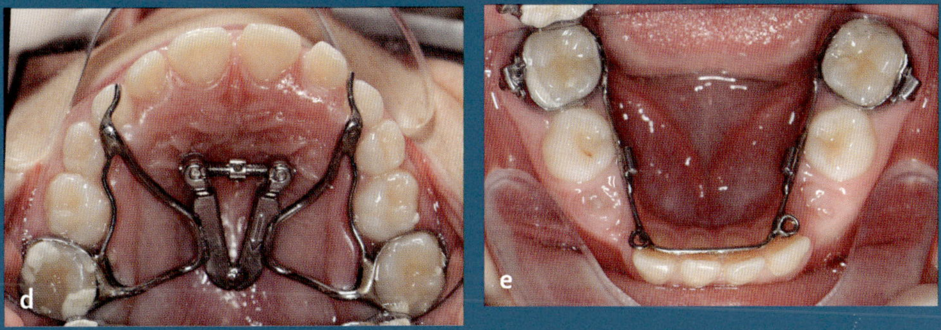

7.45 Orthodontics mechanics, fan-type RME, Lingual arch with welded eyelets.

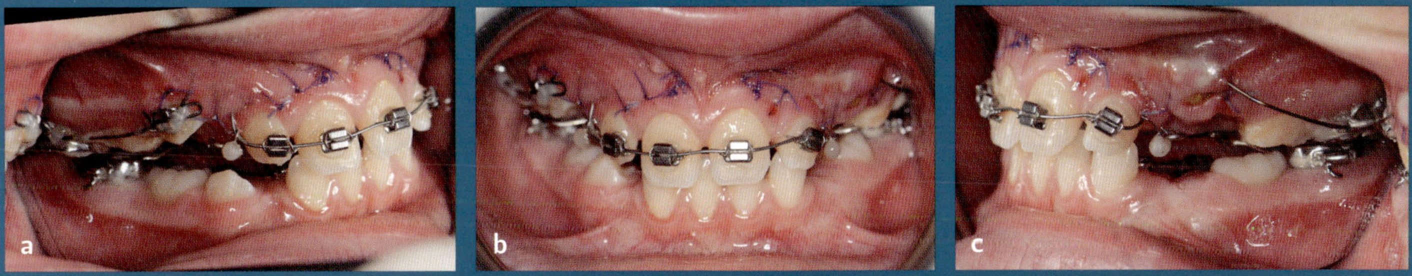

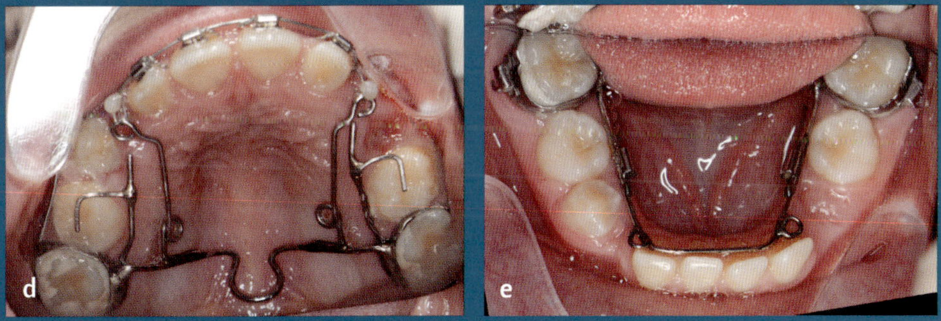

7.46 Modified (loop opened towards the incisors) Palatal Bar with loops and rests on the upper second primary teeth welded, upper .016 CuNiTi archwire, Lingual arch with welded eyelets.

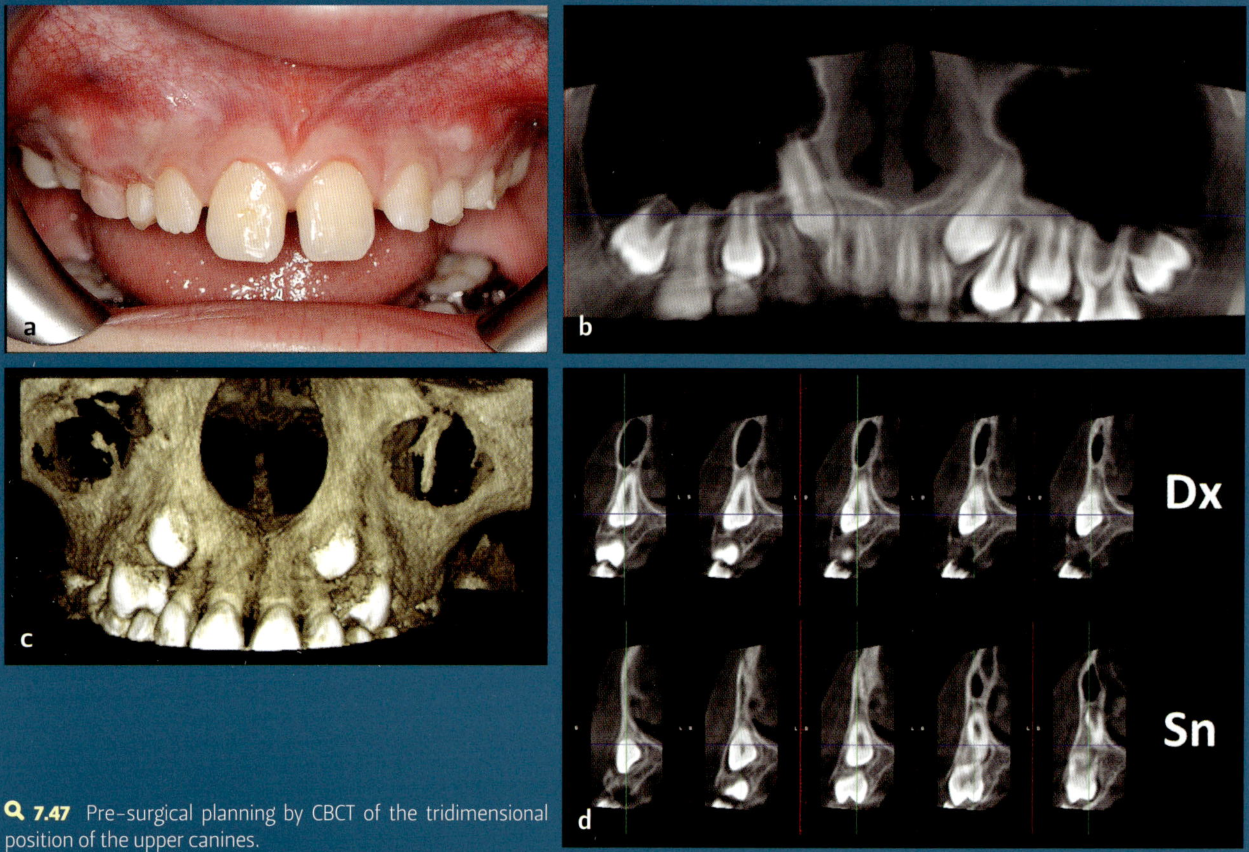

7.47 Pre-surgical planning by CBCT of the tridimensional position of the upper canines.

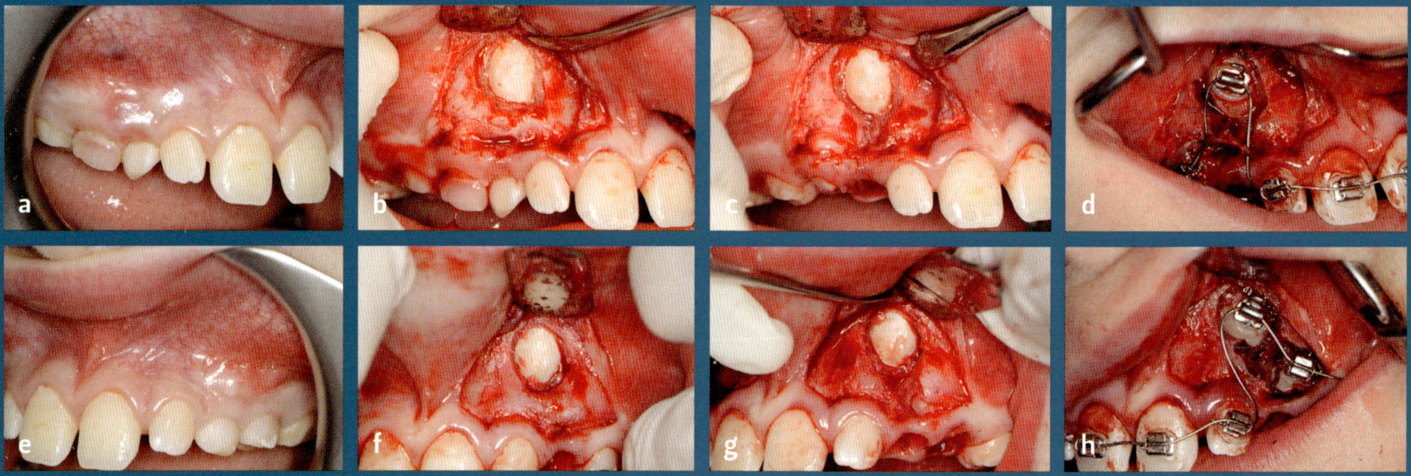

7.48 Bilateral surgery of the retained canines with intrasurgical brackets positioning and creation of the eruptive tunnel path (**c**,**g**) through the post-extraction sockets of the primary teeth.

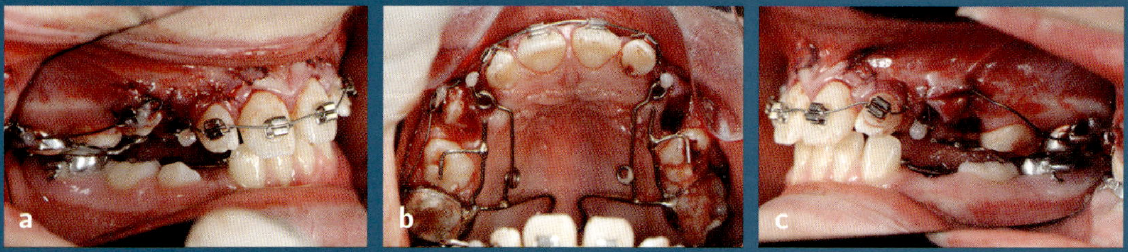

7.49 Suture and orthodontic appliance.

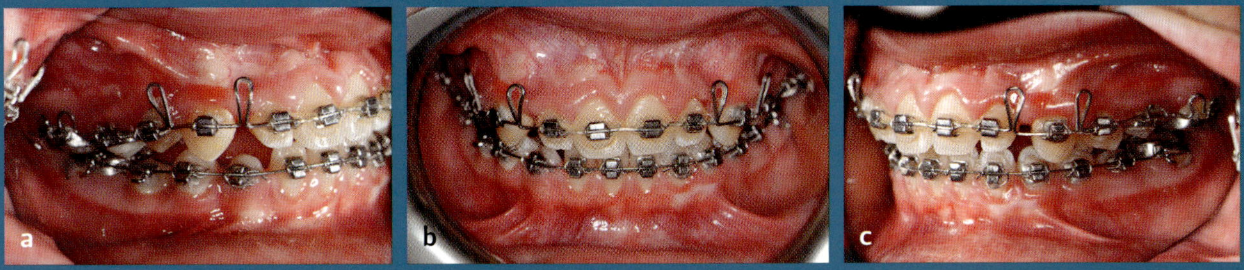
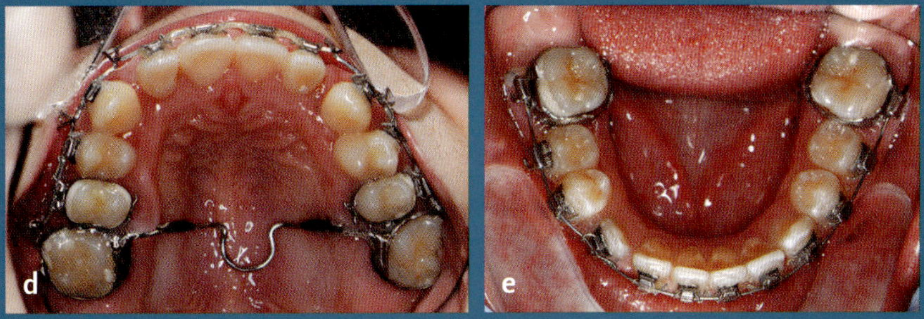

7.50 Orthodontic mechanics .018x.025ss archwire with teardrop loops for 1.3 and 2.3 check.

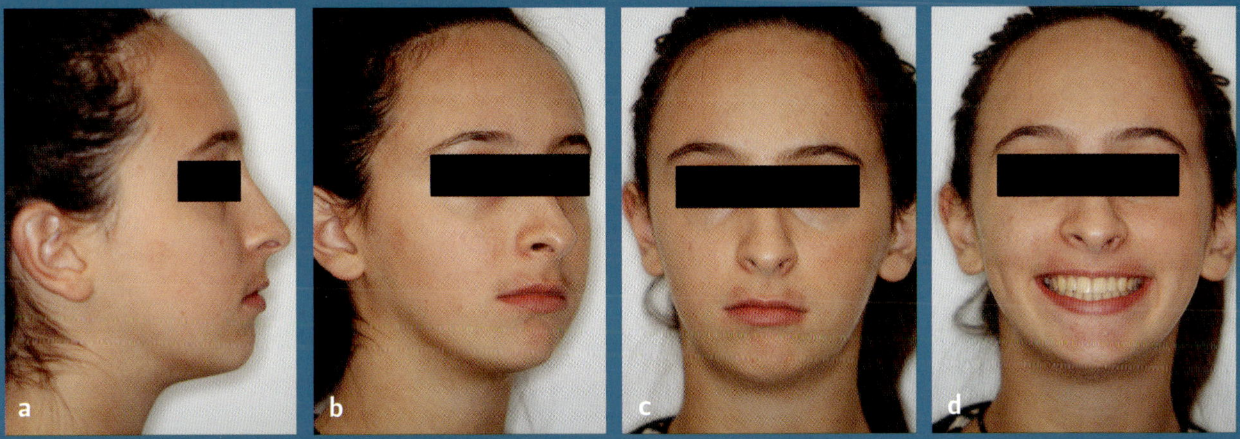

7.51 Extraoral post-treatment photos.

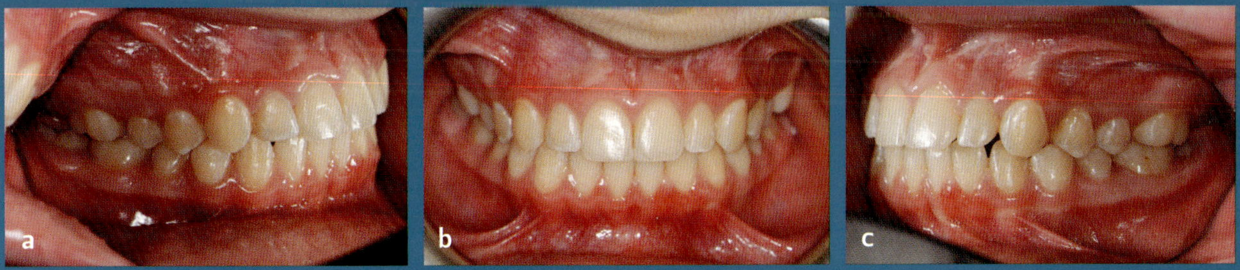
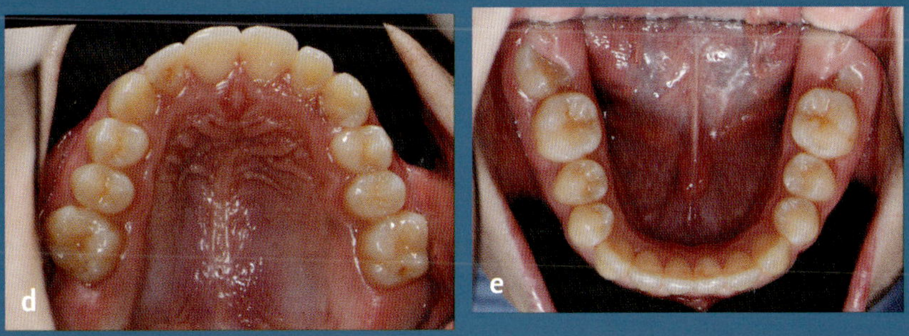

7.52 Intraoral post-treatment photos.

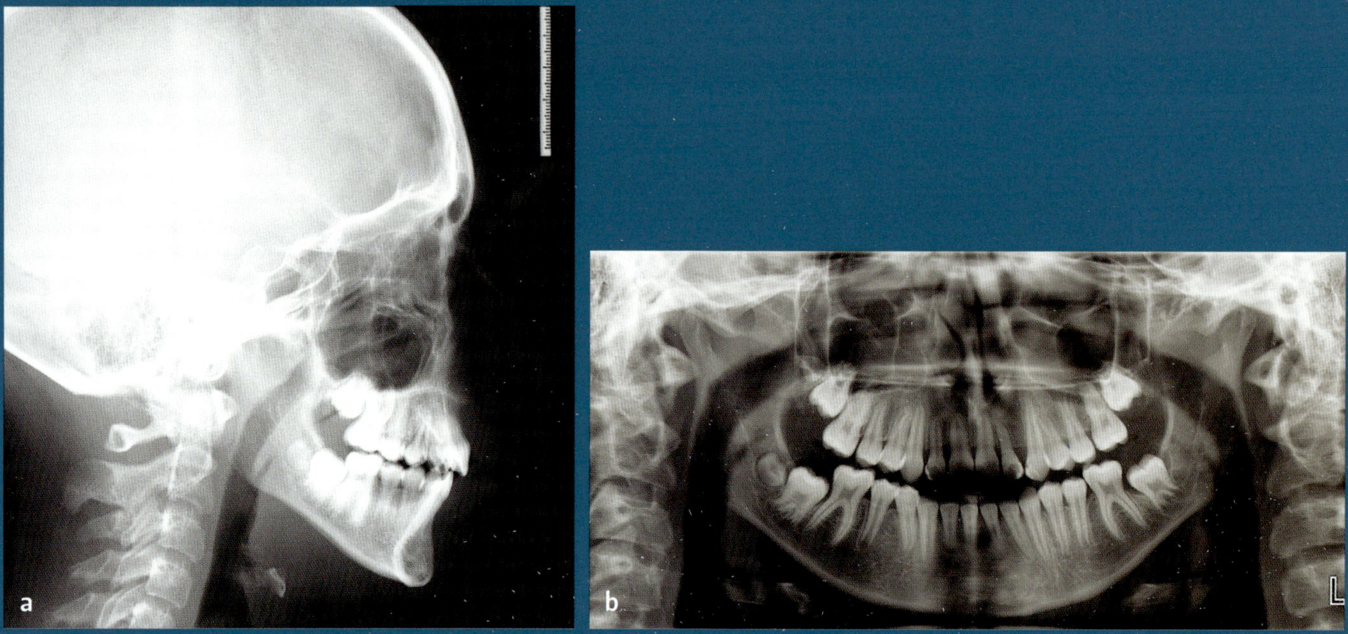

7.53 Post-treatment cephalometric Rx (**a**) and panoramic Rx (**b**).

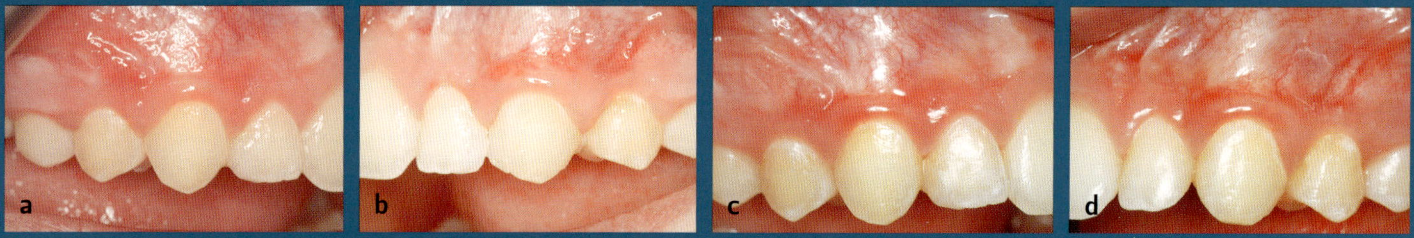

7.54 Soft tissue follow-up at the end of the treatment (**a**,**b**) and 2-year follow-up (**c**,**d**).

REFERENCES

1. Cortellini P, Bissada NF. Mucogingival conditions in the natural dentition: narrative review, case definitions, and diagnostic considerations. *J Clin Periodontol.* 2018;45 Suppl 20:S190-S198.
2. Cortellini P, Bissada NF. Mucogingival conditions in the natural dentition: narrative review, case definitions, and diagnostic considerations. *J Periodontol.* 2018;89(Suppl 1):S204-S213.
3. Cairo F, Nieri M, Cincinelli S et al. The interproximal clinical attachment level to classify gingival recessions and predict root coverage outcomes: an explorative and reliability study. *J Clin Periodontol.* 2011;38(7):661-666.
4. Zweers J, Thomas RZ, Slot DE et al. Characteristics of periodontal biotype, its dimensions, associations and prevalence: a systematic review. *J Clin Periodontol.* 2014;41(10):958-971.
5. Kao RT, Curtis DA, Kim DM et al. American Academy of Periodontology best evidence consensus statement on modifying periodontal phenotype in preparation for orthodontic and restorative treatment. *J Periodontol.* 2020;91(3):289-298.
6. Vanarsdall RL. Orthodontics and periodontal therapy. *Periodontol 2000.* 1995;9(1):132-149.
7. Renkema AM, Fudalej PS, Renkema AA et al. Gingival labial recessions in orthodontically treated and untreated

individuals: a case-control study. *J Clin Periodontol.* 2013;40(6):631-637.

8. **Renkema AM, Fudalej PS, Renkema A et al.** Development of labial gingival recessions in orthodontically treated patients. *Am J Orthod Dentofacial Orthop.* 2013;143(2):206-212.
9. **Kassab MM, Cohen RE.** The etiology and prevalence of gingival recession. *J Am Dent Assoc.* 2003;134(2):220-225.
10. **Löe H, Anerud A, Boysen H.** The natural history of periodontal disease in man: prevalence, severity, and extent of gingival recession. *J Periodontol.* 1992;63(6):489-495.
11. **Melsen B, Allais D.** Factors of importance for the development of dehiscences during labial movement of mandibular incisors: a retrospective study of adult orthodontic patients. *Am J Orthod Dentofacial Orthop.* 2005;127(5):552-625.
12. **Elkordy SA, Palomo L, Palomo JM, Mostafa YA.** Do fixed orthodontic appliances adversly affect the periodontium? A systematic review of systematic reviews. *Semin Orthod.* 2019;25(2):130-157.
13. **Tepedino M, Franchi L, Fabbro O, Chimenti C.** Postorthodontic lower incisor inclination and gingival recession - a systematic review. *Prog Orthod.* 2018;19(1):17.
14. **Aziz T, Flores-Mir C.** A systematic review of the association between appliance-induced labial movement of mandibular incisors and gingival recession. *Aust Orthod J.* 2011;27(1):33-39.
15. **Bollen AM, Cunha-Cruz J, Bakko DW et al.** The effects of orthodontic therapy on periodontal health: a systematic review of controlled evidence. *J Am Dent Assoc.* 2008;139(4):413-422.
16. **Papageorgiou SN, Eliades T.** *Clinical evidence on the effect of orthodontic treatment on the periodontal tissues.* In: Eliades T, Katsaros C. *The ortho-perio patient: clinical evidence & therapeutic guidelines.* Batavia, IL. Quintessence Publishing Co; 2019:161-173.
17. **Gebistorf M, Mijuskovic M, Pandis N et al.** Gingival recession in orthodontic patients 10 to 15 years posttreatment: A retrospective cohort study. *Am J Orthod Dentofacial Orthop.* 2018;153(5):645-655.
18. **Karring T, Nyman S, Thilander B, Magnusson I.** Bone regeneration in orthodontically produced alveolar bone dehiscences. *J Periodontal Res.* 1982;17(3):309-315.
19. **Wainwright WM.** Faciolingual tooth movement: its influence on the root and cortical plate. *Am J Orthod.* 1973;64(3):278-302.
20. **Ruf S, Hansen K, Pancherz H.** Does orthodontic proclination of lower incisors in children and adolescents cause gingival recession? *Am J Orthod Dentofacial Orthop.* 1998;114(1):100-106.
21. **Artun J, Grobéty D.** Periodontal status of mandibular incisors after pronounced orthodontic advancement during adolescence: a follow-up evaluation. *Am J Orthod Dentofacial Orthop.* 2001;119(1):2-10.
22. **Djeu G, Hayes C, Zawaideh S.** Correlation between mandibular central incisor proclination and gingival recession during fixed appliance therapy. *Angle Orthod.* 2002;72(3):238-245.
23. **Renkema AM, Navratilova Z, Mazurova K et al.** Gingival labial recessions and the post-treatment proclination of mandibular incisors. *Eur J Orthod.* 2015;37(5):508-513.
24. **Allais D, Melsen B.** Does labial movement of lower incisors influence the level of the gingival margin? A case-control study of adult orthodontic patients. *Eur J Orthod.* 2003;25(4):343-352.
25. **Joss-Vassalli I, Grebenstein C, Topouzelis N et al.** Orthodontic therapy and gingival recession: a systematic review. *Orthod Craniofac Res.* 2010;13(3):127-141.
26. **Bin Bahar BSK, Alkhalidy SR, Kaklamanos EG, Athanasiou AE.** Do orthodontic patients develop more gingival recession in anterior teeth compared to untreated individuals? A systematic review of controlled studies. *Int Orthod.* 2020;18(1):1-9.
27. **Antonarakis GS, Joss CU, Triaca A et al.** Gingival recessions of lower incisors after proclination by orthodontics alone or in combination with anterior mandibular alveolar process distraction osteogenesis. *Clin Oral Investig.* 2017;21(8):2569-2579.
28. **Kalina E, Zadurska M, Górski B.** Postorthodontic lower incisor and canine inclination and labial gingival recession in adult patients: a prospective study. *J Orofac Orthop.* 2020;10.1007/s00056-020-00263-1.
29. **Mazurova K, Kopp JB, Renkema AM et al.** Gingival recession in mandibular incisors and symphysis morphology-a retrospective cohort study. *Eur J Orthod.* 2018;40(2):185-192.
30. **Pernet F, Vento C, Pandis N, Kiliaridis S.** Long-term evaluation of lower incisors gingival recessions after orthodontic treatment. *Eur J Orthod.* 2019;41(6):559-564.
31. **Garlock DT, Buschang PH, Araujo EA et al.** Evaluation of marginal alveolar bone in the anterior mandible with pretreatment and posttreatment computed tomography in nonextraction patients. *Am J Orthod Dentofacial Orthop.* 2016;149(2):192-201.
32. **Andlin-Sobocki A.** Changes of facial gingival dimensions in children. A 2-year longitudinal study. *J Clin Periodontol.* 1993;20(3):212-218.
33. **Andlin-Sobocki A, Bodin L.** Dimensional alterations of the gingiva related to changes of facial/lingual tooth position in permanent anterior teeth of children. A 2-year longitudinal study. *J Clin Periodontol.* 1993;20(3):219-224.
34. **Engelking G, Zachrisson BU.** Effects of incisor repositioning on monkey periodontium after expansion through the cortical plate. *Am J Orthod.* 1982;82(1):23-32.
35. **Ainamo A, Bergenholtz A, Hugoson A, Ainamo J.** Location of the mucogingival junction 18 years after apically repositioned flap surgery. *J Clin Periodontol.* 1992;19(1):49-52.
36. **Wennström JL.** Mucogingival considerations in orthodontic treatment. *Semin Orthod.* 1996;2(1):46-54.
37. **Wennström JL, Lindhe J, Sinclair F, Thilander B.** Some periodontal tissue reactions to orthodontic tooth movement in monkeys. *J Clin Periodontol.* 1987;14(3):121-129.
38. **Ericsson I, Lindhe J.** Recession in sites with inadequate width of the keratinized gingiva. An experimental study in the dog. *J Clin Periodontol.* 1984;11(2):95-103.
39. **Baker DL, Seymour GJ.** The possible pathogenesis of gingival reces-

sion. A histological study of induced recession in the rat. *J Clin Periodontol.* 1976;3(4):208-219.

40. **Ericsson I, Thilander B, Lindhe J.** Periodontal conditions after orthodontic tooth movements in the dog. *Angle Orthod.* 1978;48(3):210-218.

41. **Ericsson I, Thilander B, Lindhe J, Okamoto H.** The effect of orthodontic tilting movements on the periodontal tissues of infected and non-infected dentitions in dogs. *J Clin Periodontol.* 1977;4(4):278-293.

42. **Harshita N, Kamath DG, Kadakampally D.** Perio-ortho interactions. A review. *J Pharm Sci & Res.* 2018; 10(5):1053-1056.

43. **Kim DM, Neiva R.** Periodontal soft tissue non-root coverage procedures: a systematic review from the AAP Regeneration Workshop. *J Periodontol.* 2015;86(2 Suppl):S56-S72.

44. **Johal A, Ide M.** Orthodontics in the adult patient, with special reference to the periodontally compromised patient. *Dent Update.* 1999;26(3):101-108.

45. **Yared KF, Zenobio EG, Pacheco W.** Periodontal status of mandibular central incisors after orthodontic proclination in adults. *Am J Orthod Dentofacial Orthop.* 2006;130(1):6.e1-6.e68.

46. **Lindhe J, Echeverria J.** *Consensus report of session II*, In: Lang NP, Karring T. *Proceedings of the 1st European Workshop on Clinical Periodontology.* Quintessence Ed., Berlin 1994:210-214.

47. **Johal A, Katsaros C, Kiliaridis S et al.** State of the science on controversial topics: orthodontic therapy and gingival recession (a report of the Angle Society of Europe 2013 meeting). *Prog Orthod.* 2013;14:16.

48. **Sangnes G.** Traumatization of teeth and gingiva related to habitual tooth cleaning procedures. *J Clin Periodontol.* 1976;3(2):94-103.

49. **Mandelaris GA, Neiva R, Chambrone L.** Cone-beam computed tomography and interdisciplinary dentofacial therapy: an american academy of periodontology best evidence review focusing on risk assessment of the dentoalveolar bone changes influenced by tooth movement. *J Periodontol.* 2017;88(10):960-977.

50. **Laursen MG, Rylev M, Melsen B.** The role of orthodontics in the repair of gingival recessions. *Am J Orthod Dentofacial Orthop.* 2020;157(1):29-34.

51. **Hiro T, de la Iglesia F, Andreu P.** Indirect bonding technique in lingual orthodontics: the HIRO system. *Prog Orthod.* 2008;9(2):34-45.

52. **Zucchelli G, De Sanctis M.** Treatment of multiple recession-type defects in patients with esthetic demands. *J Periodontol.* 2000;71(9):1506-1514.

53. **Zucchelli G, Mounssif I.** Periodontal plastic surgery. *Periodontol 2000.* 2015;68(1):333-368.

54. **Lundberg M, Wennström JL.** Development of gingiva following surgical exposure of a facially positioned unerupted incisor. *J Periodontol.* 1988;59(10):652-655.

55. **Andlin-Sobocki A, Persson M.** The association between spontaneous reversal of gingival recession in mandibular incisors and dentofacial changes in children. A 3-year longitudinal study. *Eur J Orthod.* 1994;16(3):229-239.

56. **Persson M, Lennartsson B.** Improvement potential of isolated gingival recession in children. *Swed Dent J.* 1986;10(1-2):45-51.

57. **Powell RN, McEniery TM.** A longitudinal study of isolated gingival recession in the mandibular central incisor region of children aged 6-8 years. *J Clin Periodontol.* 1982;9(5):357-364.

58. **Pini Prato G, Baccetti T, Magnani C et al.** Mucogingival interceptive surgery of buccally-erupted premolars in patients scheduled for orthodontic treatment. I. A 7-year longitudinal study. *J Periodontol.* 2000;71(2):172-181.

59. **Pini Prato G, Baccetti T, Giorgetti R et al.** Mucogingival interceptive surgery of buccally-erupted premolars in patients scheduled for orthodontic treatment. II. Surgically treated versus nonsurgically treated cases. *J Periodontol.* 2000;71(2):182-187.

60. **Sigler LM, Baccetti T, McNamara JA Jr.** Effect of rapid maxillary expansion and transpalatal arch treatment associated with deciduous canine extraction on the eruption of palatally displaced canines: A 2-center prospective study. *Am J Orthod Dentofacial Orthop.* 2011;139(3):e235-e244.

61. **Baccetti T, Mucedero M, Leonardi M, Cozza P.** Interceptive treatment of palatal impaction of maxillary canines with rapid maxillary expansion: a randomized clinical trial. *Am J Orthod Dentofacial Orthop.* 2009;136(5):657-661.

62. **Naoumova J, Kurol J, Kjellberg H.** Extraction of the deciduous canine as an interceptive treatment in children with palatal displaced canines - part I: shall we extract the deciduous canine or not? *Eur J Orthod.* 2015;37(2):209-218.

63. **Bazargani F, Magnuson A, Lennartsson B.** Effect of interceptive extraction of deciduous canine on palatally displaced maxillary canine: a prospective randomized controlled study. *Angle Orthod.* 2014;84(1):3-10.

64. **Baccetti T, Sigler LM, McNamara JA Jr.** An RCT on treatment of palatally displaced canines with RME and/or a transpalatal arch. *Eur J Orthod.* 2011;33(6):601-607.

65. **Baccetti T, Leonardi M, Armi P.** A randomized clinical study of two interceptive approaches to palatally displaced canines. *Eur J Orthod.* 2008;30(4):381-385.

66. **Leonardi M, Armi P, Franchi L, Baccetti T.** Two interceptive approaches to palatally displaced canines: a prospective longitudinal study. *Angle Orthod.* 2004;74(5):581-586.

67. **Armi P, Cozza P, Baccetti T.** Effect of RME and headgear treatment on the eruption of palatally displaced canines: a randomized clinical study. *Angle Orthod.* 2011;81(3):370-374.

68. **Crescini A, Baccetti T, Rotundo R et al.** Tunnel technique for the treatment of impacted mandibular canines. *Int J Periodontics Restorative Dent.* 2009;29(2):213-218.

69. **Crescini A, Clauser C, Giorgetti R et al.** Tunnel traction of infraosseous impacted maxillary canines. A three-year periodontal follow-up. *Am J Orthod Dentofacial Orthop.* 1994;105(1):61-72.

GOR (Guided Orthodontic Regeneration): orthodontics as a regenerative means

Extrusion as regeneration

The extrusion as orthodontic movement is a regenerative means that is able to stimulate the dentoalveolar complex either to expose healthy root tissue from the supracrestal tissue for future rehabilitation or to develop an implant site with an adequate three-dimensional amount of hard and soft tissues for a correct implant positioning in order to obtain a harmonious emergence profile[1-3].

Already Heithersay[4], Brown[5] and Ingber[6,7], in the early 1970s, had developed the concept of orthodontic movement in order to treat coronal-root fractures with changes in the length of the clinical crown[8], periodontal intrabony defects and displacement of gingival levels. The bone apposition on the alveolar ridge in response to the stretching of the supracrestal gingival fibers has been histologically demonstrated by Reitan et al.[9] and confirmed by Van Venrooy and Yukna[10] on animals where apical osseous apposition and sulcus depth reduction occurred in teeth with extensive periodontal destruction.

Orthodontic extrusion as a regenerative means is a pure orthodontic movement of the single tooth to be rehabilitated and, at the same time, it becomes part of a broader orthodontic treatment that involves the entire occlusion. Orthodontics is thus involved in the interdisciplinary team and offers a diagnostic and mechanical contribution for what concerns the redistribution of the spaces, the harmonization of the mucogingival and/or bone periodontal morphology, the correction of occlusal discrepancies, the changes in the crown/root ratio in order to optimize the position of teeth and abutments, the tooth shape, the vertical dimension, the occlusal references[11-13] and the stability during prosthetic rehabilitation[14], reducing invasive treatments and increasing their predictability[15].

Orthodontics in orthodontic-periodontal treatments, and in particular in orthodontic extrusion, must visualize the starting three-dimensional anatomy of hard and soft tissues and the final treatment aims. The attachment level, the mucogingival junction and the probing depth must be clear in relation to the intraoral radiographic examination. These observations must also be made during periodic re-evaluations during orthodontic mechanics. The dialogue between the orthodontist and the periodontist must be continuous because the modifications of the hard and soft tissues that are obtainable with orthodontics become an active part of the periodontal treatment, without opposing or limiting it but, on the contrary, often allowing its implementation and enhancing it. The "regenerative" advantage that is offered by orthodontics not only includes the reconstruction of a pre-implant site with a primary stability of the future implant through the increase of hard tissues, but also the improvement of soft tissues, giving the possibility to the periodontist to have a greater potential and predictability in regenerative and mucogingival surgical techniques. In the same way, the visualization of the anatomy of the remaining periodontal support of the tooth to be extruded, of the adjacent teeth and the anchorage teeth allow the orthodontist to perform movements that provide the maximum stimulation of the hard and soft tissues, aimed at periodontal regeneration.

Although there is no standard clinical protocol, in the presence of an attachment apparatus and healthy connective fibers that enable apical bone apposition and soft tissue augmentation, the maximum regenerative potential is achieved; however, even if regeneration is not complete for the presence of a compromised periodontal attachment, the resulting soft tissue improvement allows for subsequent less invasive and more predictable reconstructive surgical phases, with less morbidity, enhancing the final esthetic result[16-18].

The indications (8.1), the contraindications (8.2), the advantages (8.3), the disadvantages (8.4) and the limits (8.5) of orthodontic extrusion are described below.

Tab. 8.1 Indications to orthodontic extrusion

Treatment of subgingival or infrabony lesions between cemento-enamel junction and 1/3 coronal of the root (decays, root fractures, iatrogenic perforations, internal and external resorptions), especially in esthetic sectors
Restorations interesting the supracrestal tissue attachment
Angular bone defects and isolated periodontal pockets reduction
Implant site development
Orthodontic extraction when there is a contraindication to surgical extraction (Biphosphonate and/or radiotherapy and chemotherapy)
Bone and gingival discrepancies leveling
Orthodontic extraction for space closure on non-maintainable teeth

Tab. 8.2 Contraindications to orthodontic extrusion

Uncontrolled chronic inflammatory lesions including endo-perio lesions and fractured roots
Inability to control inflammation and acute infections that could lead to a failure of the healing and the response of the treatment
Absence of periodontal attachment (extrusion relocate only the pre-existing attachment)
Ankylosis of the tooth to be extruded
Hypercementosis
Vertical root fractures
Root proximity (especially on the molar)
If the extrusion is used for prosthetic purposes: • short roots without restoration support (crown/root ratio <1:1) • insufficient prosthetic space • furcation involvement

Tab. 8.3 Advantages to orthodontic extrusion

Conservative procedure (reduction of the prosthetic or restorative preparation of natural teeth and maintenance of teeth otherwise to be extracted; implant site development with less surgical procedures)
Bone loss reduction (compared to surgical crown lengthening or socket preservation techniques) and less risk of gingival recessions (results from soft tissue surgeries)
Relatively simple orthodontic techniques
Greater advantages in the placement of immediate loading post-extraction implants

Tab. 8.4 Disadvantages to orthodontic extrusion

Application of orthodontic appliance (esthetic problems, greater difficulties to maintain oral hygiene)
Duration of treatment (long in some cases)
Frequency of appointments
Procedures, times and costs of orthodontic treatment
Slight gingival surgical procedures to regularize gingival levels after the extrusion

Tab. 8.5 Limits to orthodontic extrusion

Severe circumferential bone loss
Horizontal bone deficit
Shape of the alveolar bone (the loss of the buccal cortical plate before and after extrusion does not allow implant placement)

Clinical application

The acronym GOR (Guided Orthodontic Regeneration) describes the orthodontic procedure either to recover healthy dental tissue for the restoration of the tooth or to regenerate hard and soft tissues for implant site development using the tooth itself as a distraction means through the tension of the periodontal ligament[19]. The GOR can be divided into:

- *Tissue modelling*: the extrusion of the tooth to recover the dental substance of the tooth itself or the extraction of the tooth to create hard and soft tissue;
- *Tissue regeneration*: development of the implant site. It is divided into:
  - *GOBR*[20] (Guided Orthodontic "Bone" Regeneration), which is mainly a bone regeneration of the implant site for immediate implant placement;
  - *GOTR*[21] (Guided Orthodontic "Tissue" Regeneration), which is mainly a tissue regeneration to increase the amount of soft tissue in order to facilitate regenerative surgical procedures with membrane (GBR) and mucogingival techniques.

Considering the amount of extrusive movement and tissue regeneration, GOR can be divided into:

- recovery of the tooth;
- extraction of the tooth without implant placement with orthodontic closure of the spaces;
- extraction of the tooth with implant placement (Implant Site Development) GOBR-GOTR.

Before starting the extrusion clinical variables (8.6) and important factors for effectiveness (8.7) must be evaluated.

Tissue modelling

GOR can be used both to model the periodontal architecture and to recover the natural healthy root system for the subsequent direct or indirect restorative treatment, and also to reshape the hard and soft tissues through the orthodontic extraction in post-extraction space closure of adjacent teeth.

Tab. 8.6 Clinical variables to be evaluated for extrusion

Amount of clinical attachment level and periodontal condition of the tooth to be extruded
Root length
Periodontal assessment of the adjacent teeth and the anchorages
Presence in the arch of periodontal problems that can be modified by orthodontics
Post-extrusion prosthetic space and final position of the roots at the end of the movement
Smile line
Gingival phenotype
Final position of the gingival margin
Patient's age and systemic conditions
Orthodontics considerations: • planning of orthodontic forces and related biomechanics • 3D prediction of the orthodontic movement • prevention of the apex/cortical plates contact • planning of the adequate anchorages

RECOVERY OF THE DENTAL STRUCTURE ("DENTAL EXTRUSION")

The recovery of the healthy dental structure to avoid the invasion of the supracrestal tissue attachment[22] (the previously called "biological width") was initially used in restorative dentistry. This technique was described in the early 1970s[4] and was applied, after careful evaluation of the residual tooth structure, to the treatment of root or coronal -root fractures, caries, root resorption, iatrogenic perforations invading the supracrestal tissue attachment, unfavourable crown/root ratios for prosthetic restoration where a clinical crown lengthening surgery would have been contraindicated[23] (8.8; 8.1) if it caused a negative crown/root relationship, an excessive lengthening of clinical crowns, a structural negative impact on the adjacent teeth or a reduction in interproximal bone with an opening of interdental spaces. In addition, orthodontic extrusion, unlike resective surgery, can involve only the tooth to be rehabilitated and, as a consequence, any post-extrusive "surgical realignments" to re-establish the correct relationships of the supracrestal tissue at-

Tab. 8.7 Factors determining the effectiveness of orthodontic extrusion

Active periodontal disease	As all orthodontic movements in the periodontal patient, active periodontal disease must be treated and completely controlled before the movement begins, to make tissue regeneration more effective
Initial conditions of teeth/tooth	Importance of endodontic evaluation for root canal therapy during extrusion and the restorative situation for anchoring the brackets; root ankylosis; hypercementosis
Force direction	Axial extrusive force along the dental axis + tipping and torque incorporation by controlling and preventing cortical plates impacts (apex)
Speed and intensity of the extrusion movement	• Slow (1 mm/month) for implant site development. Need to increase gingival and bone tissue, such as the interproximal areas where the bone must support the interdental papilla, or to correct bone defects; the dento-periodontal attachment system follows the slow movement in a better way. There is a compensatory growth of hard and soft tissues • Fast (1 mm/week) for dental extrusion. Need to extrude only the dental component leaving the gingival margin in place. The eruption, in these cases, exceeds the growth of the bone, because of the speed of movement (obtained with a high force). The gingival tissue may follow, requiring a gingivectomy localized only around the extruded root, or a fibrotomy procedure
Bone level of the adjacent tooth/teeth	Important for implant site development for possible interdental papilla deficit Possible extrusion of the adjacent tooth/teeth
Number of teeth involved	Need for periodontal bone levelling in the arch even for more than one tooth
Retention time	Stability depends on the quantity and speed of extrusion

Tab. 8.8 Contraindication to surgical crown lengthening

Periodontal reduction of the adjacent teeth (healthy tissue reduction - bone support), sacrifice of healthy periodontal attachment
Esthetic compromises and discrepancies with opening of interdental spaces
Furcations involvement
Root concavities exposure
Root hypersensitivity
Unfavorable crown/root ratio
Increase of crown/root ratio

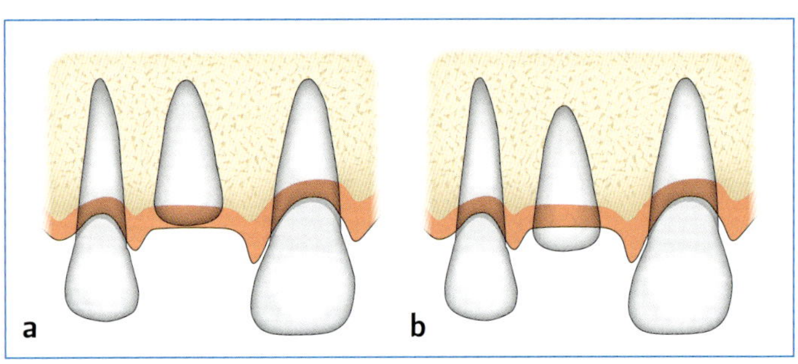

8.1 Schematic drawing of the orthodontic extrusion. Root fragment with supracrestal tissue involvement (**a**) and recovery of healthy dental tissue outside the supracrestal tissue at the end of the extrusion (**b**).

tachment become more conservative because limited only to the root that is subjected to extrusion movement[24,25]. Another indication for the use of dental extrusion is the maintenance of the alveolar bone in the upper anterior maxillary area in young patients, after trauma, to postpone the implant solution[26-28] as much as possible through the maintenance of a non-classically restorable root abutment. This strategy can also be used in the case of complicated root or coronal-root fractures, after endodontic treatment, extrusion and temporary crown reconstruction, simplifying and making more predictable the future implant treatment which will be carried out at the end of the growth, protecting the cortical bones and the alveolar dimension of the ridge[29,30]. Compared to traditional orthodontic treatment, the goal of dental orthodontic extrusion is not to change the tridimensional position of the tooth in the arch, but to maintain and preserve the root system and its periodontal attachment system[24]. Various factors must be evaluated before treatment (esthetics, clinical root length, root proximity, root morphology, furcation position, individual and relative tooth position, feasibility of tooth reconstruction)[31]. The case selection criteria for dental extrusion are summarized in 8.9.

Tab. 8.9 Case selection criteria for dental orthodontic extrusion

Level and extension of fracture/decay/perforation	At the end of the extrusion, healthy dental tissue must be present in order to re-establish a correct supracrestal attachment and a sufficient ferrule effect
Crown/root ratio	Minimum 1:1. Before starting the extrusion, evaluate the final length of the root inside the bone (very important because it is a crucial factor for the longevity of the tooth-supported restoration and a necessary condition for the implementation of this technique)
Root morphology	The endodontic space (in order to manage the spaces for a future endodontic post) and the third coronal root, which will be the part of root tissue that will form the area outside the periodontal tissues, must be evaluated. Important for the emergence profile of the subsequent restoration
Patient motivation and age	Younger patients are more motivated to use orthodontics and to maintain their teeth as an alternative to implant replacement (the average age of patients undergoing orthodontic extrusion is lower than for surgical treatment, perhaps because they are more inclined to the application of an orthodontic mechanics despite the commitment or esthetics)
Root health	There must be no periapical lesions and the root canal treatment must be excellent or it must be performed without problems. There should be no resorptions or lesions on the root surface
Residual dentition	The tooth value must be evaluated with respect to the residual dentition. In the event that other teeth that cannot be restored or cannot be maintained correctly from a hygienic or restorative point of view are present in the archwire (especially if adjacent), a broader treatment plan must be evaluated
Dental history	Teeth with previous restorations, repeated endodontic treatment, loss of tooth structure and previous root canal retentions make the tooth structurally more fragile

Two techniques of execution are reported in the literature:

1. Orthodontic extrusion with subsequent bone surgery to restore the correct gingival margin[32], to be used mainly in cases where there is a reduction of keratinized tissue which is increased by extrusion[33]. Subsequent surgical procedures are referred to as "biological width realignment procedures"[34] (see *Clinical case 2*).
2. Orthodontic extrusion with fibrotomy, to be used when the soft tissues are quantitatively and qualitatively sufficient and do not require alteration of position (see *Clinical case 1*).

The indications for fibrotomy are:

- correct pre-extrusion gingival levels (gingival levels must not be changed);
- sufficient amount of keratinized tissue width.

Fibrotomy consists in the resection of the supracrestal fibers through an intrasulcular incision with the separation of the supracrestal attachment between the cemento-enamel junction and the bone ridge, with subsequent scaling and root planing to the level of the bone ridge immediately after the fibrotomy along the entire tooth circumference[35,36]. This incision is made, according to the Authors, every 7 days[36,37] or every 14 days[38] and aims to avoid the migration of the periodontal tissue that occours with the extrusion, thus eliminating the need for subsequent osseous resective surgery[38]. In any case it is important to keep in mind that, as stated by Zenobio et al.[33], extrusion with fibrotomy may not lead to significantly different bone and tissue anatomy changes than in simple extrusion. In fact, fibrotomy does not always avoid coronal tissue migration due to the presence of supracrestal fibers that are still inserted on the root surface[1] or that reinsert quickly after fibrotomy on the wounded soft tissue[39]. Early reattachment of these fibers can be overcome by planing the root surface whenever fibrotomy is performed[1,37]. The association of the fibrotomy with the root planing is therefore able to dissociate the tooth movement from the supporting periodontal structures without altering the gingival margins[40]. Da Silva et al.[36] recommend to perform an open flap to eliminate the fibers before starting the extrusion. However, since this operation is performed only once, it does not prevent the re-attachment of the fibers (this process occurs very early after the open flap), resulting in a lower coronal migration of the gingival level compared to the one obtained with fibrotomy which is repeated regularly[36,37]. The real advantage of flap elevation before starting the extrusion (as well as with the aim of disrupting the inserted connective fibers) is to allow a better quantification of the biological width invasion[33] by the pathogenic noxa, but always at the price of additional surgery. Some Authors also recommend fibrotomy as a single procedure at the end of the movement[41,42]. In highly esthetic cases, in which the gingival margin must remain at the initial position and only a dental extrusion[36] with minimal subsequent gingival corrections[1] is required, it is also recommended to plan and carry out a gingival correction at the end of the extrusion, even if the procedure is performed with fibrotomy[37,41]. The relationship of the periodontal attachment/crestal bone related to the adjacent teeth at the beginning of the movement must be carefully evaluated, as this relationship will remain constant, since this technique takes the root out of the bone without altering bone architecture[37]. Supracrestal fibrotomy before and during forced extrusion is also recommended to reduce the reattachment process and to limit intrusive forces after the root has been positioned correctly. It is not clear, however, to what extent it reduces the stabilization time[24,43].

LIMITS OF DENTAL EXTRUSION

A limit of dental extrusion, especially in cases of high esthetic value, is the reduction of the diameter of the root conicity, which does not allow a natural emergence profile, making it difficult not to overhang the restoration and to safeguard the periodontal tissues[44]. 8.2 shows how a conical root shape after extrusion determines a reduction of the mesiodistal dimension, with a consequent increase in the emergence profile of the crown, which is not so pronounced in more cylindrical roots (8.3). In literature it is reported that, in particular with fast movement, dental extrusion may be associated with a high risk of dental ankylosis, since the ligament may tear with rapid extrusion, and also that there is a risk of root resorption, although this rarely happens if forces are controlled[41,43,45].

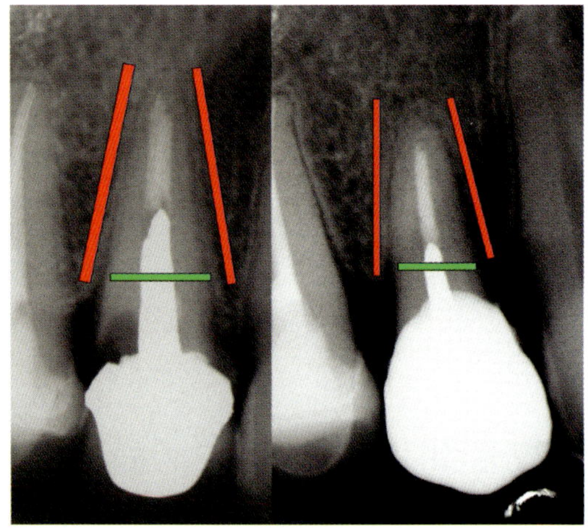

8.2 Conical root shape that after orthodontic extrusion causes a reduction of the root diameter with an increase of the emergence profile.

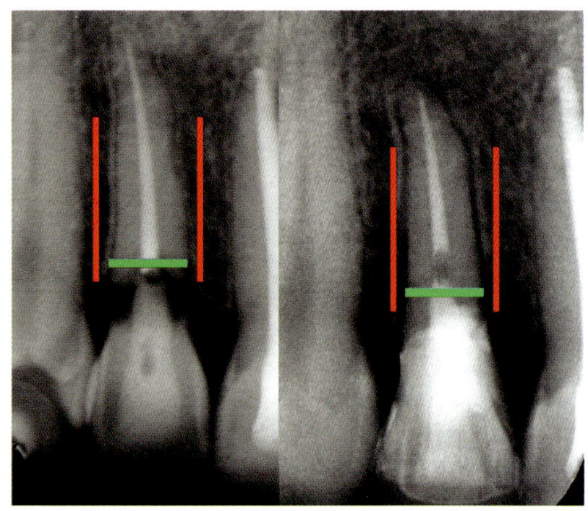

8.3 Cylindrical root shape that does not modify the root diameter after orthodontic extrusion.

ORTHODONTIC TECHNIQUE

Pre-restorative dental extrusion allows not only to reposition the root exposing healthy root tissue for restorative purposes, but also to provide better bone and gingival profiles to the tooth to be restored and to all the teeth[33]. This technique can be performed with the bonding of the entire arch or with sectional appliances[46-49]. The sectional appliance can include extrusion and stabilization mechanics at the same time. The tooth to be extruded will be provided with a classic orthodontic brackets or with a root anchorage[20]; esthetics and anchorage can also be guaranteed by temporary crowns[23,30,31]. Dental extrusion, as happens in the case of pre-implant extrusion[50], is achieved in literature in classical orthodontic mechanics, initially both with .016 Ni-Ti archwires[41] with forces lower than 70 g[33] (equal to approximately 50 g[24,40,50]), or directly with round[41] or rectangular[37,38,41,42] stain steel archwires with compensating bends so that the extrusion force is as axial as possible and centred along the root axis[37,41], and with loops or springs[41], or with Cr-Co archwires[43]; sometimes the extrusion is carried out with simple inter-arch elastics on temporary crowns[24]. The brackets is positioned on the tooth to be extruded in the most apical position with progressive restorations of the dental or root abutment, in order to be able to move the attachment more and more apically. Some Authors perform the activations every week[37,40] or every 2 weeks[33,42]. During each check, the activation of the mechanics and the elimination of any occlusal contacts are immediately carried out[37]. Dental extrusion ends when a minimum distance of 3-4 mm is reached between the bone crest and the margin that has been set as the target of the final restoration. Stabilization is carried out either with .018×.025 continuous steel archwires, or with loops[34] with passive forces for a minimum of 80[37]-90 days[33], or with .018 stain steel archwires for 8 weeks[40] or with auxiliary .017×.025 stain steel anchorage archwires. The anchorages can be inter-arch[51] or intra-arch, complete or on sectional appliance[37,38], on Hawley[24,41], on removable temporary appliances[50] or miniscrews[47]. It is important to perform periodic monthly radiographic checks and an X-ray at the end of the extrusion, before the restoration[33]. Rapid extrusion rate ranges from 1mm per week[37] to 1.5mm every 2 weeks, with fibrotomy and orthodontic activation every 2 weeks[37,38], to 4mm in 8 weeks[51].

Also in the case of dental extrusion, the priority of the orthodontic treatment objective is not the coronal levelling, but the alignment and levelling of the bone-soft tissue periodontal support, compatibly with the root positioning. The subsequent coronal reconstruction[40,51] will be the task of restorative dentistry.

Clinical protocol of dental extrusion

Our clinical protocol starts from an initial evaluation with the periodontist about the possible need for hard and soft tissue augmentation. In 8.4 a procedural summary outline for dental extrusion is described. In the case of lack of one or both types of tissue, the dental extrusion can be divided into a first phase of regenerative extrusion, in which the extrusion is slow (about 1 mm/month) and it is aimed to the regenerative remodeling of the periodontal tissue of the tooth that have to be extruded in relationship of the adjacent elements, and in a second phase, with weekly checks, in which the extrusion is fast (1 mm/week) and accompanied by fibrotomy, if necessary. In this regard, it should be re-

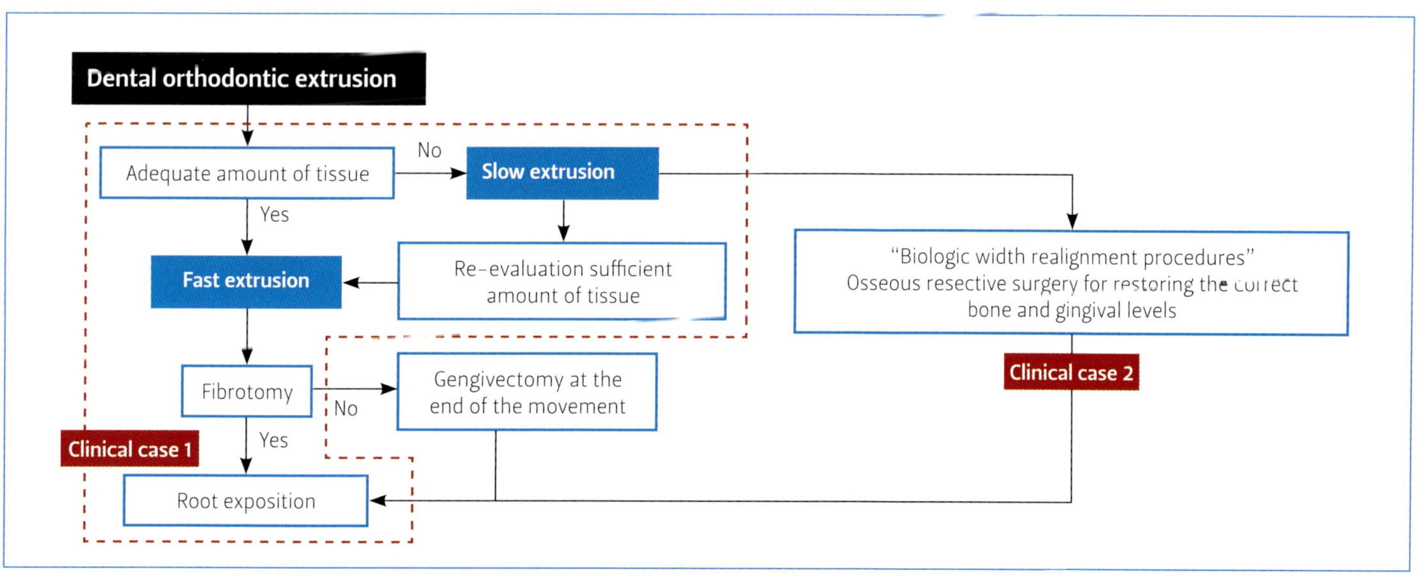

8.4 Summary diagram of diagnosis and clinical procedures for the evaluation of dental extrusion techniques.

membered that the speed of the extrusive movement[24] is of two types:

- slow (1 mm/month): need to increase the gingival and bone tissue, including the interproximal areas where the bone must support the interdental papilla, or to correct bone defects; the dento-periodontal attachment system follows slow movement in a better way. There is a compensatory growth of hard and soft tissues;
- fast (1 mm/week): need to extrude only the dental component leaving the gingival margin *in situ*, by a rapid extrusion, since the coronal migration of the tissue that supports the tooth is less pronounced as the speed of movement exceeds the physiological adaptability of tissues[41,43,45]. The extrusion in these cases exceeds the growth of the bone, because of the speed of movement[51].

In both vestibular and lingual mechanics, the protocol includes a direct or indirect bonding from the first phase with a more apical positioning of the brackets. In programming the set-up and the brackets positioning, it is important to take into account the vestibular and, more importantly, the lingual tooth morphology, the ideal center of resistance of the tooth, the real center of resistance due to the loss of periodontal support and the moment resulting from the extrusive component at the point of application of the force. If a first regenerative phase is required, the first step of the protocol is a slow extrusion, that we will see later on the implant site development. Here we will analyse the rapid extrusion aimed at exposing the restorative margin. In rapid extrusion, the first orthodontic archwire is an undersized .016 preformed CuNiTi archwire. The different and set-up position of the brackets and the activations will regulate the extrusion speed. Since fast extrusion happens with forces up to about 50 g, the anchorages and reactions on the adjacent teeth must be controlled very well. The checks are weekly and include activations, assessment of the periodontal state and any parasite movements, adjustment of the extrusion speed and control and prevention of any cortical impacts and/or occlusal contacts, also carrying out fibrotomy, where it is necessary. The following archwires, whose turnover is very fast, are β-titanium archwires, at first an undersized .016 preformed β-titanium, then a .017×.017 β-titanium, which incorporate direct extrusive steps or loops. Incremental tipping and torque loops can be inserted; the next archwire is a .017×.025 β-titanium archwire, again with extrusive steps and fibrotomy. The final archwires can be a .018×.025 stainless steel and also in this latter it is possible to add extrusion steps or loops and fibrotomy, to arrive at the stabilization with the same archwire or with an archwire with a larger dimension, such as a .019×.025 stain steel. An X-ray must be performed every 1-2 months; the X-ray at the end of the extrusion and pre-restorative one is essential (Tab. 8.10). In dental extrusion, as well as in the pre-implant regenerative one, an eventual impact of the root and in particular of the apex with the cortical plate must always be controlled and prevented; extrusive forces must be rapid,

Tab. 8.10 Clinical protocol of vestibular and lingual dental extrusion

I phase: regeneration with hard and soft tissue enhancement in case of deficit of one or both tissues
• Vestibular or lingual direct or indirect bonding - more apical positioning of the bracket - (analysis of the lingual morphology) parasite movements prevision - slot .022×.028
• .016 CuNiTi archwire
• Anchorage control TADs, if needed
• .016 β-titanium archwire -extrusive steps/loops, tipping
• .017×.017 β-titanium archwire -extrusive steps/loops, tipping, torque
Achievement of the regenerative objectives, suitable hard and soft tissue level
II phase: pure dental extrusion
• .016 CuNiTi archwire, brackets uneven positioning - fibrotomy
• .016 β-titanium archwire - extrusive steps/loops, tipping - fibrotomy
• .017×.017 β-titanium archwire - extrusive steps/loops, tipping, torque, fibrotomy
• .017×.025 β-titanium archwire - extrusive steps/loops, tipping, torque, fibrotomy
III phase: stabilization
• .017×.025 stain steel archwire -extrusive steps/loops, tipping, torque, fibrotomy if needed
• .017×.025 stain steel stabilization archwire 1 month/mm (extrusion)
Checks every 7-15 days: periodontal control/speed of extrusion, control of parasite movements on the tooth and on adjacent teeth and on anchorages, activations, hygiene, X-ray every 1-2 months

Tab. 8.11 Principles to always keep in mind during the orthodontic phase

Control and prevention of impacts of the apex to the vestibular and lingual cortical bone plates
Use of forces within 50 g slow and continuous forces for slow extrusion or quick forces for quick extrusion
Prevention of instability during tooth movement
Correlate tooth movement to gingival movement; take into consideration the residual periodontal support and the relative speed of movement
Tooth movement must be accompanied by gingival tissues in health conditions
Prevent traumatic occlusal contacts
The discomfort of the patient must be kept at the minimal possible level
The speed of movement must not have consequence on adjacent teeth
Bimonthly radiographic checks
Control and management of periodontal health, clorexidine, root planing

but always within 30-50 g; the tooth movement must be fast but must not cause instability both in the tooth to be extruded and in the adjacent teeth. In dental extrusion the tooth can be subjected to a speed movement greater than the gingival movement, always taking into account the residual periodontal support and the relative speed of movement. In dental extrusion the gingiva should not follow the tooth movement, but remain in its position in healthy conditions. Traumatizing occlusal contacts must be avoided and it is important to keep the patient in a comfortable condition. Checks should be done every week and be accompanied by fibrotomy when the gingival margin must remain in place. At each check-up, periodontal health should be evaluated and chlorhexidine applied (Tab. 8.11).

DENTAL EXTRACTION ("ORTHODONTIC EXTRACTION")

When brought to its extreme, i.e. in case of orthodontic extraction (see *Clinical case 3*), extrusion allows to create and fill the post-extraction socket with hard and soft tissue, so that the adjacent teeth can find the residual socket ready to be filled by their displacement in the extraction sockets avoiding the unpleasant clefts (linear invaginations in the interproximal gingival tissue with mesial and distal orientation, at least 1 mm deep[52]) (8.5), in which the plaque control is more complex, with a major risk for periodontal disease[53,54]. The same problem occurs in the movement in atrophic ridges[55] and this technique can be used to overcome the reduction in bone thickness after extractions[56]. The orthodontic extraction[57,58] can also be used as a means to increase the soft tissue on the edentulous site, so that it can be subsequently reshaped from the pontic of a conventional fixed denture without having to perform connective onlay grafts. The edentulous site can also be increased in conjunction with the development of the implant site if several adjacent teeth are extruded and only some of them are replaced with implants[14].

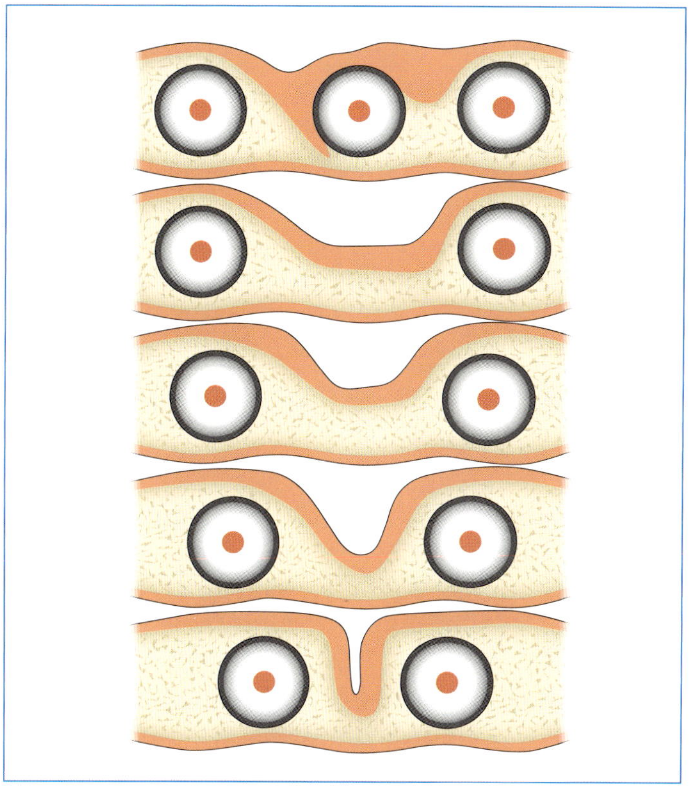

8.5 Schematic diagram where the possible cleft formation in the residual space of the post-extraction defect can be seen.

Orthodontic considerations in orthodontic extraction

The extrusive-extractive mechanics can modify the anatomy of hard and soft tissues while closing at the same time the extractive space. It is essential to evaluate the bone peaks adjacent to the lost tooth. If the bone peaks present a healthy periodontal attachment with intact cortical bone plates, the residual periodontal support of the lost tooth is used to perform a periodontal regenerative therapy by the orthodontic movement. The orthodontic extraction involves a first axial movement with a tipping component opposite to the defect that brings the interdental bone level of the lost tooth towards the peak of the adjacent tooth, then a torque movement of the residual root fragment to maintain the cortical bone and stimulate the vestibulo-lingual thickness. At the same time the space of the extraction site is closed, first with a "hyper-tipping" root movement, then with a coronal movement. On the other hand, if the attachment level of the adjacent tooth is not intact, after evaluation of the validity of the residual root support, a simultaneous extrusion of the two teeth is carried out; then, once a sufficient adjacent peak has been obtained, an extrusion sequence is carried out as previously described (see 8.91b). In the case of orthodontic extraction, the direction of the force depends on the existing periodontal support and, where possible, the extrusion/extraction mechanics proceeds parallel to the closure of the extraction space. The healthy periodontal support, for what concerns the small part that has remained on the compromised tooth, is used to mold the soft and hard tissues of the extraction site that will be subjected to the space closure during the same orthodontic extraction[19]. This technique reduces the risk of the cortical plates collapse and impingement and maintains a ridge thickness allowing for a tooth movement which is more predictable than a movement within a defect created by the collapse of the cortical plates.

Some Authors had already proposed GBR techniques with membranes with graft materials to reduce the risk of clefts which, sometimes, occur in orthodontic extraction sites even before the tooth is moved towards the extraction site and which, in addition to being esthetically disabling, can prevent or slow down a complete closure of the extractive space or cause relapse[59-66]. In some studies[60], the grafting of the post-extraction socket with heterologous materials before orthodontic movement showed some problems: compromised orthodontic movements in regenerated tissue in mice, due to the slow resorption of bovine bone; increased risk of root resorption in animals in areas treated with bone substitutes; slowing of orthodontic movement in the presence of ceramic bone (60% HA-40% β-TCP). The causes of the formation of clefts ranged from the proliferation of connective and epithelial tissue to the change of bone morphology and topography, which jeopardise the formation of transseptal fibers and physiological gingival tissue, or till to the fracture of the bone walls during dental extraction[52]. We know from literature that the tendency to develop gingival clefts, whose frequency reaches 35-100% in premolars[53,67], occurs more frequently when the onset of movement is early and in the so-called *fast movers*[59,61], but also that all the patients that undergo post-extraction space closure are at risk of producing cleft and should be monitored, as gingival cleft formation is a common occurrence after premolar extractions. In particular, adults with a thin gingival phenotype (that is a predisposing factor for their formation and severity) who develop them more severely, are more predisposed to produce cleft. The speed of closing the gap is inversely related to the cleft formation, which is more likely to happen with slow closing movements. In fast movement, in fact, the time for bone remodeling, its reduction and the reorganization of the gingival fibers complex would be less[53,61]. The advanced resorption of the alveolar ridge before starting space closure is one of the mechanisms that lead to the formation of gingival clefts[59] and this justifies, according to some Authors, the hypothesis that even a late movement in the extraction site would facilitate gingival invagination[68,69]. At an histological and histochemical level, samples taken from sites of gingival invagination show hypertrophy of the connective and epithelial tissue and, sometimes, loss of gingival collagen[70], offering an excellent site for plaque retention and being a primary risk factor for disorders of the periodontal tissue during orthodontic treatment[71]. Therefore, orthodontic extraction, as a regenerative technique, must be taken into account not only for esthetic purposes, but in particular for the protection of the patient's periodontal health[59,61], reducing the risk of loss of vestibular cortical bone, favouring the remodeling instead of the displacement of the transseptal fibers system with invagination of the gingival tissues, assumed genesis of cleft[53,61,72,73], and maintaining stable the bone architecture below the extractive site that is at risk in vestibolo-lingual[69,74] and in the interproximal dimension at the cleft level[75].

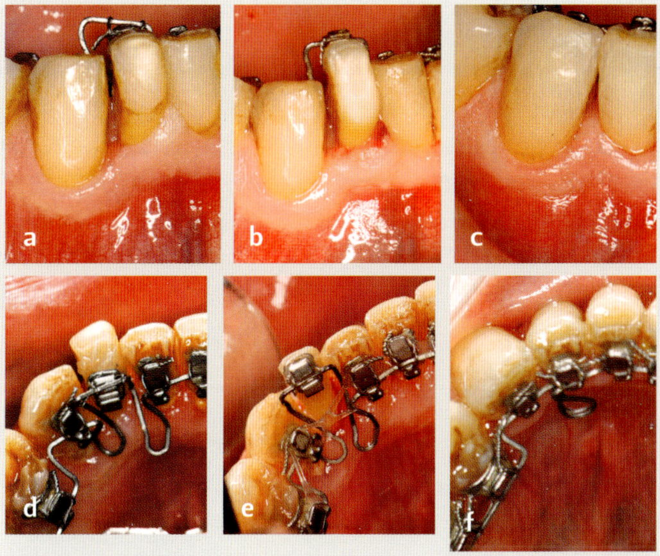

8.6* Orthodontic extraction, maintenance of the 3D volume of the post-extraction site.

Tab. 8.12 Clinical protocol of vestibular and lingual dental orthodontic extraction

• Vestibular or lingual direct or indirect bonding - positioning of the bracket with an apical tipping where the bone loss is more apical- positioning of the bracket on adjacent teeth to obtain a radicular movement which favor from the very beginning with a hyper-radicular tipping a bodily movement during the phase of space closure- slot .022×.028
• .016 CuNiTi archwire
• .016 β-titanium archwire - extrusive steps/loops, tipping
• .017×.017 β-titanium archwire - extrusive steps/loops, tipping, torque - closing loops and extrusion
• .017×.025 β-titanium archwire - extrusive steps/loops, tipping, torque - closing loops and extrusion
• .018×.025 stain steel archwire, .019×.025 stain steel archwire - closing loops, stabilization
Checks every 15 days: periodontal, occlusal control, hygiene, control of parasite movements on the tooth and on anchorages, activations, X-ray every 1-2 months

All these considerations reiterate the importance of keeping the three-dimensional volume of the extraction site stable (8.6).

Clinical protocol for vestibular orthodontics

The orthodontic protocol starts with a direct or indirect vestibular bonding. In both these choices, the positioning of the brackets on an individualized set-up of the teeth adjacent to the tooth to be extracted must be planned by positioning the brackets with an inclination that is more apical where there is a greater bone loss and that need more extrusion. This position incorporates from the very beginning a root tipping movement which will extrude and level the base of the bone defect and start a root approaching movement, reducing and simplifying the following space closure mainly by a secondary coronal movement. However, a possible risk of cortical contact and collapse must be foreseen incorporating a root torque component from the beginning to protect the maintenance of any present, even minimal, cortical bone.

With this careful approach, even the very first archwires, in round, small sized, low forces CuNiTi, incorporate a movement that is able to close the space at the root level. This mechanics will continue with a .016 β-titanium archwire first of all with a round section (.016 on .022×.028 brackets), then square (.017×.017) and then rectangular (.017×.025). In addition to an hypertipping for an early root movement of adjacent teeth, these archwires can incorporate loops which, while extruding the tooth, at the same time can correct interproximal defects and include tipping in round archwires and also torque in the square and rectangular ones, remodeling the bone deficits and thickening the soft tissues as the extraction space is closed. Incremental .017×.025, .018×.025, .019×.025 Stainless Steel archwires will be archwires for stabilization. Checks and activations are carried out every 15 days with periodontal and radiographic evaluations. Some steps can be combined or modified according to the needs of individual clinical cases (8.12).

Clinical protocol in lingual orthodontics

Orthodontic protocol for orthodontic extraction in lingual mechanics is similar to the vestibular one, always using brackets with a position with a pre-inclination with respect to the interdental bone loss.

*Reproduced from "Paolone MG, Kaitsas R. Orthodontic-periodontal interactions: Orthodontic extrusion in interdisciplinary regenerative treatments. *Int Orthod.* 2018;16(2):217-245" and "Kaitsas R, Paolone MG, Paolone G. Guided orthodontic regeneration: A tool to enhance conventional regenerative techniques in implant surgery. *Int Orthod.* 2015;13(4):539-554" ©CEO. Published by Elsevier Masson SAS. All rights reserved. With permission and "Paolone MG, Kaitsas R, Paolone G, Kaitsas V. Lingual orthodontics and forced eruption: a means for osseous and tissue regeneration. *Prog Orthod.* 2008;9(2):46-57" with permission by SIDO.

Particular attention should be paid to lingual morphology and awareness of cortical bone ridges integrity on counter-torque movements. The interbrackets distance must be compensated with the use of very light super-elastic alloys such as the pre-formed CuNi-Ti archwires, then the sequence continues with round .016 β-titanium archwires, where steps and teardrop loops can be inserted for tipping and then insert torque information as soon as it is possible to apply .017×.017 then .017×.025 β-titanium archwires. Also in the lingual protocol, it is possible to combine some steps in relation to the clinics of the single patient (see 8.12).

Tissue regeneration

The extrusive movement can be used as a regenerative means to develop the implant site as a no-surgical approach, making the implant placement easier and more predictable (8.7). Although a wide variety of surgical hard and soft tissue improvement techniques have been developed[76,77], sometimes unpredictable results and esthetic compromises are inevitable, and many of these implant-related esthetical imperfections cannot be fully corrected[78]. The use of orthodontics, therefore, can avoid or reduce the need for further, more invasive surgical procedures[79], which are at greater risk of esthetic failures and defeats (8.13).

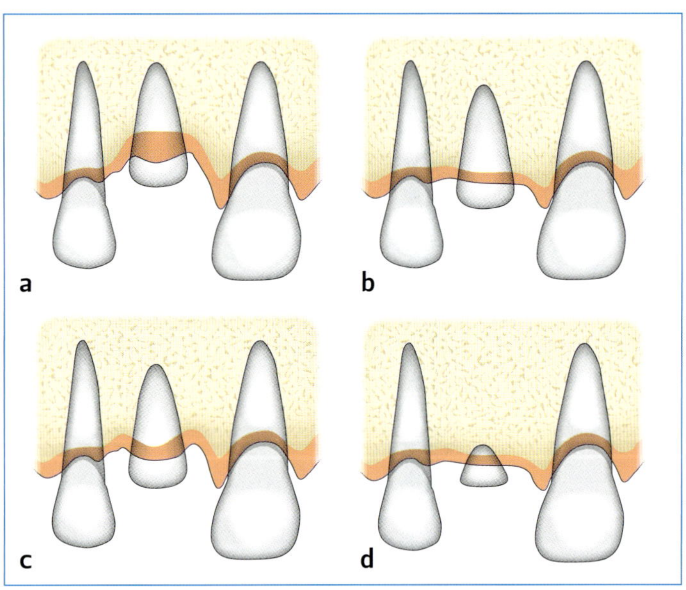

8.7 Schematic diagram that shows orthodontic extrusion as implant site development.

Tab. 8.13 Clinical situation for the use of orthodontic extrusion as implant site development

Hopeless periodontal compromised tooth
Extended decay or internal/external resorption or serious endo-perio compromised teeth without recovery of the tooth
Root fractures beyond both horizontal and vertical 1/3 coronal
Severe mucogingival defects associated with bone loss
Unfavorable crown/root ratio

GOR is the orthodontic procedure that regenerates hard and soft tissue for the development of the implant site using the tooth itself as a distraction means by the tension of the periodontal ligament [19]. This ability of the tooth allows tissue regeneration by modifying the site three-dimensionality. This procedure was previously called Orthodontic Extrusion[19], Forced Orthodontic Eruption[80], Orthodontic Extraction[81], Forced Eruption[51], Dynamic Orthodontic Extraction[82], Biodynamic Orthodontic Modelling[82], but in this volume it will be called Guided Orthodontic Regeneration (GOR) as the orthodontic movement achieves a regeneration of hard and soft tissues. The ability of a tooth to directly influence the periodontium orthodontically depends on the amount of residual attachment present on the tooth itself and on its periodontal health, and it is usable even in extreme cases. "Using a *hopeless* tooth for regenerative purposes is a unique possibility", said Zachrisson[83], as it achieves several objectives by modifying the morphology of the defect, improving the appearance of soft tissues, leveling the bone defects and the implant site adjacent to the natural teeth, assuming an enormous value in the esthetic sector[81].

The first Authors that introduced the orthodontic extrusion technique as pre-implant tissue and bone modelling were the Salama[81] brothers, who defined it as Orthodontic Extrusive Remodeling. Using this technique, a tooth that could not be used from a restorative point of view was extruded to its complete extraction using the regenerated soft and hard tissue to facilitate implant placement. Mantzikos and Shamus[84], introducing the name of Biodynamic Orthodontic Modeling, studied the effects that extrusive

Tab. 8.14 Effects on soft tissue

Stage 1	Time 0. Start of extrusive movement
Stage 2	Redness of the gingival collar
Stage 3	Red patch
Stage 4	Soft tissue keratinization

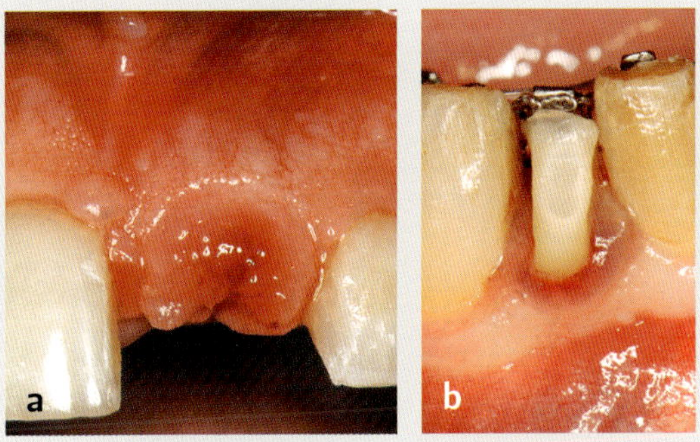

8.8* Red patch after the gingival sulcus extroflession.

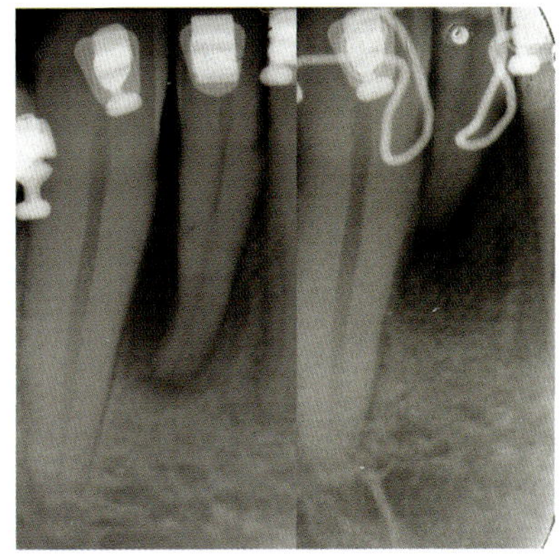

8.9* Bone remodeling after orthodontic extrusion.

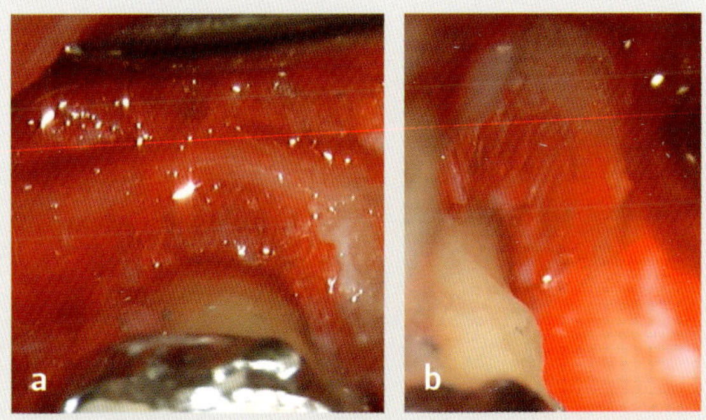

8.10 After flap elevation it can be seen the new stretched bone fibers that are created after the extrusion at the root level.

movement has on bone and soft tissue, demonstrating how orthodontics dynamically models tissues. The effects on soft tissues[85] were summarized in four phases (8.14). The extrusion of the root fragment destined to extraction determines at a soft tissue level an eversion of the sulcular tissue which appears with a redness of gingival collar, the so-called *red patch* (immature tissue resulting from the eversion of the sulcular epithelium), that requires 28-47 days for its complete keratinization[41] (8.8); there is a subsequent maturation of the soft tissues and an increase in the width and thickness of keratinized gingiva, also at the interdental level; the height of the papilla in contact with the *hopeless* tooth increases only in the case of a healthy periodontal attachment on the adjacent tooth[80].

The effects on hard tissues[82] (8.15), have been outlined in three phases. Like soft tissues, hard tissues also change during movement starting with a phase of bone remodeling (8.9) until its complete mineralization after the stabilization phase (8.10). The stabilization period after extrusion is very important. If this period is not observed, tissue relapse may occur because of incomplete tissue remodeling and lack of soft tissue stabilization[15]. Bone regeneration with native autologous tissue obtained by extrusion is better than the one obtained with heterologous bone grafts, due to the presence of osteocytes in bone gaps within living bone[86]. It is important to correctly plan the dental extrusive vector in relation to the relationship between root and alveolar morphology[16,87]. The quantification of tissue response to extrusion in relation to the development of the implant site was studied by Amato et al.[88]. Among the values analyzed, the most important are: for an average extrusion movement of 6.2 mm we have: a) a bone gain of 4 mm (also confirmed by Conserva et al.[89] [4.63 mm]) (8.11); for Van Venrooy and Yukna[10] the gain is slightly reduced (from 1.3 to 1.8 mm), scored on average 0.69 to 1 mm of bone apposition for each vertical extrusive millimeter

Tab. 8.15 Effects on hard tissue

Stage 1	Time 0. Start of extrusive movement
Stage 2	Biodynamic and biomechanical bone remodeling
Stage 3	Alveolar stabilization

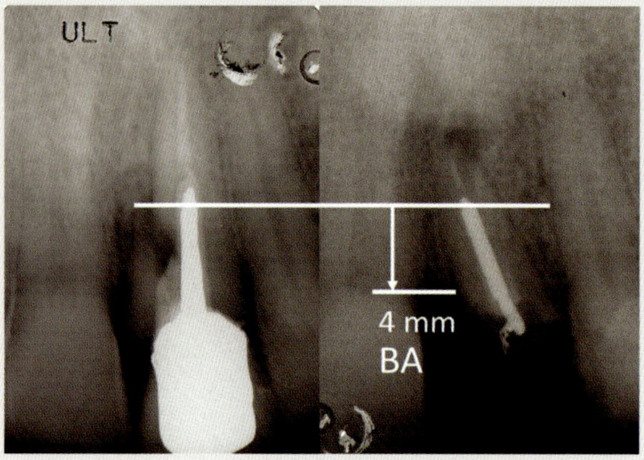

8.11* Mean bone augmentation after extrusion. BA: Bone Augmentation.

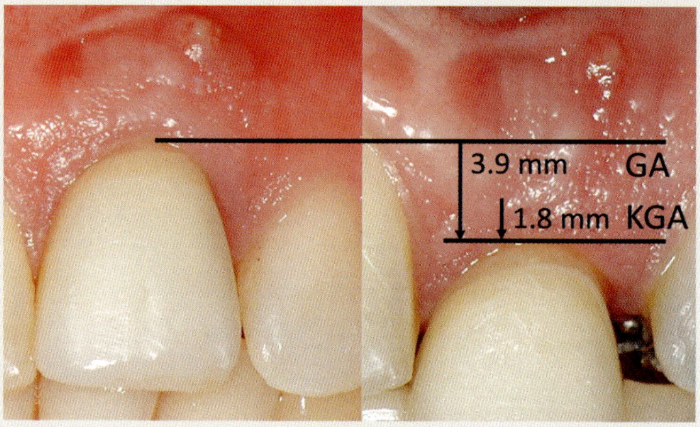

8.12* Mean gingival tissue augmentation after extrusion. GA: Gingival Augmentation; KGA: Keratinized Gingival Augmentation.

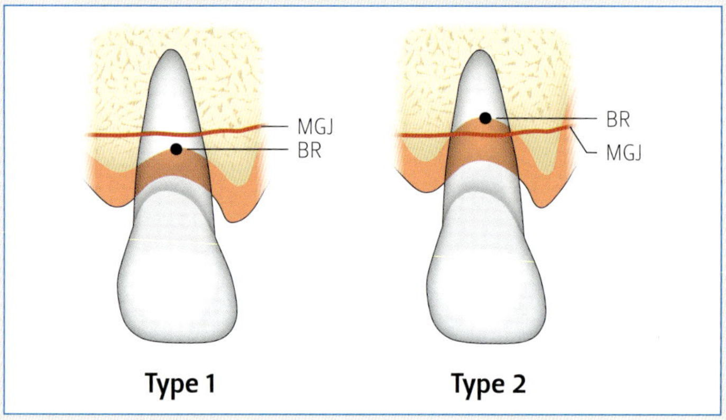

8.13 Schematic diagram the show the relationship between mucogingival junction and bone ridge in type 1 and 2. BR: Bone Ridge; MGJ: Mucogingival junction.

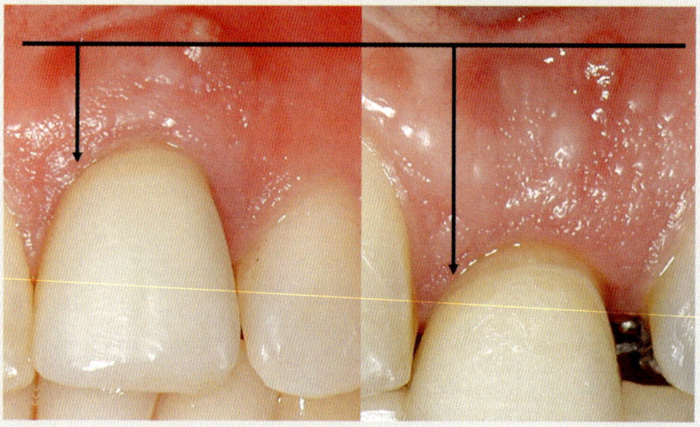

8.14* Modification of the soft tissue in type 1.

in relation to the direction and intensity of force[80]; b) a displacement of the mucogingival junction of 2.1 mm; c) an increase in gingival tissue of 3.9 mm; d) an increase in keratinized tissue of 1.8 mm (8.12).

In order to standardize the clinical procedure, Hochman et al.[90] have drawn up a diagnostic protocol to make the bone and tissue response predictable and the additional surgical procedures at the end of the extrusion movement. Three parameters must be evaluated: 1) probing depth before the start of the extrusion movement; 2) position of the mucogingival junction; 3) bone crest probing (*bone sounding*[91,92]) to determine the position of the bone crest in relation to the overlying tissues. Three types of soft tissue response are possible after orthodontic extrusion depending on the relationship of the mucogingival line to the top of the bone crest (8.13):

- type 1: *increase of the width of the keratinized gingiva and overall soft tissues width.* During movement, the soft tissue increases and the mucogingival line remains at the initial level, resulting in an increase in the width of keratinized tissue at the end of the extrusion. This occurs when the mucogingival line is attached to the underlying bone surface and the keratinized gingiva is connected to both bone and root surface (8.14);
- type 2: *increased overall soft tissue width with no effect on the keratinized gingiva.* During the movement, the soft tissue increases and the mucogingival line follows the movement with an unaltered extension of the width of keratinized tissue at the end of the extrusion. This occurs when the mucogingival junction is connected to the root surface and not to the bone surface (e.g. bone dehiscence, altered passive eruption, history of bone loss) (8.15);

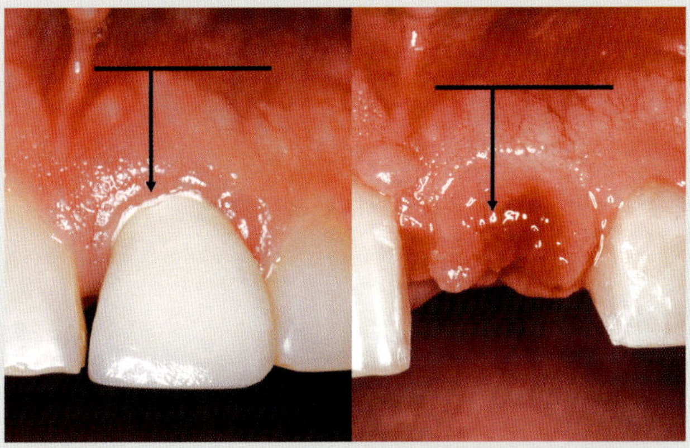

8.15* Modification of the soft tissue in type 2.

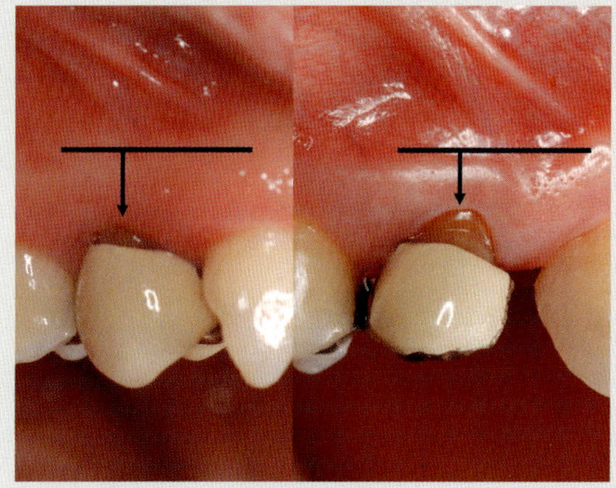

8.16 Modification of the soft tissue in type 3.

- type 3: *overall width of soft tissue and width of keratinized gingiva remain unchanged.* During movement, the soft tissue and the keratinized gingiva show no movement, remaining in the initial position. This occurs when there is loss of periodontal attachment on the root surface with the presence of a circumferential periodontal pocket. In this situation, both the mucogingival junction and the keratinized gingiva are not connected to the root surface. Therefore, in order to modify the soft tissue, the periodontal pocket must first be eliminated by means of an extrusive movement with eversion of the base of the pocket (8.16).

Comparison with other regenerative techniques

Although there is no general protocol[93], extrusion as implant site development is a viable alternative compared to other conventional surgical techniques, being equally effective, even in the esthetic zone[8]; since neither method is superior to the other, the clinician's preferences prevail[8]. Tissues increase in a directly proportional relationship to orthodontic movement[88] (8.16). Additional bone and tissue augmentation surgery is not always needed[93] and it is not related to biomechanical aspects of orthodontic extraction, but to the quality of the hard and soft tissues present at the start of the treatment. However, some parameters remain controversial and it is not possible to establish a complete and detailed clinical protocol (traction axis, level of adhesion of attachment, stabilization period)[94]. Although it is possible to regenerate bone tissue, it may happen that in the implant site it is necessary to slightly increase and optimize bone volume with small bone grafts[2]. The technique would seem to be affected by the height of the bone of the adjacent teeth and the periodontal and endodontic conditions of the tooth[8]. The time required for extrusion depends on the tooth-bone attachment of the tooth to be extruded. A tooth with dense bone will take a longer time than a tooth with minimal residual bone[16].

Tab. 8.16 Tissue improvement in relation with orthodontic movement (%)[88]

Measurement	Mean	SD	Range
Bone improvement/ orthodontic movement	68.9	17.3	10-97
Gingival improvement/ orthodontic movement	65.2	19.9	28-100

Initial amount of apical attachment

There is no evidence on the minimal necessary quantity of bone support that tooth must have before starting orthodontic extrusion[8]. Van Venrooy and Yukna[10] demonstrated bone apposition with a periodontal attachment to approximately mid-root. Zuccati and Bocchieri[95] affirm that in order to develop bone and gingiva in the vertical direction there must be from 1/4 to 1/3 of an intact periodontal attachment, up to a few millimeters present only on the palatal aspect without vestibular attachment. Joo et al.[96] and Gonzalez Lopez et al.[97] consider 1/3 of intact periodontal attachment around the apical third of the tooth as a prerequisite. Chou et al.[98] confirm this data and recommend endodontic treatment, if a lesion is present, to reduce apical bone destruction. Korayem et al.[93], in their systematic review, described cases with residual supporting bone ranging from 1/3 apical root to a minimum of 10%.

Three-dimensional root movement

The ability to develop the implant site through the extrusion of the root fragment knowing the bone defect to be regenerated, allows, with the three-dimensional movement of the root, to add hard and soft tissue where it is necessary, relocating the pre-existing attachment[99]. The morphology of the bone ridge, in fact, can be enhanced by the orthodontic movement either in the coronal direction or at the bucco-lingual level, by implementing a combined movement of extrusion and torque if the healthy periodontal attachment is present only on one surface including apical or root ones[95,100] and also at the mesio-distal level[101]. The effectiveness of this type of movement depends on the activity of the periodontal disease, the initial condition of the tooth, the speed, the amount and direction of the force and the condition of the bone support of the adjacent teeth; finally, it also depends on the retention time[102]. Various methods have been reported in the literature. The most used is the vestibular torque of the root[79,95,99,100]. Uribe et al.[101] described in a clinical case how, by the mesial tipping of the root in the direction of the existing angular bone defect, the root fragment regenerated the bone tissue that was lost because of periodontal disease, with an increase in the volume of the alveolar bone and simultaneous improvement of the height of the interproximal papilla. This method allows to exploit a greater surface area of periodontal ligament through the orthodontic movement to regenerate tissue compared to simple vertical extrusion, which acts on root surface always more apically reduced. Therefore, by changing the direction of the force and tipping the tooth in order to extrude it in a greater quantity where the defect is most apical, the amount of bone formation itself can be changed. Watanabe et al.[103] moved the root to the palatal position during the extrusion to regenerate the resorbed buccal cortical bone. Ziskind et al.[12] studied the lateral movement of root fragment following vertical extrusion, quantifying it from 0.44 to 0.8 mm of lateral movement for each millimeter of vertical movement. This movement must be controlled and used for the benefit of the three-dimensional regeneration of the site. Even simple vertical extrusion offers an advantage on the bone site. In fact, as soon as the root is extruded, the depth and diameter of the pocket are reduced. This creates a better environment for the immediate implant placement, minimizing the gap between the implant and surrounding tissue[16,80,89,103,104]. In this perspective, the fundamental prerequisites are those of a healthy periodontal attachment around the apex of the tooth to be extruded and the bone relationship with the neighboring teeth[98,104]. This level dictates the limit of the quantity of extrusion[105].

Conclusions

Orthodontic extrusion seems to be a reliable alternative to conventional surgical procedures for augmentation and development of an implant site (even if it was not possible to make a direct comparison with conventional surgical methods and, therefore, a conclusion of its relative effectiveness[93]) and it is currently the only non-surgical tissue management technique able to enhance the ultimate success of an implant rehabilitation[94]. The reduction of subsequent interventions decreases the scar tissues, with improvement in esthetics[11,15]. Soft tissue modeling also makes it easier to perform additional regeneration techniques that may be required, such as GBR[21,41], GBR+VISTA technique[29], peri-implant bone grafts[16] or SMART technique[106]. It can be used not only in highly esthetical areas, but also in posterior areas to reduce more invasive surgical techniques for bone augmentation, such as sinus floor elevation, GBR or block bone grafts[107]. While keeping in mind the eventual complications, such as bone dehiscence, tissue recessions, unsuitable bone site and incorrect regeneration for ideal implant placement[79], the orthodontic use of *hopeless* teeth used for extraction allows to offer a conservative rehabilitation contribution to the patient's tissues. This is of particular relevance in lingual orthodontics where esthetics is guaranteed. Before starting extrusion, it is necessary to carry out some measurements which are summarized in 8.17.

Tab. 8.17 Measurements to be made before orthodontic extrusion

Analysis of the position and the relationship of the mucogingival junction related to the underlying bone
Periodontal attachment on the root
Periodontal probing
Underlying bone morphology
Periodontal attachment of the adjacent teeth
Quality and amount of keratinized tissue
Site esthetics
Prosthetic space and occlusal evaluations
Complete orthodontic evaluation

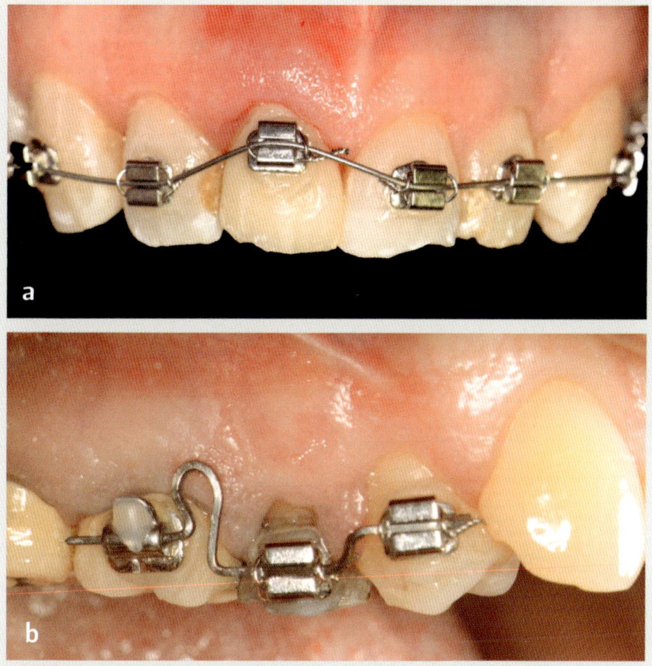

8.17 Extrusion with fixed continuous and sectional mechanics.

ORTHODONTIC TECHNIQUE

Despite the variety of treatment protocols reported and the absence of an univocal consensus on the clinical protocol, the literature reports clinically applicable protocols[93] (Tab. 8.18) that recommend the use of light, continuous, extrusive forces of 15 g for the anterior teeth and 50 g for the posterior teeth, a constant and slow speed of 2 mm/month, possible incorporations of torque and tipping components, a stabilization of about 1 mm/month, anchorage mechanics and control of the tipping reactions of the adjacent teeth[93,94]. In literature there are clinical cases treated in fixed and removable mechanics, with fixed vestibular mechanics, sectional techniques included[46] (Fig. 8.17), with simple elastics on temporary prosthetic appliances[1,11,31,45,90,97] (Fig. 8.18) or NiTi springs on temporary bridges[81,89] or elastic chains or simple elastics on removable Hawley appliances[24] and clinical cases treated with fixed lingual appliances[108] (Fig. 8.19). In conventional orthodontics, extrusion can be applied on a single tooth or can be part of complete orthodontic treatments[107]. According to the literature, the most used mechanics for orthodontic extrusion, in the 92% of cases, is a fixed bi-maxillary (17%), or single arch (50%) or sectorial (33%) appliances, with vestibular or lingual bonding or traction on post and splint if the root fragments do not allow a complete adhesion on the brackets and an exclusive axial movement of the tooth is required, being a critical success factor of orthodontic extrusion[94]. In literature, the mechanics is realized with light archwires in twisted steel[82,84,85,105] or simple undersized round[40] or β-titanium or undersized superelastic NiTi wires[81,88,107,109,110]. The initial pure axial extrusion movements and, subsequently, the tipping and torque can be obtained according to conventional mechanics also by adding loops in steel wires[84,88,98,107] or inset compensation bends[2], or in β-titanium[19,88], cobalt-chromium[103,111], or by repositioning the brackets on an always more apical position[11] and managing any restoration to put the brackets more

Tab. 8.18 Guidelines that are clinical applicable for orthodontic regenerative extrusion for implant site development[93]

Low continuous extrusive forces, 15 g anterior teeth, 50 g posterior teeth
Constant and low speed about 2 mm/month
During extrusive phase a torque/tipping component can be incorporated
Stabilization must be about 1 mm/month
Anchorage
Control tipping/torque reactions on adjacent teeth
Knowledge and choice of the archwire composition: properties, advantages and limits
Preserve cortical bone plate integrity

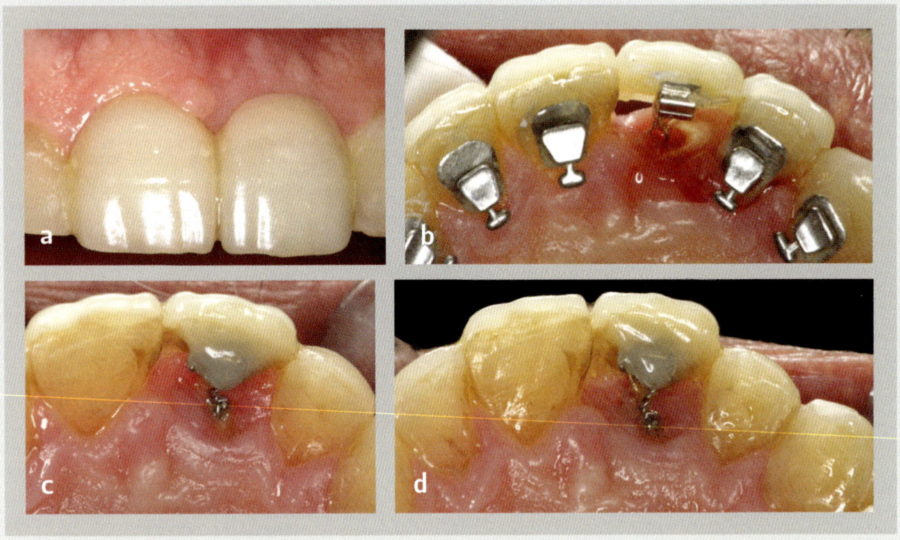

8.18* Extrusion with elastic wire on post and provisional veneer.

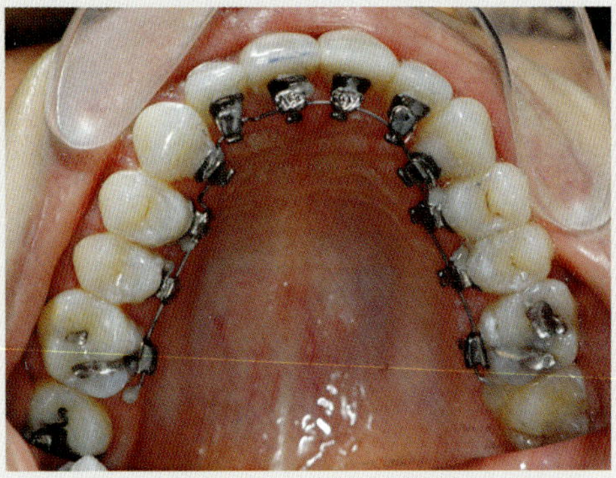

8.19 Extrusion with fixed lingual mechanics.

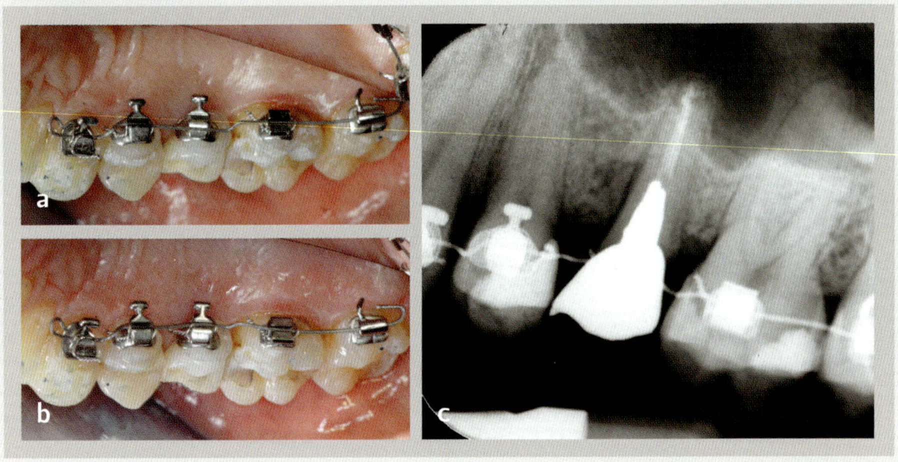

8.20 1-2 mm/month activations.

apically. The frequency of orthodontic checks reported in the literature varies every 15, 30 or 60 days; however, the importance of a monthly periodontal check-up, for plaque control, as well as an X-ray and a detailed occlusal check to eliminate occlusal contacts and jiggling, is common to all publications[94]. The recommended forces in the literature are 15 g for incisors and 60 g for molars, within 30 g for a slow extrusion and even over 50 g for a fast extrusion[9,41,93,110,112,113]. The amount of force must overcome the ligament tension and ensure an optimal tissue response[82]. The speed in the regenerative extrusion must be kept slow and constant and must not exceed 1 mm, maximum 2 mm, each month[93,102] (8.20). The direction of the force, at first, should be conducted along the major axis to facilitate a vertical movement that is parallel along the major axis of the root. Great caution should be taken to avoid parasite lingual, vestibular movements or uncontrolled torque or tipping forces which could result in contact of the root apex with the buccal or lingual cortical plate with a consequent loss of the cortical plate itself: it is very important to always keep intact the cortical plate during all the orthodontic mechanics[9,80,87,100,101,106,114,115]. For this reason, from the very first moments of the extrusion, we prefer to immediately incorporate a root counter-torque information to counterbalance the parasite root-vestibular torque component due to the pure extrusive vertical force of the activations that are increased because of the apical displacement of the center of resistance in

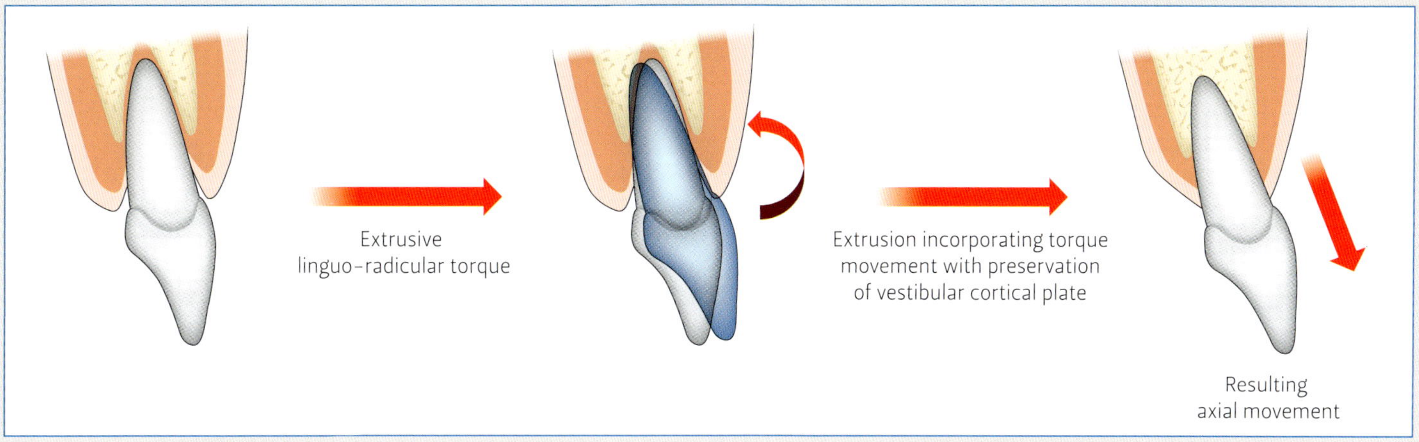

8.21 Incorporation of the radiculo-lingual torque information to counteract the radiculo-vestibular parasite torque component due to the pure vertical extrusive force (grater in periodontal bone support loss).

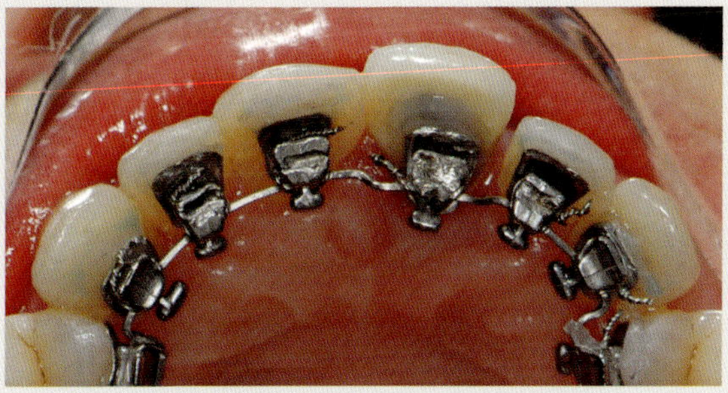

8.22* Incorporation of the radiculo-lingual torque bending in extrusion.

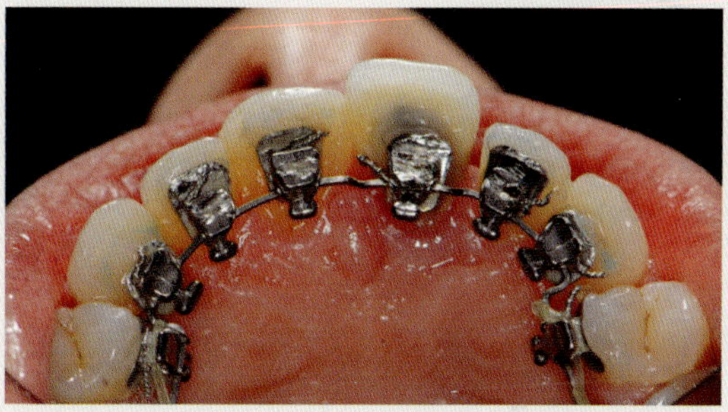

8.23* Incorporation of the bending torque + extrusion.

teeth that have lost periodontal bone support (8.21 and 8.22). This is more evident in buccal mechanics than in lingual, as described in Chapter 5. If a root-lingual torque is not incorporated, extrusion creates a clockwise moment which is, with respect to the center of resistance of the tooth, closer to the tooth apex, in cases with reduction of periodontal support. This moment moves the apex towards a vestibular direction. It is therefore important to use a counter-torque moment that immediately has a root-lingual torque that reduces the risk of fenestration or dehiscence on the buccal cortical plate. This strategy allows for coronal tissue movement, remodeling of the interproximal papilla and improvement of keratinized tissue[2]. Once a first axial traction has been made, other movements can be incorporated. According to several Authors, in fact, the use of a vestibular-root controlled torque to guide the apical bone position can increase the vestibulo-lingual thickness and modify the implant site. The feasibility of this technique depends on the fact that the vestibular cortical plate is intact at the start of the movement and is kept intact throughout the movement[79,95,100]. In fact, in all the phases of the orthodontic movement, it is essential not to impact against the cortical plates, especially at the apical level, always bearing in mind that the cortical plates are often very thin, in particular on the vestibular aspect[94]. The application of a root-vestibular torque in a context of forced eruption forms a neo-apposed bone that goes coronally and buccally from the palatal side visible in the extraction site, relocating a pre-existing attachment and obviously not creating a new one, with an increase in hard and soft tissues, including the width of keratinized tissues in particular clinical conditions[99]. Torque can be achieved according to all conventional mechanics, by positioning a preformed brackets turned upside-down in an apico-coronal direction, or by adding the information on the archwire

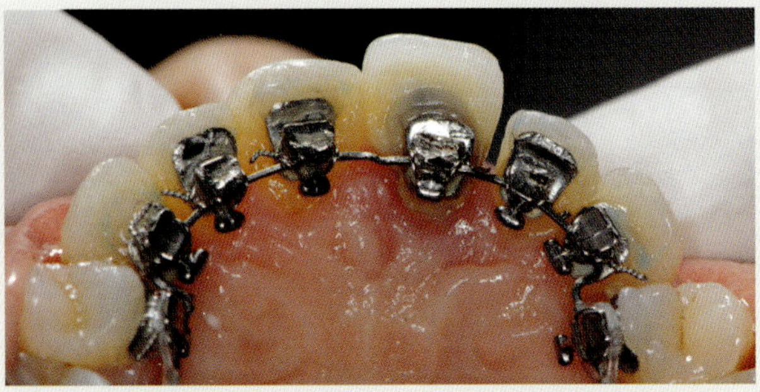

8.24* Incorporation of the bending tipping + extrusion.

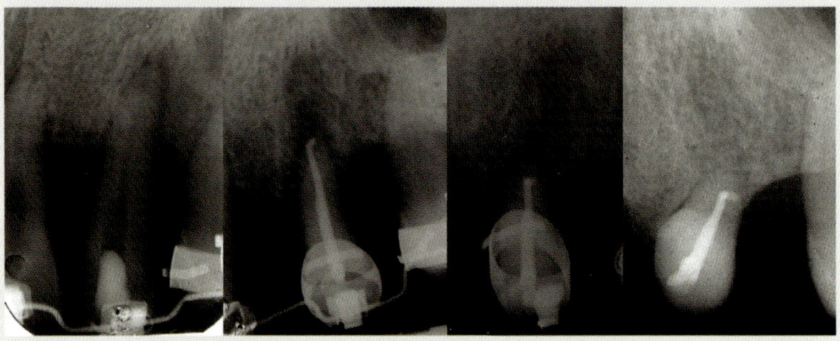

8.25 Adding to extrusion a tipping movement of a conical root, the oval oblique section can be exploited and the extrusion area is greater with respect to a conical axial apical pure movement with round section.

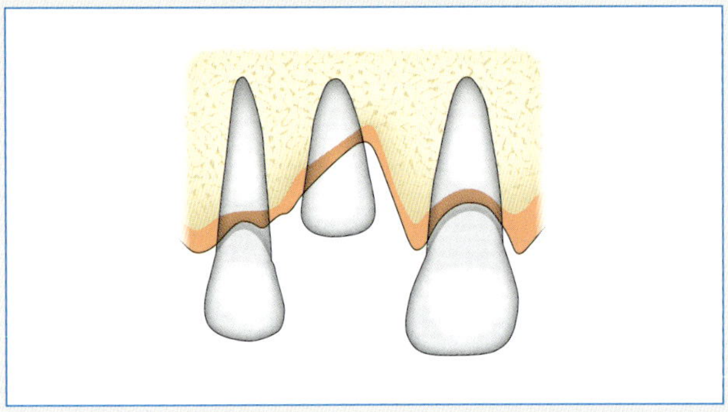

8.26 Schematic diagram which shows a bone defect that needs a post-extraction regeneration or alveolar preservation techniques for implant placement.

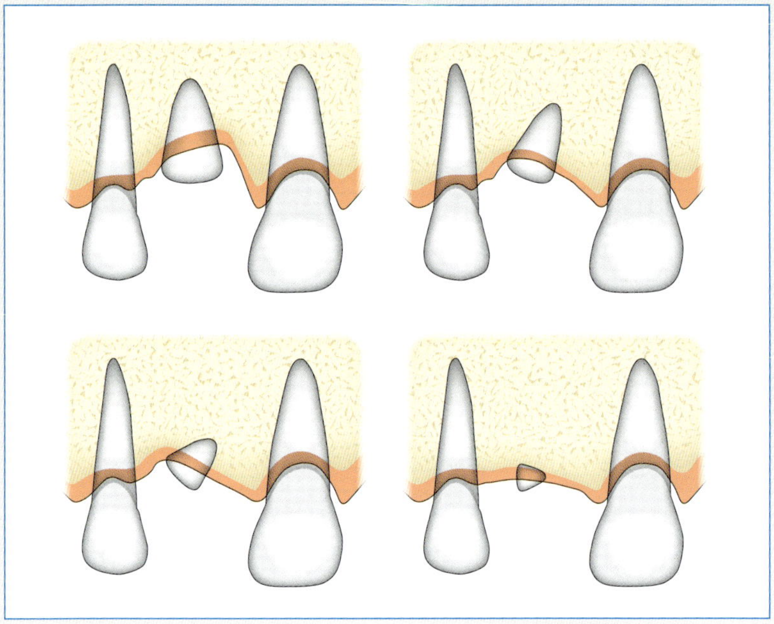

8.27 Schematic diagram which represents the 3D movement of the root fragment to regenerate bone, where it is necessary, in order to develop a correct site for implant placement.

directly (8.23) or with loops[1]. Lingual mechanics allows this realization both during the first axial extrusion and during the torque phase, guaranteeing esthetics throughout the treatment[19,108]. In the same way, the extrusion technique can maintain an adequate bucco-lingual or mesio-distal width. Mechanics may involve the tipping of a tooth (8.24) in the direction of the angular defect, resulting in an increase in the volume of the alveolar bone in the implant area, and a simultaneous improvement in the height of the interproximal papilla can also be expected; the tipped root fragment can, therefore, have a potential for the development of the papilla[50,81,82,101]. Let us imagine the root of a tooth that must be extruded as a cone: if we exploit an oblique section by tilting the extrusive area, we obtain a large area of periodontal tissue stimulation which is greater than with a pure conical apical axial movement[80] (8.25). If, on the other hand, we visualize the intact periodontal support area, a three-dimensional combined tipping and radicular torque movement, which has a direction from this deeper periodontal area that is still intact by extruding the defect, stimulates the formation of hard and soft tissues and modifies the anatomy of periodontal damage, leveling it (8.26 and 8.27). It is always important to check parasite tipping and torque movements of the teeth adjacent to the element to be extruded; such reactions must be predicted, quantified and taken into account[12]. A mesio-distal or buccal collapse of the adjacent elements can compromise the

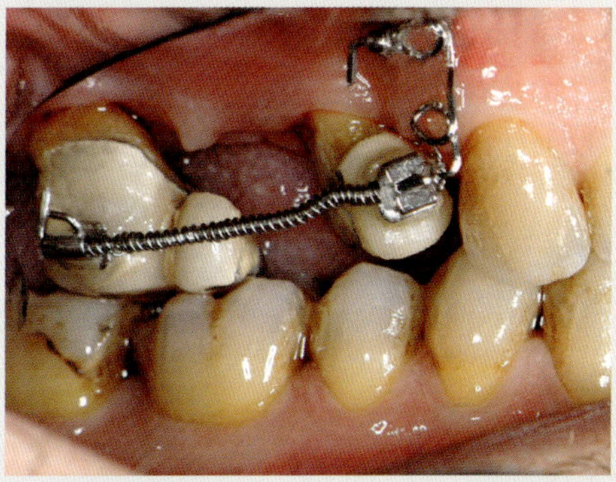

8.28 Anchorage with TAD of a sectional for extrusion and mesialisation.

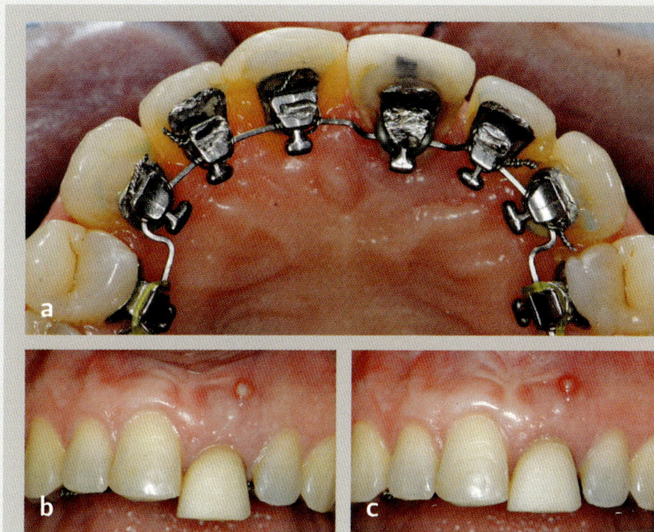

8.29* Elimination of occlusal contacts during extrusion.

orthodontic regeneration and the periodontal tissues of the contiguous teeth[106]; consequently the anchorage of the adjacent teeth is fundamental, as it is the knowledge of their periodontal anatomy, avoiding uncontrolled tilting movements, which would compromise the extrusion of the tooth of the site to be regenerated and the cortical plates of the adjacent elements[96]; on the other hand, the movements that correct and implement the periodontal situation of the adjacent teeth must be strengthened. The choice of the mechanics, in addition to being subjective, is influenced by the bone height of the adjacent teeth, the periodontal conditions of the tooth and also by the quantity and direction of the forces[8,50]. All the Authors reiterate the importance of the application of anchorage[111], including continuous or segmented techniques of additional anchorage archwires[33,41,109-111,116]. The control of the anchorage concerns, in fact, both the teeth adjacent to the extrusion and the general anchorage of the complete orthodontic treatment[16] and assumes greater importance when the extrusion is applied to more than one tooth[106,117]. The anchorage, whatever it is, is important to limit parasite movements on adjacent teeth and in general on the entire occlusion. These anchorages, in literature, include continuous archwires, segmented ones, palatal bars, miniscrews, implants[100,118]. Temporary Anchorage Devices (TADs) can enhance conventional anchorages[2] (8.28). The choice of the type, section and positioning of the miniscrews depends on the recipient site, which can be easily evaluated with the new 3D radiological techniques, and depends on the need for individual anchorage aimed at the extrusion only or at a complete treatment. In this regard, since lingual mechanics is by definition a self-anchoring mechanics, in which the anchorage is innate in the same mechanics, the conventional lingual treatment plan and the sequence itself provide a suitable and sufficient anchorage. In this technique, the inter-bracket's distance makes it necessary to use very light NiTi or β-titanium or steel archwires with loops[19,20].

Throughout the whole extrusion, careful control must be applied to the occlusal contact of the extruded tooth. The tooth must not be in contact, but must be free of occlusion and must not have jiggling movement (8.29). For this reason, generally in the literature, for what concerns the bracket's location, an apical positioning seems to be preferred, as gingival as possible on the tooth to be extruded, because it allows an immediate and progressive grinding of the tooth to avoid occlusal contacts[16,41,85,94,110,116,119]. The adhesion of the brackets on prosthetic restorations requires a surface pre-treatment with hydrofluoric acid and silane[16]. When the crown morphology does not allow the application of a brackets and the use of a radicular post allows an anchorage[44] (8.30), it must al-

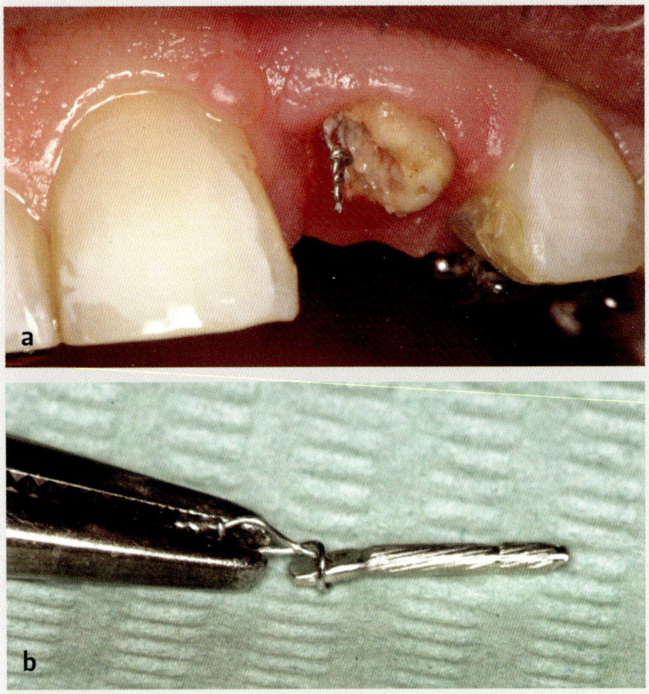

8.30 Anchorage on cemented endodontic post.

ways be kept in mind that this mechanism has the disadvantage of a small control of the extrusive direction, therefore there is a greater risk of a contact with the cortical bone plates, as accessory movements and as direct compressive movements due to excessive vertical forces[94,120]. All the movement must take place with a careful hygiene control, in the absence of inflammation, under periodontal checks and local application of chlorhexidine by the patient. Any endodontic treatment, if the pulp reaction makes it necessary, is imperative. It is necessary to carry out periodically, at least every 2 months, an X-ray check, always keeping in mind that bone maturation occurs after calcification of the osteoid. An apparent delay in the clinical effect of extrusion, in reality, is due to the eversion of the non-keratinized sulcular epithelium and should not cause alarm; in fact, the deeper the pocket, the longer it will take for the eversion of the sulcular epithelium to reveal; this phenomenon is clinically evident as red patch[84,101,116]. As far as stabilization is concerned, on average a month of retention is required for each millimeter of active extrusion, before proceeding with the extraction; this stabilization time ranges from zero up to 6[81] or 12 weeks[16,82,89]. In general, the literature supports that a retention phase is necessary for the maturation of apical bone apposition, in order to prevent relapse of the intrusion[8,102]. Stabilization must allow the deposition of the bone at the apical level and avoid the risk of re-intrusion[102]. According to some Authors, the adequate retention time is 6 months to prevent relapse, because the re-intrusion results from the reorganization of the orientation of the fibers which, at first, are oriented obliquely because of the coronal extrusion movement and then afterwards go back to the original orientation 6 months later[2,29,82,98,102]; however, the length of the retention is subjective and is generally performed with orthodontic mechanics or with lingual fixed retainer[94]. Stabilization can sometimes be complicated by excessive mobility of the element due to the reduction of the remaining tissue[106]. According to some Authors, 2 days before implant placement, after stabilization, a rapid extrusive final force can be applied to increase the width of the periodontal ligament and thus make the extraction simpler and less traumatic[88]. An overcompensation beyond the limits of the desired hard and soft tissue objectives is also recommended and a coronal overcorrection of 2-3 mm should be programmed to the ideal final position of the gingival margin and with respect to the level of the contralateral tooth in the Aesthetic zone, to compensate for a recession of the gingival margin during implant-prosthetic rehabilitation[1,16,88,96,106].

In general, extrusion should allow expression of the associated gingival movement; the tooth must be moved slowly in order not to have instability and during the extrusion a possible antagonist contact must be always checked. It is worth remembering once again that, whatever mechanics we choose to use, the patient's well-being must be promoted, periodontal health maintained and inflammation controlled throughout the orthodontic phase, as animal experiments confirm clinical, radiographic and histological positive changes even in conditions of extensive loss of periodontal support and advanced periodontal disease[10].

Principles to always keep in mind during the orthodontic phase

The extrusion speed should be based on the following principles (see 8.11): first of all, the tooth must not move too quickly to reduce the risk of instability and trauma to the residual periodontal attachment; the tooth must have a movement speed that allows the gingiva to follow the movement itself; the gingiva must remain in a healthy condition; the speed of the movement in question must not have consequences on the adjacent teeth, neither in terms of position, nor in terms of root or bone resorption; pathological occlusal contacts must be avoided and prevented and the patient's comfort must be protected as much as possible in terms of pain control, esthetics (lingual orthodontics), minimum mechanical encumbrance. Furthermore, especially in the presence of endodontically treated teeth, the risk of ankylosis is greater and the possible presence of even partial ankylosis or root resorption must be taken into consideration in modulating the force or speed of extrusion. The same speed of movement and the amount of force can cause ankylosis[121,122] or endodontic or periodontal damage[123,124].

Vestibular clinical orthodontic protocol

The orthodontic protocol provides for a direct or indirect vestibular bonding, in both of these choices the positioning of the bracket on an individualized set-up of the tooth must be programmed as apical as possible: the objective of the first phase is to obtain a first pure axial movement controlling the parasite components of torque and tipping to prevent apical contacts that could lead to loss of cortical bone in relation to the morphology of the residual periodontal support. The first archwires are light archwires with very low strength, round, undersized, in .016 CuNiTi, preformed for lingual technique, which we use in vestibular mechanics as well and very light, for greater control of parasite movements. The round NiTi archwires, including the 37° heat-activated superelastic NiTi archwires[16], due to the low load-deflection ratio and the metallic ultrastructure allow continuous, light, constant and long-lasting forces, but do not allow a control of the torque and require a progressive repositioning of the brackets. The NiTi archwires are excellent initial archwires that can also have transition temperatures between the austenitic phase and the martensitic phase equivalent to the temperature of the oral cavity, guaranteeing at the same time elasticity and anchorage[125]. Subsequently, the extrusion is carried out with incremental rectangular archwires in β-titanium or stainless steel; this allows to incorporate the three orders information with progressive increments and detailed control of three-dimensional movements such as torque and tipping with incremental steps or loops[88,98] with or without repositioning of the brackets[94]. These millimetric progressive activations allow low forces that can be activated regularly and continuously, in order to have a physiological action on the periodontal ligament[94]. Therefore, the extrusion sequence always proceeds with β-titanium alloy archwires, first with a round section (.016 on .022×.028 brackets), then square (.017×.017) and then rectangular (.017×.025). These alloys contain, among other elements, molybdenum and copper and therefore have a strength/modulus ratio double than the 18-8 austenitic stainless steel and offer, for the same section, lighter forces per unit of displacement (2.2 times less than steel), with large deformations. The allotropic transition temperature from compact hexagonal structure to centered cubic structure can be lowered by ions such as copper. These archwires permit, like steel, to carry out simple extrusion steps and to incorporate torque and tipping steps in the rectangular sections that allow, during the extrusion phase, to control the apical impact against the cortical plates, the leveling of adjacent bone peaks and the torque for site stimulation. If the single step is insufficient, teardrop, T, and L loops can be incorporated and the point of application of the force can be moved with respect to the center of rotation. In the last phases we use .017×.025 stainless steel archwire with simple extrusive steps or with teardrop, T, L-shaped loops. The stainless steel one is also our stabilization archwire with incremental sections .018×.025, .019×.025. Some phases can be omitted, merged or adapted in relation to the needs of the individual clinical case.

During the entire extrusive orthodontic treatment, checks should preferably be carried out every 15 days, with the control of the patient's level of oral hygiene, periodontal evaluation, activation, possible grinding in case of occlusal contact or when a jiggling can happen, the management and prevention of parasitic move-

Tab. 8.19 Clinical vestibular and lingual protocol for the implant site development

• Vestibular or lingual direct or indirect bonding - more apical positioning of the bracket - slot .022×.028 • .016 CuNiTi archwire • anchorage control - TADs if necessary • .016 β-titanium archwire - extrusive steps, tipping • .017×.017 β-titanium archwire - extrusive steps/loops, tipping, torque and radicular control movement • .017×.025 β-titanium archwire - extrusive steps/loops, tipping control, torque • .018×.025 stain steel archwire, .019×.025 stain steel archwire - extrusive steps/loops, tipping, torque, stabilization 1 month/mm
Checks every 15 days: periodontal, occlusal control, hygiene, control of parasite movements on the tooth and on anchorages, activations, X-ray every 1-2 months

ments on the tooth itself and on the anchorages, an intraoral X-ray every month or bimonthly. The movements must be slow (1-2 mm/month) and any possible rebonding must take into account 3D parasite movements (8.19).

Lingual clinical orthodontic protocol

The orthodontic protocol is realized with a direct or indirect lingual bonding; also in lingual mechanics the positioning of the bracket must be programmed as apical as possible and is carried out on an individualized set-up, such as the Hiro-System©[126] (8.31): the control of the anchorage and lingual mechanics must obtain, in this very first moment, a pure axial movement, preventing any tipping and torque, and compensating for the various morphology of the lingual surface of the tooth and the relative distance from the center of resistance. The morphology of the residual periodontal support and the situation of the vestibular or lingual cortical bone plates also influence the control of the three-dimensional movement of the extrusion, which in this first phase is, in fact, axial. At the beginning, round light undersized archwires, in very light .016 CuNiTi, preformed for lingual technique, are applied. After a first initial levelling, a different titanium alloy is applied, such as a round, undersized, preformed for lingual technique .016, β-titanium, always with great attention so that the movement is axial. The need to incorporate tipping and torque movements requires the initial use of .017×.017 β-titanium archwire, then .017×.025 always β-titanium. These alloys allow simple extrusive steps or more complex loops with tipping information to level the interproximal defects or torque corrections in order to prevent apico-cortical impacts and to obtain vestibulo-lingual stimulations. When incorporating torque movements, inset or offset compensating steps must be inserted in order to preserve cortical apical impacts, to move the lever arm to the point of application of the torque force (8.32 and 8.33). This information can be repeated on .017×.025 stainless steel stabilization archwires. Also in this case, some phases can be modified in relation to the needs of the single clinical case (see 8.19). In 8.34 it can be seen the regenerative advantages and the increases of the tissues that can be obtained with orthodontics and the possible subsequent modifications that can be obtained with periodontal surgery. The application of the techniques will be described in the presentation of the different clinical cases.

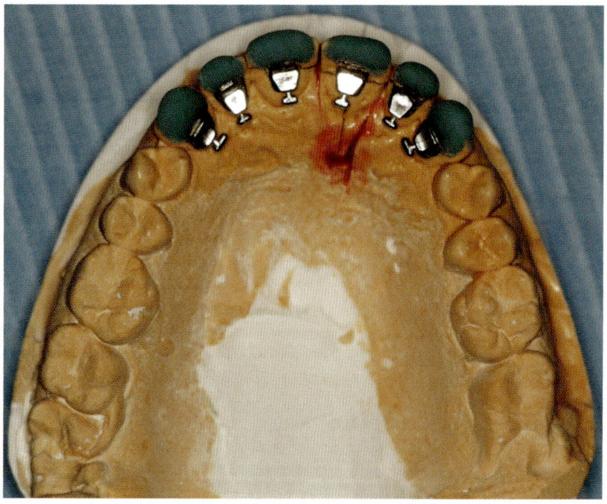

8.31 Lingual indirect bonding on extrusive set-up on 2.1.

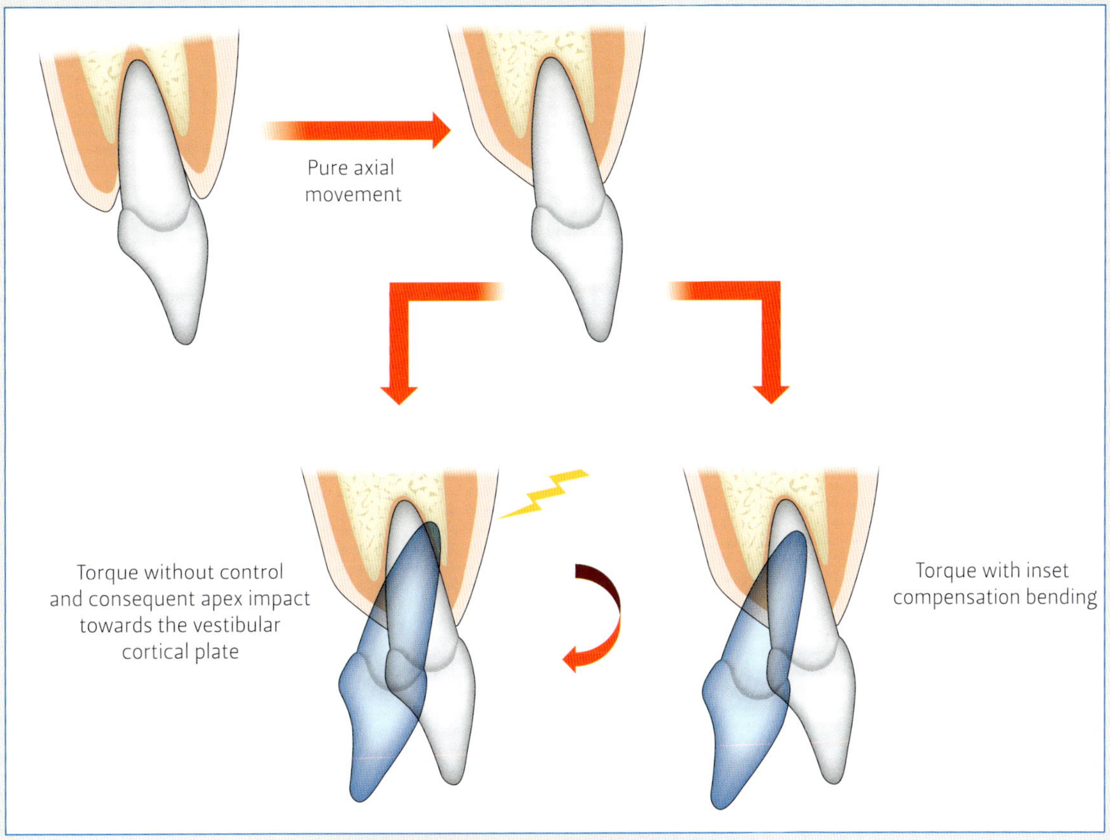

8.32 Incorporation of inset compensation bending to relocate the lever arm to the application point of the torque and extrusion forces.

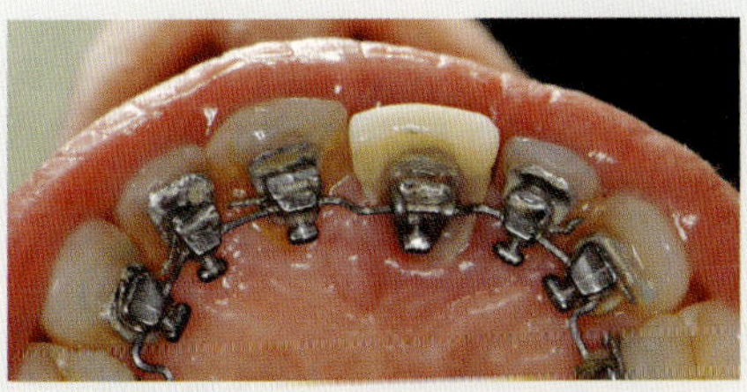

8.33* Incorporation of inset bending in extrusion.

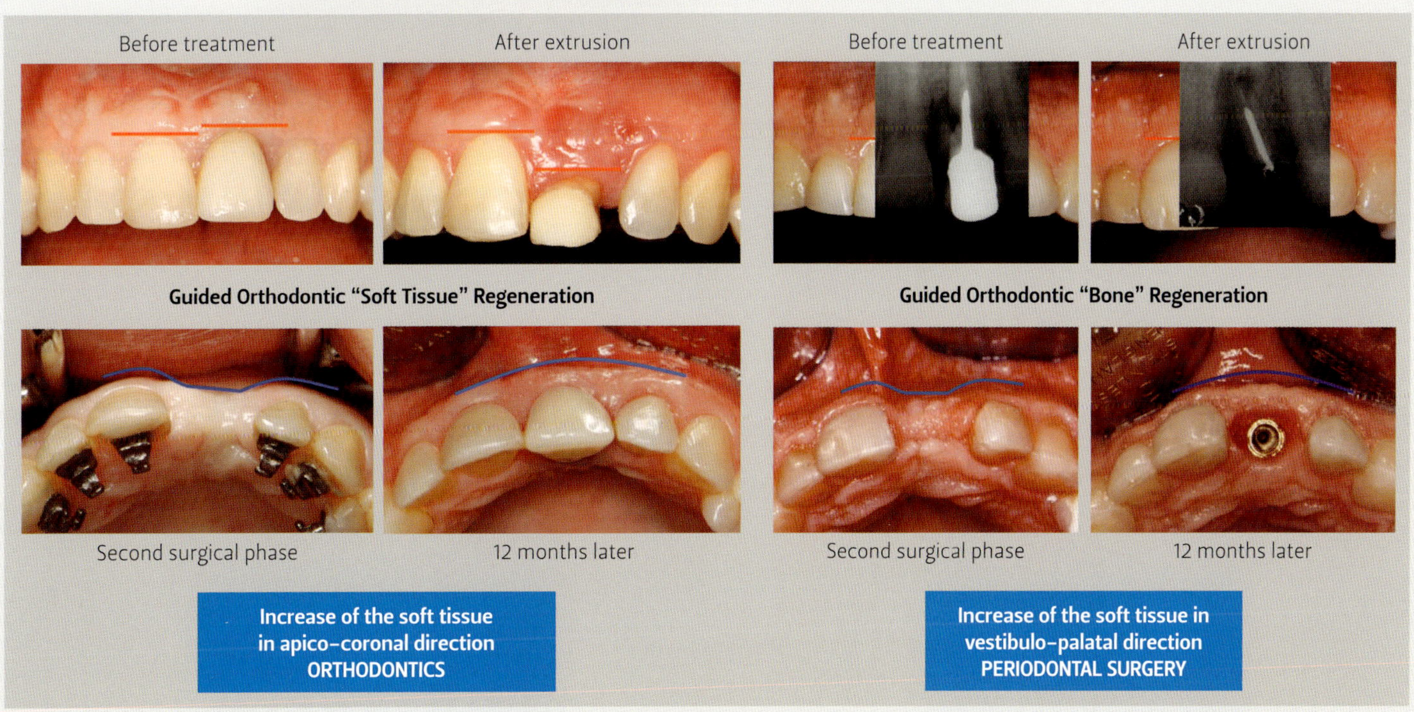

8.34* Summary table of the GOR (GOBR-GOTR) as implant site development.

Clinical case 1 (dental extrusion - anterior sector)

A 42-year old patient asks for the restoration of a hypothetical cervical decay on 1.2 (8.35). At the radiographic examination (8.36) it is observed an external cervical resorption which is the consequence of a previous trauma, when the patient was 16 years old. Taking into consideration the highly esthetic area, various therapeutic options are evaluated in order to try to rehabilitate the tooth instead of its extraction and implant replacement. These treatments include conservative restoration, prosthetic restoration alone or with a possible surgical crown lengthening or a dental orthodontic extrusion. After evaluating if the amount of dental residual substance were sufficient to restore the element, the periodontal situation is studied. The extent of the resorption presents an invasion of the supracrestal tissue attachment and it is therefore necessary to re-establish its correct width (8.37a). Taking into account the shape of the root of the tooth (cylindrical without future alteration of the emergence prosthetic profile), a dental orthodontic extrusion is performed with a subsequent restoration (8.37b).

The patient has no skeletal, functional or occlusal contraindications to orthodontic therapy, which aims only at the dental extrusion of the right upper lateral incisor (8.38 and 8.39). Orthodontic therapy is performed with a lingual technique (Kurz 7th Generation®, Ormco). The indirect bonding (Hiro-System©[126]) is prepared with a sectorial set-up of 1.2 to obtain an extrusive step, in order to directly incorporate from the very beginning a first axial extrusive movement. Slow controlled extrusion is achieved with a .016 CuNi-Ti archwire during the first month, then a .016 β-titanium archwire with extrusive steps (8.40). The objective of the movement after a first incisor derotation (8.41), is a mainly axial movement along the major axis of the tooth.

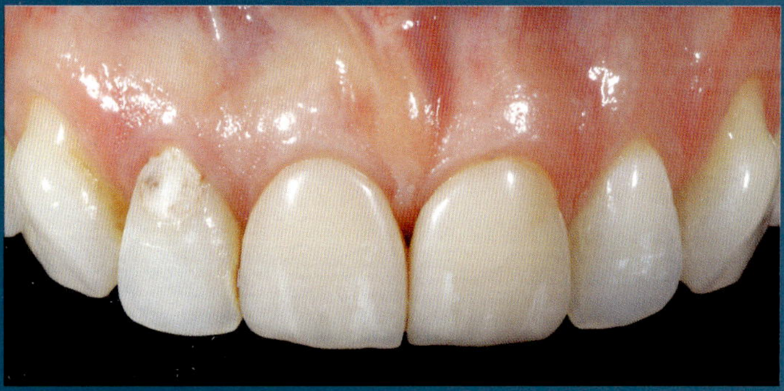

8.35 Vestibular view of the cervical lesion of 1.2.

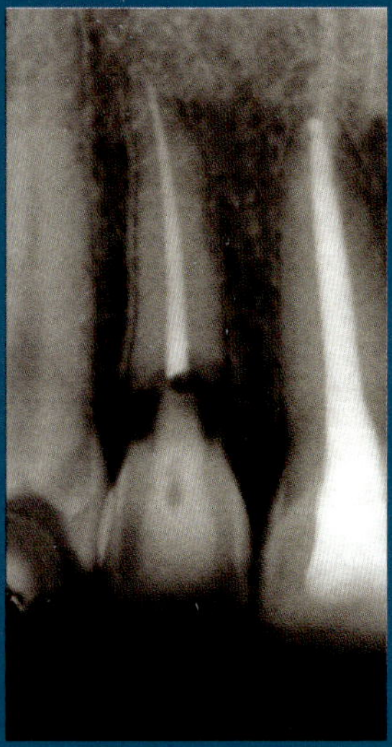

8.36 X-ray that shows the cervical resorption with almost complete break of the tooth integrity. (Reproduced from "Paolone MG, Kaitsas R. Orthodontic-periodontal interactions: Orthodontic extrusion in interdisciplinary regenerative treatments. *Int Orthod.* 2018;16(2):217-245" ©CEO. Published by Elsevier Masson SAS. All rights reserved. With permission.)

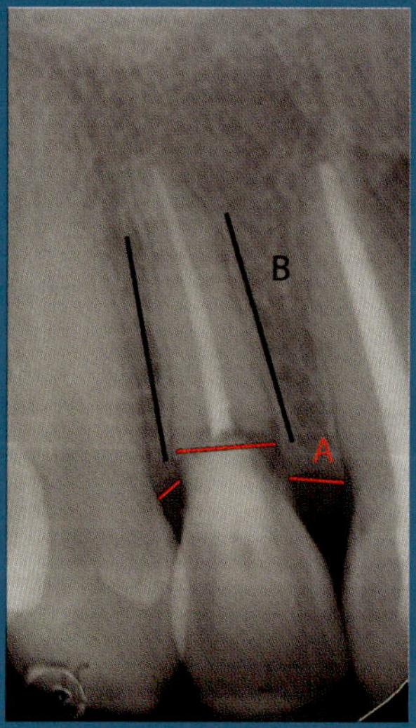

8.37 Supracrestal tissue attachment invasion (A) of the resorption with root cylindrical-form (B).

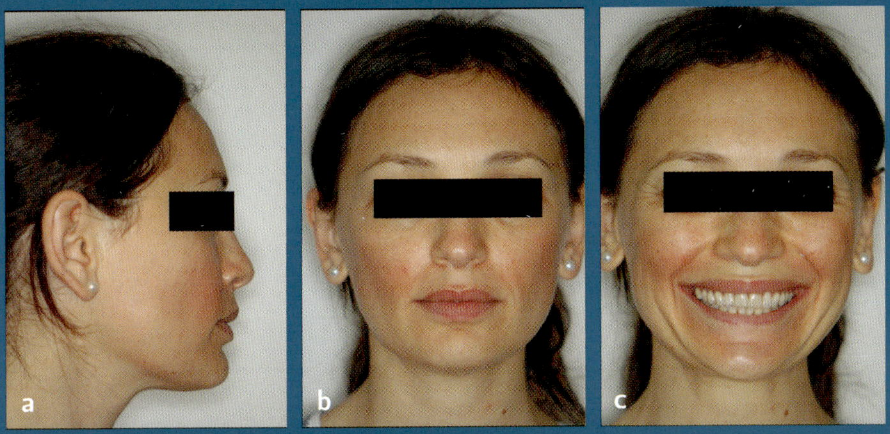

8.38 Extraoral pre-orthodontic treatment photos.

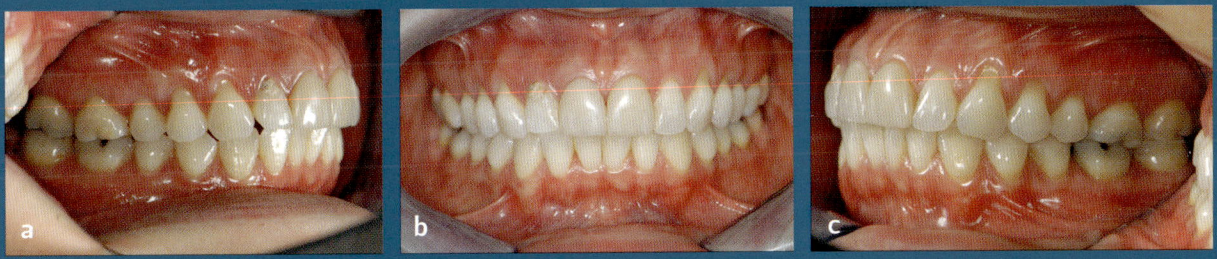

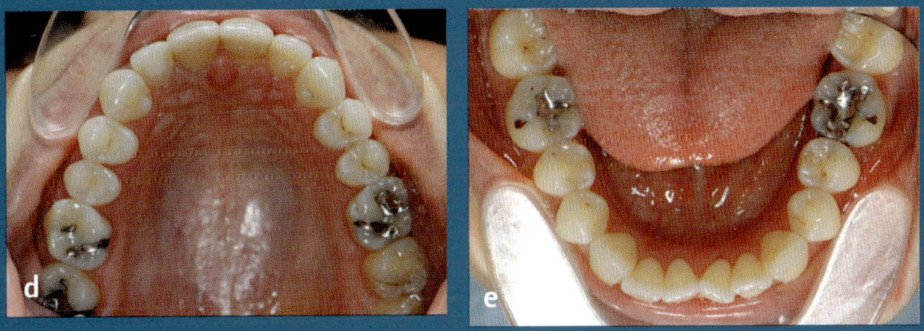

8.39 Intraoral pre-orthodontic treatment photos.

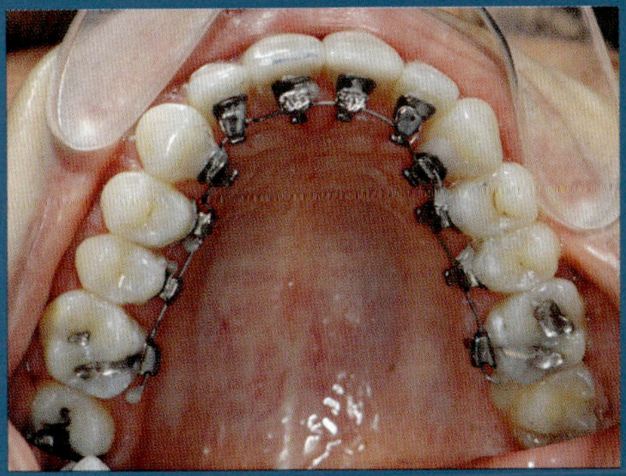

8.40 .016 β-titanium archwire with extrusive steps.

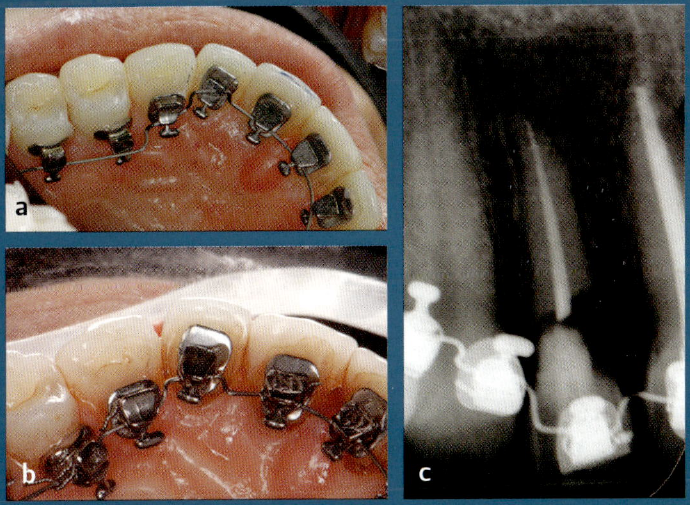

8.41 .016 β-titanium archwire with extrusive steps and derotation. (Reproduced from "Paolone MG, Kaitsas R. Orthodontic-periodontal interactions: Orthodontic extrusion in interdisciplinary regenerative treatments. *Int Orthod.* 2018;16(2):217-245" ©CEO. Published by Elsevier Masson SAS. All rights reserved. With permission.)

During this first phase the extrusion is slow to take advantage from the regenerative capacity of the periodontal ligament overcorrecting soft and hard tissues. When the amount of soft tissue is overcorrected of 2 mm with respect to the final objective, as previously described in the literature, the treatment is continued with a fast extrusion with fibrotomy (8.42 and 8.43). Throughout all the extrusion movement the tooth is removed from occlusal contact by grinding (8.44). The tooth is then stabilized for 3 months at first with the same .016 β-titanium archwire (8.45), then with a .017×.017 β-titanium archwire for detailed control, finally with a .017×.025 in β-titanium archwire.

At this point, at the end of the extrusion (8.46), a flap is elevated in order to isolate the tooth and, after applying the rubber dam (8.47), the element is restored with a fiber post and composite cement. The tooth is prepared for a feldspatic ceramic veneer cemented with composite cement (thanks to Dr. G. Paolone for the restorative contribution) (8.48 and 8.49). 8.50 shows the newly cemented restoration and the 8.51 and 8.52 the end-treatment check. The following figures show a 10-year follow-up in which it can be seen the perfect integration of the tissues around the restoration (8.53) and a perfect esthetic integration (8.54). At 8.55 and 8.56 the patient can be observed 10 years after treatment.

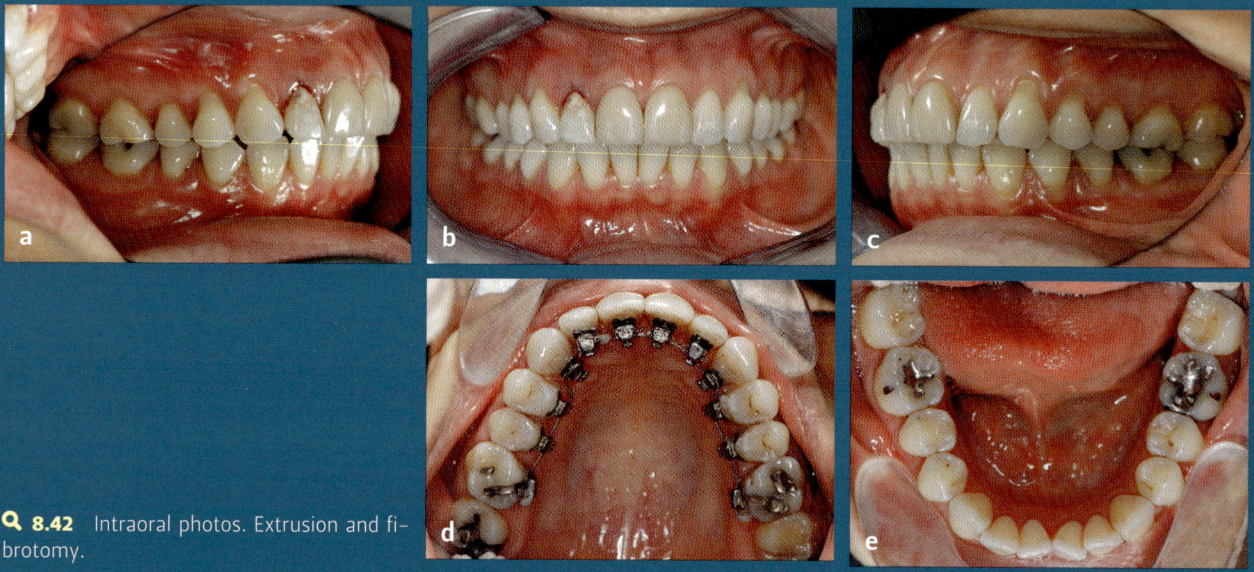

8.42 Intraoral photos. Extrusion and fibrotomy.

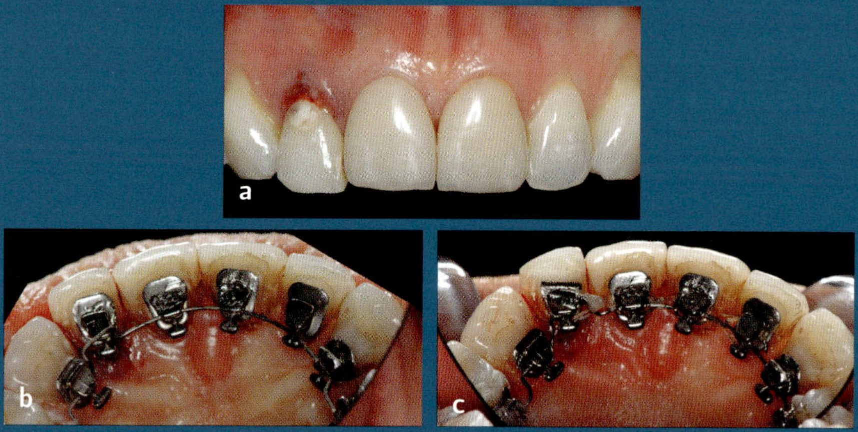

8.43 Fast extrusion with fibrotomy.

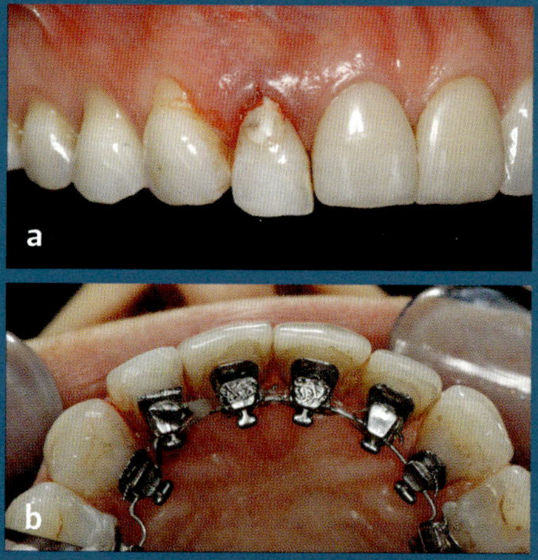

8.44 Circumferential fibrotomy after the "regenerative" extrusion as it is shown in scheme in 8.4.

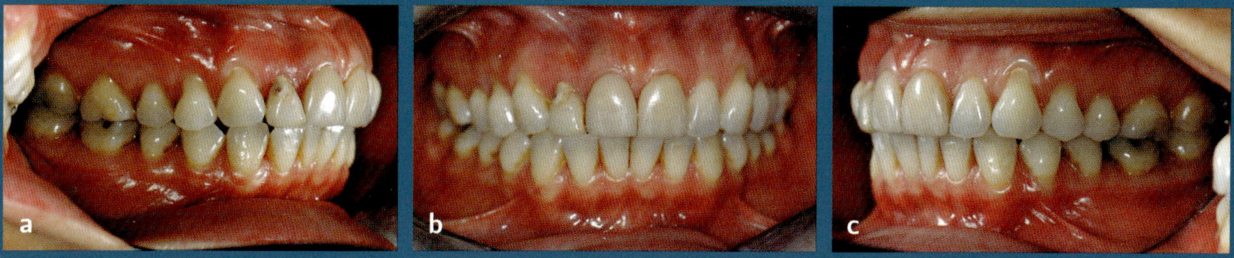

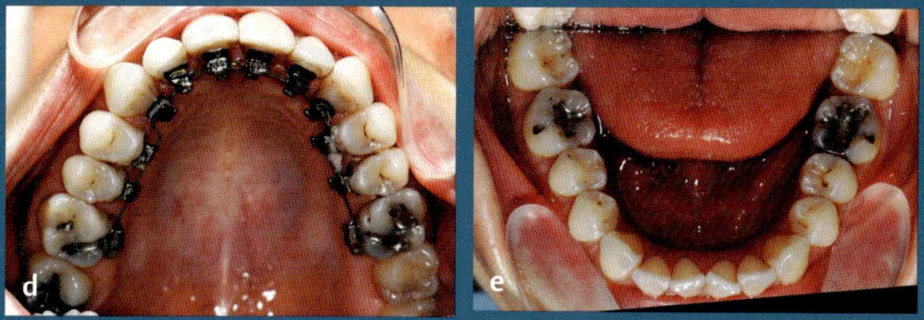

8.45 Intraoral photos. Orthodontic stabilization.

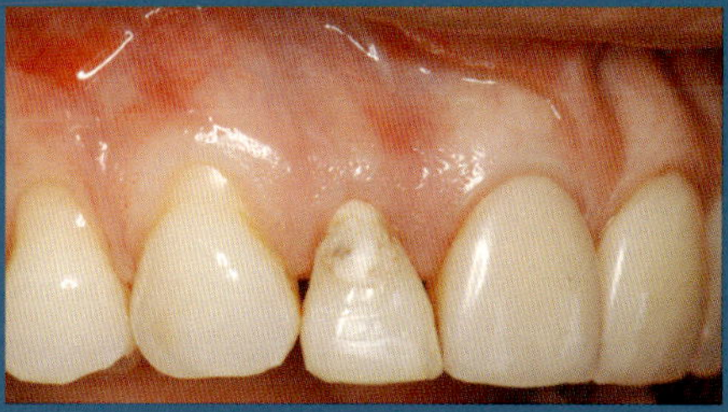

8.46 View of the tissue and tooth at the end of the orthodontic treatment before the restorative treatment. (Reproduced from "Paolone MG, Kaitsas R. Orthodontic-periodontal interactions: Orthodontic extrusion in interdisciplinary regenerative treatments. *Int Orthod*. 2018;16(2):217-245" ©CEO. Published by Elsevier Masson SAS. All rights reserved. With permission.)

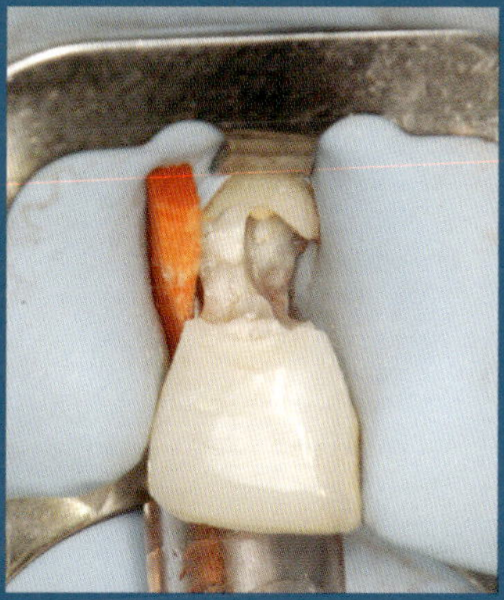

8.47 Rubber dam application and isolation of the external resorption. (Reproduced from "Paolone MG, Kaitsas R. Orthodontic-periodontal interactions: Orthodontic extrusion in interdisciplinary regenerative treatments. *Int Orthod*. 2018;16(2):217-245" ©CEO. Published by Elsevier Masson SAS. All rights reserved. With permission.)

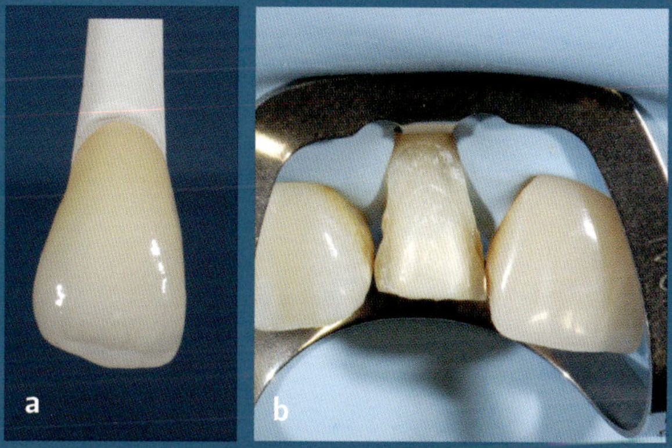

8.48 Ceramic veneer and rubber dam before cementation. (Reproduced from "Paolone MG, Kaitsas R. Orthodontic-periodontal interactions: Orthodontic extrusion in interdisciplinary regenerative treatments. *Int Orthod*. 2018;16(2):217-245" ©CEO. Published by Elsevier Masson SAS. All rights reserved. With permission.)

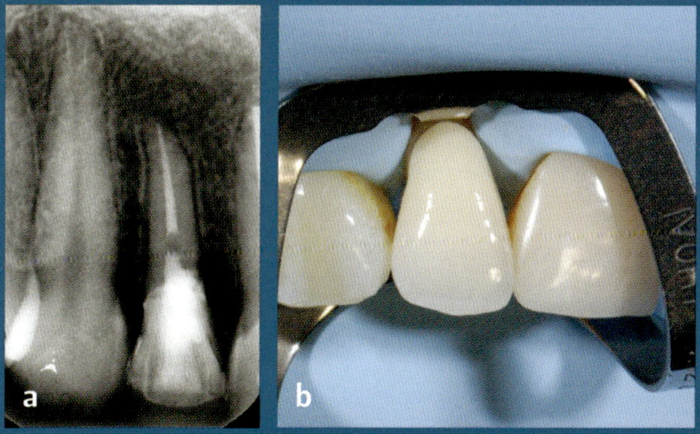

8.49 Veneer just cemented and X-ray check after the cementation (thanks to Dr. Gaetano Paolone for the restorative contribution). (Reproduced from "Paolone MG, Kaitsas R. Orthodontic-periodontal interactions: Orthodontic extrusion in interdisciplinary regenerative treatments. *Int Orthod*. 2018;16(2):217-245" ©CEO. Published by Elsevier Masson SAS. All rights reserved. With permission.)

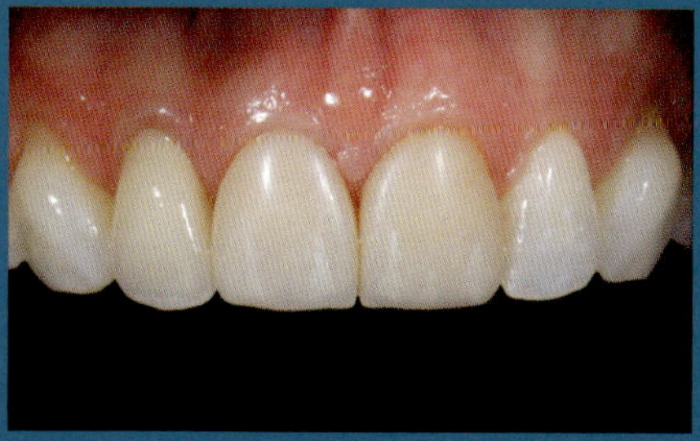

8.50 Control of the tissue at the end of the treatment. (Reproduced from "Paolone MG, Kaitsas R. Orthodontic-periodontal interactions: Orthodontic extrusion in interdisciplinary regenerative treatments. *Int Orthod*. 2018;16(2):217-245" ©CEO. Published by Elsevier Masson SAS. All rights reserved. With permission.)

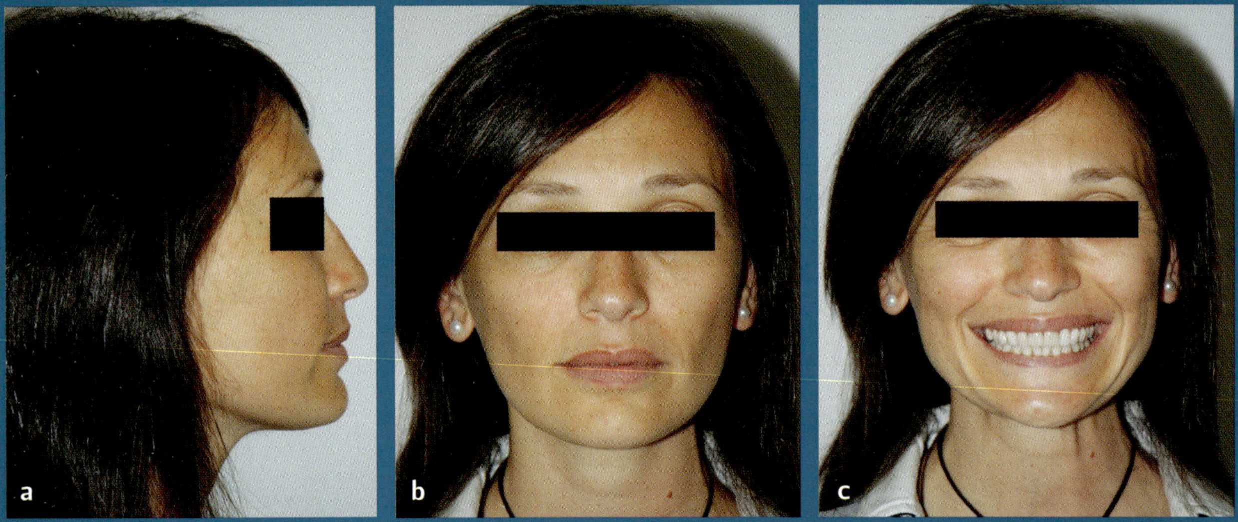

8.51 Extraoral photos at the end of the treatment.

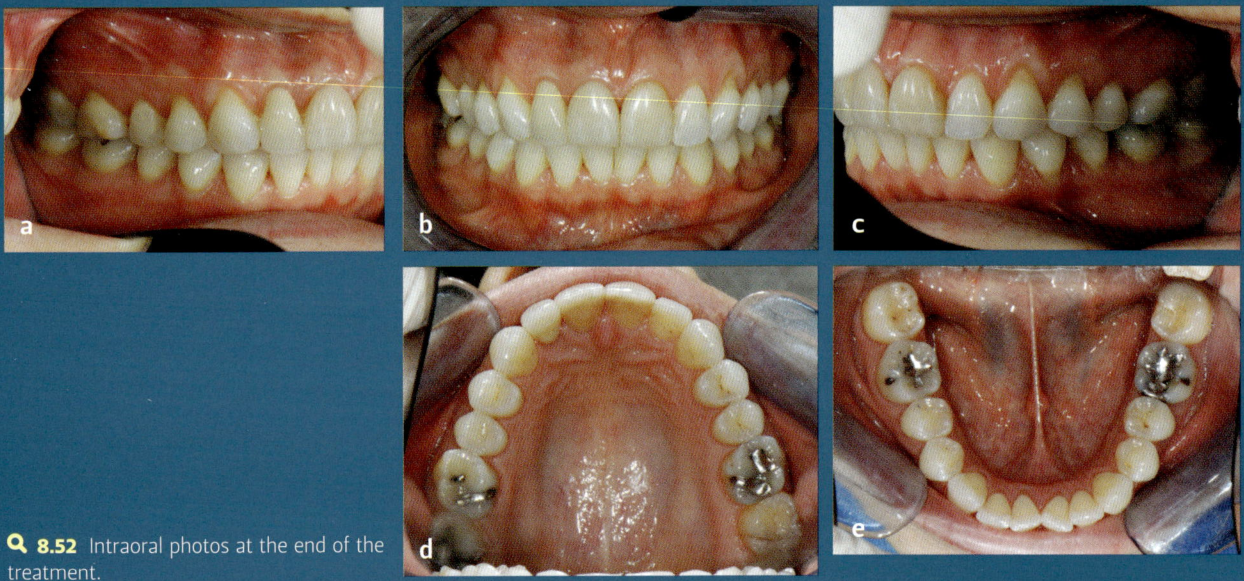

8.52 Intraoral photos at the end of the treatment.

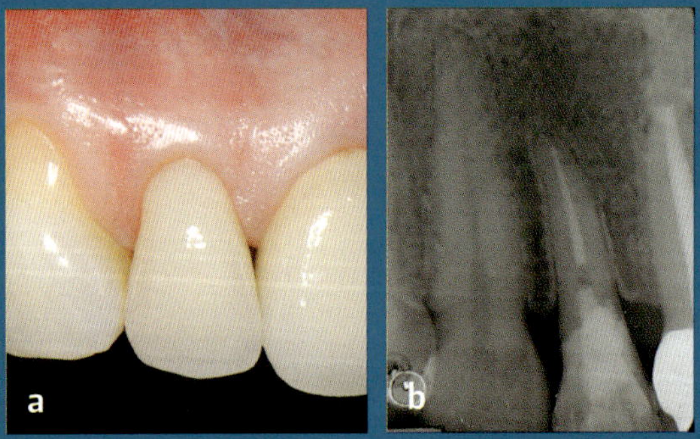

8.53 Clinical and X-ray 10-year follow-up.

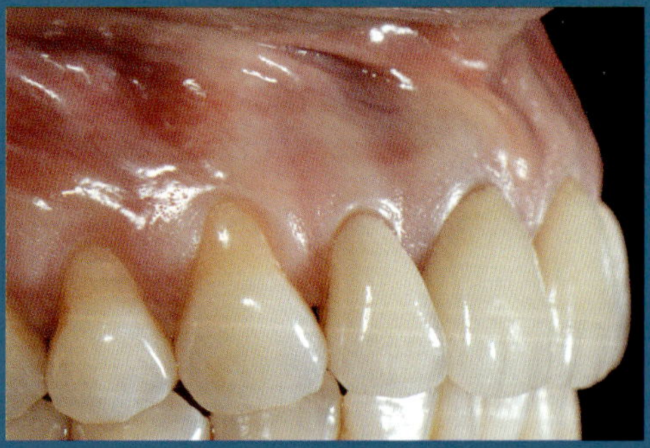

8.54 10-year follow-up.

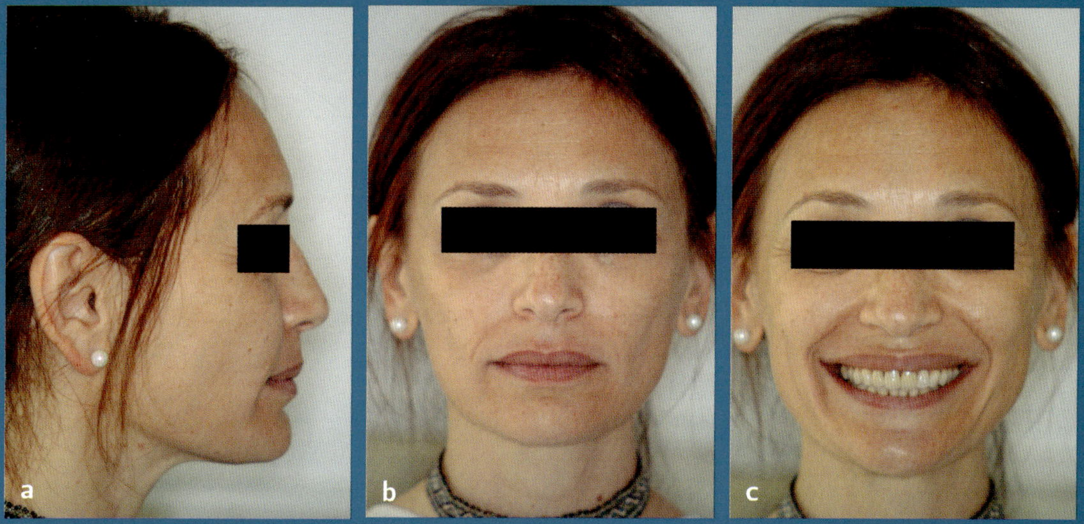

8.55 10-year extraoral photos.

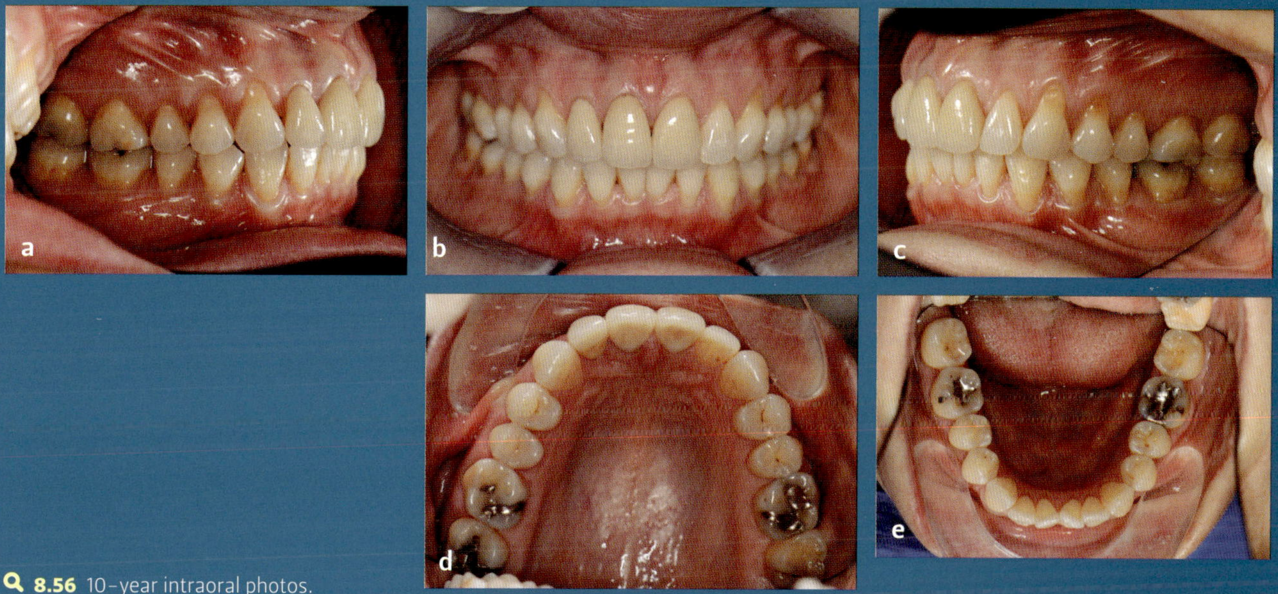

8.56 10-year intraoral photos.

Clinical case 2 (dental extrusion - posterior sector)

The patient, 46 years old, complains about discomfort and slight mobility of 1.4 (8.57). After an X-ray examination (8.58) a decay is detected below the prosthetic restoration. After having evaluated the various alternatives (implant rehabilitation included) and considered the remaining dental structure and the crown/root ratio sufficient to be used as a prosthetic abutment for a new restoration, a dental extrusion of the root is carried out to allow the creation of an appropriate prosthetic ferrule. A fibrotomy is not performed, but surgical biological width realignment procedures to increase the width of keratinized tissue around the new prosthetic restoration; this amount would have remained unchanged if fibrotomy had been performed.

The extrusion is carried out with vestibular mechanics by means of a 1.7-1.3 sectional with Tweed® brackets .022×.028 with a .016 CuNiTi archwire and apical brackets positioning on the tooth to be extruded (8.59). The extrusion is completed with sequential increments of the extrusive steps with vertical bends on a .017×.022 stainless steel sectional for the first month and then a .018×.025 stain steel (8.60 and 8.61), with continuous follow-ups and grinding to eliminate the occlusal contact on the tooth, and finally a .019×.025 stainless steel (8.62). This sectional is also used for the last 4 months of stabilization (8.63). Every month a radiography is taken (8.64).

At the end of the orthodontic extrusion in order to restore the correct gingival levels, a surgical "Realignment of biological width"[34] is performed (8.65-8.69). After the maturation of the tissues and after the stabilization phase (8.70), the restoration is finalized with a full zirconia crown (8.71-8.75). The 2-year follow-up can be observed at 8.76 and 8.77.

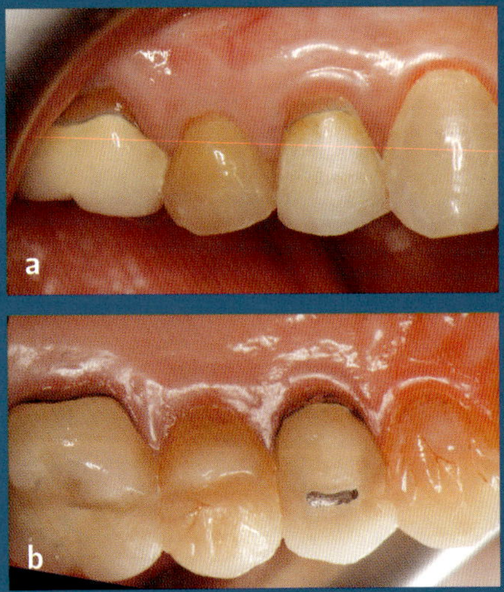

8.57 Vestibular and palatal view of 1.4.

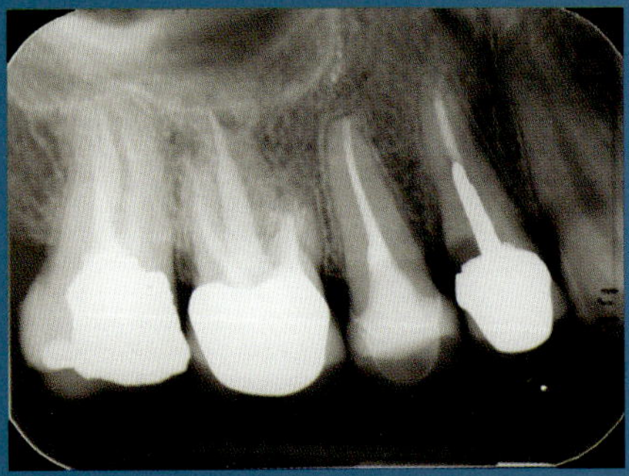

8.58 X-ray where it can be seen the distal decay of 1.4.

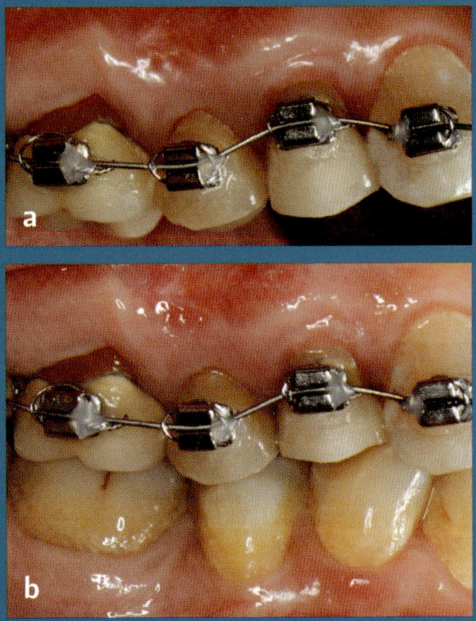

8.59 CuNiTi .016 and apical positioning of the brackets on the tooth that must be extruded.

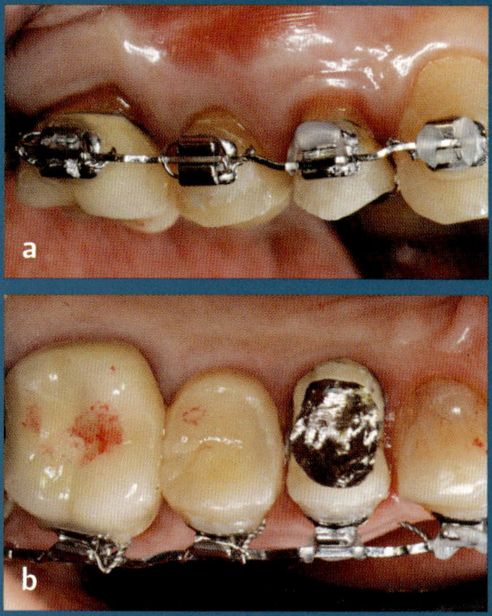

8.60 .018x.025 stainless steel, extrusive step, occlusal grinding.

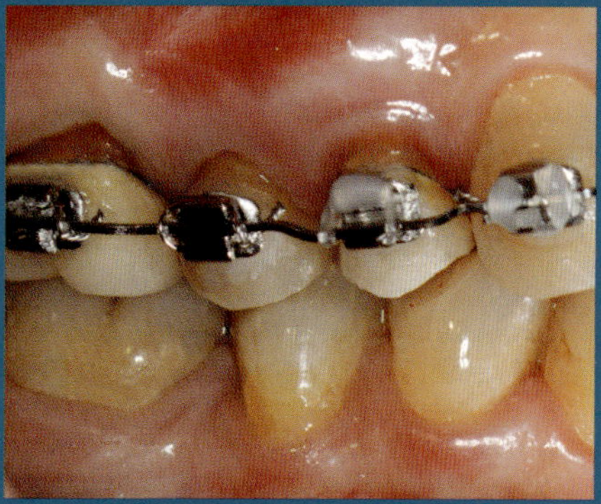

8.61 .018x.025 stainless steel, extrusive step, occlusal grinding.

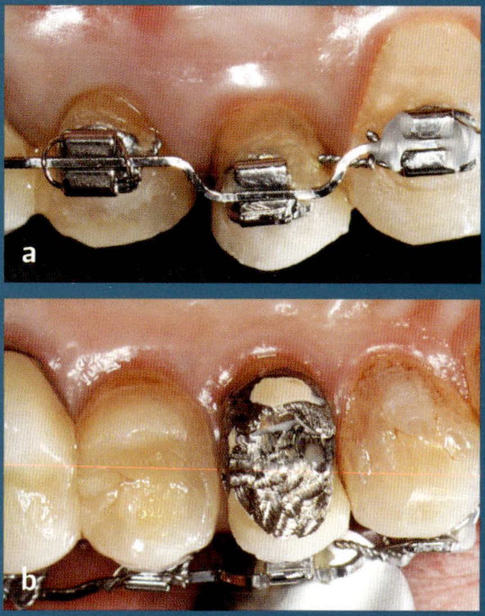

8.62 .019x.025 stainless steel, increase in extrusive step.

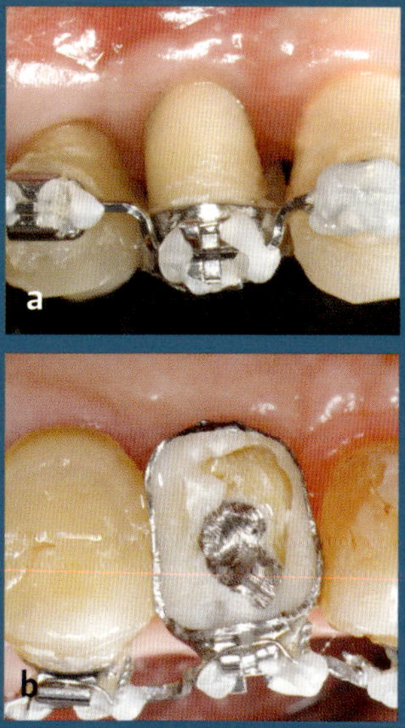

8.63 Orthodontic stabilization.

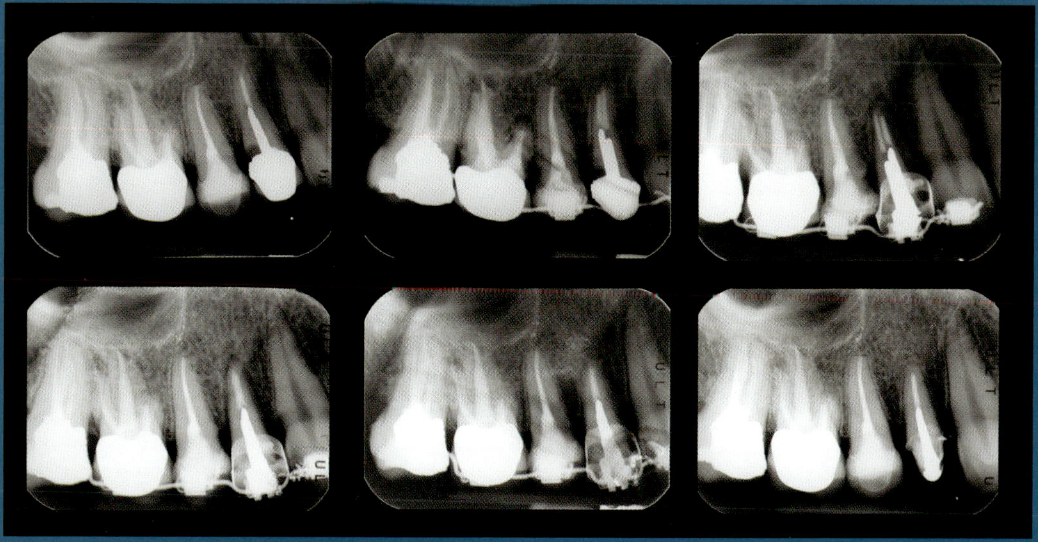

8.64 Extrusion, radiographic monthly check.

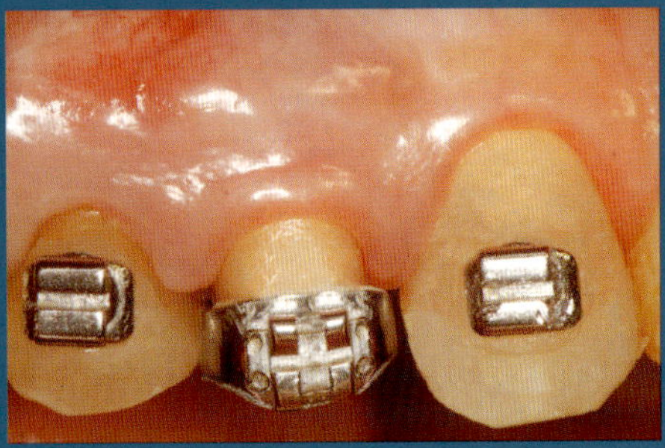

8.65 Vestibular view of the tissue at the end of the dental extrusion before the surgical crown lengthening.

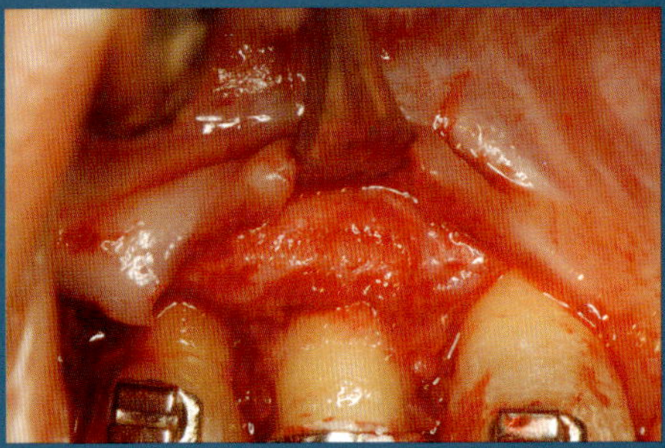

8.66 Vestibular view of the bone levels gained with extrusion. It can be seen the neo-apposition of the fibers.

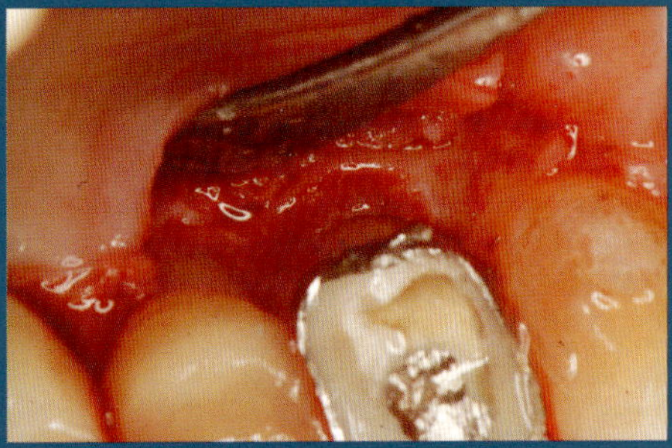

8.67 Palatal view of the bone levels gained with extrusion. It can be seen the neo-apposition of the fibers.

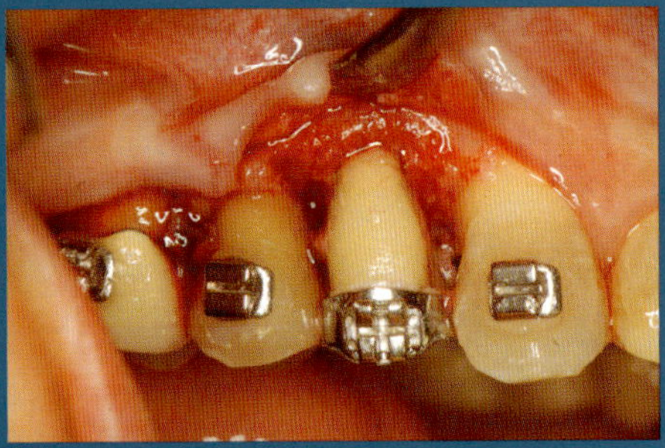

8.68 New bone margin.

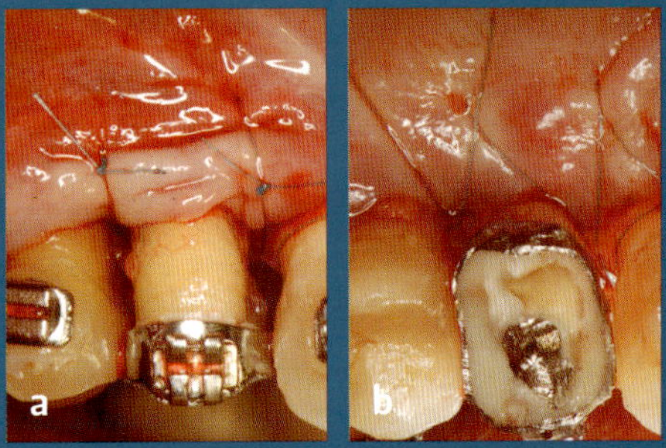

8.69 Apically repositioned flap and vestibular vertical and palatal horizontal mattress suture.

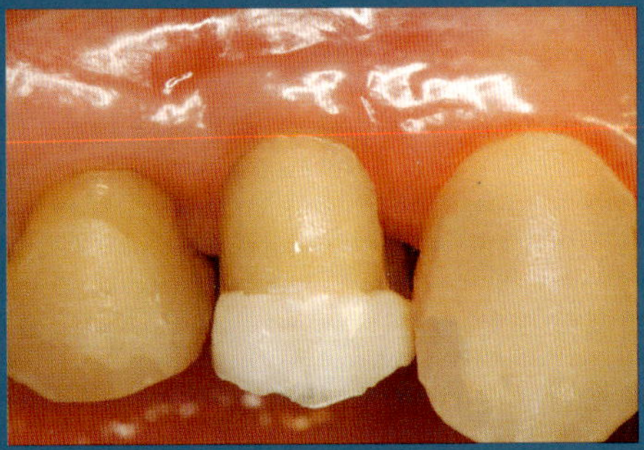

8.70 Clinical view of the tissues after healing.

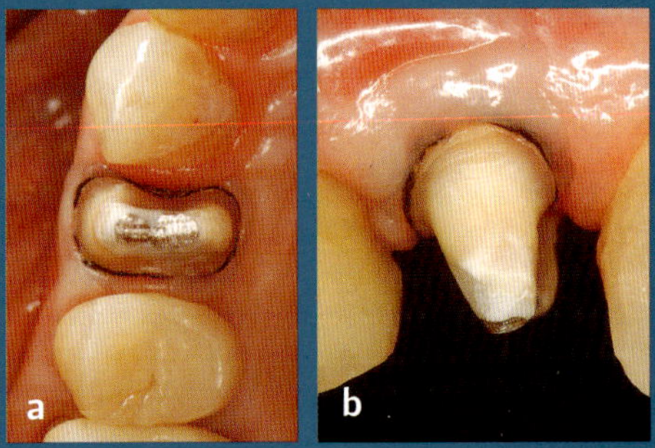

8.71 Definitive impression.

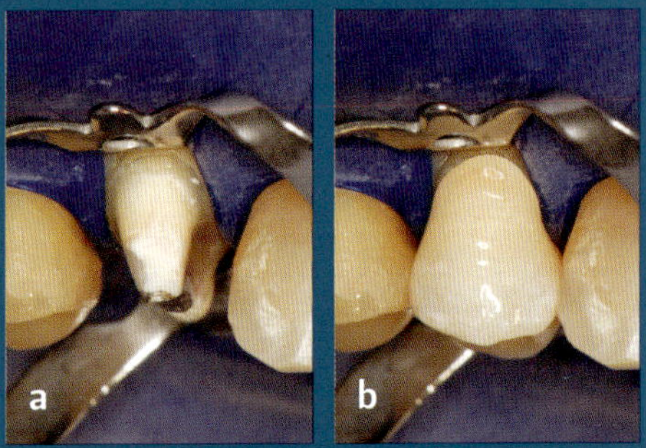

8.72 Definitive cementation of the zirconia crown under rubber dam.

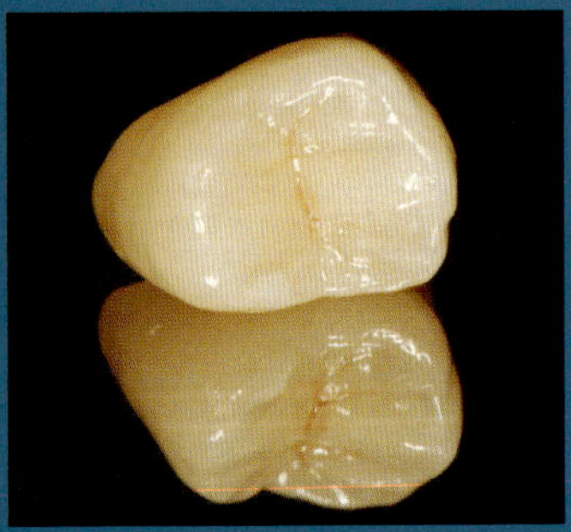

8.73 Definitive zirconia crown.

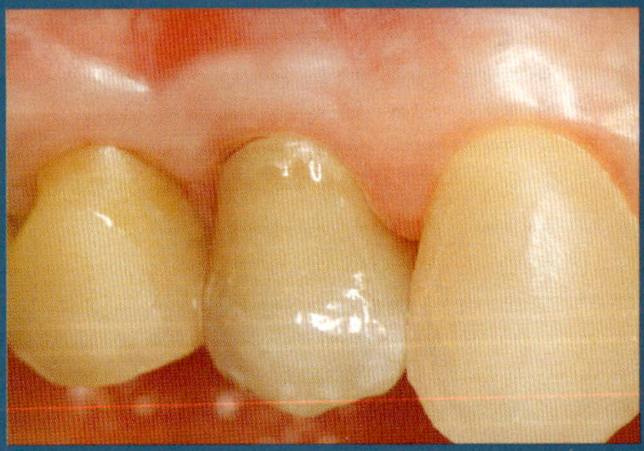

8.74 End-therapy tissue view.

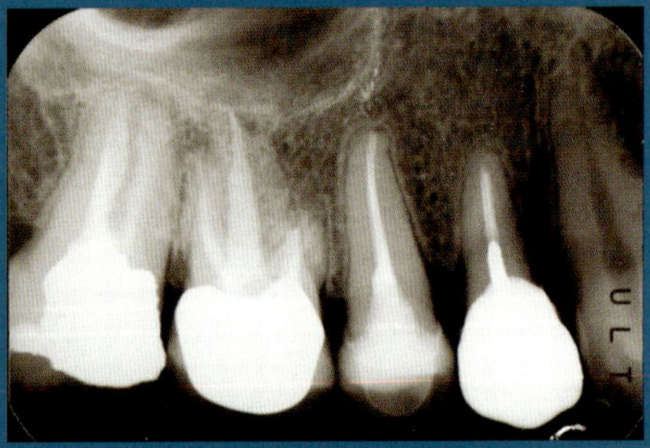

8.75 X-ray check of the definitive crown.

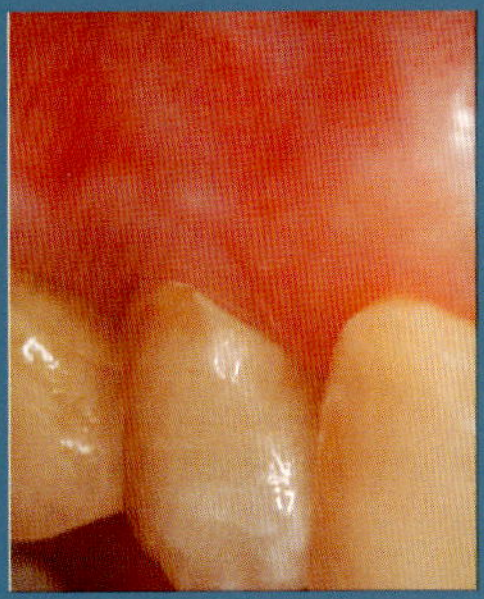

8.76 2-year vestibular view of the tissue.

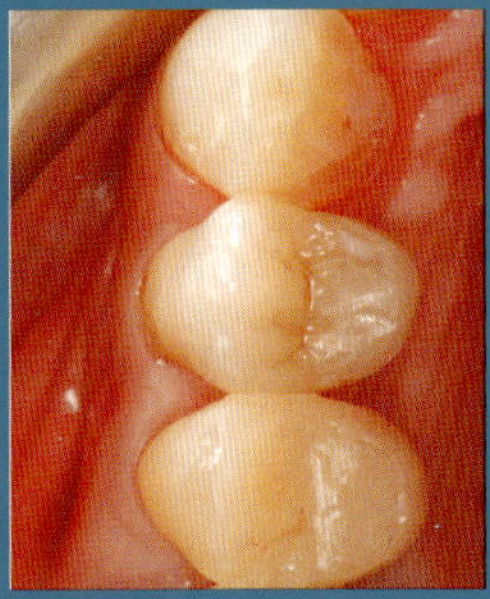

8.77 2-year occlusal view of the tissue.

Clinical case 3 (orthodontic extraction)

The patient comes to our observation for recurrent abscesses on 4.2. The tooth is positive at the vitality test, and shows an intrabony defect along the disto-vestibulo-lingual area that is confirmed at the periodontal probing and at the radiographic examination (8.78). There are many therapeutic alternatives, including GTR, extraction, implant rehabilitation with or without GTR and implant rehabilitation with orthodontic extrusion. The patient also complains of an esthetic problem related to the lower crowding and requires a complete rehabilitation (the complete case will be discussed in Chapter 11, *Clinical case 1*; here we will focus only on the tooth in question). After the initial periodontal therapy at the 3 month re-evaluation (8.79) taking into account the patient's need of the crowding resolution and the fact that the probing reduction is small and the BOP is still high, the regenerative periodontal surgical alternative is excluded. An orthodontic solution is therefore proposed with the extraction of the 4.2 to solve the crowding of the lower anterior teeth. The tooth, however, is extracted in an unconventional way: an orthodontic extraction is performed with tissue regeneration through an extrusive movement, preventing the collapse of the cortical plates and the bone ridge and remodeling the tissues simultaneously with the space closure. This decision is taken after the periodontal evaluation of 4.3, which has the mesial periodontal attachment adjacent to the defect sufficient to close the post-extrusion space maintaining the integrity of the periodontal attachment of the adjacent teeth.

A complete lingual appliance (Kurz 7th Generation®, Ormco) is applied on the lower arch, with the aim of remodeling hard and soft tissues during extraction and trying to reduce the risk of clefts after the extraction of a such a periodontally compromised tooth. Initially 4.2 is extruded providing a vertical axial component to level its distal interproximal defect to the mesial level of 4.3. The sectorial set-up already incorporates a first axial extrusive component in the bonding. In this first phase the mechanics is realized with an .016 CuNi-Ti archwire (8.80) for the first month and then with a .016 β-titanium archwire with progressive extrusive steps on the arch and with loops (8.81 and 8.82). During the extrusion, the tooth is removed from the occlusal contact by grinding (8.83) until root canal therapy is required.

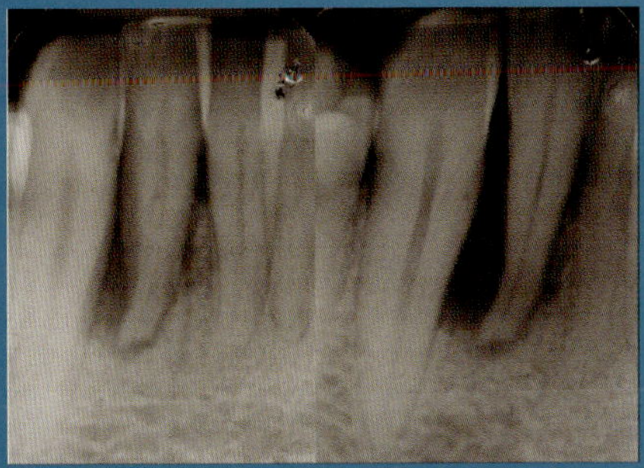

8.78 X-ray, the periodontal defect at 4.2 can be seen.

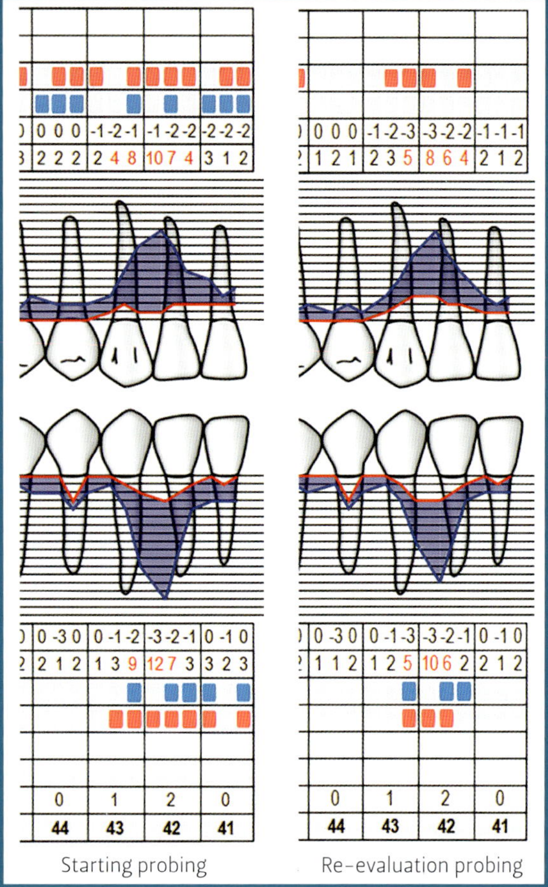

8.79 Detail of the starting and re-evaluation periodontal probing limited to the bone defect. In this phase, it is important to evaluate the clinical attachment level of the adjacent teeth next to the tooth that must be extracted by extrusion. (Online periodontal charting tool, www.perio-tools.com). The complete periodontal probing is shown in the *Clinical case 1* of Chapter 11.

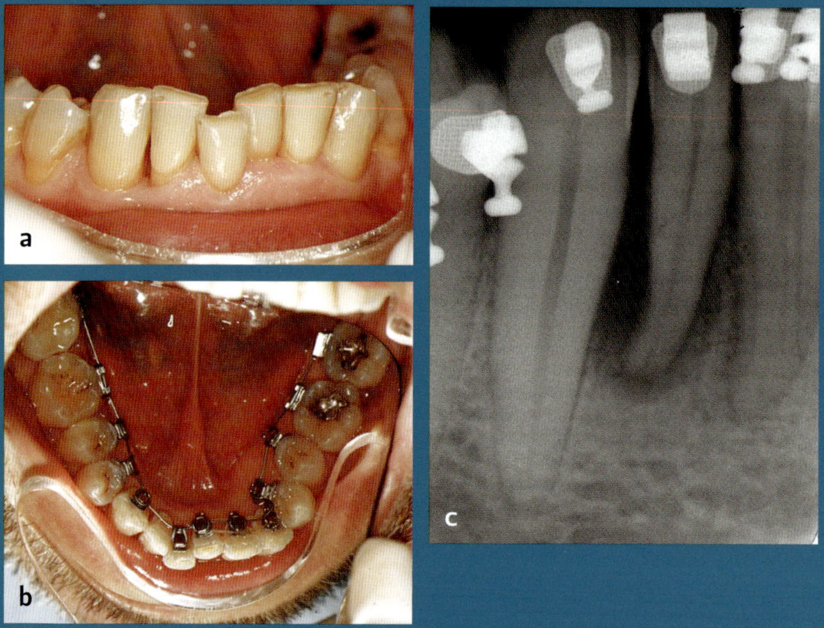

8.80 .016 CuNiTi archwire. (Reproduced from "Paolone MG, Kaitsas R. Orthodontic-periodontal interactions: Orthodontic extrusion in interdisciplinary regenerative treatments. *Int Orthod.* 2018;16(2):217-245" ©CEO. Published by Elsevier Masson SAS. All rights reserved. With permission.)

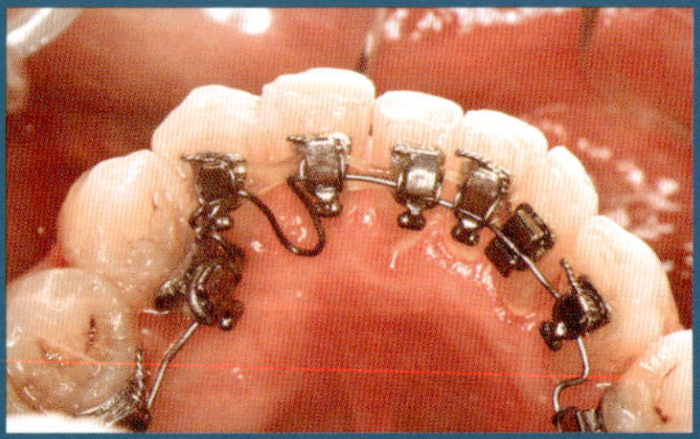

8.81 .016 β-titanium archwire, loops, extrusive bending.

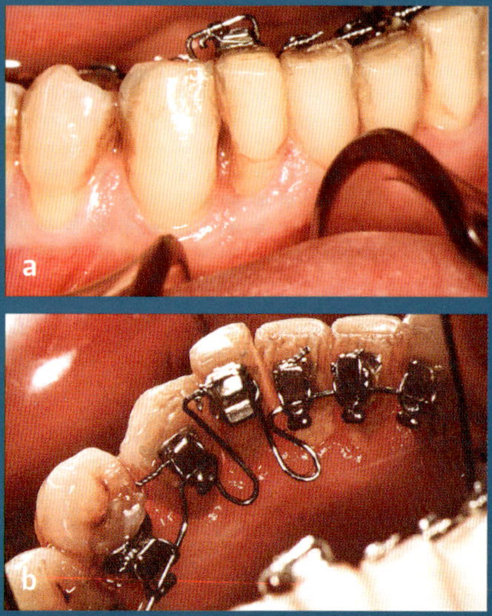

8.82 .016 β-titanium archwire, loops, extrusive bending.

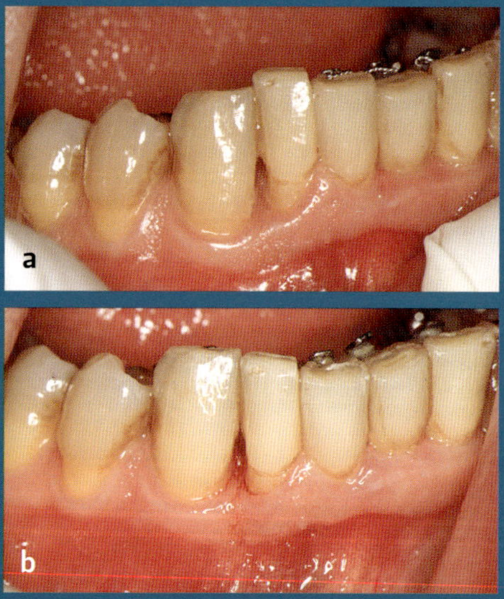

8.83 Grinding to reduce the occlusal contact with the antagonist.

The extrusion continues at first with a .017×.017 β-titanium archwire (8.84 and 8.85) and then with a .017×.025 β-titanium archwire (8.86), always with loops with activations of about 1 mm. The insertion of the loops allows the possibility of a progressive activation with controlled extrusive tipping movements of the distal margin of 4.2 to the mesial level of 4.3. Extrusion is slow and activations and checks take place every 15 days. The direction of the movement and the consequent information on the archwire derive from the visualization of the three-dimensional view of the periodontal defect that has been diagnosed by the surgeon and referred to the orthodontist. The modification of the bone defect by extrusion and the final goal of the treatment need periodically periodontal re-evaluation shared with the orthodontist. Since the 4.2 bone defect is disto-bucco-lingual, with a greater loss on the buccal site than on the lingual one, a radiculo-lingual torque is incorporated in addition to the tipping movement in order to reduce the risk of root impact on the vestibular cortical plate and to protect the health of hard and soft tissues as much as possible. This procedure is realized being conscious of the reduction in the torque moment expression using a .017×.017 in β-titanium archwire in the .022×.028 slot with a light force-effect. In a second time a radiculo-vestibular torque is used, trying to reduce the formation of vestibular clefts and favor the stimulation of hard and soft tissues (8.86 and 8.87). The extrusion is pushed until the complete extraction of the tooth is realized. The same .017×.017 β-titanium archwire (8.88) and .017×.025 β-titanium archwire are then used to complete the closure of the residual space and for the stabilization. The mechanics is summarized in 8.89-8.91a. In 8.91b and 8.92 the closure of the space and the follow-up at the end of the treatment can be seen.

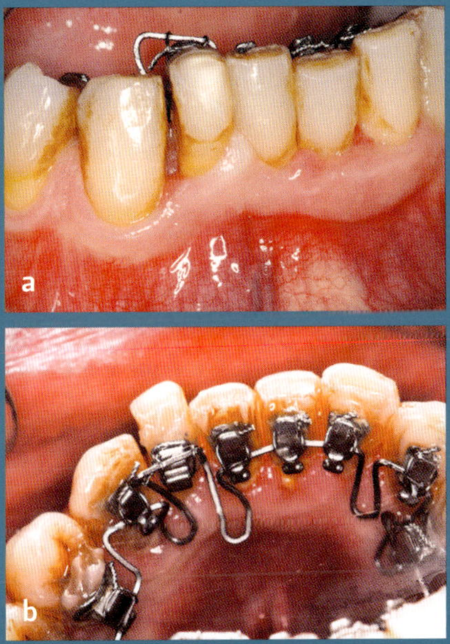

8.84 .017x.017 β-titanium archwire, loops, extrusive bending.

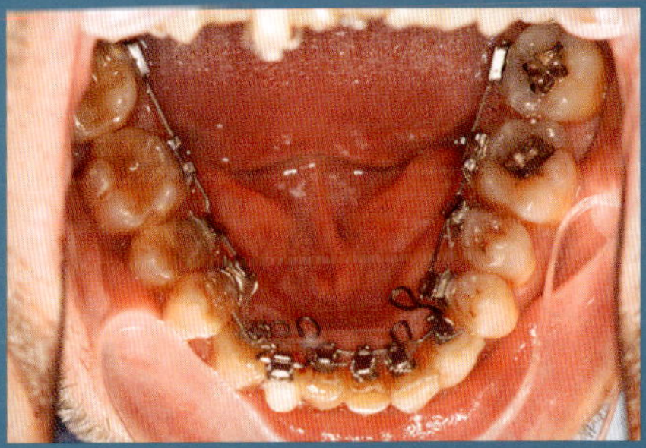

8.85 .017x.017 β-titanium archwire, loops, extrusive bending.

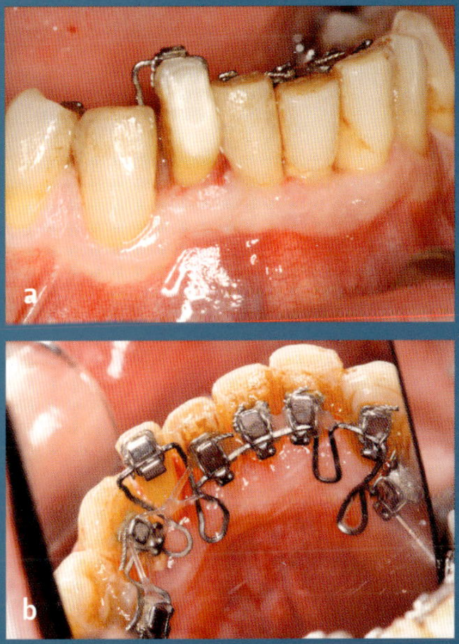

8.86 .017x.025 β-titanium archwire, loops, extrusive bending, root canal treatment.

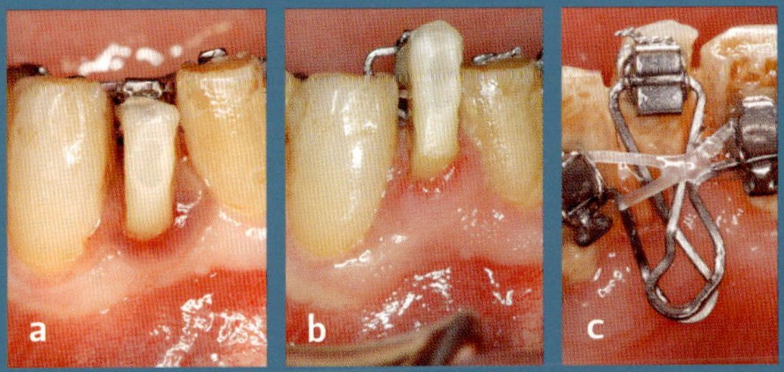

8.87 .017x.025 β-titanium archwire, loops, extrusive bending.

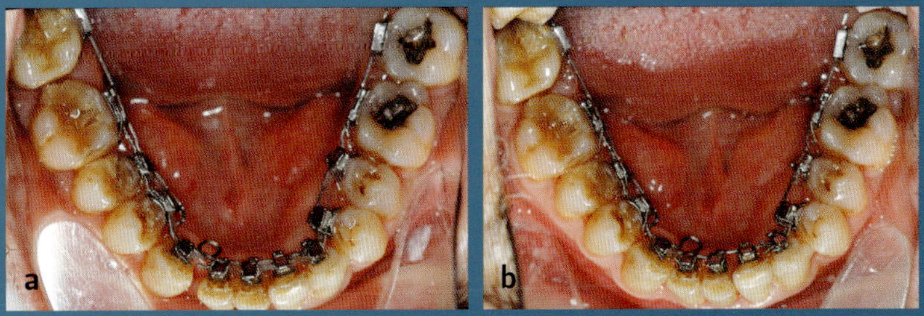

8.88 .017x.017 β-titanium archwire, closing loops.

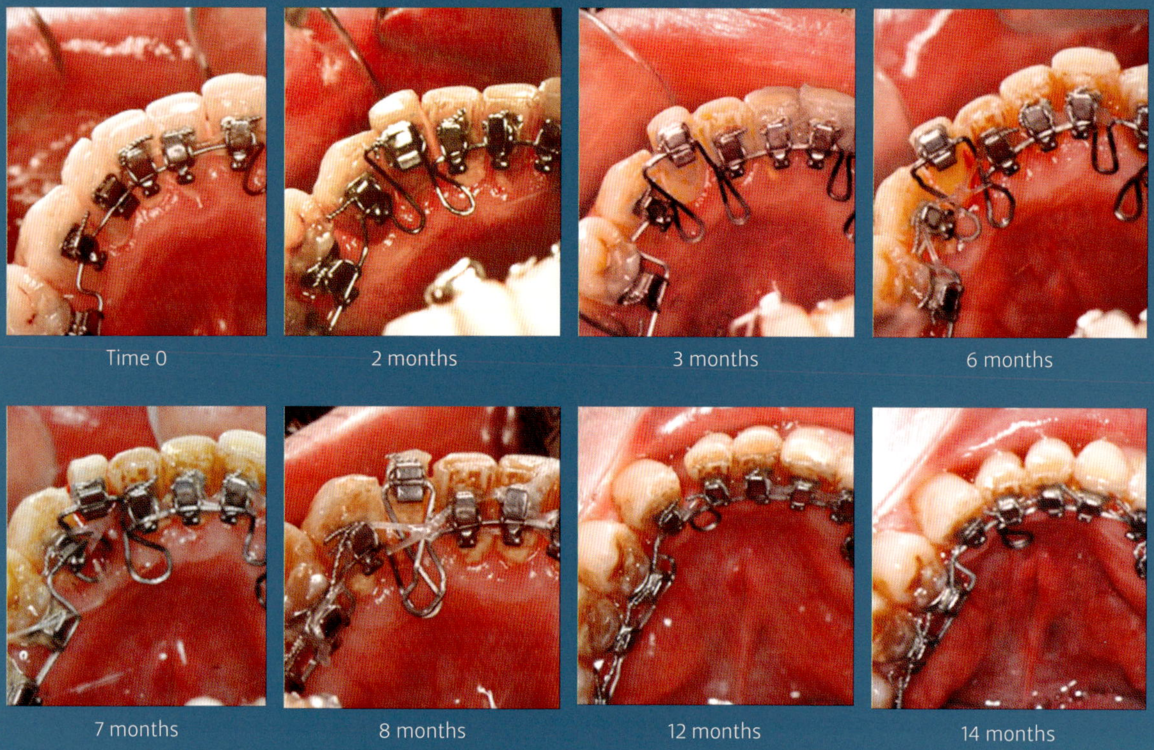

8.89 Orthodontic mechanics, occlusal view. (Reproduced from "Paolone MG, Kaitsas R. Orthodontic-periodontal interactions: Orthodontic extrusion in interdisciplinary regenerative treatments. *Int Orthod.* 2018;16(2):217-245" ©CEO. Published by Elsevier Masson SAS. All rights reserved. With permission.)

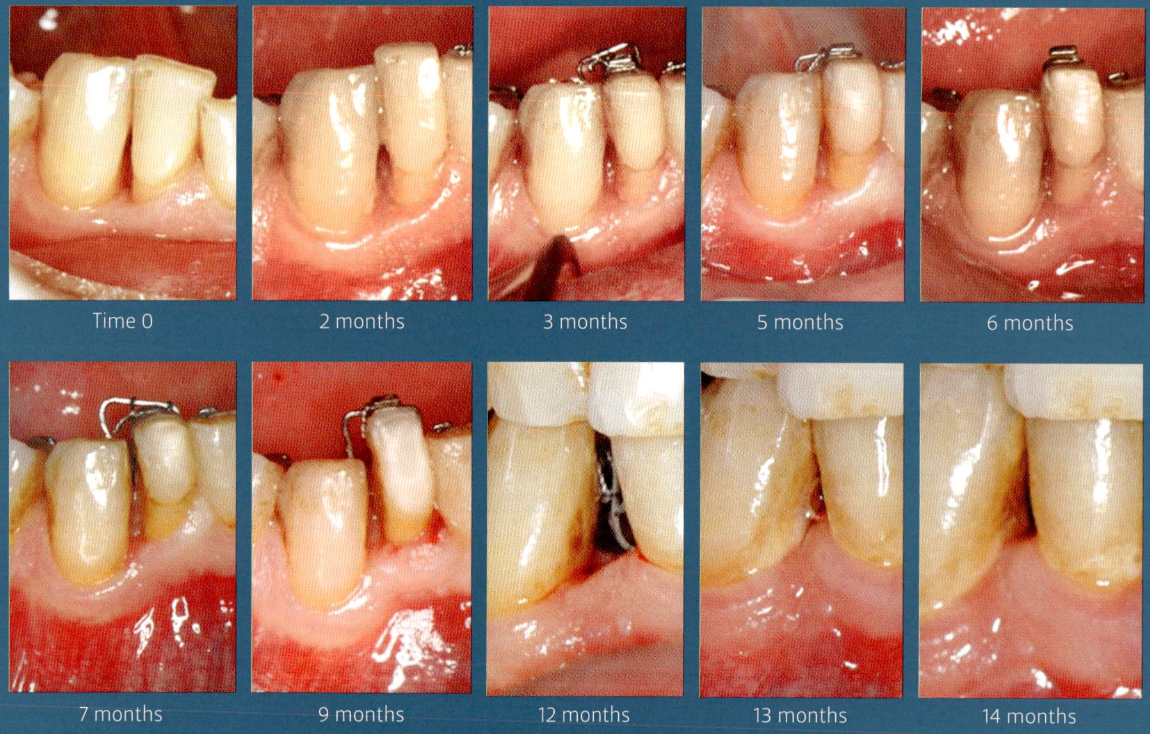

8.90 Orthodontic mechanics, vestibular view. (Reproduced from "Paolone MG, Kaitsas R. Orthodontic-periodontal interactions: Orthodontic extrusion in interdisciplinary regenerative treatments. *Int Orthod.* 2018;16(2):217-245" ©CEO. Published by Elsevier Masson SAS. All rights reserved. With permission.)

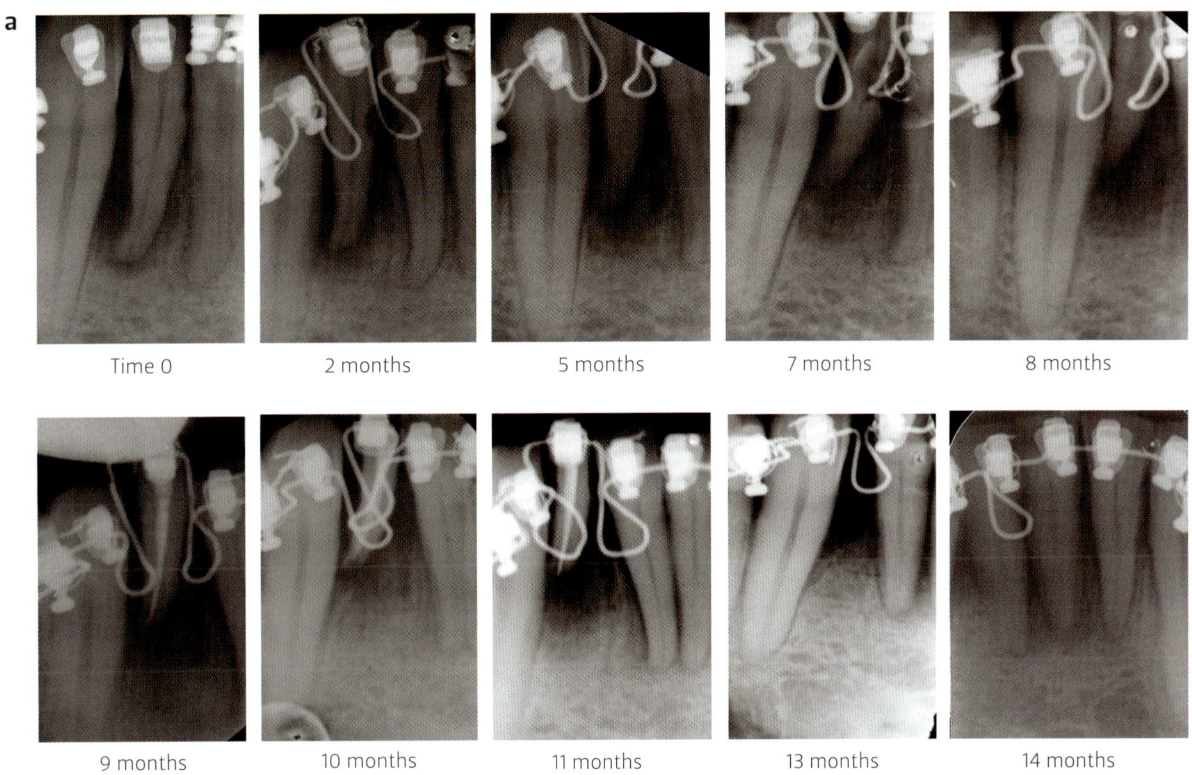

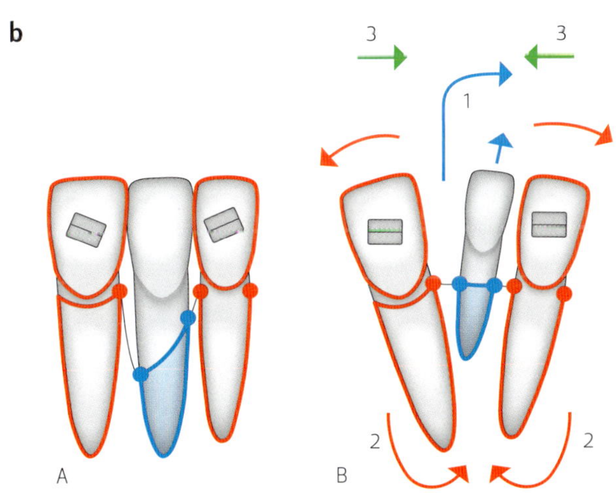

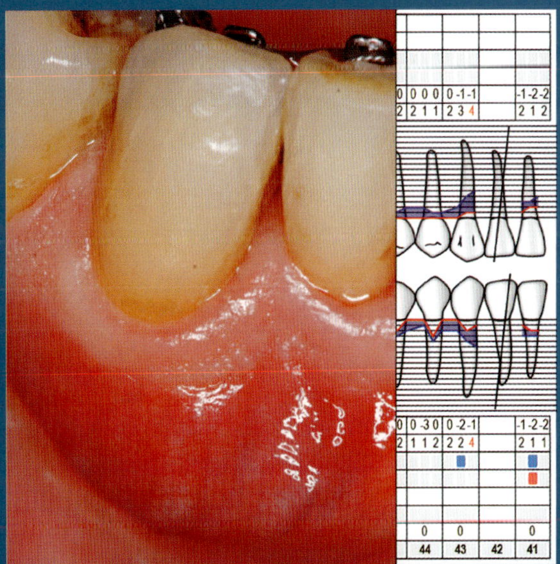

8.91 (**a**) Orthodontic mechanics, X-rays (reproduced from "Paolone MG, Kaitsas R. Orthodontic-periodontal interactions: Orthodontic extrusion in interdisciplinary regenerative treatments. *Int Orthod.* 2018;16(2):217-245" ©CEO. Published by Elsevier Masson SAS. All rights reserved. With permission). (**b**) Schematic diagram of the dental extraction. Drawing of the bone peaks levelling (1) and of the contextual hypertipping root movement with brackets hypertipping positioning, (2) and then coronal movement (3) of the adjacent teeth.

8.92 End of the closure of the extraction space. (reproduced from "Paolone MG, Kaitsas R. Orthodontic-periodontal interactions: Orthodontic extrusion in interdisciplinary regenerative treatments. *Int Orthod.* 2018;16(2):217-245" ©CEO. Published by Elsevier Masson SAS. All rights reserved. With permission) and detail of the end-treatment periodontal probing limited to the defect area (Online periodontal charting tool, dal sito www.perio-tools.com).

Clinical case 4 (GOBR - Guided Orthodontic "Bone" Regeneration)

The patient, 57 years old, asks for the rehabilitation of 2.1, who has an old metal-ceramic crown that had been temporarily cemented elsewhere after a new trauma (as it can be observed from the amount of cement emerging along the gingival sulcus, 8.93). The tooth had various traumatic injuries over the years that have led to a restoration with a gold post and core and a fixed metal-ceramic crown. At the clinical examination, the crown shows a coronal displacement of the incisal margin and a vestibular displacement of the entire crown (8.94). At the radiographic examination, a root fracture (8.95) at the middle third is observed and, at the periodontal probing, a 9 mm mesio-vestibular defect on the mesial aspect and of 5 mm on the vestibular aspect is found; on the palatal aspect, the defect extension is 6 mm. The diagnostic-therapeutic evaluation allows the consideration of various alternatives, including a simple prosthetic restoration with or without surgical crown lengthening or with dental orthodontic extrusion, socket preservation techniques, immediate post-extraction implant and delayed implant placement with GBR. The radiographic examination confirms the impossibility of restoring the fractured root by a new post using a conventional fixed crown. A surgical crown lengthening could lead to disabling esthetic consequences. The residual root fragment is almost useless, therefore an orthodontic root recovery with a dental ex-

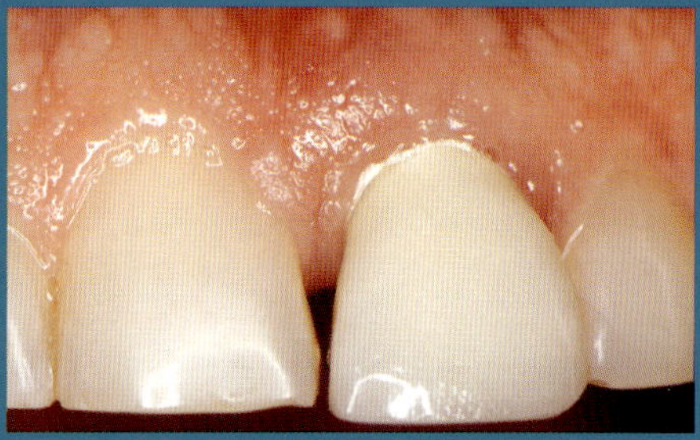

8.93 Vestibular view of 2.1 where the uneven incisal margin and cement extrusion on the gingival edge can be seen. (Reproduced from "Paolone MG, Kaitsas R. Orthodontic-periodontal interactions: Orthodontic extrusion in interdisciplinary regenerative treatments. *Int Orthod.* 2018;16(2):217-245" ©CEO. Published by Elsevier Masson SAS. All rights reserved. With permission.)

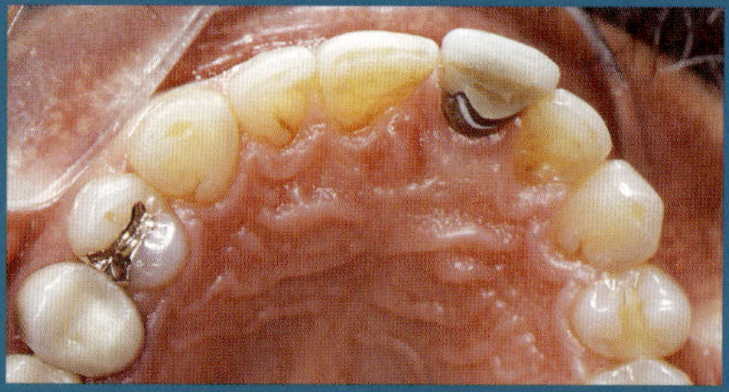

8.94 Palatal view of the vestibularization of 2.1. (Reproduced from "Paolone MG, Kaitsas R, Paolone G, Kaitsas V. Lingual orthodontics and forced eruption: a means for osseous and tissue regeneration. *Prog Orthod.* 2008;9(2):46-57" with permission by SIDO.)

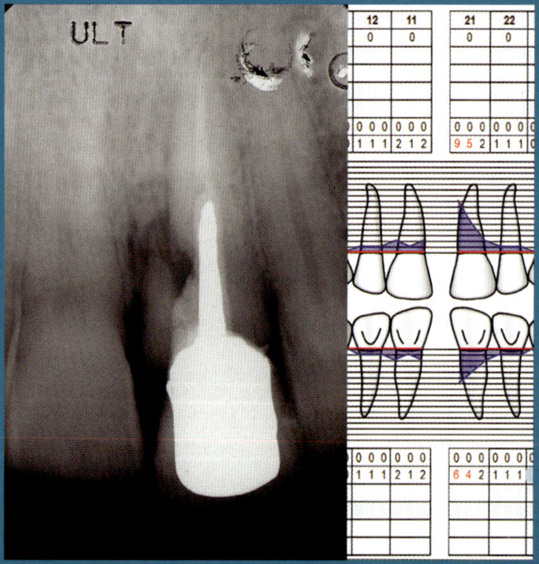

8.95 X-ray view of the root fracture with the totally displaced unrecoverable fragment. (Reproduced from "Paolone MG, Kaitsas R, Paolone G, Kaitsas V. Lingual orthodontics and forced eruption: a means for osseous and tissue regeneration. *Prog Orthod.* 2008;9(2):46-57" with permission by SIDO and "Paolone MG, Kaitsas R. Orthodontic-periodontal interactions: Orthodontic extrusion in interdisciplinary regenerative treatments. *Int Orthod.* 2018;16(2):217-245" ©CEO. Published by Elsevier Masson SAS. All rights reserved. With permission) with the detail of the initial periodontal probing limited to the bone defect. (Online periodontal charting tool, dal sito www.perio-tools.com).

trusion must be excluded due to an unfavorable crown/root ratio. After choosing the implant substitution for the rehabilitation, the choice is to extrude the root fragment in order to develop the implant site, to avoid the insertion of grafts and membranes with complex surgical management, aimed to prevent the collapse of the soft tissues in the bone defect. This choice involves the complete elimination of the bone defect and the simultaneous increase of the amount of soft tissue. After initial periodontal therapy and periodontal re-evaluation, orthodontic therapy is started.

The patient's request is limited just to the rehabilitation of the fractured left upper incisor only, choosing to exclude a complete class II ortho-surgical treatment. The patient has a class II profile with a retrognathic mandible (8.96). At the intraoral examination there is an increase in OVJ and OVB and a canine and molar class I on the right and a molar class I and canine class II on the left (8.97). The cephalometric values confirm a class II with a reduced sagittal mandibular dimension (8.98; 8.20).

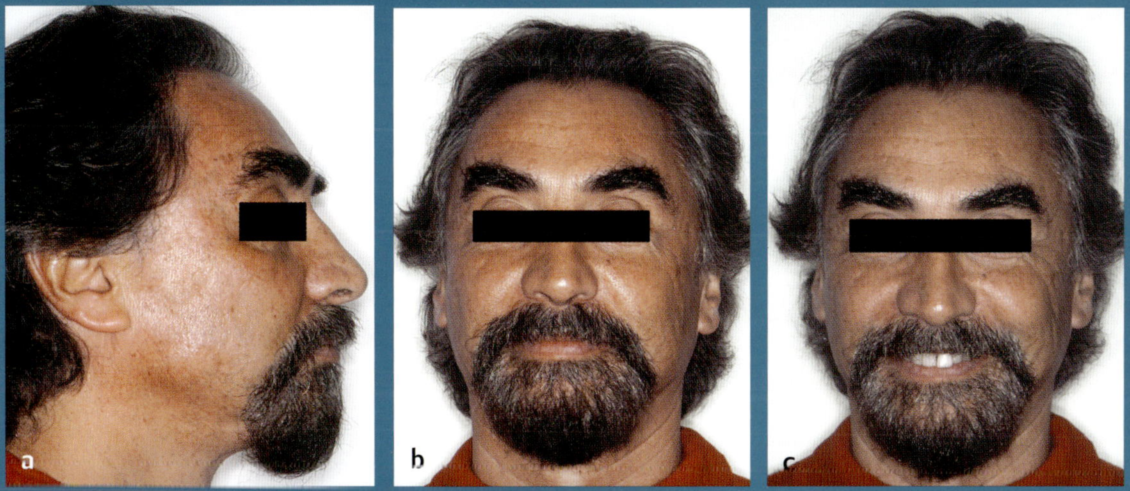

8.96 Extraoral pre-treatment photos. (Reproduced from "Paolone MG, Kaitsas R, Paolone G, Kaitsas V. Lingual orthodontics and forced eruption: a means for osseous and tissue regeneration. *Prog Orthod.* 2008;9(2):46-57" with permission by SIDO.)

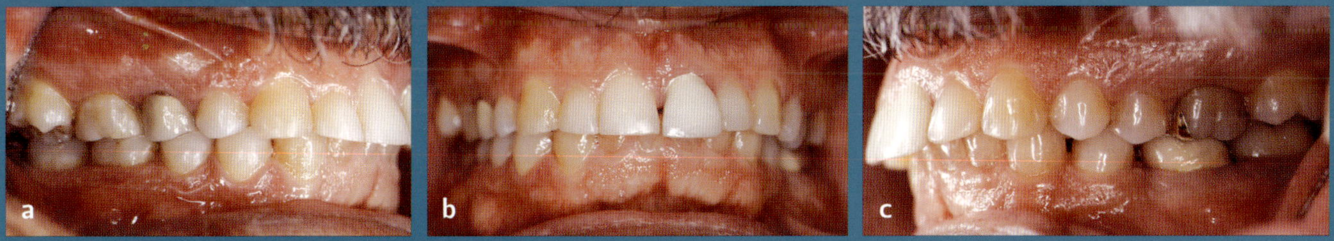

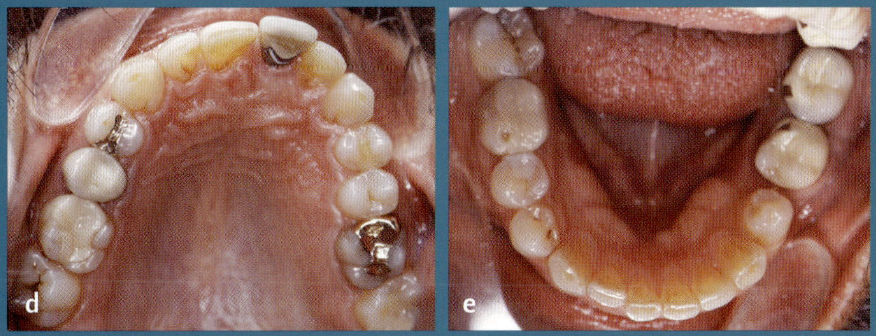

8.97 Intraoral pre-treatment photos. (Reproduced from "Paolone MG, Kaitsas R, Paolone G, Kaitsas V. Lingual orthodontics and forced eruption: a means for osseous and tissue regeneration. *Prog Orthod.* 2008;9(2):46-57" with permission by SIDO.)

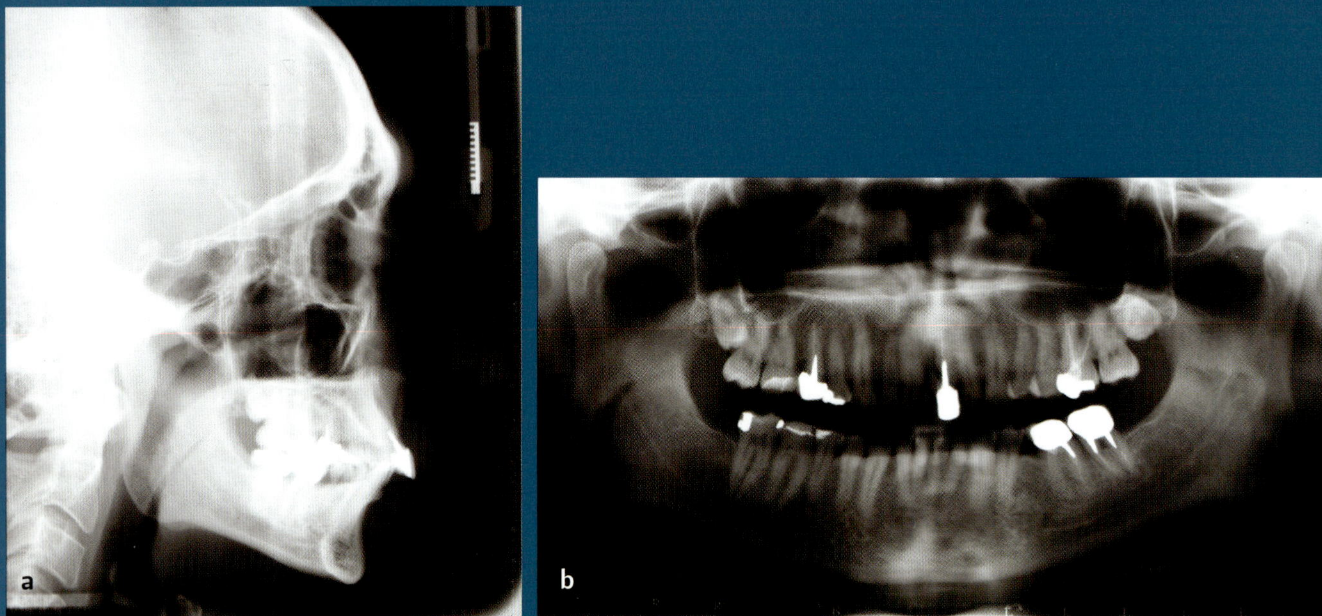

8.98 Pre-treatment cephalometric Rx (**a**) and panoramic Rx (**b**). (Reproduced from "Paolone MG, Kaitsas R, Paolone G, Kaitsas V. Lingual orthodontics and forced eruption: a means for osseous and tissue regeneration. *Prog Orthod*. 2008;9(2):46-57" with permission by SIDO.)

Tab. 8.20 Cephalometric values

Sagittal skeletal relationships	Pre-treatment	Post-treatment	Mean	DS
Maxillary sagittal relationship SNA	79°	80°	82°	3.5°
Mandibular sagittal relationship SNPg	71°	72°	80°	3.5°
Intermaxillary sagittal relationship ANPg	8°	8°	2°	2.5°
Vertical skeletal relationships				
Maxillary vertical relationship SN / ANS-PNS	10°	10°	8°	3.0°
Mandibular vertical relationship SN / Go-Gn	32°	32°	33°	2.5°
Intermaxillary vertical relationship ANS-PNS / Go-Gn	22°	22°	25°	6.0°
Dento-basal relationships				
Upper incisor inclination $\underline{1}$ - ANS-PNS	108°	110°	110°	6.0°
Lower incisor inclination $\overline{1}$ - Go-Gn	102°	103°	94°	7.0°
Lower incisor compensation $\overline{1}$ - A-Pg (mm)	+2	+2	2	2.0
Dental relationships				
Overjet (OVJ, mm)	3	2	3,5	2.5
Overbite (OVB, mm)	3	2	2	2.5
Interincisal angle $\underline{1}$ / $\overline{1}$	112°	115°	132°	6.0°

When treating upper incisors, esthetic priority is essential during orthodontic therapy. The orthodontic extrusion is therefore carried out with lingual orthodontic therapy (Kurz 7th Generation®, Ormco) on the upper anterior teeth including the first premolars; the control of occlusal stability is achieved with composite rests. The information of a first extrusive component is inserted in the indirect bonding positioning apically the 2.1 brackets, on an individualized extrusive set-up. The ceramic crown is prepared for the bonding using a hydrofluoric acid (HF) and then a silane before proceeding to the ordinary bonding sequence. The first archwire that is applied is a .016 CuNiTi archwire (8.99) and after 1 month a .016 β-titanium archwire (8.100 and 8.101) with incremental extrusive steps (8.102) incorporating a tipping to extrude mainly the mesial interproximal area, where there is the defect due to the fracture, with the aim of leveling the defect to the mesial peak of 1.1 (8.103). All these precautions, including the apical positioning of the brackets, allow a controlled extrusion without detachments. The extrusive steps, including the tipping movement, are incorporated in the sequence of successive .017×.017 and .017×.025 β-titanium rectangular archwires with 1 mm/month slow extrusive movements. The conventional sequence of lingual mechanics achieves controlled extrusion by preventing uncontrolled components of radiculo-buccal torque of 2.1 or parasite movements of the adjacent teeth, which could impact and compromise the thin buccal cortical plate. The 15-day check, in addition to the orthodontic activation, include periodontal re-evaluation, plaque control and motivation for the management of home oral hygiene. The tooth is constantly removed from the occlusion and the brackets is progressively repositioned more apically, until, when the residual dimension of the dental crown does not allow a suitable adhesion and the esthetics is no longer acceptable, an extrusive mechanics is created combining endodontic and restorative solutions (8.104). This interdisciplinary solution combines endodontic retention with an endodontic post that has been modified with a milled hole to accommodate a ligature before the zinc oxyphosphate cementation (thanks to Prof. Vasilios Kaitsas for the contribution) (8.105) for the orthodontic traction on a veneer bonded to the vestibular surface of the remaining incisors in composite resin 1.2-1.1-X-2.2 (8.106); this restorative solution simultaneously guarantees esthetics, anchorage and orthodontic traction of the element (8.107-8.109). The eversion of the non-keratinized sulcular epithelium is visible in the red patch (8.110). Once hypercorrection and over-extrusion are completed, the root fragment is stabilized for 6 months (1 month for each millimeter of extrusion), with the aim of reducing relapse and allowing hard and soft tissue maturation of the extrusion site before proceeding with extraction and implant placement. During the entire treatment, intraoral X-ray check is taken every month.

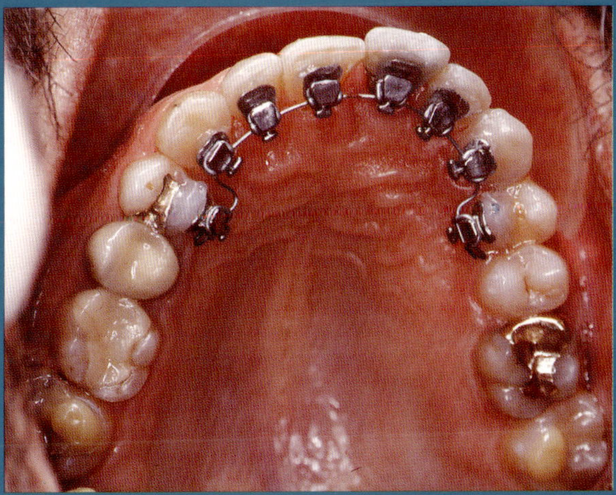

8.99 .016 in CuNiTi archwire. (Reproduced from "Paolone MG, Kaitsas R, Paolone G, Kaitsas V. Lingual orthodontics and forced eruption: a means for osseous and tissue regeneration. *Prog Orthod.* 2008;9(2):46-57" with permission by SIDO.)

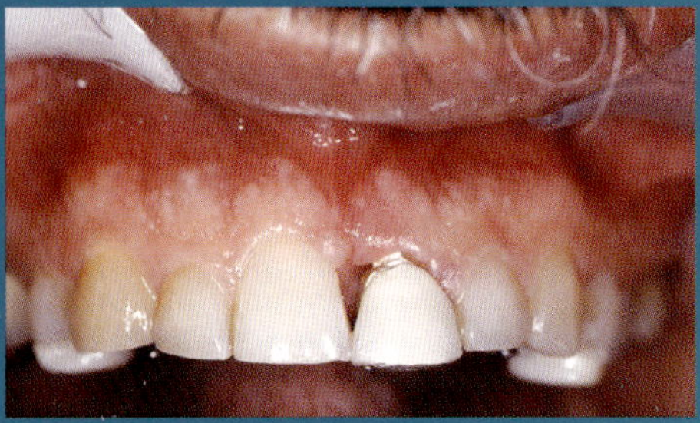

8.100 .016 β-titanium archwire, extrusive steps. (Reproduced from "Paolone MG, Kaitsas R, Paolone G, Kaitsas V. Lingual orthodontics and forced eruption: a means for osseous and tissue regeneration. *Prog Orthod.* 2008;9(2):46-57" with permission by SIDO.)

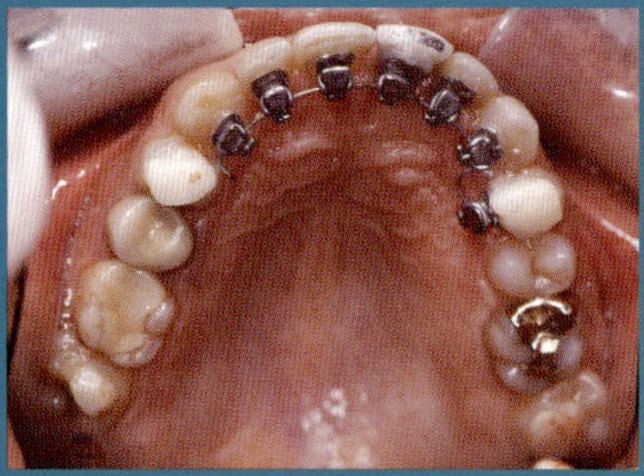

8.101 .016 β-titanium archwire, extrusive steps. (Reproduced from "Paolone MG, Kaitsas R, Paolone G, Kaitsas V. Lingual orthodontics and forced eruption: a means for osseous and tissue regeneration. *Prog Orthod.* 2008;9(2):46-57" with permission by SIDO.)

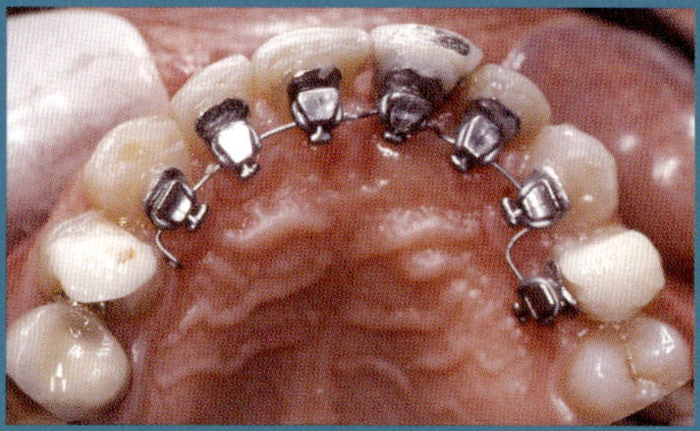

8.102 .016 β-titanium archwire, extrusive steps, grinding. (Reproduced from "Paolone MG, Kaitsas R. Orthodontic-periodontal interactions: Orthodontic extrusion in interdisciplinary regenerative treatments. *Int Orthod.* 2018;16(2):217-245" ©CEO. Published by Elsevier Masson SAS. All rights reserved. With permission.)

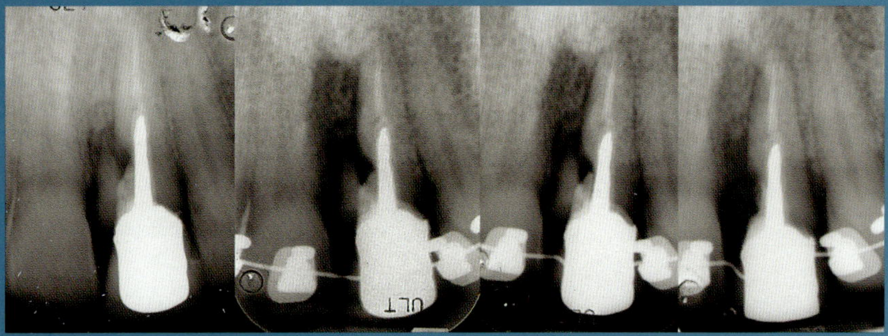

8.103 Orthodontic extrusion, X-ray checks, tipping to level at the mesial peak of 1.1. (Reproduced from "Paolone MG, Kaitsas R, Paolone G, Kaitsas V. Lingual orthodontics and forced eruption: a means for osseous and tissue regeneration. *Prog Orthod.* 2008;9(2):46-57" with permission by SIDO and "Paolone MG, Kaitsas R. Orthodontic-periodontal interactions: Orthodontic extrusion in interdisciplinary regenerative treatments. *Int Orthod.* 2018;16(2):217-245" ©CEO. Published by Elsevier Masson SAS. All rights reserved. With permission.)

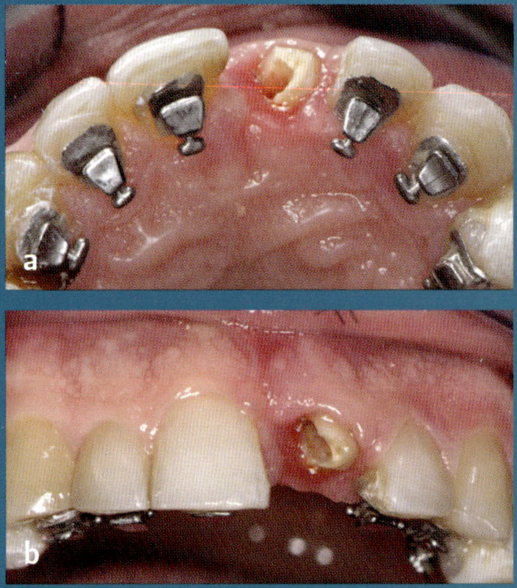

8.104 Root fragment prepared for endodontic anchorage. (Reproduced from "Paolone MG, Kaitsas R, Paolone G, Kaitsas V. Lingual orthodontics and forced eruption: a means for osseous and tissue regeneration. *Prog Orthod.* 2008;9(2):46-57" with permission by SIDO.)

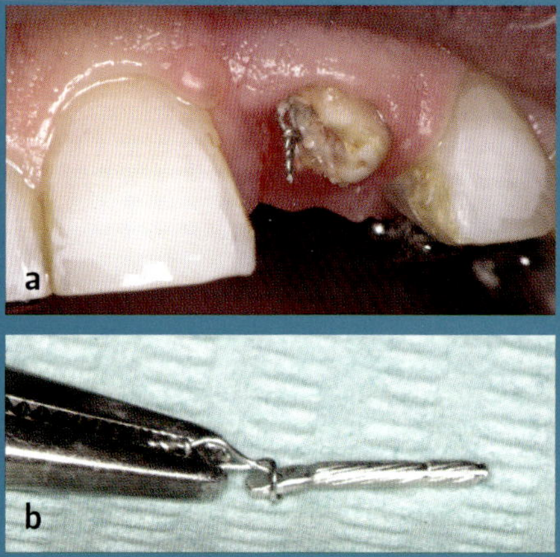

8.105 Endodontic retention. (Thank to Prof. Vasilios Kaitsas for the contribution.)

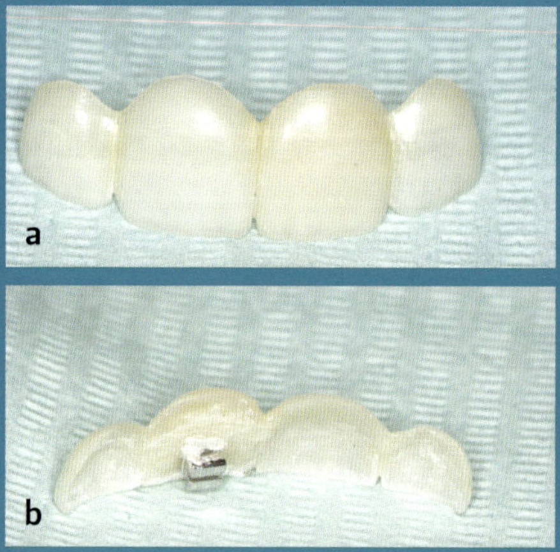

8.106 Veneer 2112 for anchorage and esthetic appearance. (Reproduced from "Paolone MG, Kaitsas R, Paolone G, Kaitsas V. Lingual orthodontics and forced eruption: a means for osseous and tissue regeneration. *Prog Orthod.* 2008;9(2):46-57" with permission by SIDO and "Paolone MG, Kaitsas R. Orthodontic-periodontal interactions: Orthodontic extrusion in interdisciplinary regenerative treatments. *Int Orthod.* 2018;16(2):217-245" ©CEO. Published by Elsevier Masson SAS. All rights reserved. With permission.)

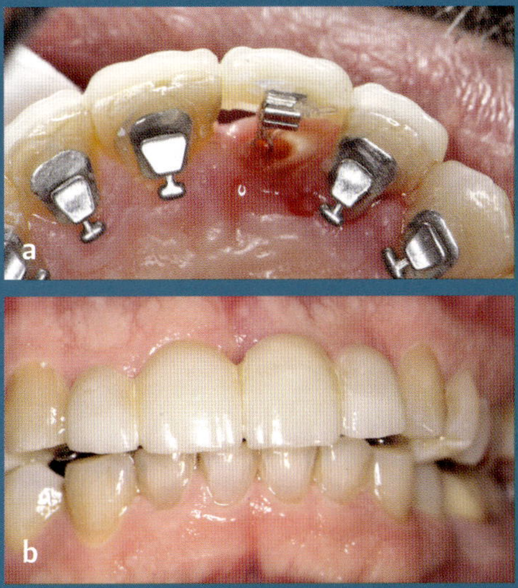

8.107 Orthodontic traction on endodontic post.

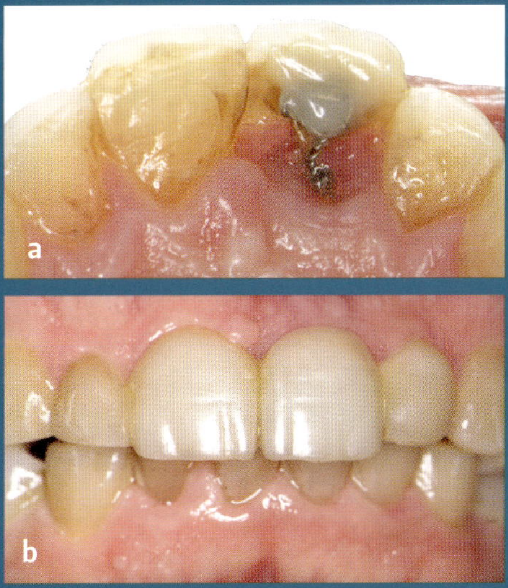

8.108 Orthodontic traction on endodontic post and veneer. (Reproduced from "Paolone MG, Kaitsas R, Paolone G, Kaitsas V. Lingual orthodontics and forced eruption: a means for osseous and tissue regeneration. *Prog Orthod.* 2008;9(2):46-57" with permission by SIDO.)

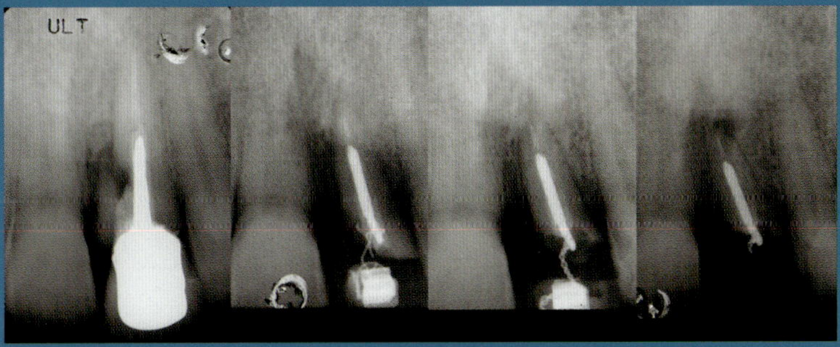

8.109 X-ray check of the orthodontic extrusion with endodontic anchorage. (Reproduced from "Paolone MG, Kaitsas R, Paolone G, Kaitsas V. Lingual ortho dontics and forced eruption: a means for osseous and tissue regeneration. *Prog Orthod.* 2008;9(2):46-57" with permission by SIDO and "Paolone MG, Kaitsas R. Orthodontic-periodontal interactions: Orthodontic extrusion in interdisciplinary regenerative treatments. *Int Orthod.* 2018;16(2):217-245" ©CEO. Published by Elsevier Masson SAS. All rights reserved. With permission.)

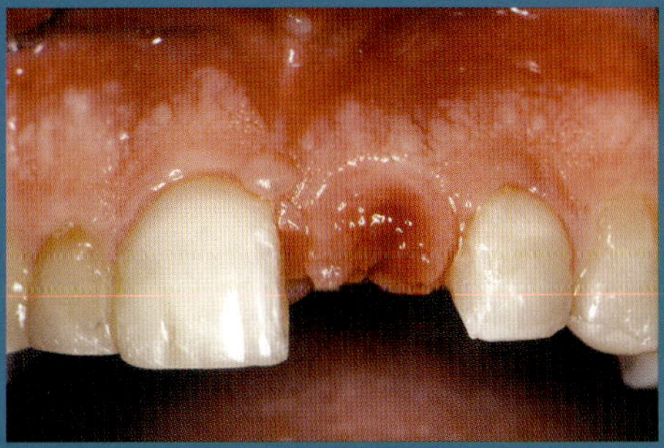

8.110 Red patch. Tissue view at the beginning of the first surgical phase. (Reproduced from "Paolone MG, Kaitsas R, Paolone G, Kaitsas V. Lingual orthodontics and forced eruption: a means for osseous and tissue regeneration. *Prog Orthod.* 2008;9(2):46-57" with permission by SIDO and "Paolone MG, Kaitsas R. Orthodontic-periodontal interactions: Orthodontic extrusion in interdisciplinary regenerative treatments. *Int Orthod.* 2018;16(2):217-245" ©CEO. Published by Elsevier Masson SAS. All rights reserved. With permission.)

After the stabilization period of the extrusion (8.110 and 8.111), a full-thickness trapezoidal flap is elevated with an intrasulcular incision from 1.2 to 2.3. The root fragment is extracted in an atraumatic way (8.112) in order not to damage the regenerated bone walls. Observing the post-extraction socket (8.113), we can appreciate the complete elimination of the bone defect that was present at the beginning of the extrusion (8.114) and the complete regeneration of the whole mesio-vestibulo-palatal bone area with autologous orthodontic bone without use of xenografts, an advantage that leads us, as previously stated, to the realization of the GOBR (Guided Orthodontic "Bone" Regeneration).

After checking the insertion axis, the fixture (4.5/15 mm Frialit-2®, Dentsply) is placed into the post-extraction socket (8.115 and 8.116). With this regenerative technique, the implant placement switches from a possible peri-implant bone regeneration (even if of a reduced size) to an immediate post-extraction implant placement with a greater treatment predictability. The flap is sutured with 4-0 e-PTFE and 5-0 polyglycolic acid on the vertical relief incisions (8.117). After 4 months, the second surgical phase is performed in which, using the soft tissue gained with orthodontic extrusion, the peri-implant tissues are increased to enhance the longevity and esthetics of the case (8.118) by a partial thickness envelope flap with an intrasulcular incision and a crestal incision at the level of the edentulous ridge (8.119). After the osseointegration check (8.120), to increase the amount of vestibular tissue, a bilaminar connective tissue graft is performed using the same surgical site as the recipient site, harvesting the connective tissue from the thinning of the palatal flap (8.121 and 8.122) and suturing it to the vestibular flap (8.123). A healing abutment is then inserted and the flap is sutured with a ramp mattress suture[127] (8.124) to coronally displace the buccal flap and to compress the palatal flap. After 4 months, a temporary crown built on a cus-

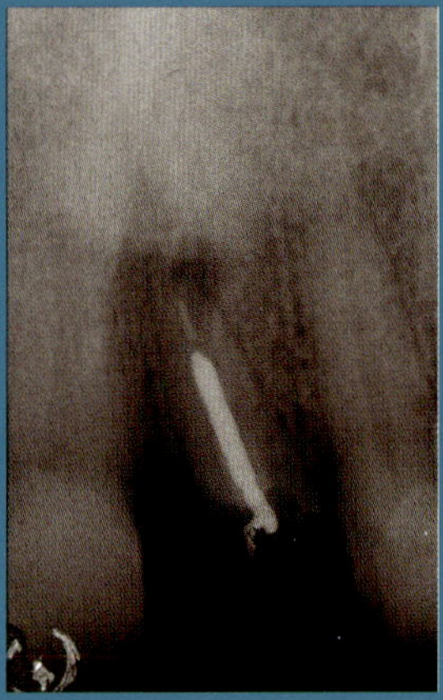

8.111 X-ray check at the end of orthodontic extrusion and the beginning of the first surgical phase. (Reproduced from "Paolone MG, Kaitsas R, Paolone G, Kaitsas V. Lingual orthodontics and forced eruption: a means for osseous and tissue regeneration. *Prog Orthod.* 2008;9(2):46-57" with permission by SIDO and "Paolone MG, Kaitsas R. Orthodontic-periodontal interactions: Orthodontic extrusion in interdisciplinary regenerative treatments. *Int Orthod.* 2018;16(2):217-245" ©CEO. Published by Elsevier Masson SAS. All rights reserved. With permission.)

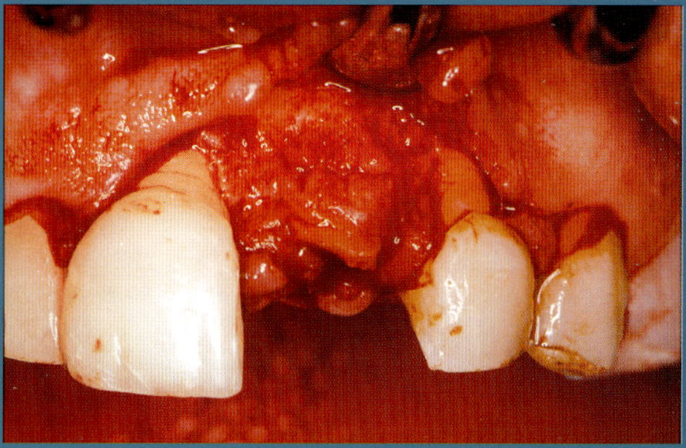

8.112 Extraction of the root fragment.

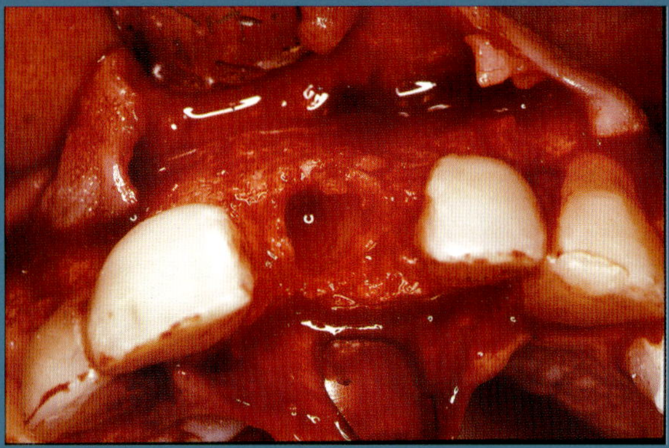

8.113 Post-extraction socket. (Reproduced from "Paolone MG, Kaitsas R, Paolone G, Kaitsas V. Lingual orthodontics and forced eruption: a means for osseous and tissue regeneration. *Prog Orthod.* 2008;9(2):46-57" with permission by SIDO and "Paolone MG, Kaitsas R. Orthodontic-periodontal interactions: Orthodontic extrusion in interdisciplinary regenerative treatments. *Int Orthod.* 2018;16(2):217-245" ©CEO. Published by Elsevier Masson SAS. All rights reserved. With permission.)

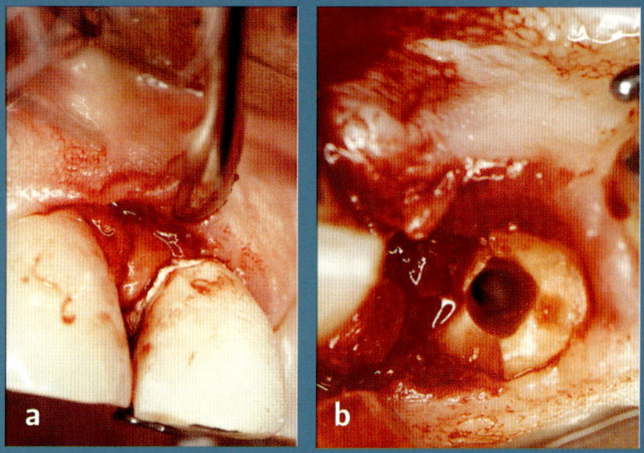

8.114 Pre-extrusion bone defect (**a**) at the removal of the fragment (**b**) in relationship to the bone regeneration of 8.113 after extrusion.

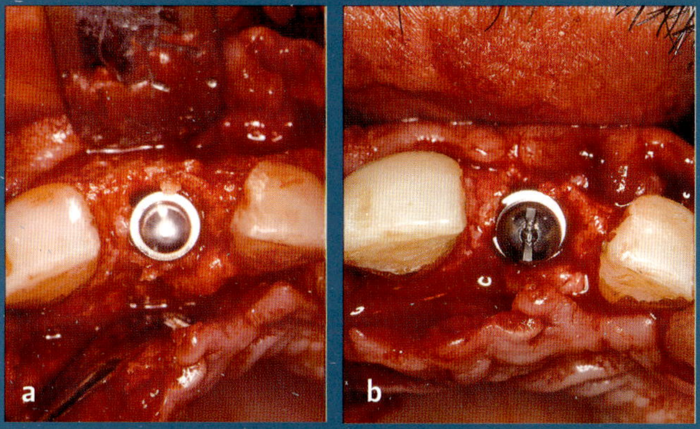

8.115 Implant placement in the post-extraction socket. (Reproduced from "Paolone MG, Kaitsas R, Paolone G, Kaitsas V. Lingual orthodontics and forced eruption: a means for osseous and tissue regeneration. *Prog Orthod.* 2008;9(2):46-57" with permission by SIDO.)

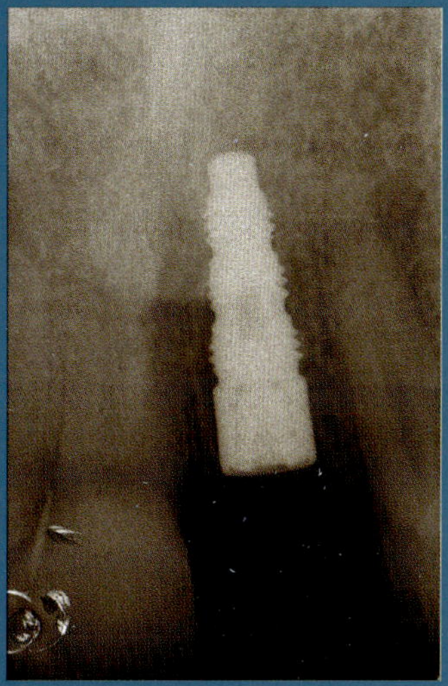

8.116 X-ray check (Reproduced from "Paolone MG, Kaitsas R, Paolone G, Kaitsas V. Lingual orthodontics and forced eruption: a means for osseous and tissue regeneration. *Prog Orthod.* 2008;9(2):46-57" with permission by SIDO.)

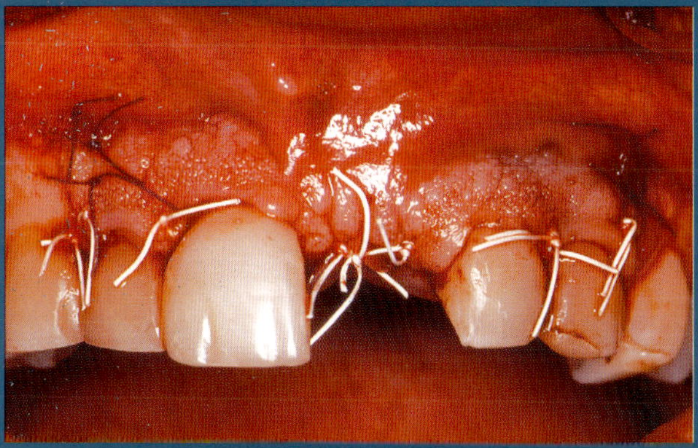

8.117 Flap suture.

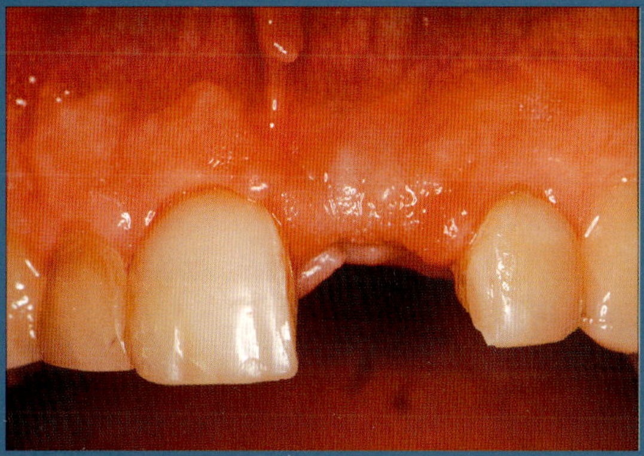

8.118 Tissue aspect before the second surgical phase.

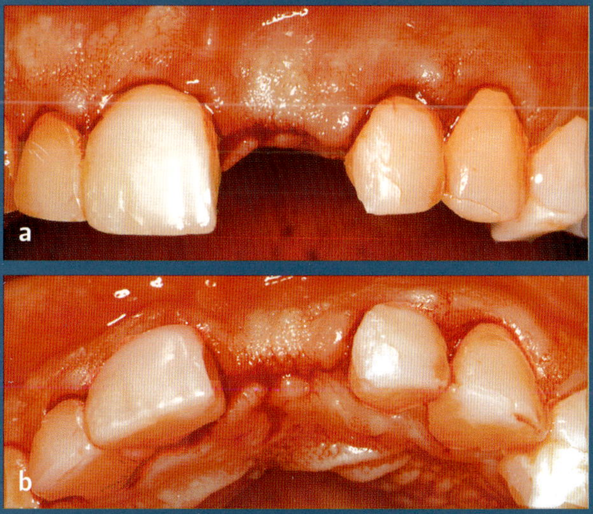

8.119 Partial thickness envelope flap, dental and crestal intrasulcular incision (**a**) at the edentulous ridge level (**b**). (Reproduced from "Paolone MG, Kaitsas R, Paolone G, Kaitsas V. Lingual orthodontics and forced eruption: a means for osseous and tissue regeneration. *Prog Orthod.* 2008;9(2):46-57" with permission by SIDO.)

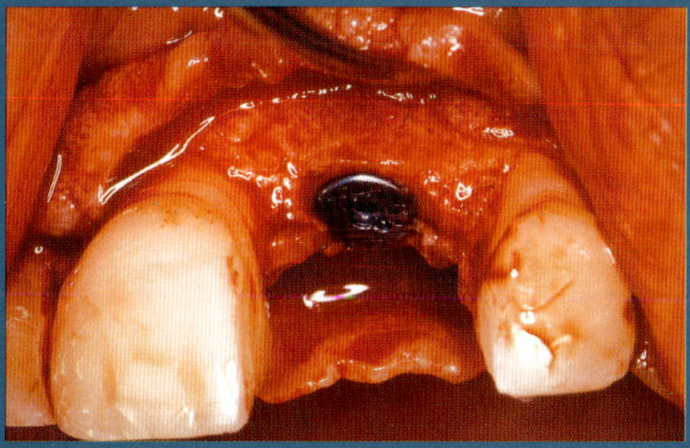

8.120 Osseointegration check.

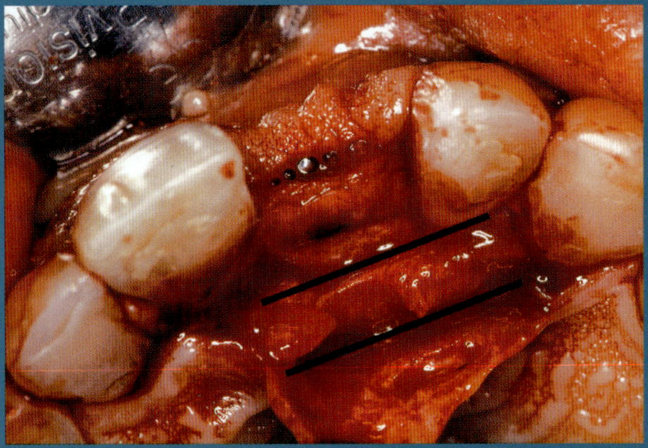

8.121 Palatal intraoral connective tissue donor site in the same surgical site.

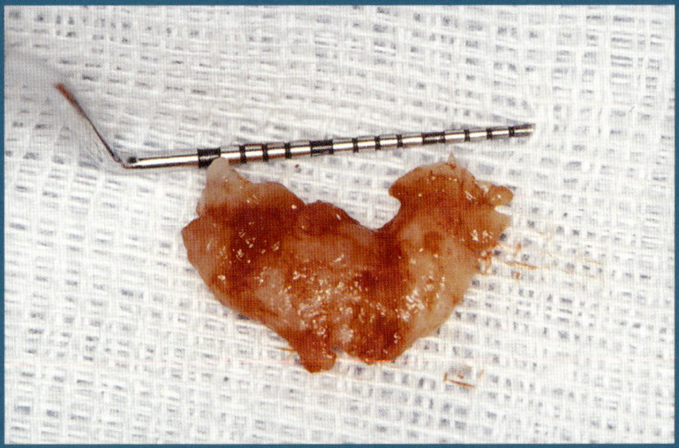

8.122 View of the connective graft.

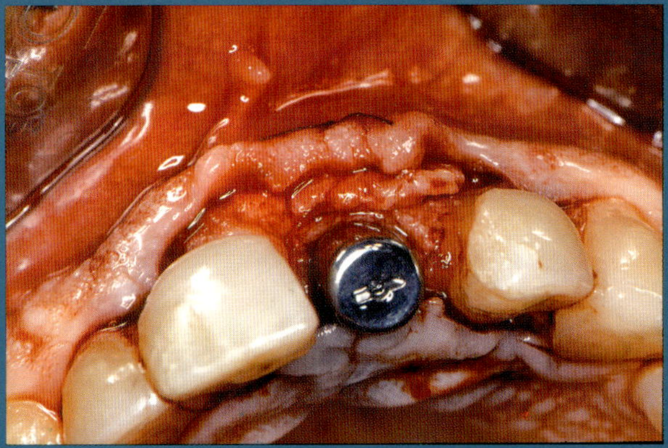

8.123 Placement of the connective graft and suture to improve the width of the soft tissue. (Reproduced from "Paolone MG, Kaitsas R, Paolone G, Kaitsas V. Lingual orthodontics and forced eruption: a means for osseous and tissue regeneration. *Prog Orthod.* 2008;9(2):46-57" with permission by SIDO and "Paolone MG, Kaitsas R. Orthodontic-periodontal interactions: Orthodontic extrusion in interdisciplinary regenerative treatments. *Int Orthod.* 2018;16(2):217-245" ©CEO. Published by Elsevier Masson SAS. All rights reserved. With permission.)

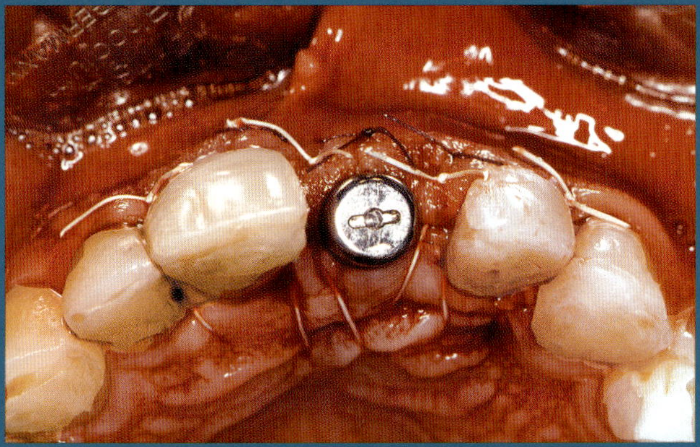

8.124 Ramp mattress suture after healing abutment placement.

tomized titanium milled abutment (8.125 and 8.126) is cemented in order to guide the tissue maturation. The temporary crown is recontoured for other 8 months (check and maturation of the soft tissue can be observed in 8.127 and 8.128) and after 12 months from the second surgical phase the soft tissue information obtained by the modifications of the temporary crown is transferred to the laboratory (8.129) and an all-ceramic crown is realized on an esthetic ceramic abutment (8.130-8.136). In 8.137-8.139 the patient can be observed at the end of treatment (see 8.20). In 8.140 and 8.141, an 8-year follow-up can be seen, with maintenance of integration, soft tissue thickness and X-ray check (8.142).

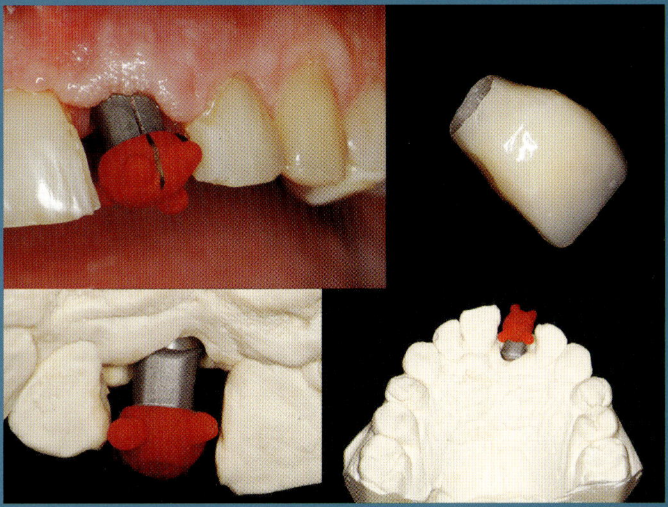

◀ **8.125** Customized temporary crown that guides the tissue development during the healing phases with its cast. (Reproduced from "Paolone MG, Kaitsas R, Paolone G, Kaitsas V. Lingual orthodontics and forced eruption: a means for osseous and tissue regeneration. *Prog Orthod.* 2008;9(2):46-57" with permission by SIDO.)

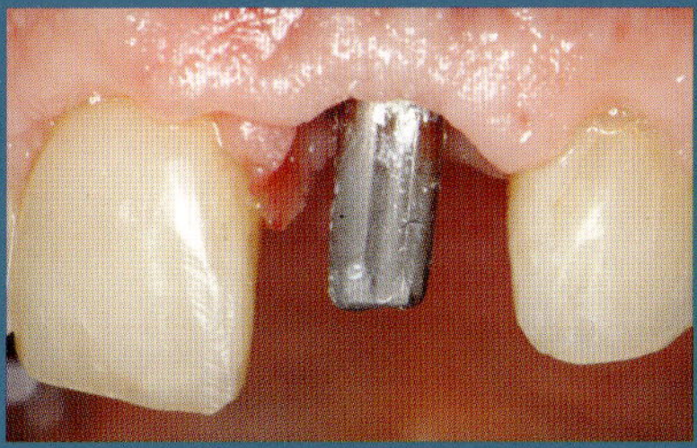

8.126 Customized abutment *in situ.* (Reproduced from "Paolone MG, Kaitsas R, Paolone G, Kaitsas V. Lingual orthodontics and forced eruption: a means for osseous and tissue regeneration. *Prog Orthod.* 2008;9(2):46-57" with permission by SIDO.)

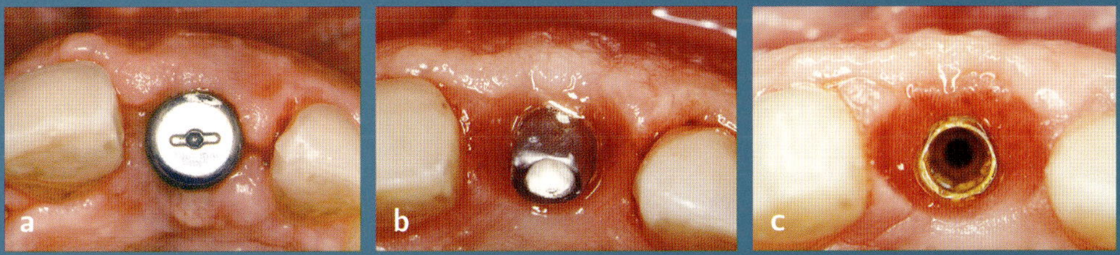

8.127 Occlusal view, tissue check.

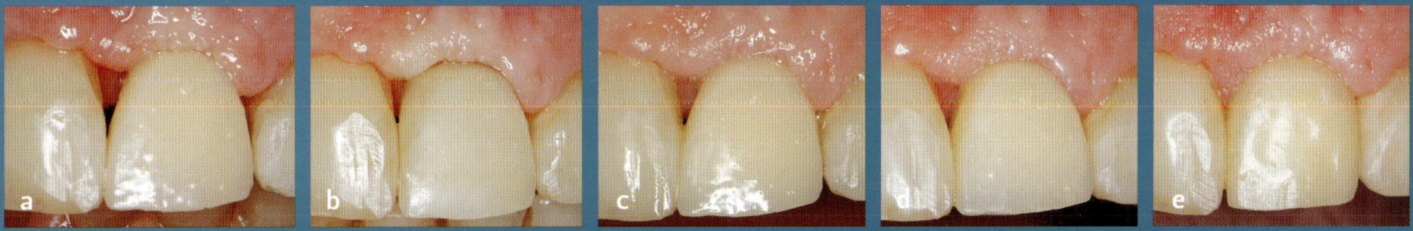

8.128 Vestibular tissue check and interproximal papillae guidance.

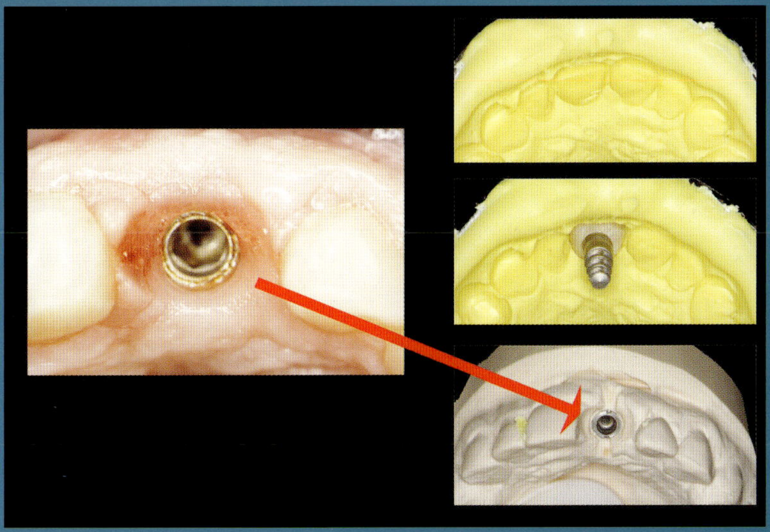

8.129 Soft tissue information transfer to the laboratory. (Reproduced from "Paolone MG, Kaitsas R, Paolone G, Kaitsas V. Lingual orthodontics and forced eruption: a means for osseous and tissue regeneration. *Prog Orthod.* 2008;9(2):46-57" with permission by SIDO.)

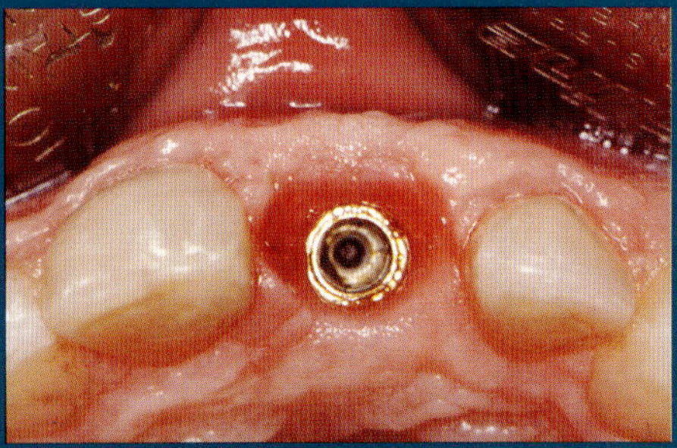

8.130 View of the vestibular improvement at the cementation. (Reproduced from "Paolone MG, Kaitsas R, Paolone G, Kaitsas V. Lingual orthodontics and forced eruption: a means for osseous and tissue regeneration. *Prog Orthod.* 2008;9(2):46-57" with permission by SIDO and "Paolone MG, Kaitsas R. Orthodontic-periodontal interactions: Orthodontic extrusion in interdisciplinary regenerative treatments. *Int Orthod.* 2018;16(2):217-245" ©CEO. Published by Elsevier Masson SAS. All rights reserved. With permission.)

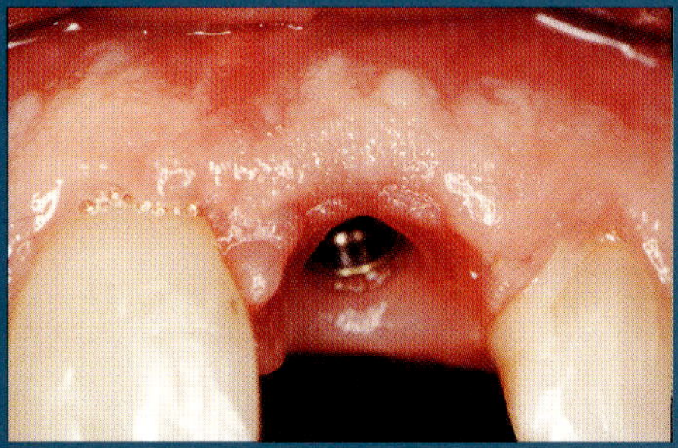

8.131 Check of the inteproximal papillae in definitive position.

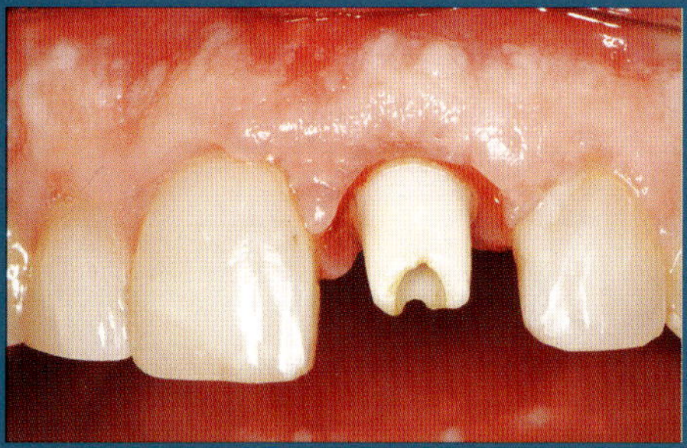

8.132 Zirconia esthetic abutment. (Reproduced from "Paolone MG, Kaitsas R, Paolone G, Kaitsas V. Lingual orthodontics and forced eruption: a means for osseous and tissue regeneration. *Prog Orthod.* 2008;9(2):46-57" with permission by SIDO and "Paolone MG, Kaitsas R. Orthodontic-periodontal interactions: Orthodontic extrusion in interdisciplinary regenerative treatments. *Int Orthod.* 2018;16(2):217-245" ©CEO. Published by Elsevier Masson SAS. All rights reserved. With permission.)

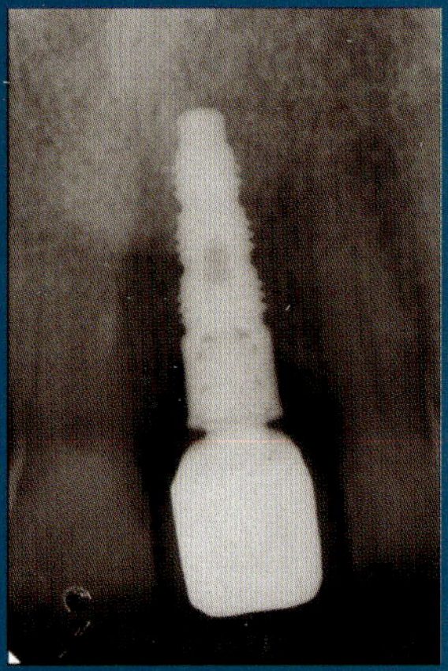

8.133 X-ray check after cementation. (Reproduced from "Paolone MG, Kaitsas R, Paolone G, Kaitsas V. Lingual orthodontics and forced eruption: a means for osseous and tissue regeneration. *Prog Orthod.* 2008;9(2):46-57" with permission by SIDO and "Paolone MG, Kaitsas R. Orthodontic-periodontal interactions: Orthodontic extrusion in interdisciplinary regenerative treatments. *Int Orthod.* 2018;16(2):217-245" ©CEO. Published by Elsevier Masson SAS. All rights reserved. With permission.)

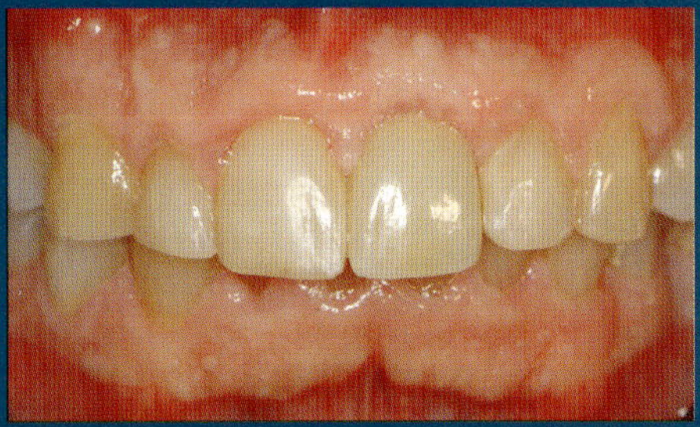

8.134 Definitive crown just cemented. (Reproduced from "Paolone MG, Kaitsas R, Paolone G, Kaitsas V. Lingual orthodontics and forced eruption: a means for osseous and tissue regeneration. *Prog Orthod.* 2008;9(2):46-57" with permission by SIDO.)

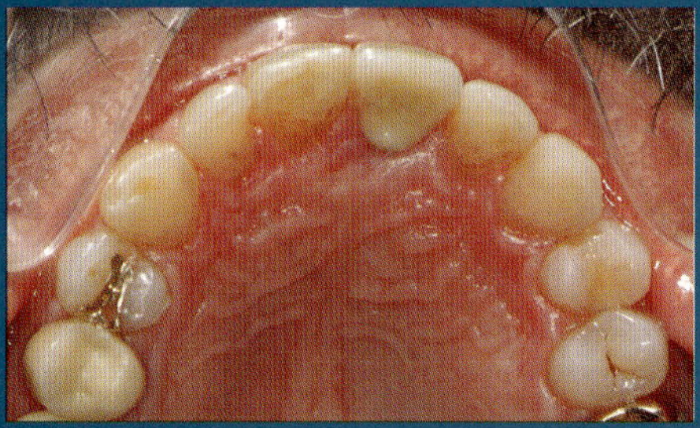

8.135 Palatal view. (Reproduced from "Paolone MG, Kaitsas R, Paolone G, Kaitsas V. Lingual orthodontics and forced eruption: a means for osseous and tissue regeneration. *Prog Orthod.* 2008;9(2):46-57" with permission by SIDO.)

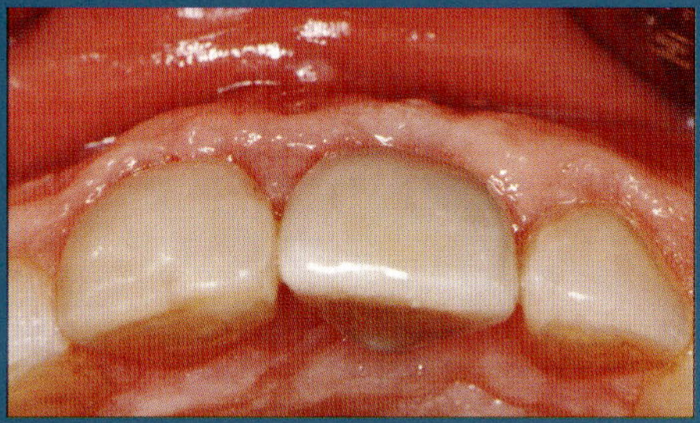

8.136 Occlusal view.

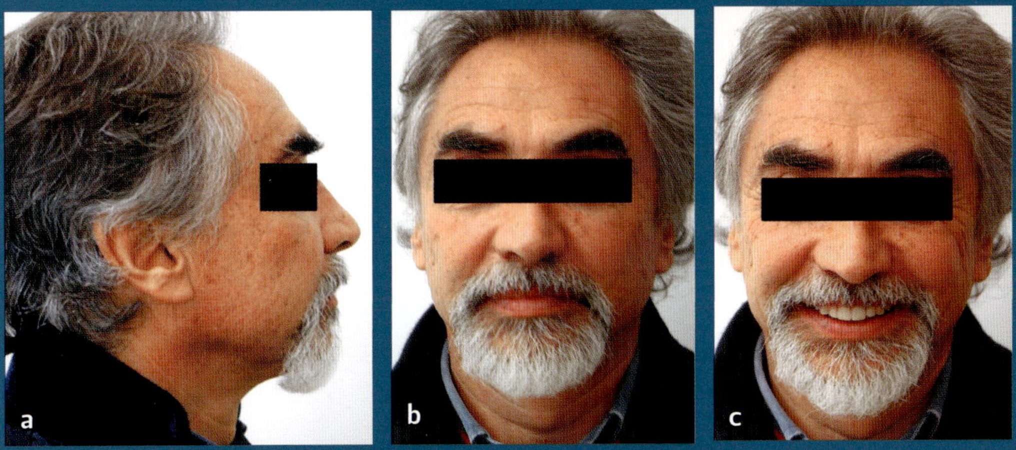

8.137 Extraoral post-orthodontic treatment photos.

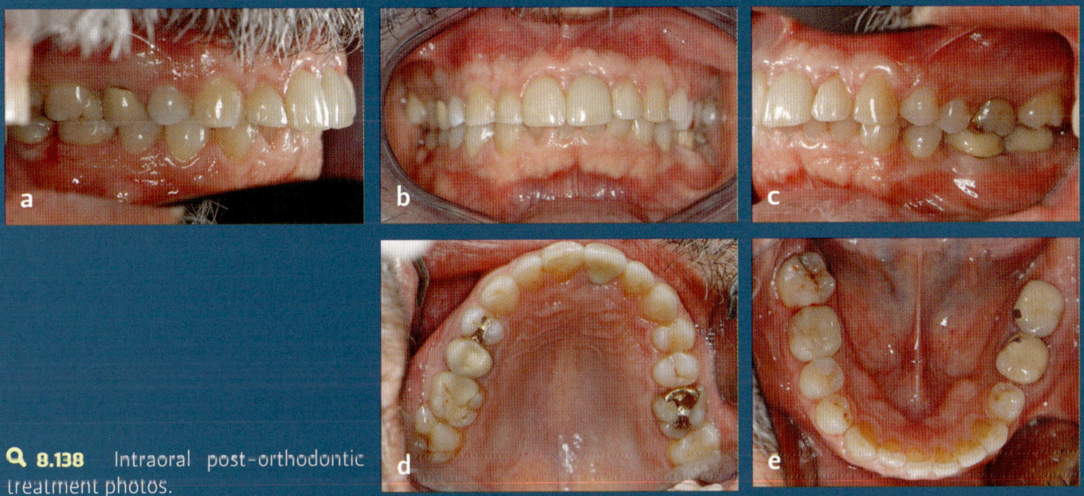

8.138 Intraoral post-orthodontic treatment photos.

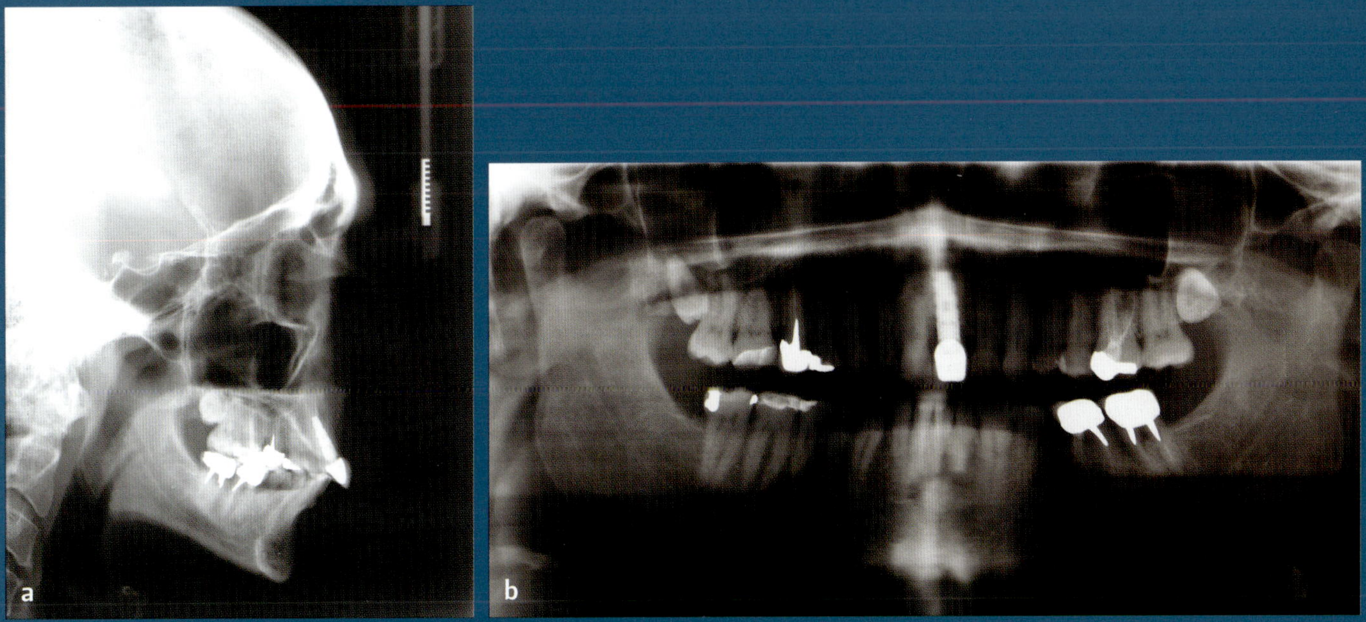

8.139 Post-treatment cephalometric Rx (**a**) and panoramic Rx (**b**). (Reproduced from "Paolone MG, Kaitsas R, Paolone G, Kaitsas V. Lingual orthodontics and forced eruption: a means for osseous and tissue regeneration. *Prog Orthod.* 2008;9(2):46-57" with permission by SIDO.)

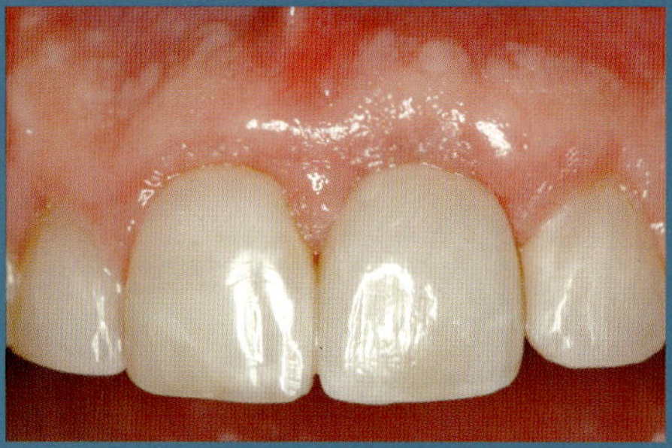

8.140 8-year follow-up. (Reproduced from "Paolone MG, Kaitsas R, Paolone G, Kaitsas V. Lingual orthodontics and forced eruption: a means for osseous and tissue regeneration. *Prog Orthod.* 2008;9(2):46-57" with permission by SIDO and "Paolone MG, Kaitsas R. Orthodontic-periodontal interactions: Orthodontic extrusion in interdisciplinary regenerative treatments. *Int Orthod.* 2018;16(2):217-245" ©CEO. Published by Elsevier Masson SAS. All rights reserved. With permission.)

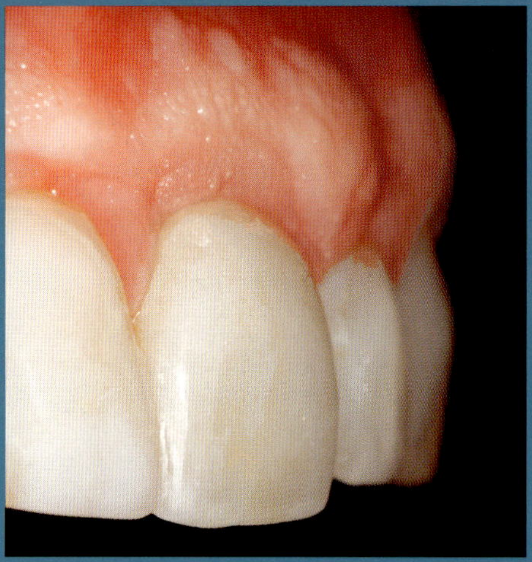

8.141 Vestibular tissues. 8-year follow-up.

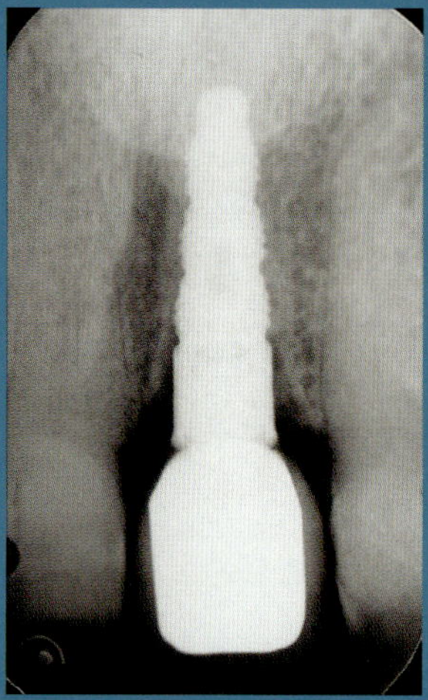

8.142 X-ray 8-year follow-up.

Clinical case 5 (GOTR - Guided Orthodontic "Tissue" Regeneration)

The patient comes to our attention for a slight pain on 2.1, reporting repeated trauma on this tooth. At the clinical observation (8.143), a redness of the tissues at the palatal level and a 5 mm horizontal probing are observed; the radiographic examination confirms the diagnostic hypothesis of a huge external resorption present at the root level (8.144). The patient does not want to extract the tooth to place an implant, so a flap is elevated and the defect is isolated and restored with a composite filling to postpone the implant treatment (8.145-8.147). After another new trauma, the tooth becomes symptomatic presenting a sinus tract and pain with a hyperemic response to the vitality test on the left lateral upper incisor (8.148). At this point the tooth is unrecoverable, therefore the choice is to place an implant. The tooth shows a large bone destruction at the palatal level, that is confirmed by the periodontal probing (8.149 and 8.150). The problem now is to use a regenerative technique that is suitable for this bone destruction. The "classical" techniques impose a delayed or contextual treatment to the implant placement (i.e. socket preservation techniques, GBR with delayed or contextual placement of the implant). In all the cases, the main need is to have enough soft tissue to cover the graft and the membrane to increase the predictability of the regenerative surgery. Orthodontics helps us to increase the amount of soft tissue, exploiting the residual tooth through extrusion, in order not only to regenerate bone tissue (in this case the extrusion would be contraindicated due to the presence of an active apical lesion), but also mainly to increase the amount of soft tissue in order to be able to cover the membrane without risk of dehiscence increasing the surgical predictability. Hence the name of GOTR (Guided Orthodontic "Tissue" Regeneration).

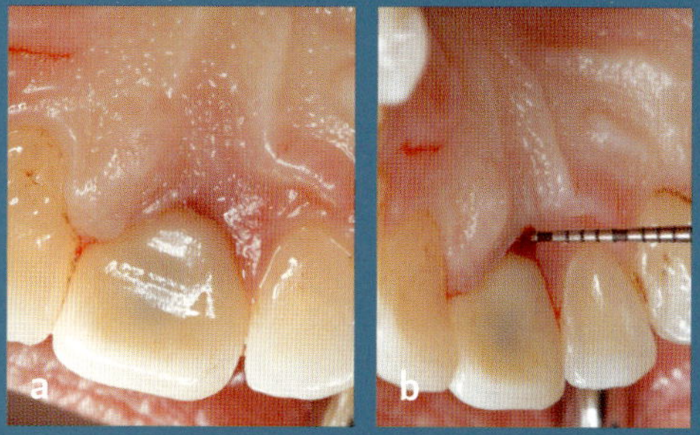

8.143 Palatal view of the inflammation at the prosthetic margin and 5-mm probing.

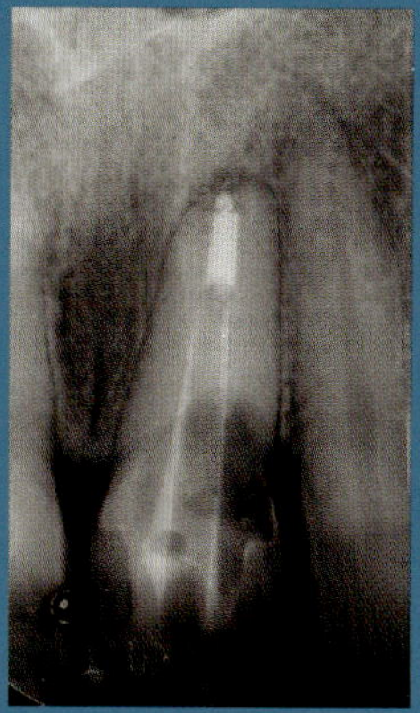

8.144 Root external resorption. (Reproduced from "Paolone MG, Kaitsas R. Orthodontic-periodontal interactions: Orthodontic extrusion in interdisciplinary regenerative treatments. *Int Orthod.* 2018;16(2):217-245" and "Kaitsas R, Paolone MG, Paolone G. Guided orthodontic regeneration: A tool to enhance conventional regenerative techniques in implant surgery. *Int Orthod.* 2015;13(4):539-554" ©CEO. Published by Elsevier Masson SAS. All rights reserved. With permission.)

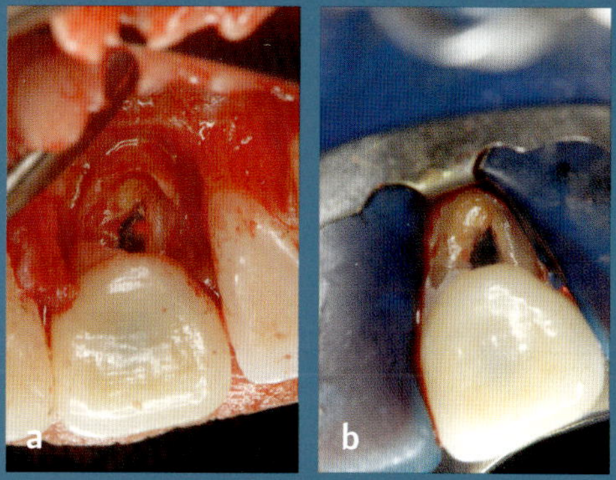

8.145 Palatal flap elevation and defect isolation for the restoration.

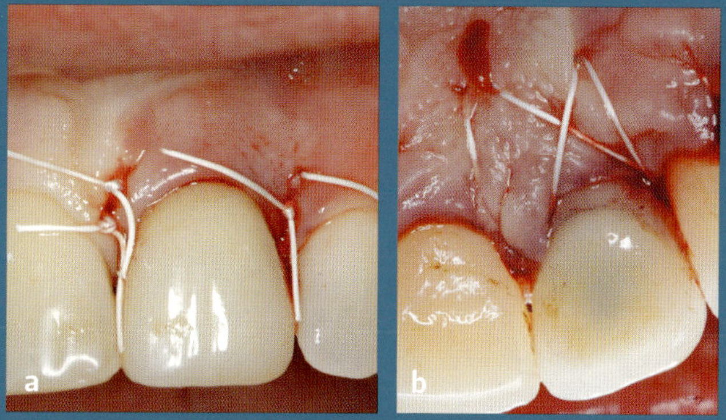

8.146 Palatal flap suture.

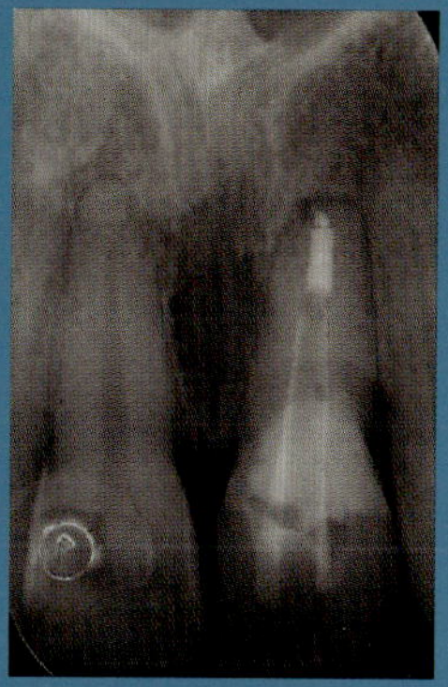

8.147 X-ray check of the palatal restoration.

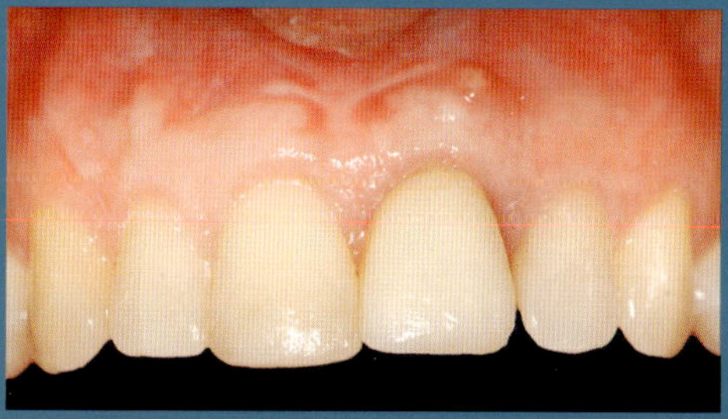

8.148 Clinical examination of 2.1 that shows the tooth dislocation and the apical sinus tract. (Reproduced from "Paolone MG, Kaitsas R. Orthodontic-periodontal interactions: Orthodontic extrusion in interdisciplinary regenerative treatments. *Int Orthod.* 2018;16(2):217-245" and "Kaitsas R, Paolone MG, Paolone G. Guided orthodontic regeneration: A tool to enhance conventional regenerative techniques in implant surgery. *Int Orthod.* 2015;13(4):539-554" ©CEO. Published by Elsevier Masson SAS. All rights reserved. With permission.)

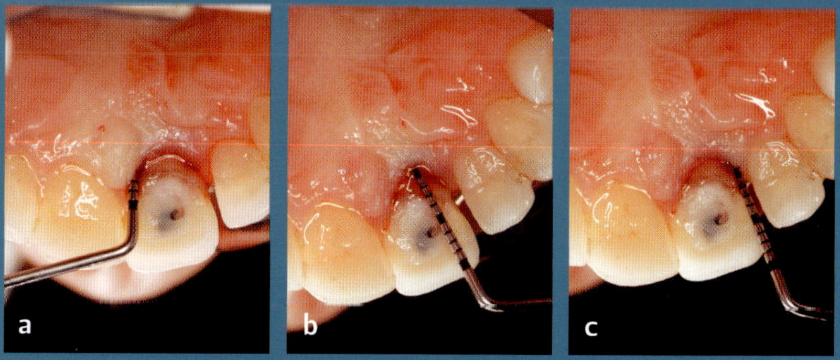

8.149 Palatal periodontal probing that shows the bone defect that must be regenerated. (Reproduced from "Paolone MG, Kaitsas R. Orthodontic-periodontal interactions: Orthodontic extrusion in interdisciplinary regenerative treatments. Int Orthod. 2018;16(2):217-245" and "Kaitsas R, Paolone MG, Paolone G. Guided orthodontic regeneration: A tool to enhance conventional regenerative techniques in implant surgery. *Int Orthod.* 2015;13(4):539-554" ©CEO. Published by Elsevier Masson SAS. All rights reserved. With permission.)

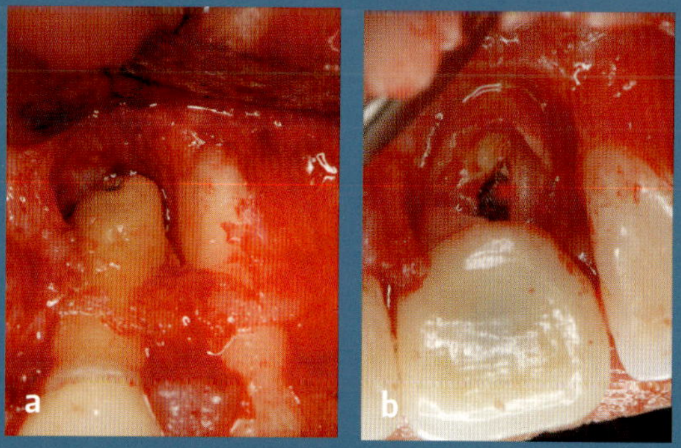

8.150 Surgical view of the bone defect. Vestibular and palatal aspect. (Reproduced from "Paolone MG, Kaitsas R. Orthodontic-periodontal interactions: Orthodontic extrusion in interdisciplinary regenerative treatments. *Int Orthod.* 2018;16(2):217-245" and "Kaitsas R, Paolone MG, Paolone G. Guided orthodontic regeneration: A tool to enhance conventional regenerative techniques in implant surgery. *Int Orthod.* 2015;13(4):539-554" ©CEO. Published by Elsevier Masson SAS. All rights reserved. With permission.)

The patient has facial symmetry, harmonic profile with labial competence (8.151), dental class I, normal OVJ and OVB (8.152), skeletal normodivergent class I (8.153; 8.21). The orthodontic treatment is carried out with an orthodontic lingual appliance (Kurz 7th Generation®, Ormco) on the entire upper arch. The brackets on the incisor to be extruded is positioned more apically using a Hiro-System©[126] indirect bonding with a set-up that includes an extrusive step (8.154). The first applied archwire is a pre-formed .016 CuNiTi lingual archwire; this arch expresses a continuous and light force. Checks are carried out every 15 days (8.155) with strict periodontal control and apical repositioning of the attachment (8.156). After one month a .016 β-titanium archwire is applied, for lingual technique; in the second month a 017×.017 β-titanium archwire is used at first, then a .017×.025 β-titanium archwire (8.157) is applied to incorporate the first bends. After a first pure axial movement, aimed at levelling the mesial peak on the adjacent defect, the tooth is subjected to tipping, to extrude the more severe distal bone defect, and then to torque (8.158). The tooth is tipped first distally, then mesially and it is finally torqued following the guide of the periodontist and based on the visualization of the endo-perio bone lesion to hypercorrect and guarantee interproximal bone peaks in order to create a GBR on the implant and, at the same time, a GTR on left upper lateral incisor, which showed signs of hyper-

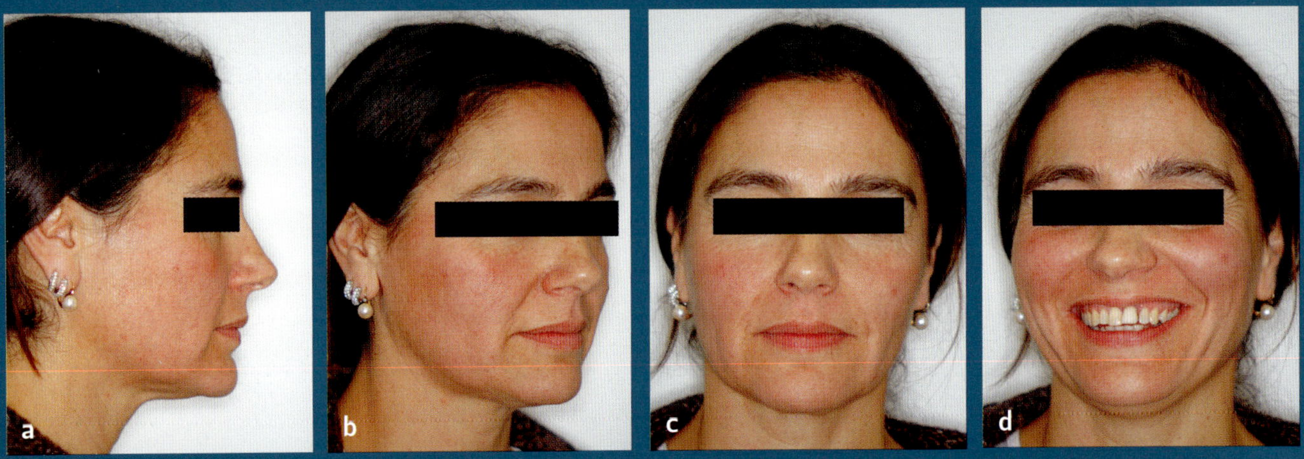

8.151 Extraoral pre-orthodontic treatment photos.

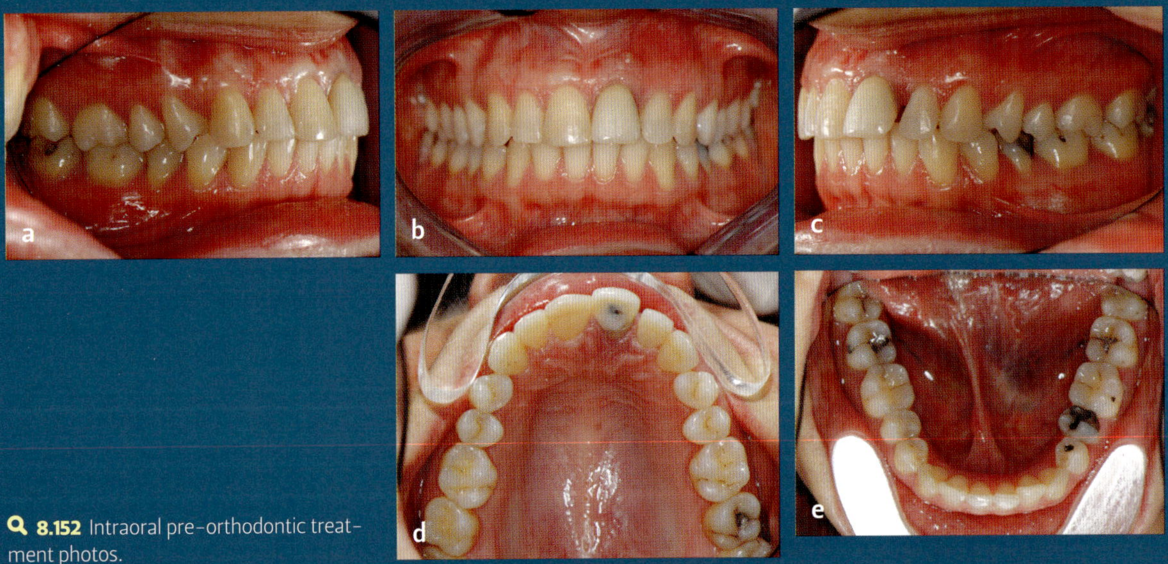

8.152 Intraoral pre-orthodontic treatment photos.

emia. Subsequently, it is important to perform a buccal root torque by simultaneously including in the archwire a compensating lingual inset bend, which, on the one hand, enhances the lingual coronal torque, and on the other hand reduces the risk of apical vestibular impaction. The steps are incremental (8.159). The use of the .017×.025 β-titanium archwire allows to obtain through bends the detailed three-dimensional control of the extrusion with light forces and also the control and prevention of any parasite movements of the teeth adjacent to the 2.1. In particular, an attempt is made to obtain a lingual root torque movement of 2.2, which presents from the start of the treatment a pulpar hyperemia, in order to control and minimize the impact with the

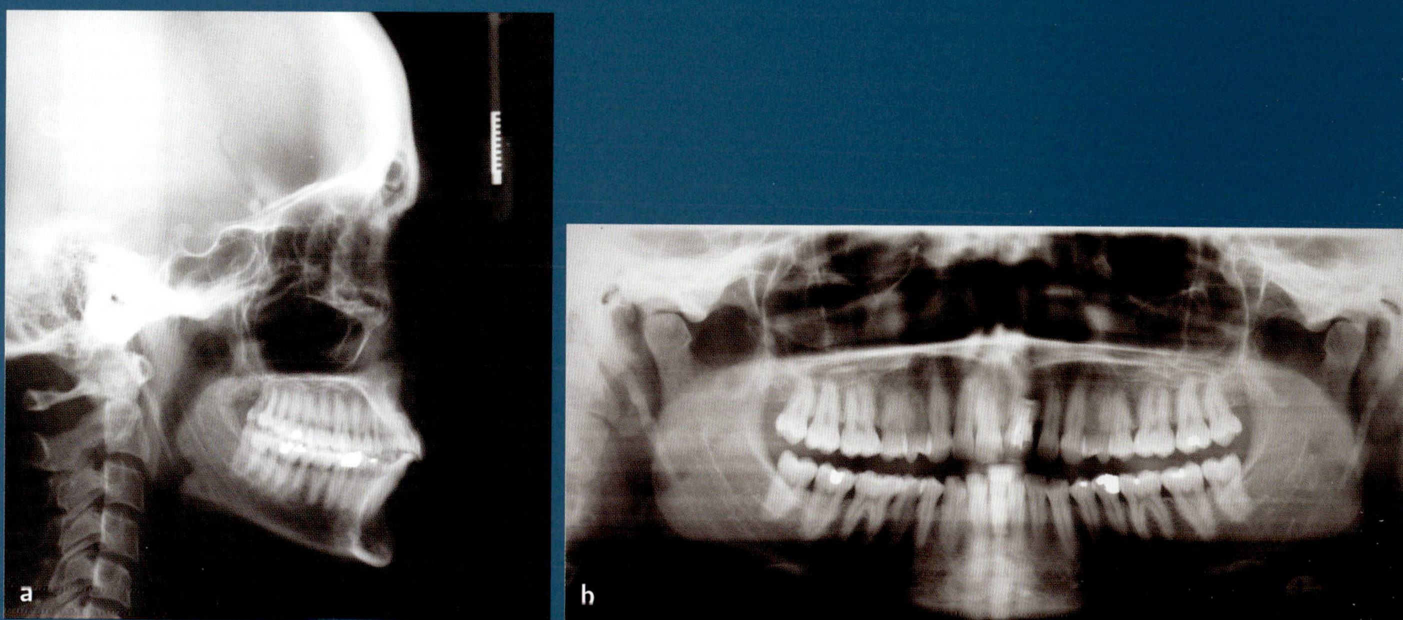

8.153 Pre-treatment cephalometric Rx (**a**) and panoramic Rx (**b**).

Tab. 8.21 Cephalometric values

Sagittal skeletal relationships	**Pre-treatment**	**Post-treatment**	**Mean**	**DS**
Maxillary sagittal relationship SNA	75°	75°	82°	3.5°
Mandibular sagittal relationship SNPg	76°	76°	80°	3.5°
Intermaxillary sagittal relationship ANPg	-1°	-1°	2°	2.5°
Vertical skeletal relationships				
Maxillary vertical relationship SN / ANS-PNS	11°	10°	8°	3.0°
Mandibular vertical relationship SN / Go-Gn	30°	30°	33°	2.5°
Intermaxillary vertical relationship ANS-PNS / Go-Gn	21°	20°	25°	6.0°
Dento-basal relationships				
Upper incisor inclination $\underline{1}$ - ANS-PNS	123°	120°	110°	6.0°
Lower incisor inclination $\overline{1}$ - Go-Gn	105°	104°	94°	7.0°
Lower incisor compensation $\overline{1}$ - A-Pg (mm)	+3	+2	2	2.0
Dental relationships				
Overjet (OVJ, mm)	3	2	3,5	2.5
Overbite (OVB, mm)	3	2	2	2,5
Interincisal angle $\underline{1}$ / $\overline{1}$	112°	115°	132°	6.0°

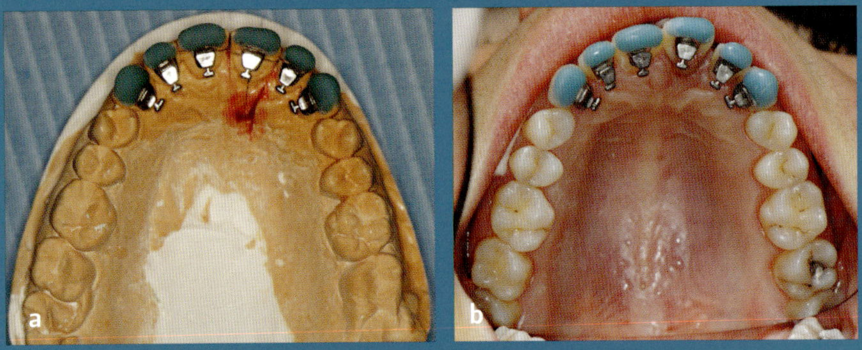

8.154 Indirect lingual bonding with extrusive set-up of 2.1.

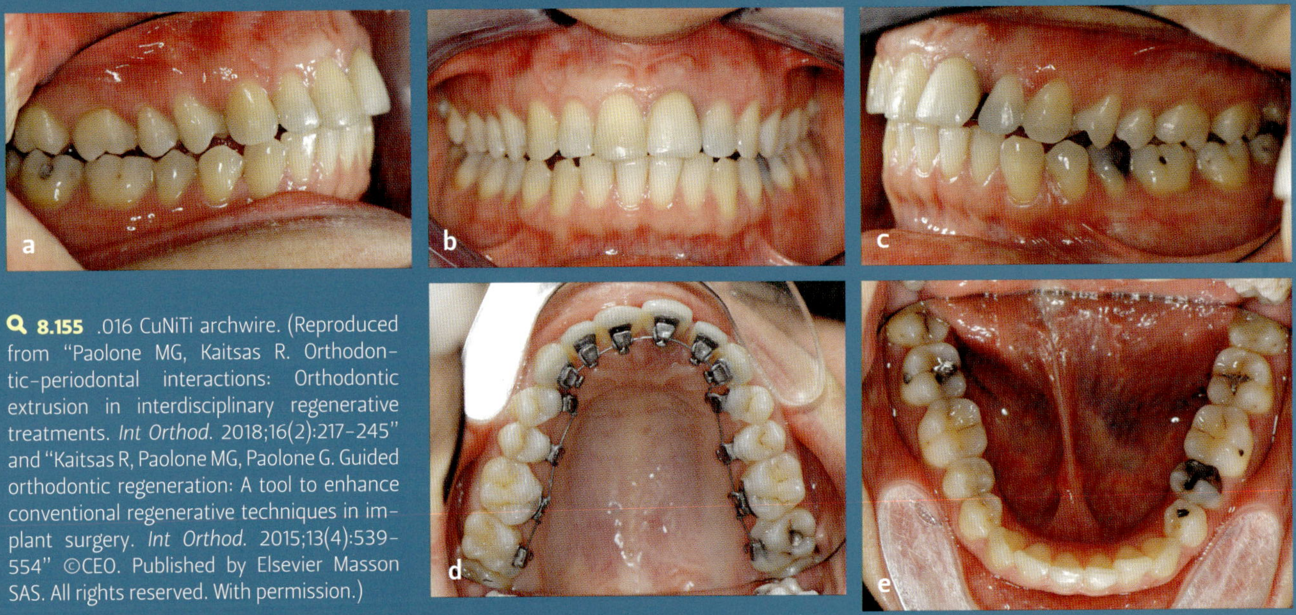

8.155 .016 CuNiTi archwire. (Reproduced from "Paolone MG, Kaitsas R. Orthodontic-periodontal interactions: Orthodontic extrusion in interdisciplinary regenerative treatments. *Int Orthod.* 2018;16(2):217-245" and "Kaitsas R, Paolone MG, Paolone G. Guided orthodontic regeneration: A tool to enhance conventional regenerative techniques in implant surgery. *Int Orthod.* 2015;13(4):539-554" ©CEO. Published by Elsevier Masson SAS. All rights reserved. With permission.)

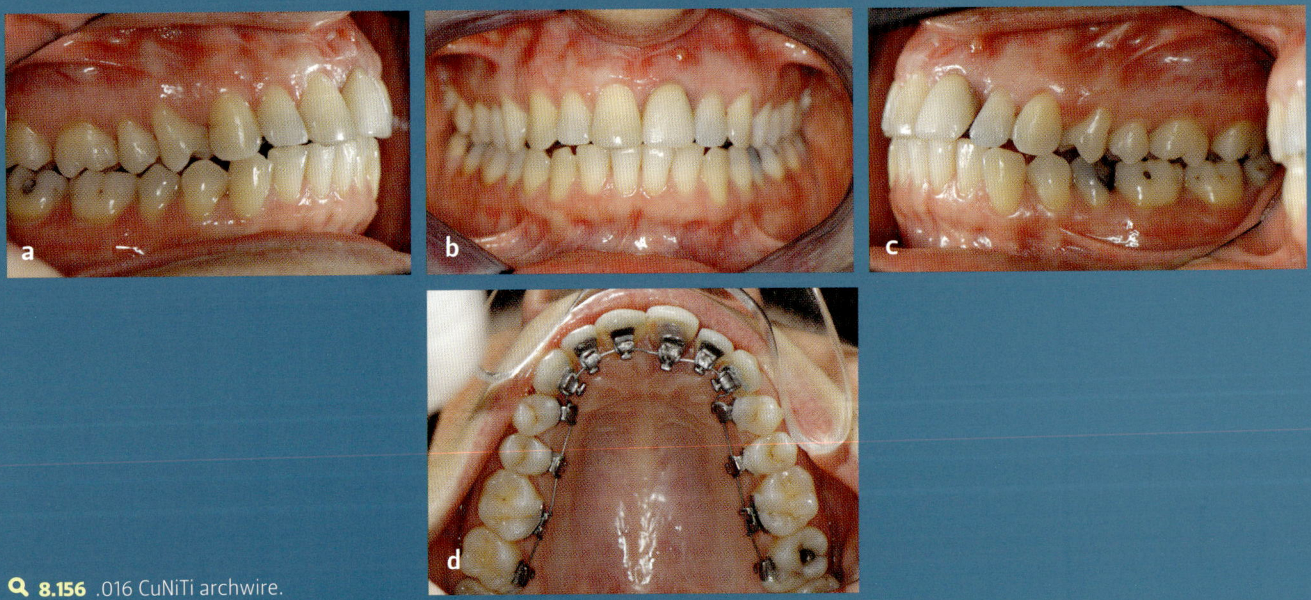

8.156 .016 CuNiTi archwire.

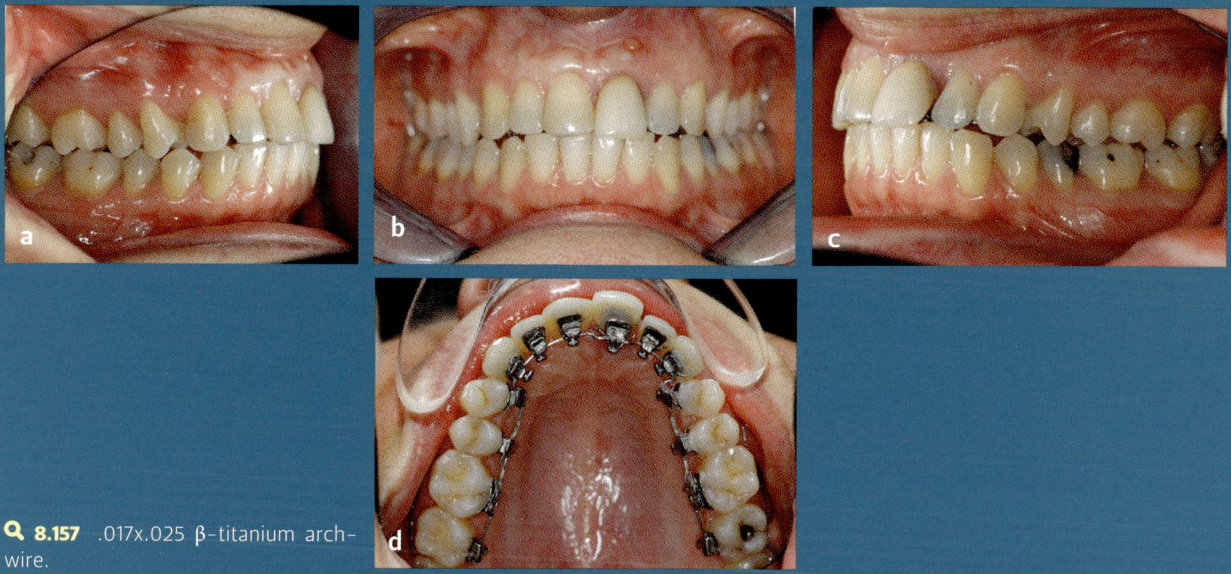

8.157 .017x.025 β-titanium archwire.

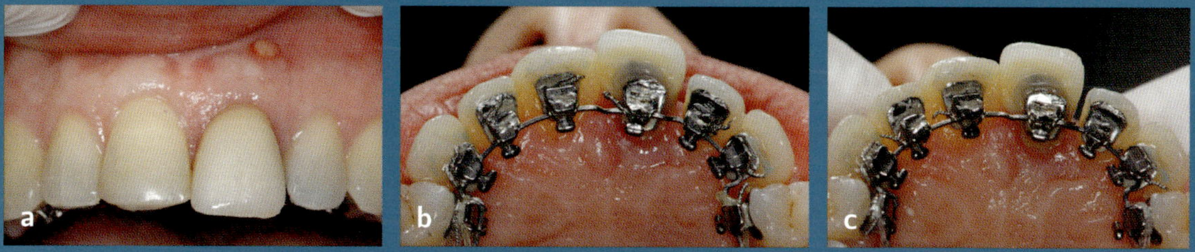

8.158 .017x.025 β-titanium archwire, tipping and torque bends, incremental extrusive steps.

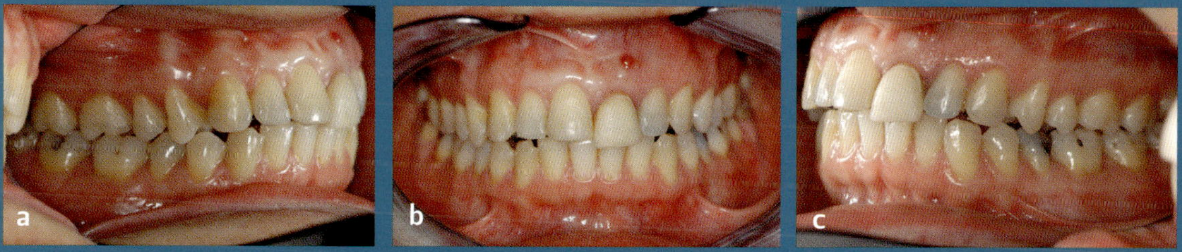

8.159 Intermediate phase of the extrusion.

buccal cortical plate. The use of conventional elastic chains or of the *double over tie* technique, which allows a maximum accommodation of the archwire in the lingual technique (8.160), allows the reading of the mechanical information inserted on the archwire to direct the extrusion in order to obtain an extrusive tipping and a coronal-lingual torque at the same time, since the tooth has the greatest part of the healthy periodontal attachment in the apico-palatal area (8.161). Every 15 days, in addition to extrusive activations, the tooth is grinded to avoid occlusal contacts and jiggling (8.162 and 8.163). Further activation can be achieved by repositioning the brackets more apically in combination with the restoration (8.164). To enhance the torque component and to reduce the risk of contact of the apex with the cortical plates, an inset is carried out on the same torque bends to bring the tooth more palatally, trying to reduce cortical impact (8.165 and 8.166; see 8.32). Then, when it is no longer possible to provide the patient with sufficient esthetics, an aligner is made that contains a vestibular resin veneer, thus guaranteeing esthetics and an easy access to lingual mechanics (8.167) even in the orthodontic stabilization phase (8.168).

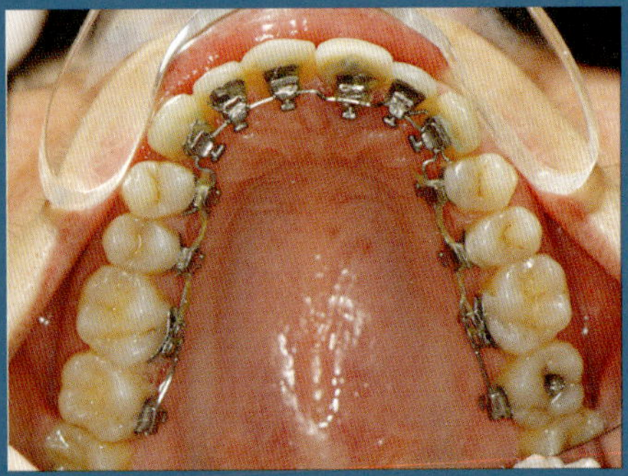

8.160 .017x.025 β-titanium archwire, tipping and torque bends, incremental extrusive steps, *double over tie*.

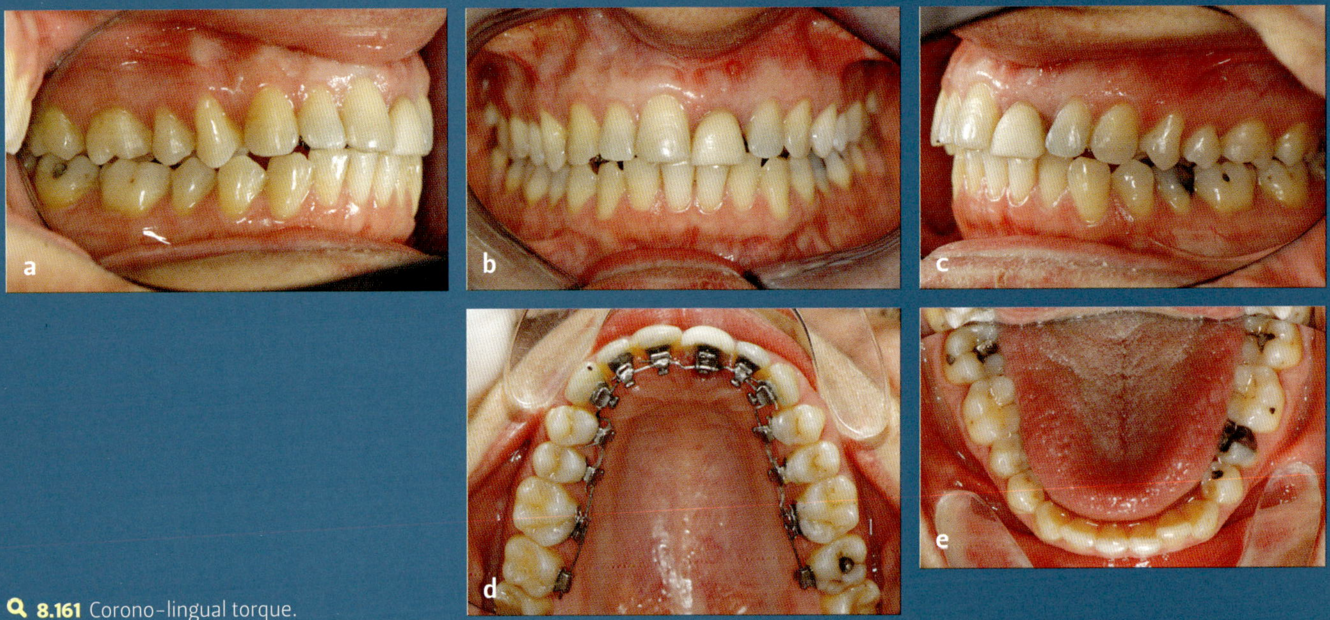

8.161 Corono-lingual torque.

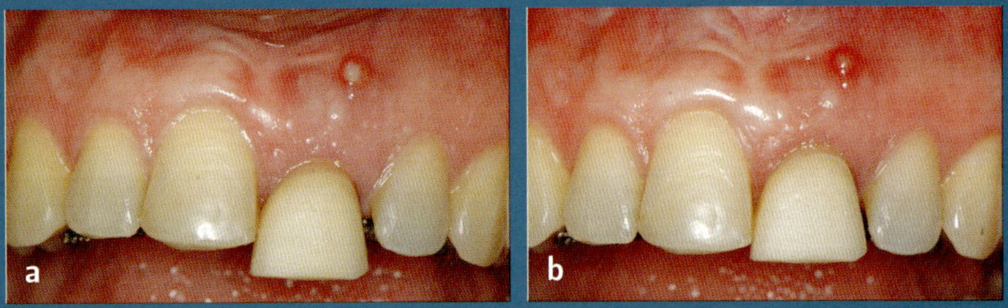

8.162 Grinding.

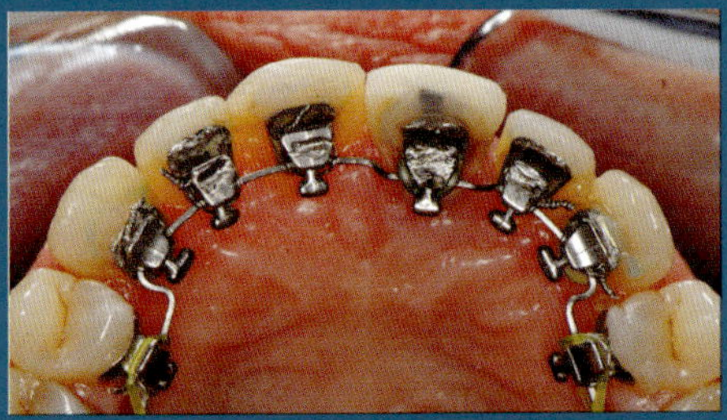

8.163 Grinding, occlusal view.

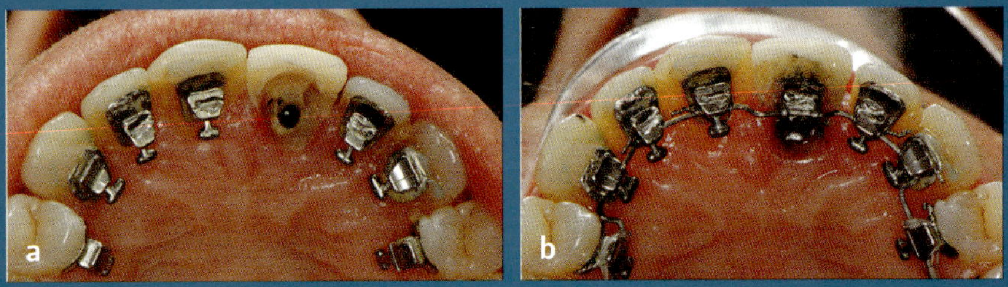

8.164 Apical repositioning of the brackets.

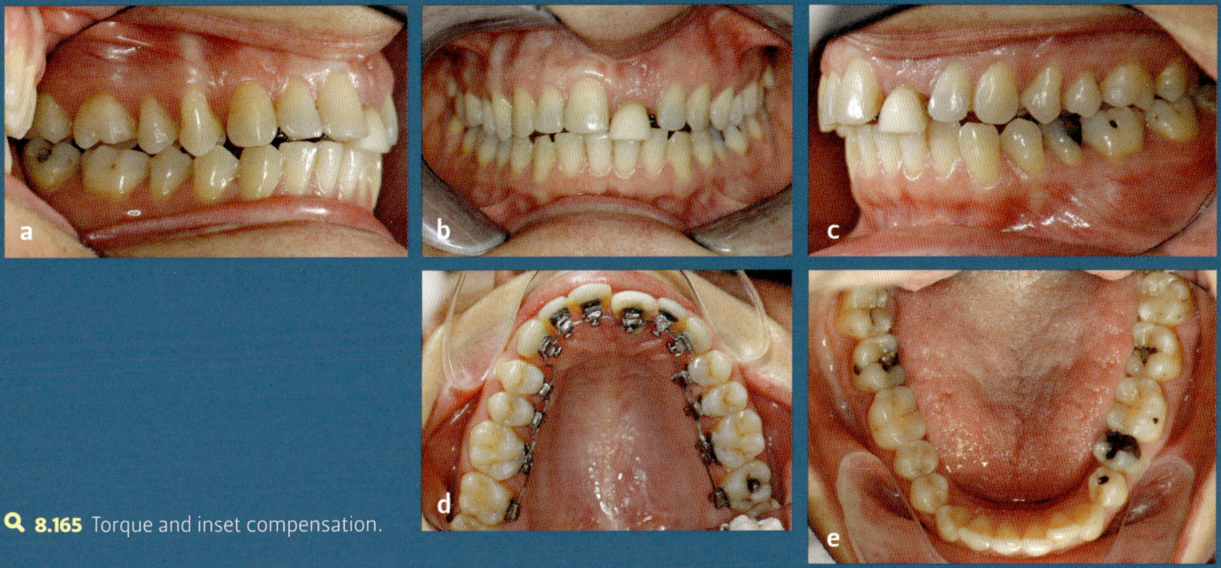

8.165 Torque and inset compensation.

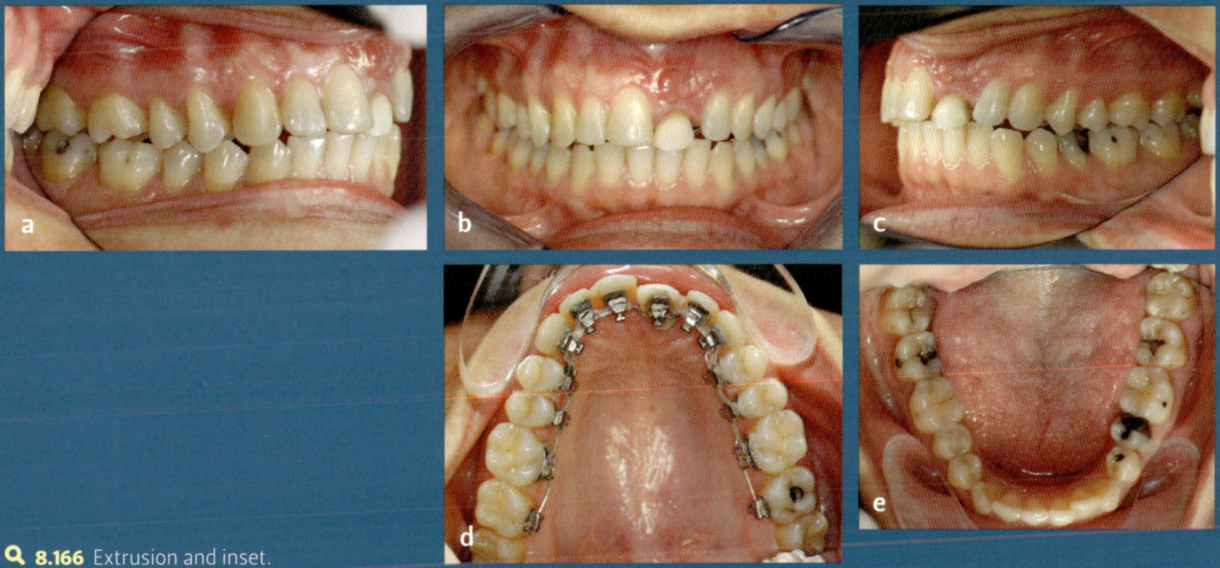

8.166 Extrusion and inset.

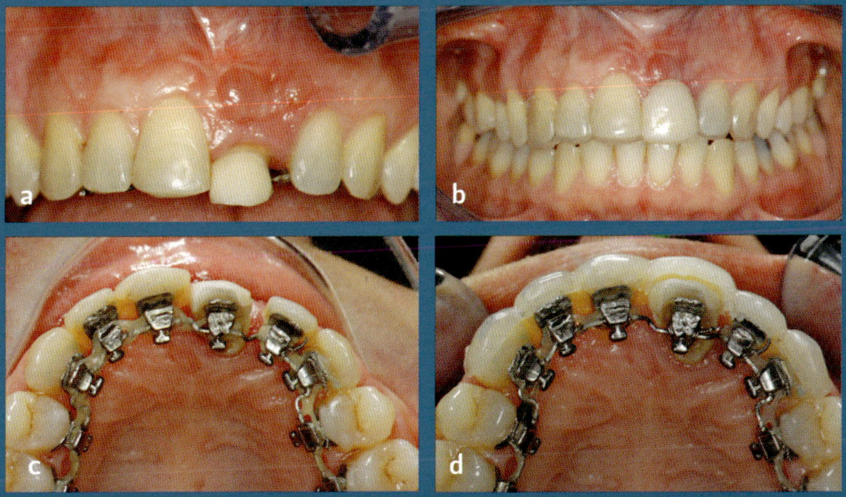

8.167 Aligner with vestibular composite veneer.

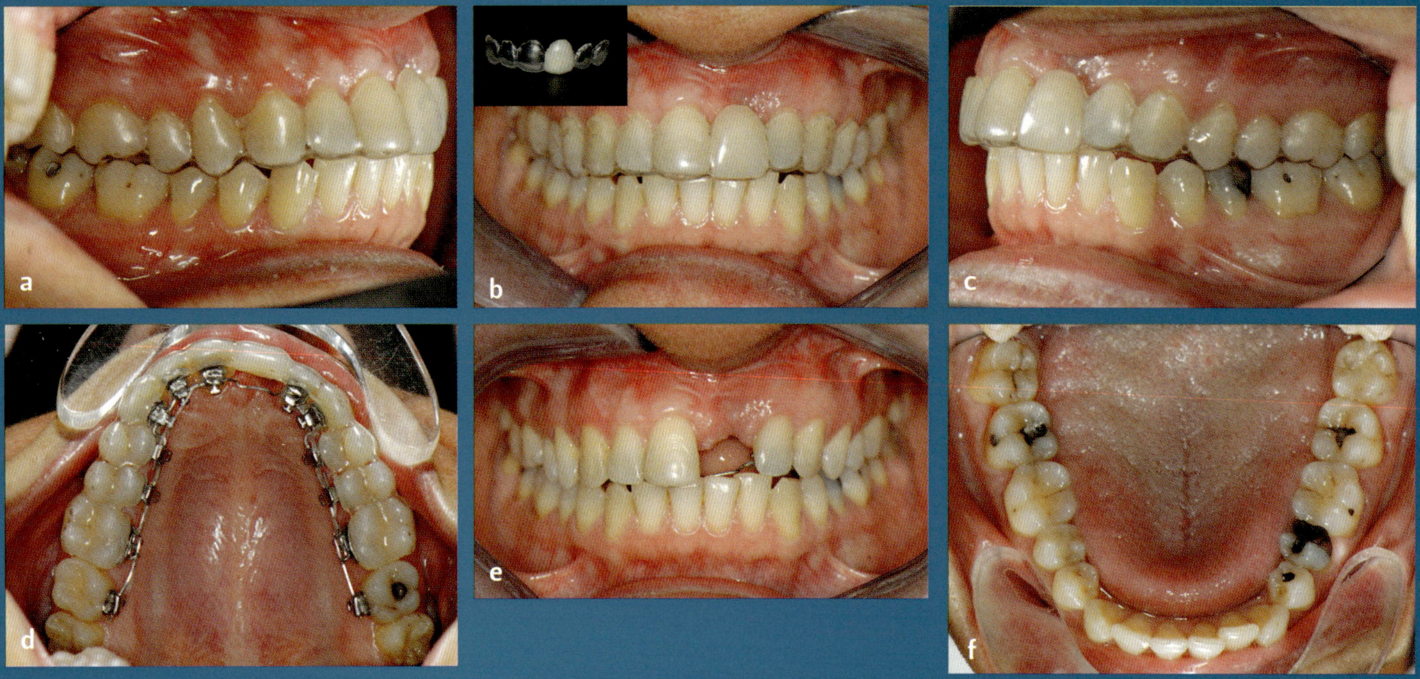

8.168 Stabilization archwires after first surgery.

Orthodontic stabilization after implant and temporary crown placement involves keeping the mechanics with passive archwires that control the teeth adjacent to the implant for another 6 months after the application of the temporary crown (8.169 and 8.170). With this in mind, GOR realizes a classical extrusion to protect the bone peaks for the future surgical bone regeneration (GBR) at the level of both hard and soft tissues (GOTR) (8.171–8.173). In 8.173 the first axial and slight distal tipping movement of the initial 2 months can be observed and, subsequently, the mesial tipping and then, from the fourth month of extrusion, the torque movement can be seen.

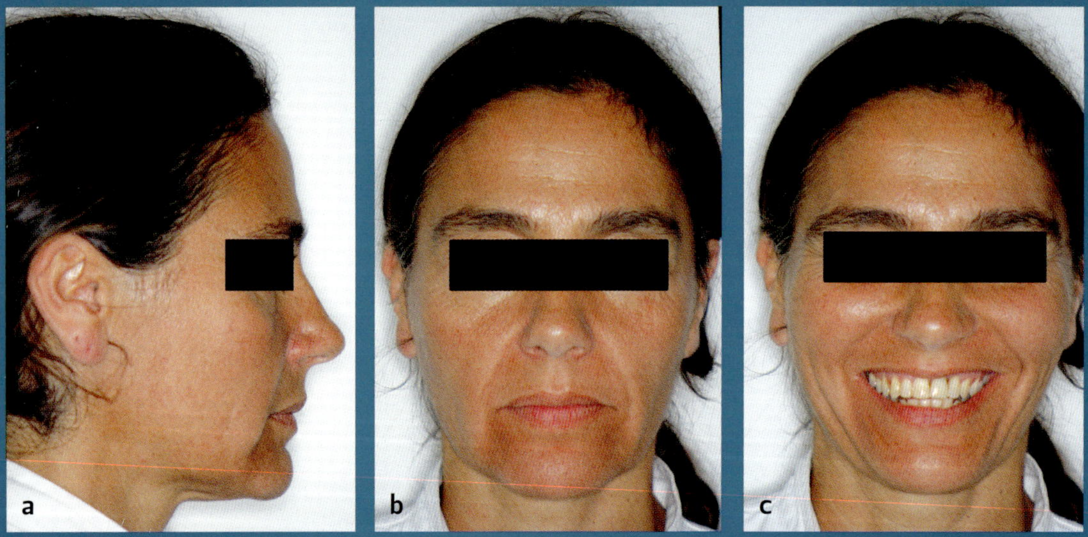

8.169 Extraoral post-orthodontic treatment photos, stabilization with temporary crown.

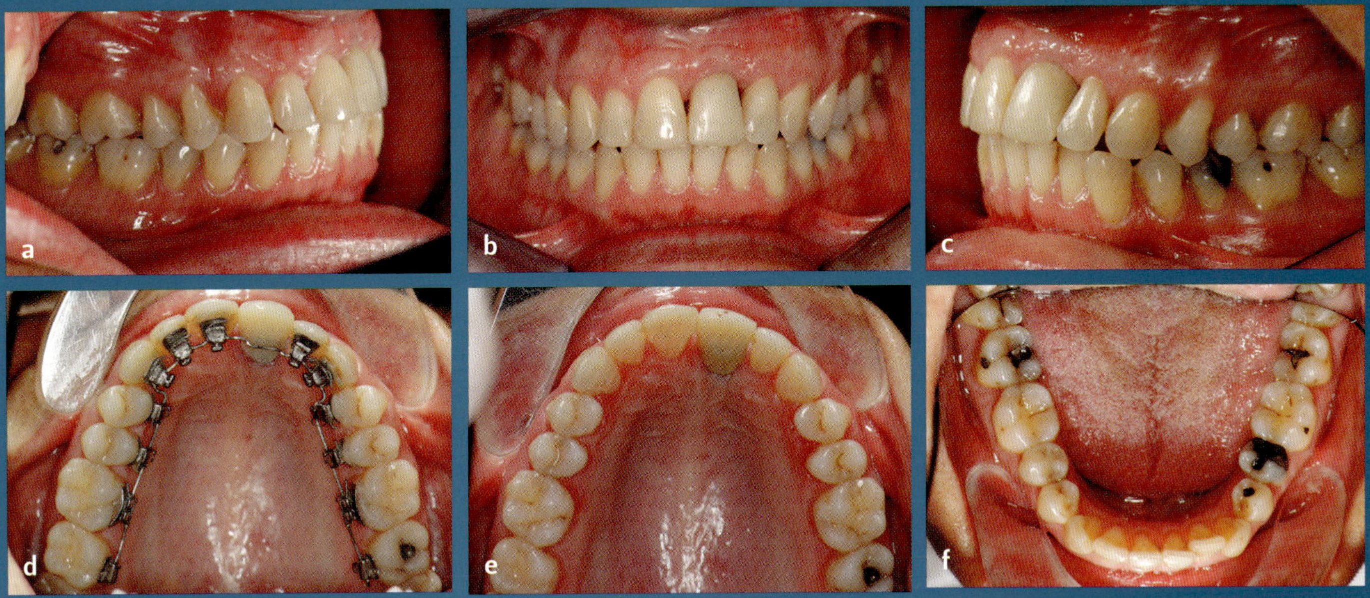

8.170 Intraoral post-orthodontic treatment photos, stabilization with temporary crown.

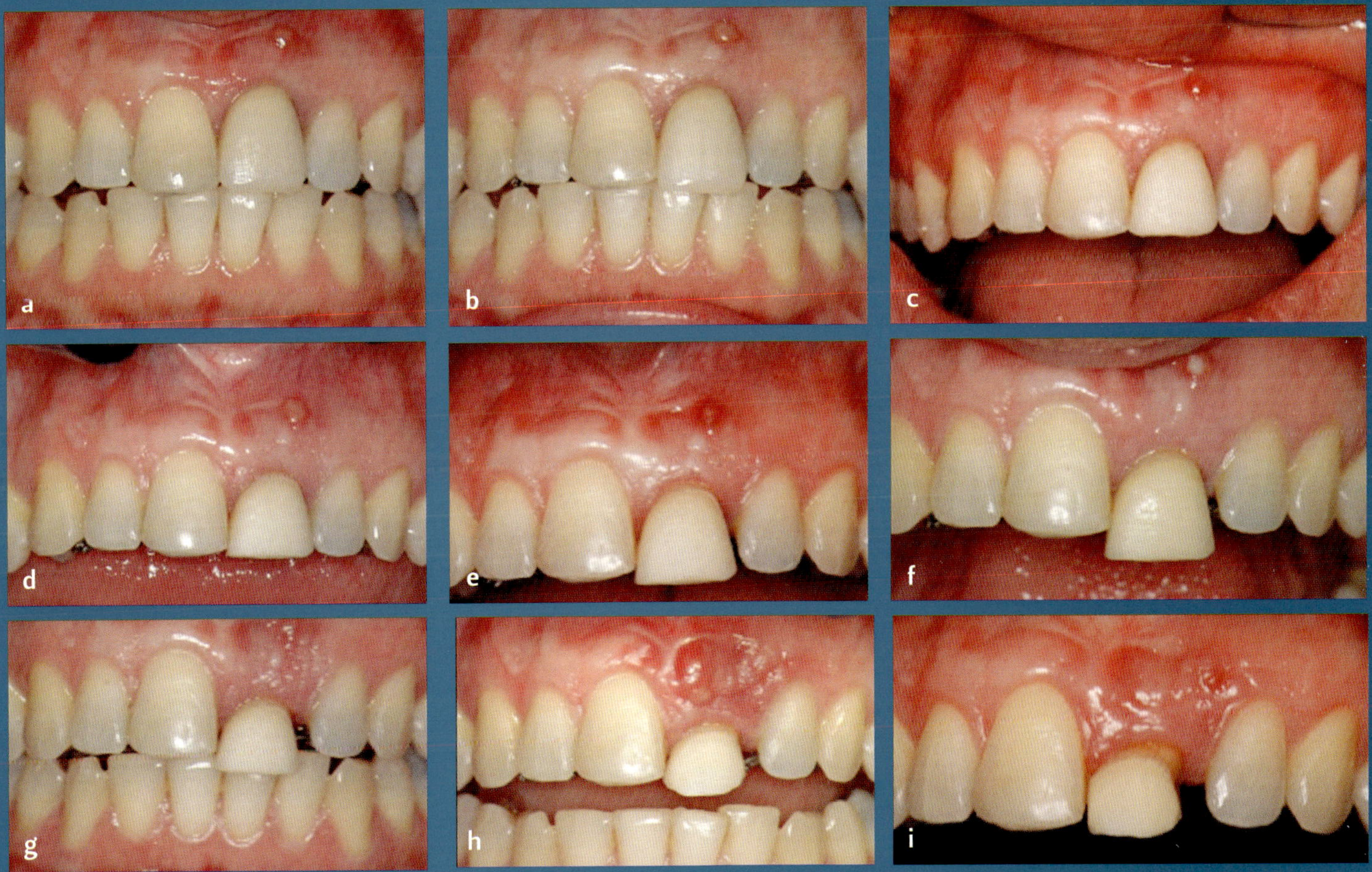

8.171 Summary of the extrusion phases: vestibular view (time: 0-6 months). (Reproduced from "Paolone MG, Kaitsas R. Orthodontic-periodontal interactions: Orthodontic extrusion in interdisciplinary regenerative treatments. *Int Orthod.* 2018;16(2):217-245" and "Kaitsas R, Paolone MG, Paolone G. Guided orthodontic regeneration: A tool to enhance conventional regenerative techniques in implant surgery. *Int Orthod.* 2015;13(4):539-554" ©CEO. Published by Elsevier Masson SAS. All rights reserved. With permission.)

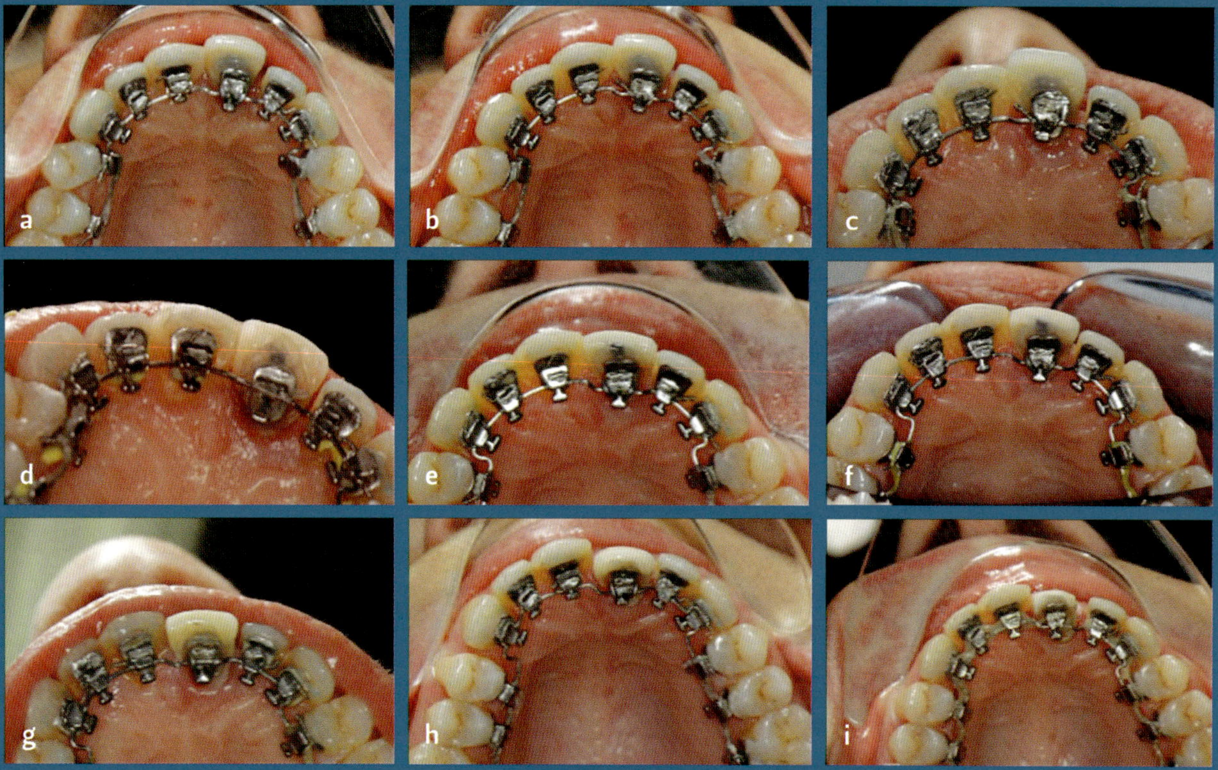

8.172 Summary of the extrusion phases: occlusal view (time: 0–6 months). (Reproduced from "Paolone MG, Kaitsas R. Orthodontic-periodontal interactions: Orthodontic extrusion in interdisciplinary regenerative treatments. *Int Orthod.* 2018;16(2):217-245" and "Kaitsas R, Paolone MG, Paolone G. Guided orthodontic regeneration: A tool to enhance conventional regenerative techniques in implant surgery. *Int Orthod.* 2015;13(4):539-554" ©CEO. Published by Elsevier Masson SAS. All rights reserved. With permission.)

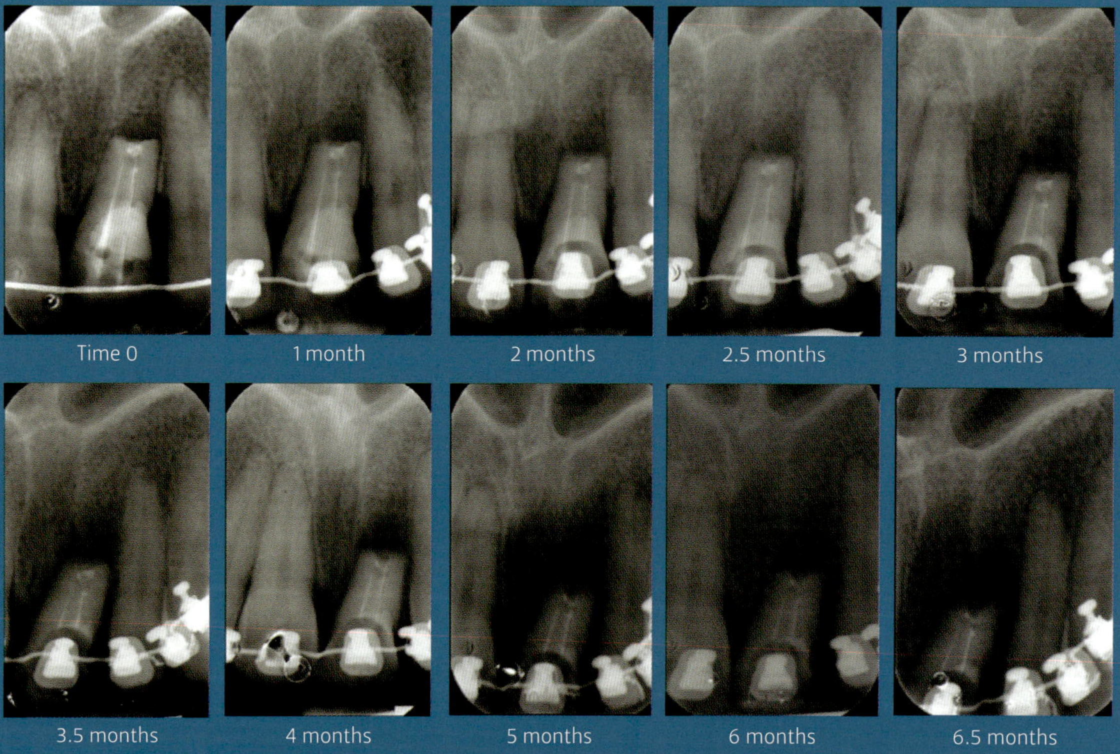

8.173 Summary of the extrusion phases: X-rays. (Reproduced from "Paolone MG, Kaitsas R. Orthodontic-periodontal interactions: Orthodontic extrusion in interdisciplinary regenerative treatments. *Int Orthod.* 2018; 16(2):217-245" and "Kaitsas R, Paolone MG, Paolone G. Guided orthodontic regeneration: A tool to enhance conventional regenerative techniques in implant surgery. *Int Orthod.* 2015;13(4):539-554" ©CEO. Published by Elsevier Masson SAS. All rights reserved. With permission.)

After the orthodontic stabilization period, the site is ready to perform the surgical phase. The huge amount of soft tissue obtained with orthodontic extrusion can be observed, now sufficient to cover the membrane increasing the predictability of regenerative surgery (8.174). The further advantage, being a type 1[90], is the increased width of keratinized gingiva, an element that allows to reduce subsequent mucogingival surgery in the second surgical phase. Comparing the two X-rays (8.175) it can be seen the coronal displacement of the bone peaks associated with the extruded element, which will facilitate the predictability of GBR. A full-thickness trapezoidal flap is elevated with "hockey stick" relief incision[128] (8.176) at the level of 1.1 and 2.2, with an intrasulcular incision at the level of the teeth. The root fragment is extracted in atraumatic way, taking care not to damage the newly formed tissue (8.177). After the removal of root fragment, it can be seen the bone defect in the extraction area around the non-recoverable fragment and the bone dehiscence at the level of the root of element 2.2 (8.178). The complete lack of the vestibular cortical plate can be observed from the occlusal view (8.179). After the measurement of the bone defect (8.180) the bone regeneration obtained with the orthodontic movement by GOR can be observed on the mesial aspect of 2.2 (8.181). Periosteal relief incisions are performed and the complete mobility of the flap is controlled in order to completely cover the site to be regenerated (8.182). The insertion axis is checked using the aligner, worn for the entire period of orthodontic treatment by the patient, as a surgical guide (8.183).

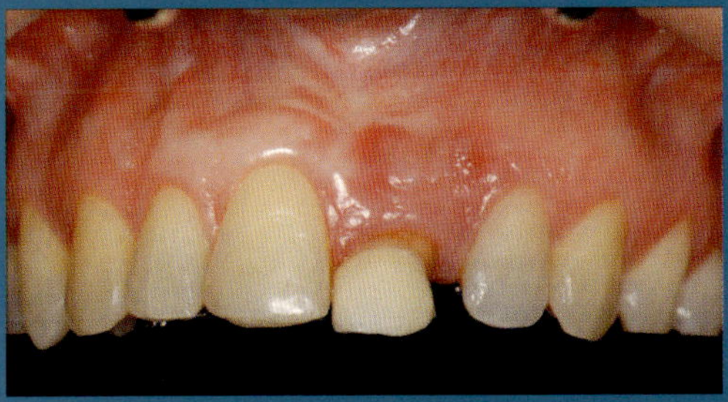

8.174 Soft tissue after extrusion. (Reproduced from "Paolone MG, Kaitsas R. Orthodontic-periodontal interactions: Orthodontic extrusion in interdisciplinary regenerative treatments. *Int Orthod.* 2018;16(2):217-245" and "Kaitsas R, Paolone MG, Paolone G. Guided orthodontic regeneration: A tool to enhance conventional regenerative techniques in implant surgery. *Int Orthod.* 2015;13(4):539-554" ©CEO. Published by Elsevier Masson SAS. All rights reserved. With permission.)

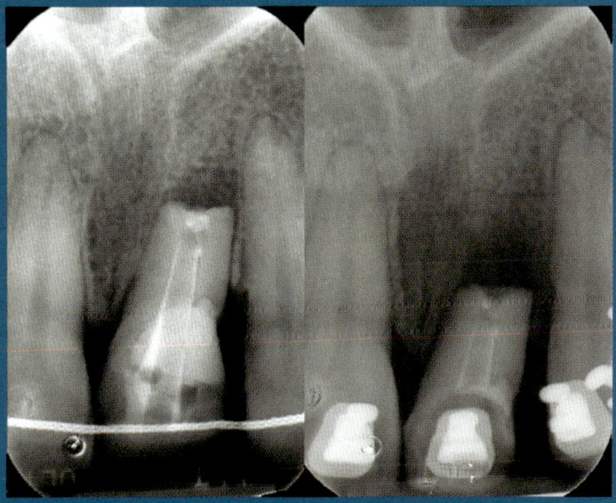

8.175 X-ray comparison of the bone peaks.

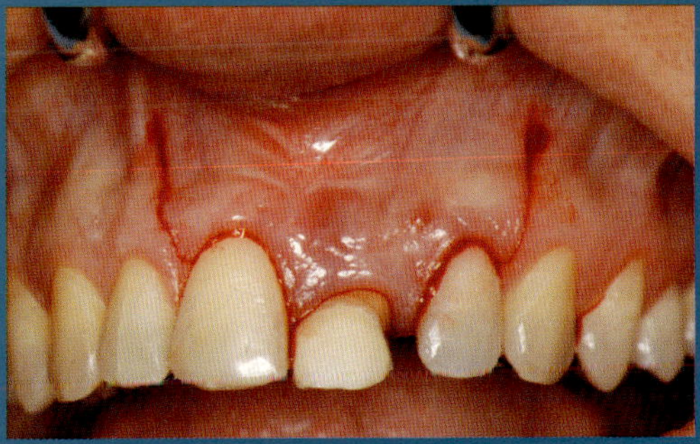

8.176 Trapezoidal full-thickness flap with hockey-stick relief vertical incisions. (Reproduced from "Kaitsas R, Paolone MG, Paolone G. Guided orthodontic regeneration: A tool to enhance conventional regenerative techniques in implant surgery. *Int Orthod.* 2015;13(4):539-554" ©CEO. Published by Elsevier Masson SAS. All rights reserved. With permission.)

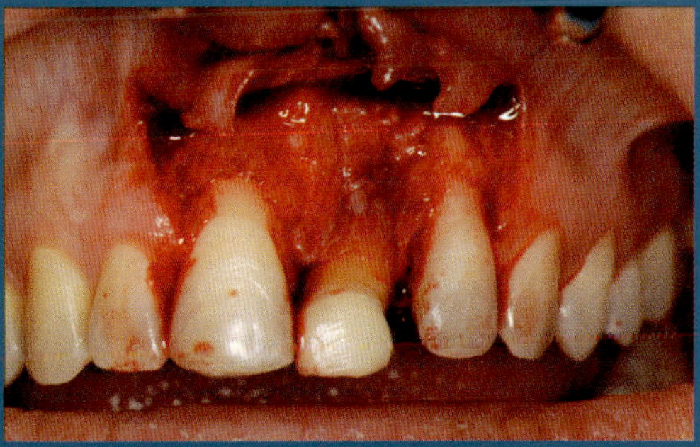

8.177 Flap elevation with the root fragment *in situ*. (Reproduced from "Paolone MG, Kaitsas R. Orthodontic-periodontal interactions: Orthodontic extrusion in interdisciplinary regenerative treatments. *Int Orthod.* 2018;16(2):217-245" and "Kaitsas R, Paolone MG, Paolone G. Guided orthodontic regeneration: A tool to enhance conventional regenerative techniques in implant surgery. *Int Orthod.* 2015;13(4):539-554" ©CEO. Published by Elsevier Masson SAS. All rights reserved. With permission.)

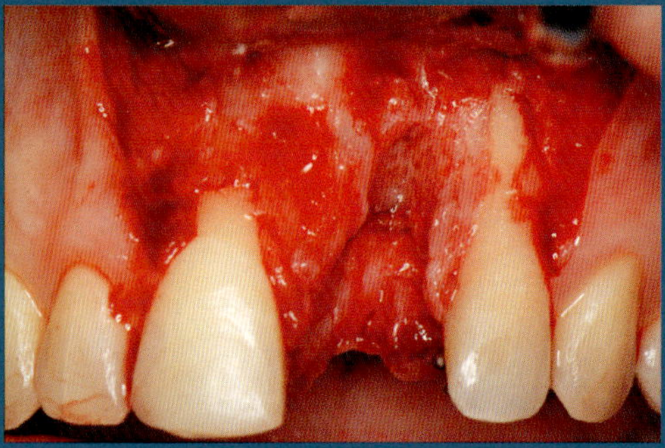

8.178 Residual bone defect after the fragment extraction. The bone dehiscence on the 2.2, cause of the hyperemia can be observed.

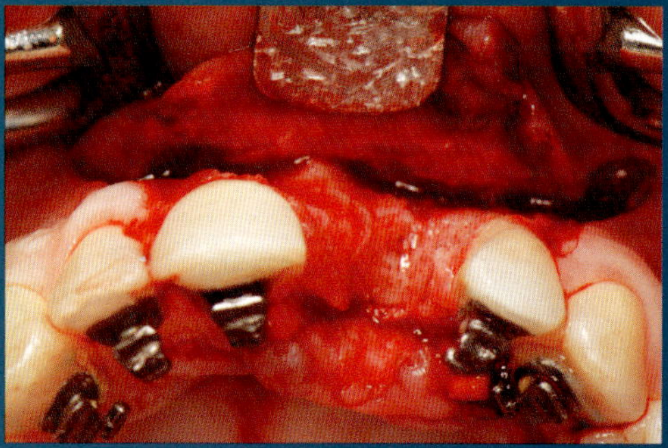

8.179 Occlusal view of the bone defect where the lack of the vestibular cortical plate can be seen.

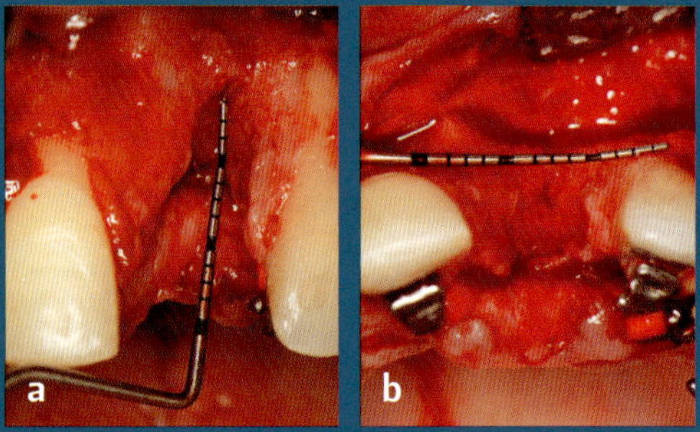

8.180 Measurement of the bone defect.

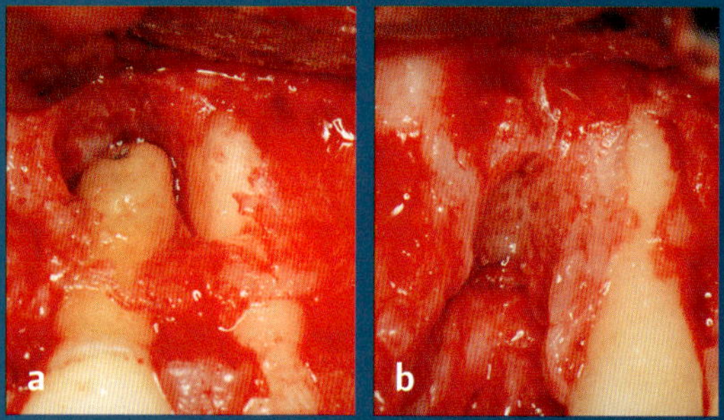

8.181 Comparison of the pre- and post-extrusion bone amount. The complete regeneration of the bone level on the mesial surface of 2.2 can be seen.

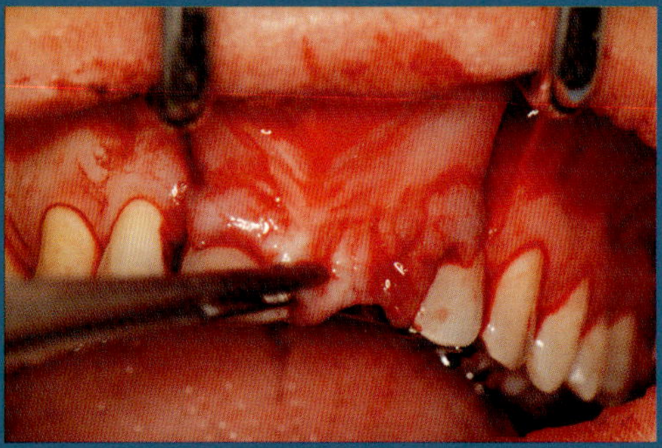

8.182 Control of the flap passivation after the execution of the periosteal relief incisions.

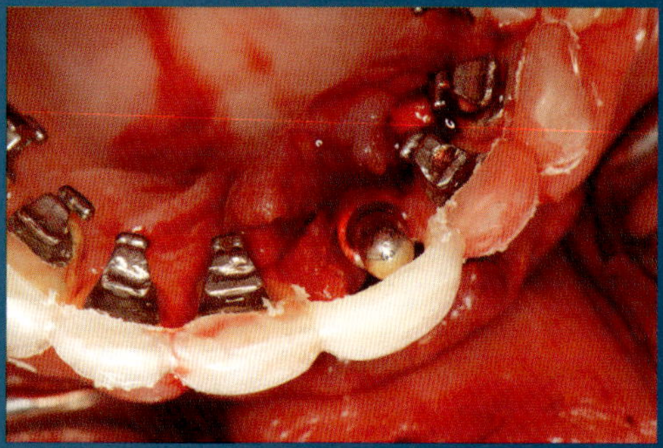

8.183 Control by probe of the insertion axis using the esthetic aligner of the patient as surgical template.

After implant placement (4.5/15 mm Frialit-2®, Dentsply) (8.184), the peri-implant bone defect is grafted with particulate autologous bone collected in the same surgical site by a bone scraper, covering also the vestibular dehiscence at the level of 2.2 (8.185-8.188). After cortical bone perforations performed to increase the vascularization of the graft, the defects are covered with a non-resorbable titanium-reinforced e-PTFE membrane previously adapted to the defects to be regenerated and fixed with a single titanium pin at the apical level, extending at vestibular dehiscence of 2.2 to simultaneously perform a GTR for the adjacent tooth tissues (8.189). The flap is sutured at the crestal level with a double line of resorbable 5-0 polyglycolic acid sutures by horizontal mattress and interrupted sutures, and by 5-0 e-PTFE interrupted sutures along the vertical incision. The flap is stabilized with an apical e-PTFE 5-0 Cornick suture (8.190 and 8.191). During the healing period, the tissues are followed up to avoid areas of uncovering and infections of the membrane and underlying graft (in 8.192, the first 4 months of healing of the soft tissue, the most critical period for GBR sites can be seen). After 12 months (8.193 and 8.194) the second surgical phase is performed, to increase the vestibulo-palatal thickness of the soft tissues by a Roll Flap Technique[129]. A full thickness trapezoidal flap is elevated with "hockey stick" relief incisions[128] at 1.1 and 2.2 level, following the same flap design as in the first surgical phase (8.195). It is created in the edentulous site, after an intrasulcular incision at 1.1 and 2.2 level, the palatal pedicle (8.196) which, after de-epithelialization (8.197), is reflected on the vestibular site. After elevating the flap, the membrane with a perfectly integration and without any sign of inflammation can be observed (8.198). After the removal of the membrane, taking care to remove it completely without leaving residues, the bone tissue regeneration around the implant and on the vestibular surface of 2.2 is checked (8.199 and 8.200). In particular, the regenerated bone tissue can be observed on the vestibular surface, at the level of

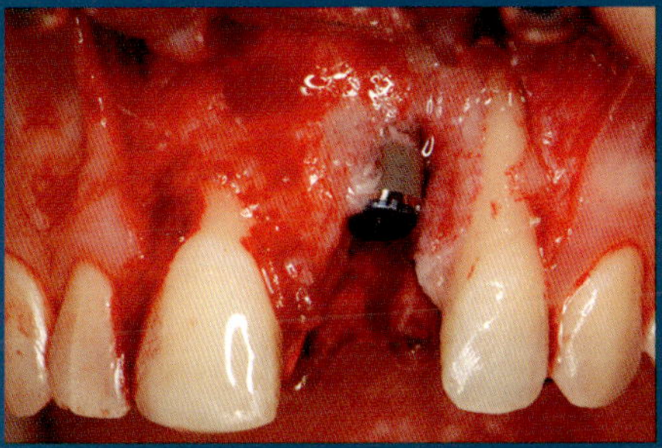

8.184 Implant placement. (Reproduced from "Paolone MG, Kaitsas R. Orthodontic-periodontal interactions: Orthodontic extrusion in interdisciplinary regenerative treatments. *Int Orthod.* 2018;16(2):217-245" and "Kaitsas R, Paolone MG, Paolone G. Guided orthodontic regeneration: A tool to enhance conventional regenerative techniques in implant surgery. *Int Orthod.* 2015;13(4):539-554" ©CEO. Published by Elsevier Masson SAS. All rights reserved. With permission.)

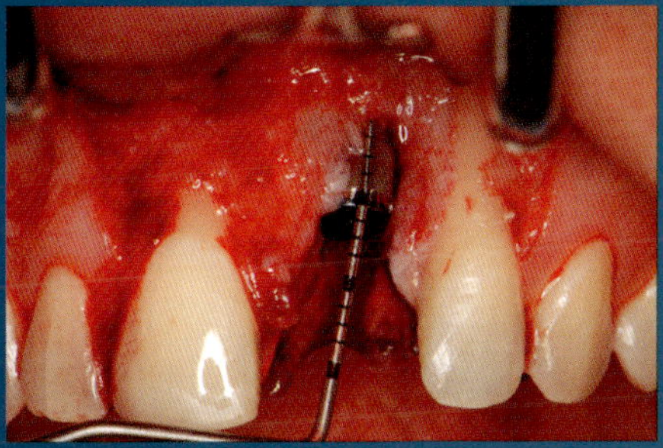

8.185 Measurement of the peri-implant vestibular defect. Apico-coronal extension.

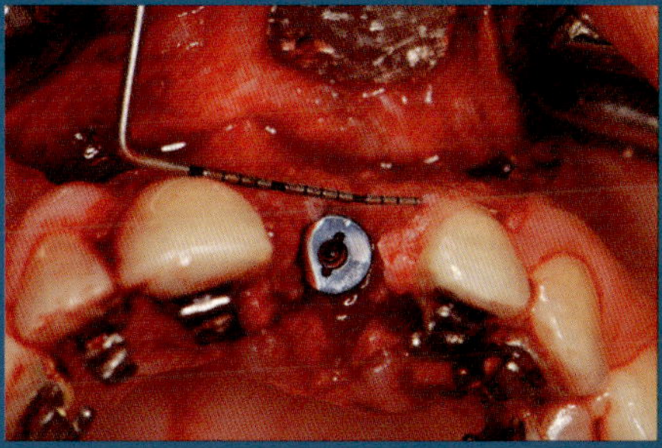

8.186 Measurement of the peri-implant vestibular defect. Mesio-distal extension.

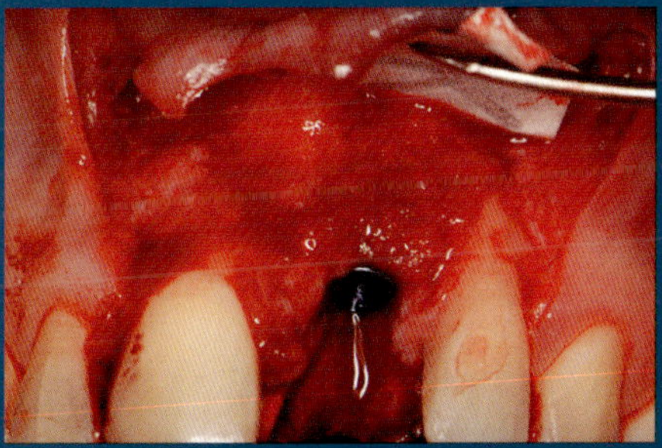

8.187 Filling of the peri-implant defect with autologous bone. (Reproduced from "Paolone MG, Kaitsas R. Orthodontic-periodontal interactions: Orthodontic extrusion in interdisciplinary regenerative treatments. *Int Orthod.* 2018;16(2):217-245" and "Kaitsas R, Paolone MG, Paolone G. Guided orthodontic regeneration: A tool to enhance conventional regenerative techniques in implant surgery. *Int Orthod.* 2015;13(4):539-554" ©CEO. Published by Elsevier Masson SAS. All rights reserved. With permission.)

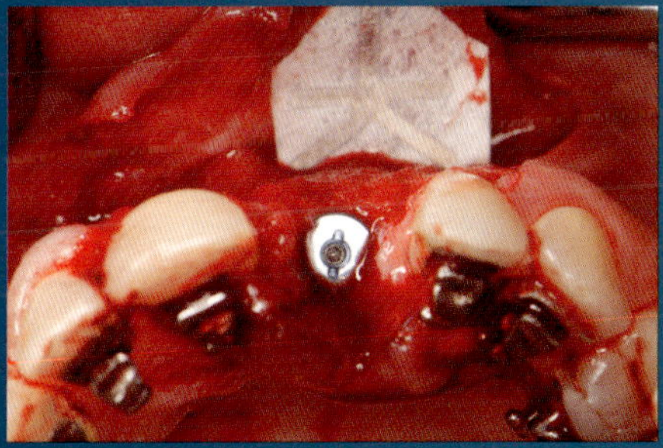

8.188 Occlusal view of the defect with autologous bone graft.

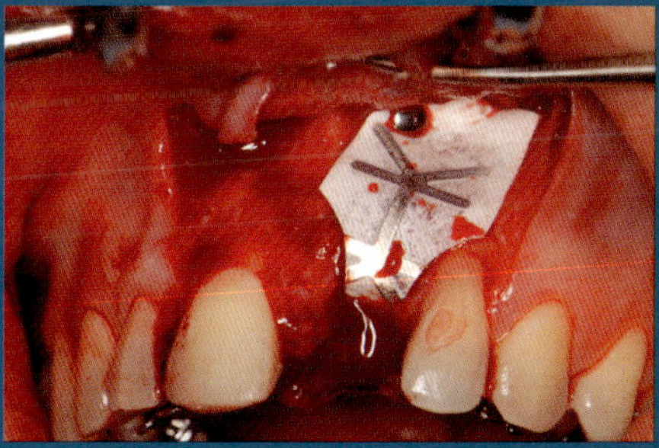

8.189 Fixation of the non-resorbable titanium-reinforced membrane with a pin *in situ*. (Reproduced from "Paolone MG, Kaitsas R. Orthodontic-periodontal interactions: Orthodontic extrusion in interdisciplinary regenerative treatments. *Int Orthod.* 2018;16(2):217-245" and "Kaitsas R, Paolone MG, Paolone G. Guided orthodontic regeneration: A tool to enhance conventional regenerative techniques in implant surgery. *Int Orthod.* 2015;13(4):539-554" ©CEO. Published by Elsevier Masson SAS. All rights reserved. With permission.)

the implant head and on the root of 2.2 (8.201). In 8.202 it can be seen how the GBR on the implant on 2.1 site and the GTR of 2.2 are combined with the GOR in the same site. After placing the healing abutment, a ramp mattress suture[127] is performed to stabilize the soft tissues, with interrupted sutures along the relief incisions and an apical Cornick suture to stabilize the flap with 4-0 Polypropylene suture (8.203 and 8.204). From the occlusal view it is possible to observe the vestibular augmentation of the soft tissues obtained with the second surgical phase (8.205).

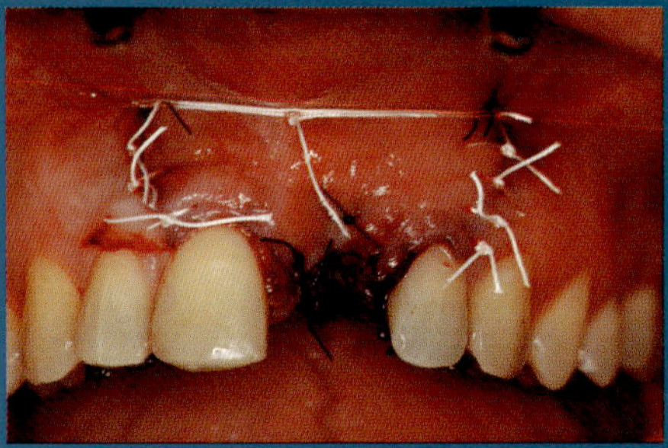

8.190 Flap suture. (Reproduced from "Kaitsas R, Paolone MG, Paolone G. Guided orthodontic regeneration: A tool to enhance conventional regenerative techniques in implant surgery. *Int Orthod.* 2015;13(4):539-554" ©CEO. Published by Elsevier Masson SAS. All rights reserved. With permission.)

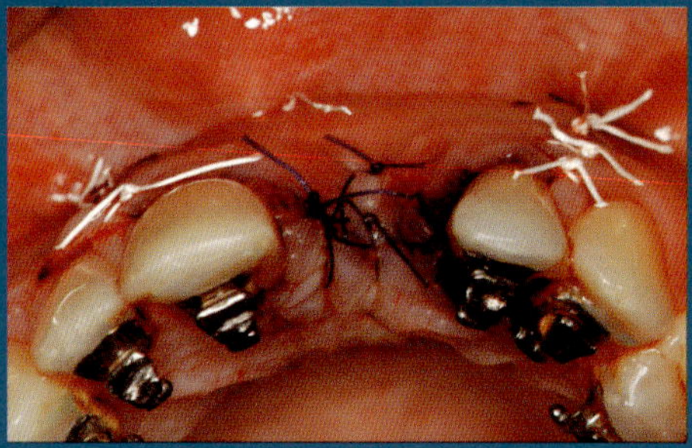

8.191 Occlusal view of the flap suture where the double line of suture in the crestal zone can be seen.

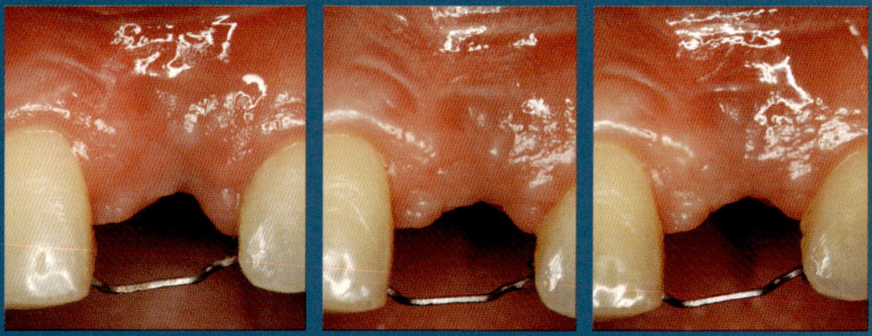

8.192 Tissue follow-up during the healing phase (3-6-9 months).

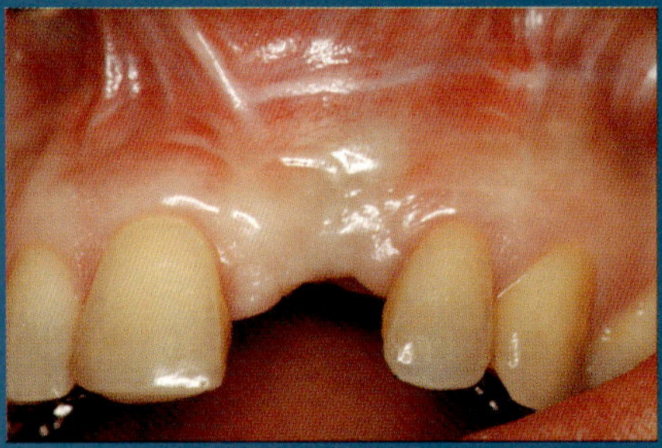

8.193 Tissue aspect during the second surgical phase (12 months). (Reproduced from "Paolone MG, Kaitsas R. Orthodontic-periodontal interactions: Orthodontic extrusion in interdisciplinary regenerative treatments. *Int Orthod.* 2018;16(2):217-245" and "Kaitsas R, Paolone MG, Paolone G. Guided orthodontic regeneration: A tool to enhance conventional regenerative techniques in implant surgery. *Int Orthod.* 2015;13(4):539-554" ©CEO. Published by Elsevier Masson SAS. All rights reserved. With permission.)

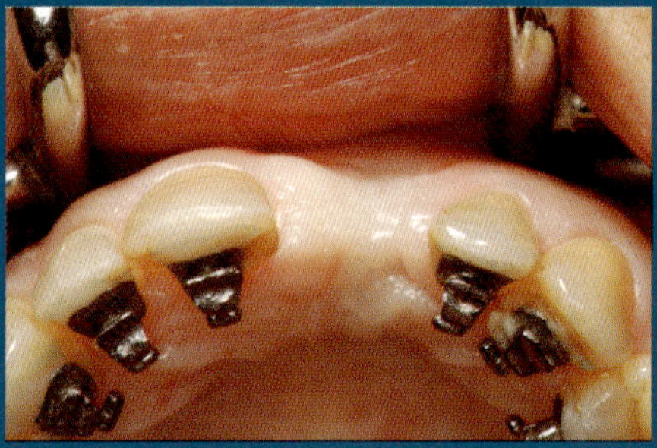

8.194 Tissue aspect during the second surgical phase. Occlusal view.

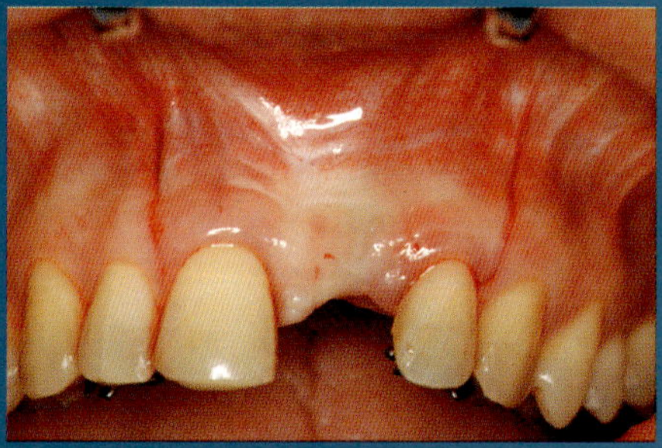

8.195 Flap design for the second surgical phase. Vertical relief incisions. (Reproduced from "Kaitsas R, Paolone MG, Paolone G. Guided orthodontic regeneration: A tool to enhance conventional regenerative techniques in implant surgery. *Int Orthod.* 2015;13(4):539-554" ©CEO. Published by Elsevier Masson SAS. All rights reserved. With permission.)

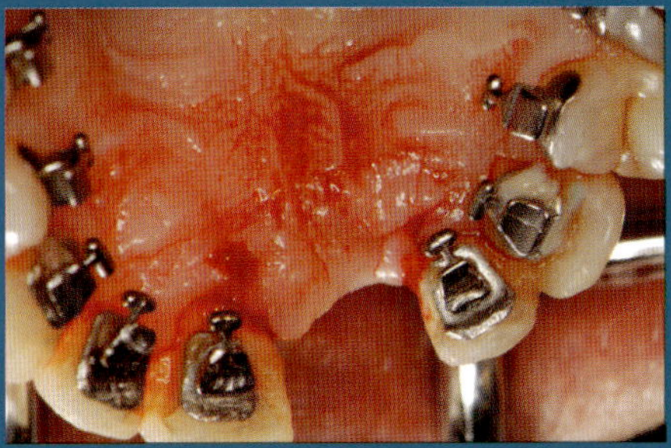

8.196 Preparation of the palatal pedicle. (Reproduced from "Kaitsas R, Paolone MG, Paolone G. Guided orthodontic regeneration: A tool to enhance conventional regenerative techniques in implant surgery. *Int Orthod.* 2015;13(4):539-554" ©CEO. Published by Elsevier Masson SAS. All rights reserved. With permission.)

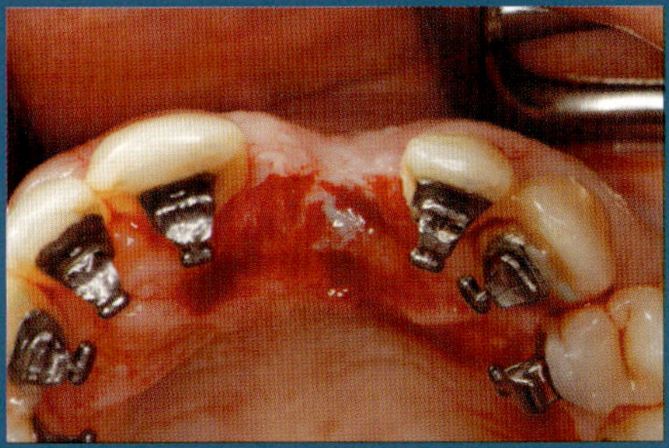

8.197 Disepithelization of the palatal pedicle. (Reproduced from "Kaitsas R, Paolone MG, Paolone G. Guided orthodontic regeneration: A tool to enhance conventional regenerative techniques in implant surgery. *Int Orthod.* 2015;13(4):539-554" ©CEO. Published by Elsevier Masson SAS. All rights reserved. With permission.)

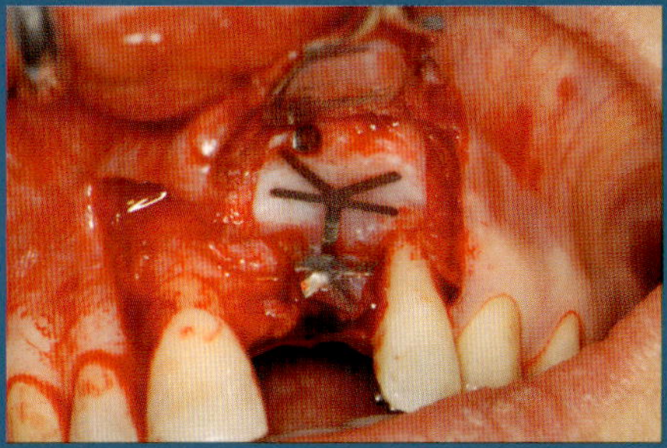

8.198 Flap elevation and membrane check without any inflammation signs. (Reproduced from "Paolone MG, Kaitsas R. Orthodontic-periodontal interactions: Orthodontic extrusion in interdisciplinary regenerative treatments. *Int Orthod.* 2018;16(2):217-245" and "Kaitsas R, Paolone MG, Paolone G. Guided orthodontic regeneration: A tool to enhance conventional regenerative techniques in implant surgery. *Int Orthod.* 2015;13(4):539-554" ©CEO. Published by Elsevier Masson SAS. All rights reserved. With permission.)

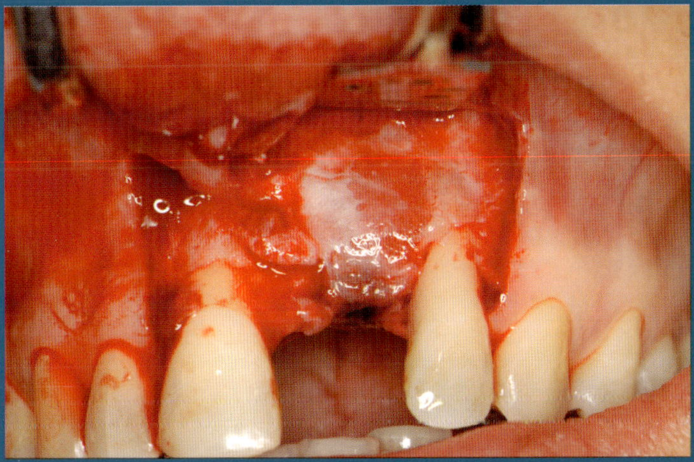

8.199 Membrane removal and checks of the neo-formed bone around the implant and root surface of 2.2. (Reproduced from "Paolone MG, Kaitsas R. Orthodontic-periodontal interactions: Orthodontic extrusion in interdisciplinary regenerative treatments. *Int Orthod.* 2018;16(2):217-245" and "Kaitsas R, Paolone MG, Paolone G. Guided orthodontic regeneration: A tool to enhance conventional regenerative techniques in implant surgery. *Int Orthod.* 2015;13(4):539-554" ©CEO. Published by Elsevier Masson SAS. All rights reserved. With permission.)

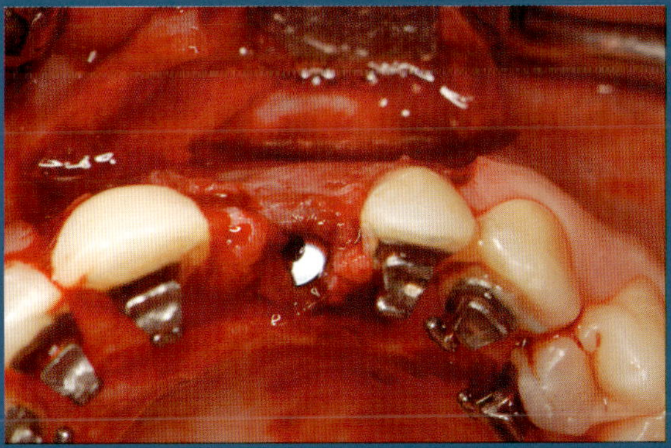

8.200 Occlusal view of the new-formed tissue around the implant.

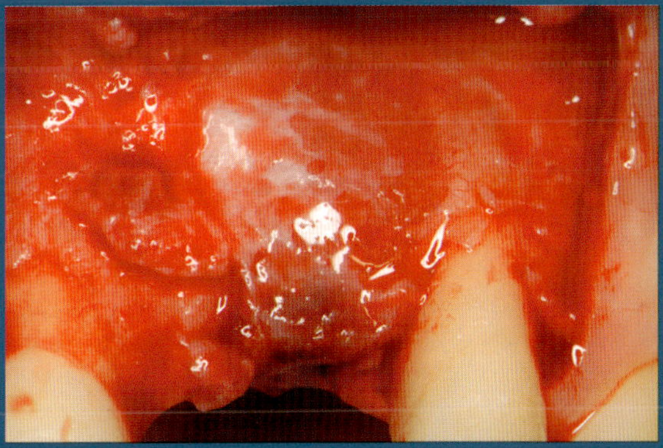

8.201 Detail of the new-formed bone.

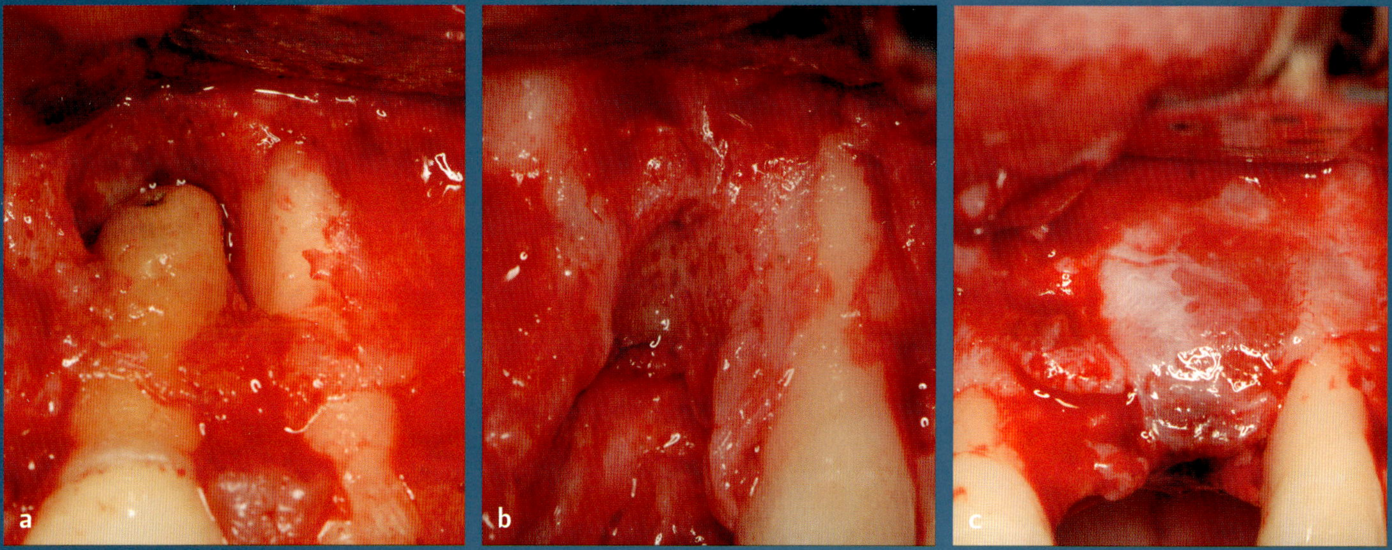

8.202 Comparison of the initial bone volume (**a**), post-extrusion (**b**) and post-regeneration by GBR (**c**).

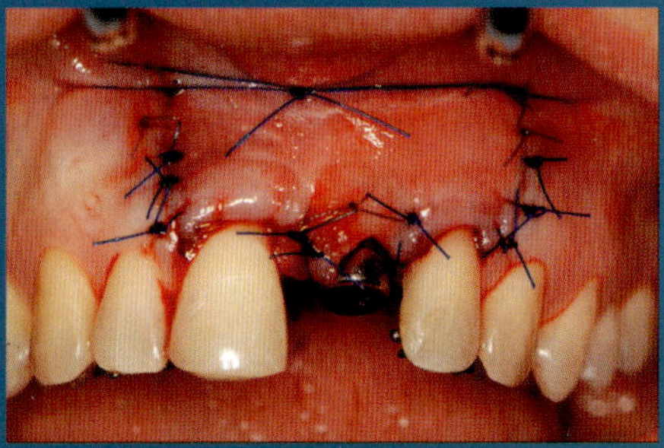

8.203 Flap suture after healing abutment placement and vestibular roll flap. (Reproduced from "Kaitsas R, Paolone MG, Paolone G. Guided orthodontic regeneration: A tool to enhance conventional regenerative techniques in implant surgery. *Int Orthod.* 2015;13(4):539-554" ©CEO. Published by Elsevier Masson SAS. All rights reserved. With permission.)

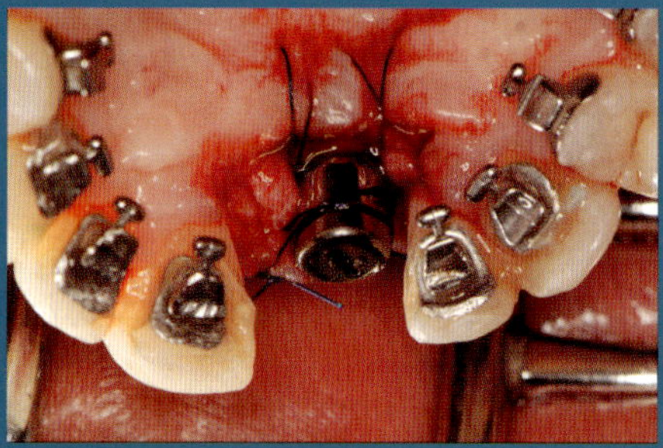

8.204 Detail of the ramp mattress suture.

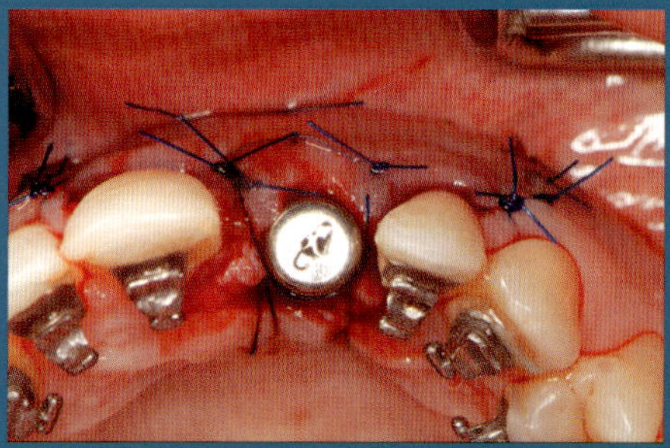

8.205 Occlusal view of the suture where the thickening of the tissue after roll flap can be seen. (Reproduced from "Paolone MG, Kaitsas R. Orthodontic-periodontal interactions: Orthodontic extrusion in interdisciplinary regenerative treatments. *Int Orthod.* 2018;16(2):217-245" and "Kaitsas R, Paolone MG, Paolone G. Guided orthodontic regeneration: A tool to enhance conventional regenerative techniques in implant surgery. *Int Orthod.* 2015;13(4):539-554" ©CEO. Published by Elsevier Masson SAS. All rights reserved. With permission.)

After 4 months, a temporary crown built on a customized titanium milled abutment is cemented to guide tissue maturation as described in *Clinical case 4* (8.206 and 8.207). The temporary crown is recontoured for 8 months and, 12 months after the second surgical phase, the soft tissue information is transferred to the laboratory and a metal-ceramic crown is packaged on a customized abutment. In 8.208-8.212 it can be seen the aspect of the soft tissues before the final cementation, the shape of the gingival scalloping, the definitive crown just cemented, the X-ray check and the amount of vestibulo-palatal soft tissues. In the following photographs, the 3-year (8.213 and 8.214) and 10-year (8.215-8.221; see 8.21) follow-up can be seen, in which the integration between the implant-prosthetic and soft tissue rehabilitation can be appreciated.

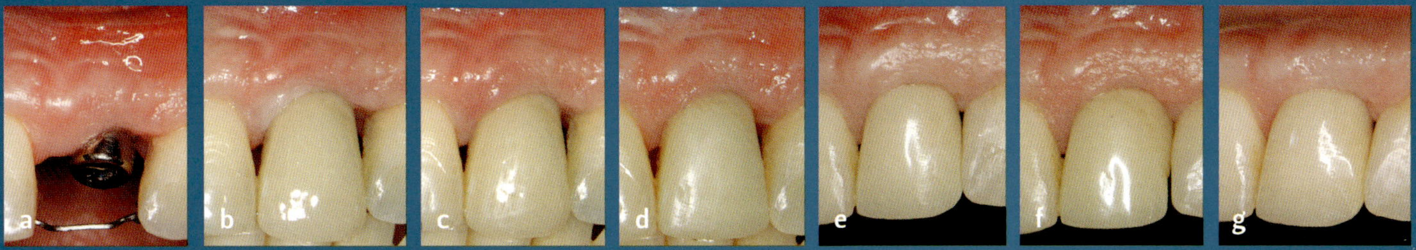

8.206 Control of the tissue healing guided by customized temporary crown.

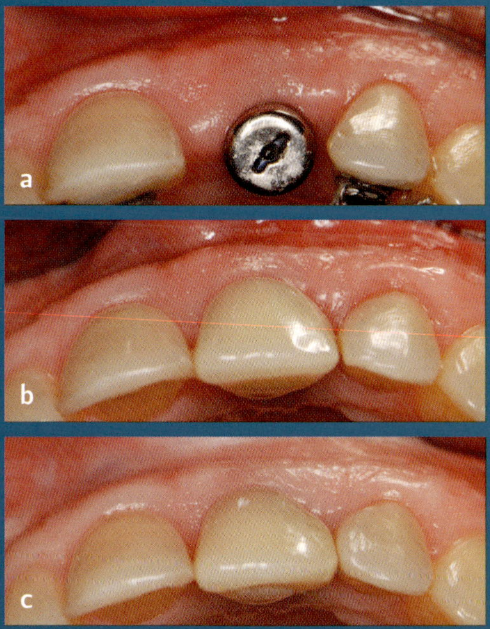

8.207 Occlusal view of the vestibular tissue maturation at 3 (**a**), 6 (**b**) and 12 months (**c**).

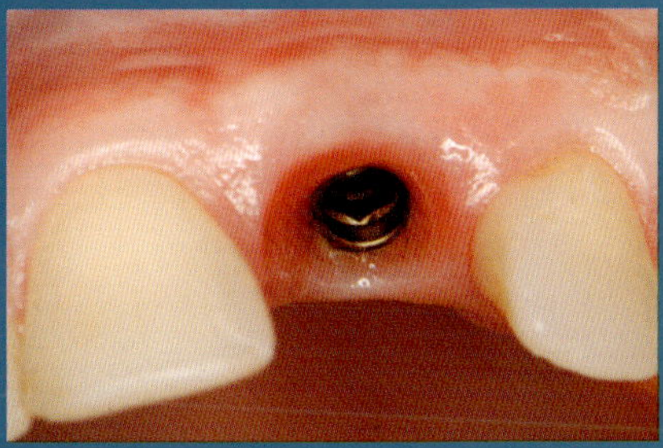

8.208 Tissue aspect 12 months, at the cementation time.

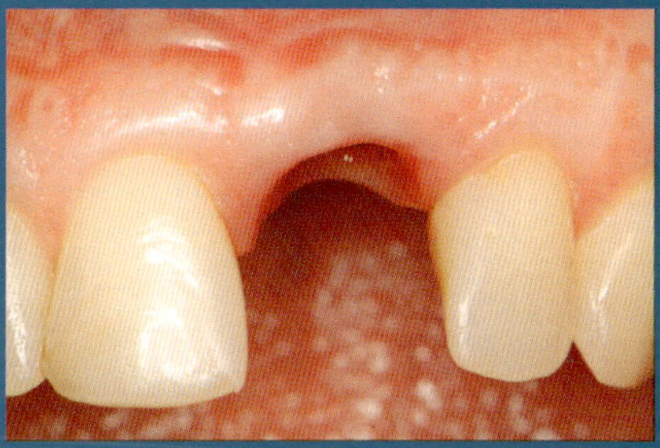

8.209 View of the gingival scallop guided by the customized temporary crown.

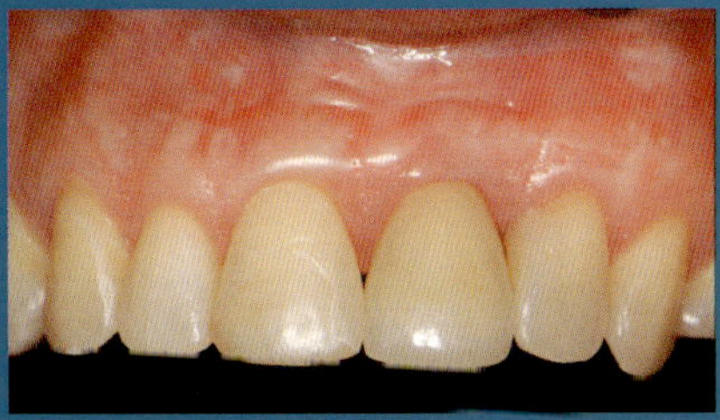

8.210 Zirconia crown, just cemented.

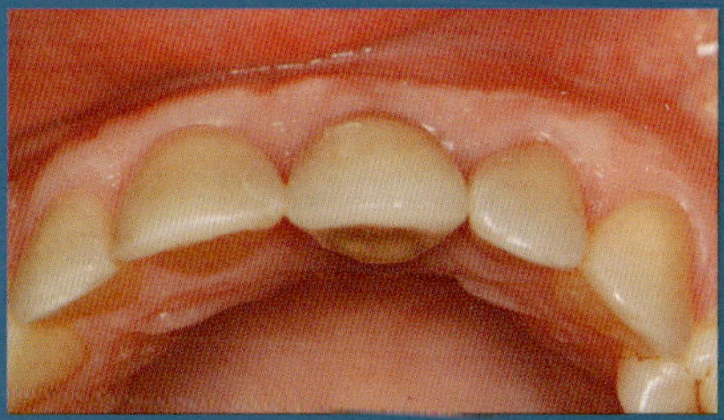

8.211 Occlusal view of the thickening of the vestibular tissue.

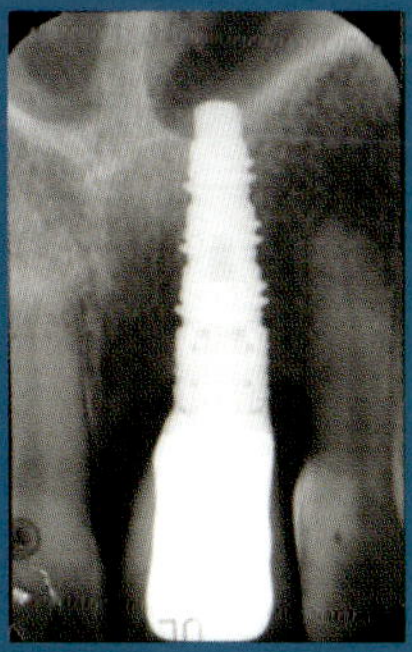

8.212 X-ray check after cementation.

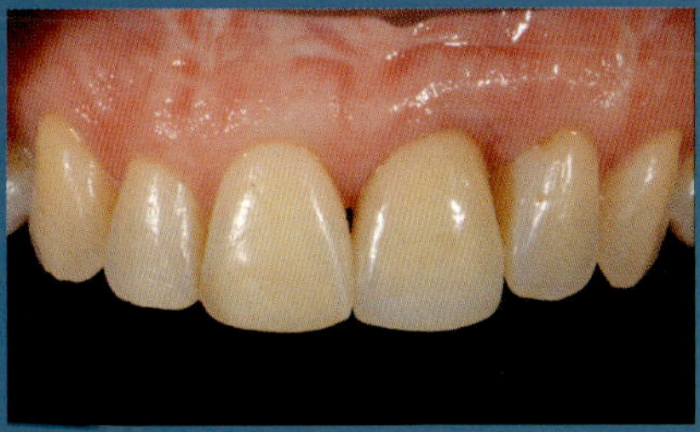

8.213 3-year follow-up. (Reproduced from "Paolone MG, Kaitsas R. Orthodontic-periodontal interactions: Orthodontic extrusion in interdisciplinary regenerative treatments. *Int Orthod.* 2018;16(2):217-245" and "Kaitsas R, Paolone MG, Paolone G. Guided orthodontic regeneration: A tool to enhance conventional regenerative techniques in implant surgery. *Int Orthod.* 2015;13(4):539-554" ©CEO. Published by Elsevier Masson SAS. All rights reserved. With permission.)

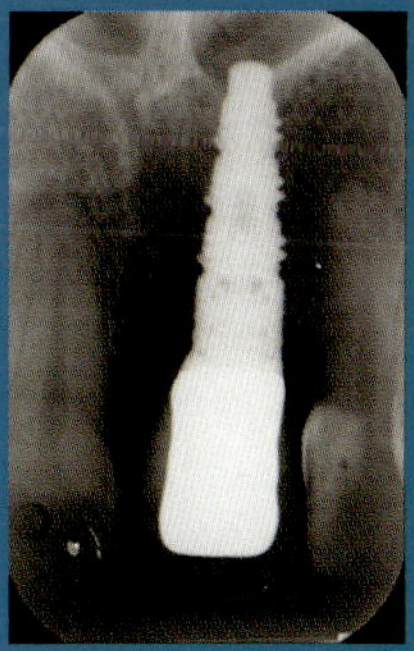

8.214 3-year X-ray follow up. (Reproduced from "Paolone MG, Kaitsas R. Orthodontic-periodontal interactions: Orthodontic extrusion in interdisciplinary regenerative treatments. *Int Orthod.* 2018;16(2):217-245" and "Kaitsas R, Paolone MG, Paolone G. Guided orthodontic regeneration: A tool to enhance conventional regenerative techniques in implant surgery. *Int Orthod.* 2015;13(4):539-554" ©CEO. Published by Elsevier Masson SAS. All rights reserved. With permission.)

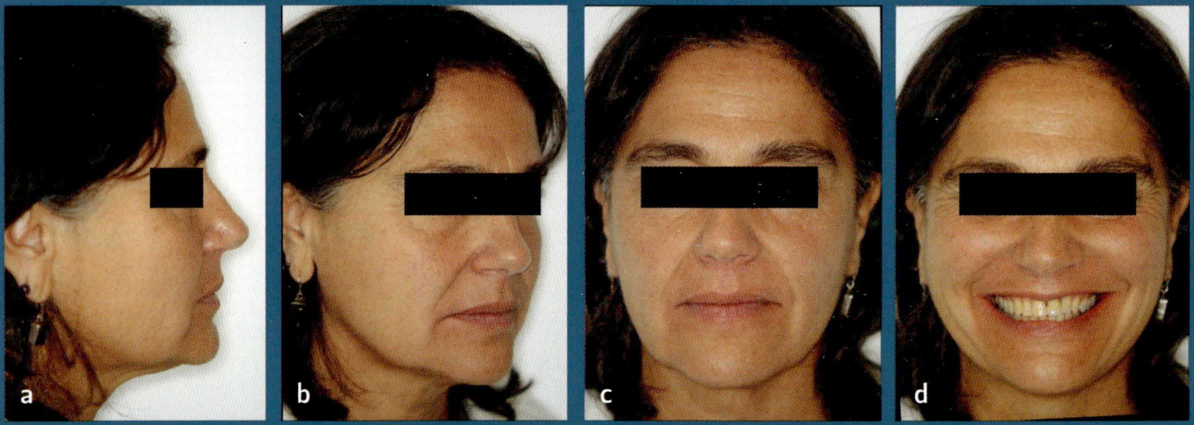

8.215 10-year follow-up extraoral photos.

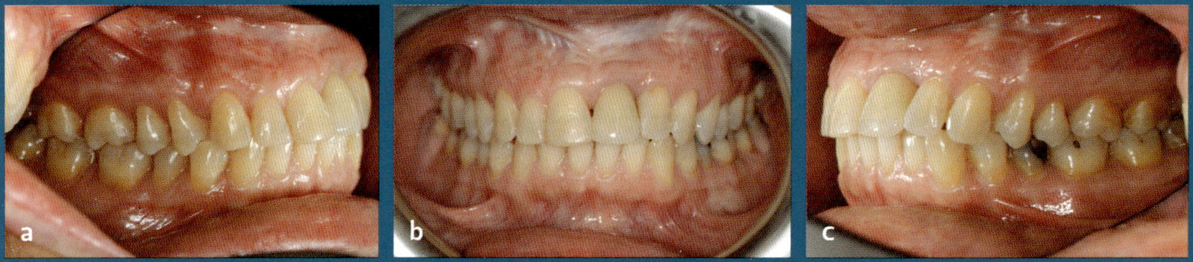

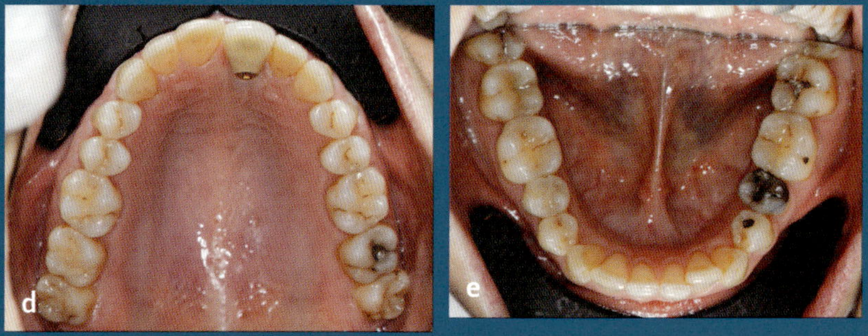

8.216 10-year follow-up intraoral photos.

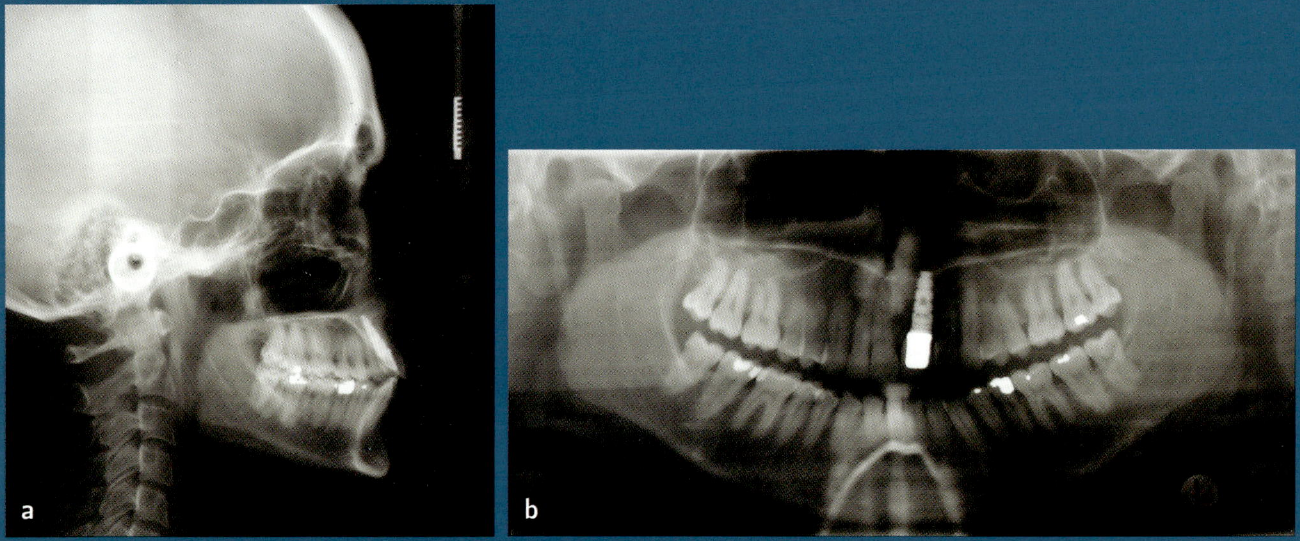

8.217 10-year follow-up cephalometric Rx (**a**) and panoramic Rx (**b**).

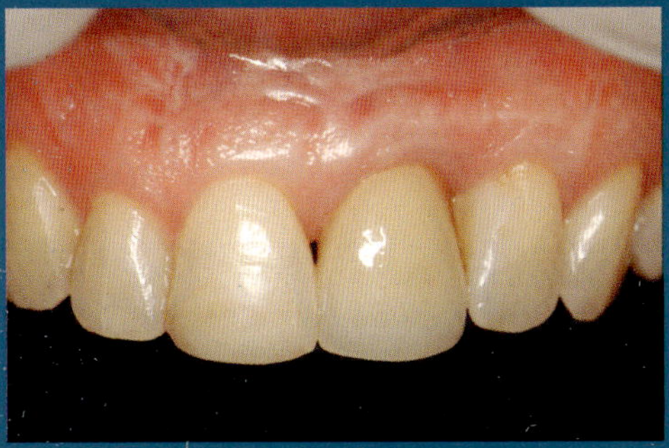

8.218 10-year follow-up.

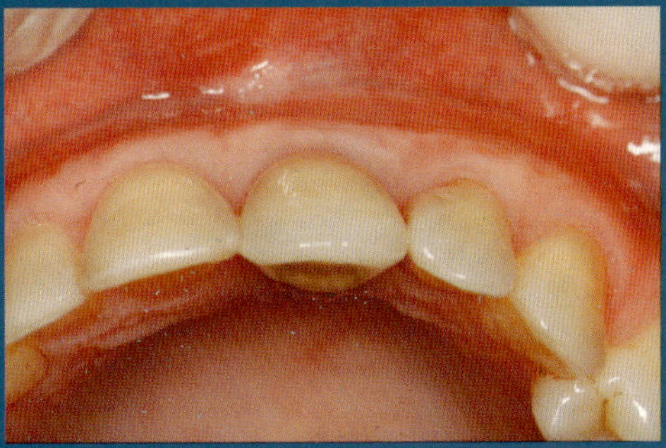

8.219 10-year follow-up occlusal view.

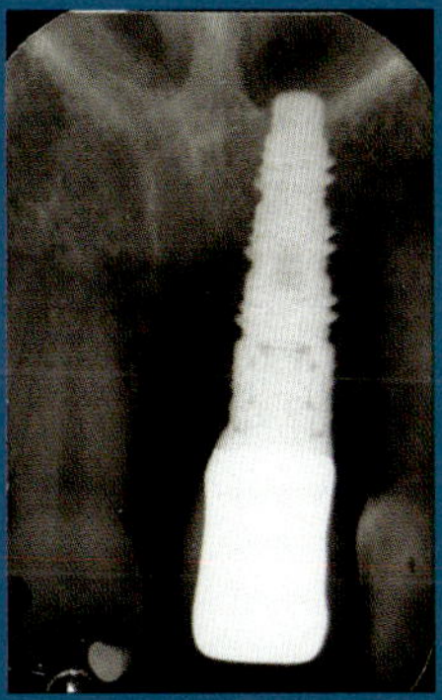

8.220 10-year X-ray follow-up.

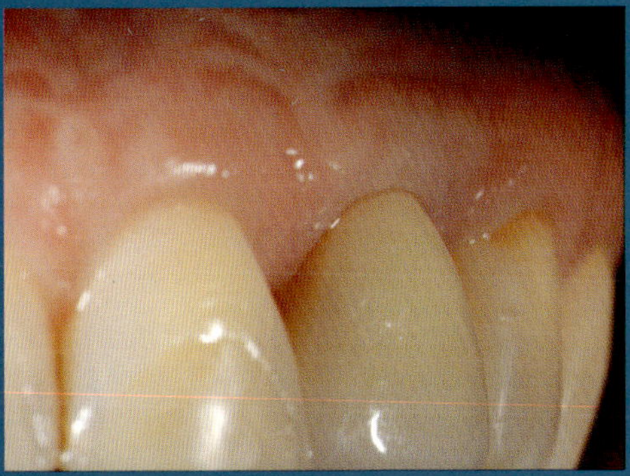

8.221 10-year volumetric maintenance and integration of the soft tissue around the prosthetic restoration.

Clinical case 6 (GOR with immediate loading)

An important indication to pre-implant orthodontic extrusion is its application in immediate loading post-extraction implant placement procedures, where an excellent primary stability is required for implant placement and an adequate amount of soft tissue is important to obtain good esthetics. In this case the amount of soft and hard tissue that is obtainable with the extrusion is sufficient to achieve primary and esthetic stability, reducing additional surgery and therefore the morbidity of the intervention. In this case the patient presents a vertical fracture on 2.5, a mesial bone defect along the root and a vestibular cortical plate resorption (8.222-8.224). The patient's main request is not to have temporary edentulousness (even if the tooth is relatively posterior). Then the option of performing a post-extraction implant with immediate loading is evaluated. In order to increase the predictability of the intervention, a GOR is performed to increase the amount of hard and soft tissue.

In this case the lingual mechanics is limited to the upper left lateral sector only (Kurz 7th Generation®, Ormco). The patient undergoes monthly X-ray and periodontal checks. The extrusion steps are carried out in a sectorial lingual orthodontic mechanics, at first with a .016 β-titanium sectional wire with an uneven 1.5 mm position of the brackets on the 2.5 tooth (8.225-8.228), and subsequently with a rectangular .017×.017 β-titanium (8.229) with steps of 1 mm/month and an axial component along the major axis. The brackets is applied using a pre-treatment with hydrofluoric acid (HF) and then a silane on the tooth with successive apically repositioning. When the adhesion becomes unfeasible a band is applied, with a vestibulo-lingual inset bend to compensate the vestibulo-lingual root anatomy that is reduced when compared to the coronal, and also in order to center the root fragment in the alveolar ridge. Great attention is paid to the canine, the final mesial element of the sectional appliance which requires a root torque control (8.230). In 8.231 the monthly X-ray follow-up can be observed.

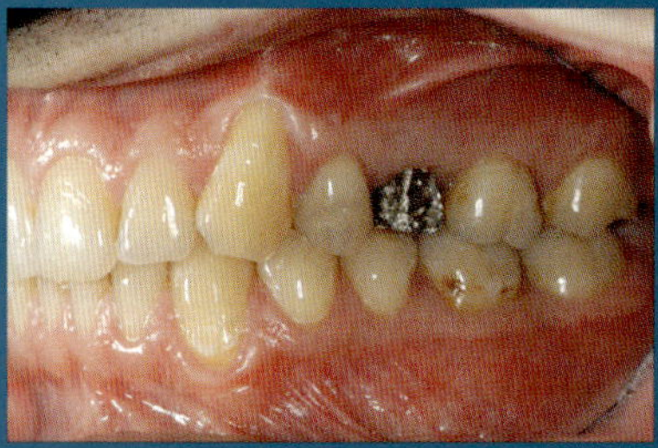

8.222 Vestibular intraoral view of 2.5.

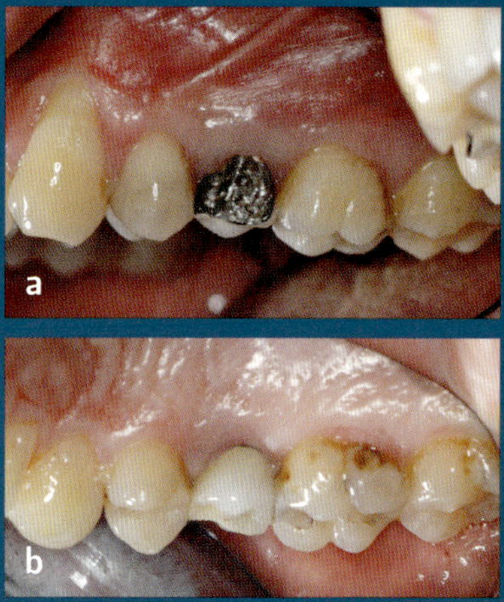

8.223 Intraoral view of 2.5. Vestibular and palatal view.

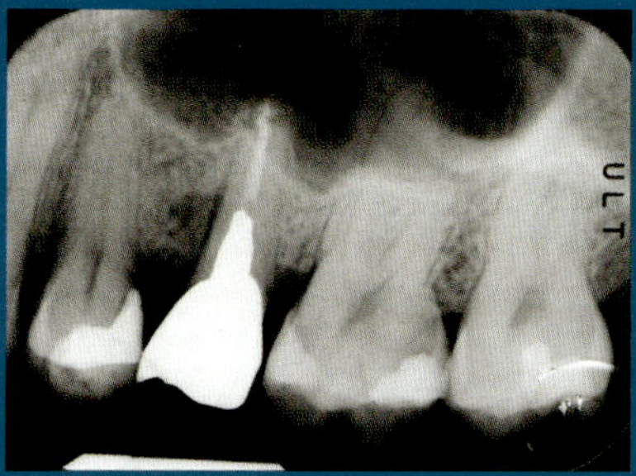

8.224 X-ray of 2.5 where the mesial bone defect due to the root fracture can be seen.

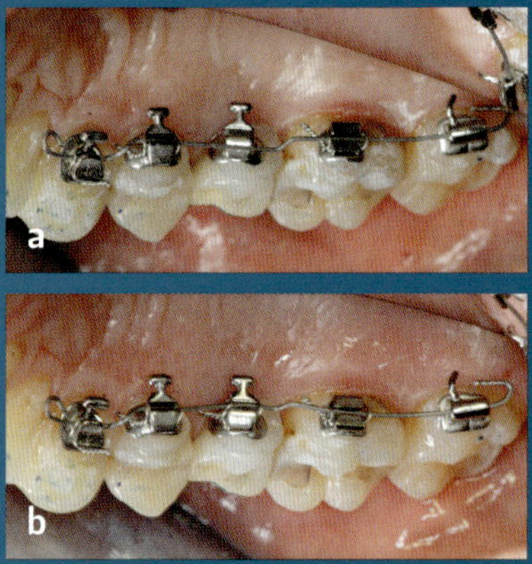

8.225 Lingual mechanics, .016 β-titanium sectional, extrusive steps.

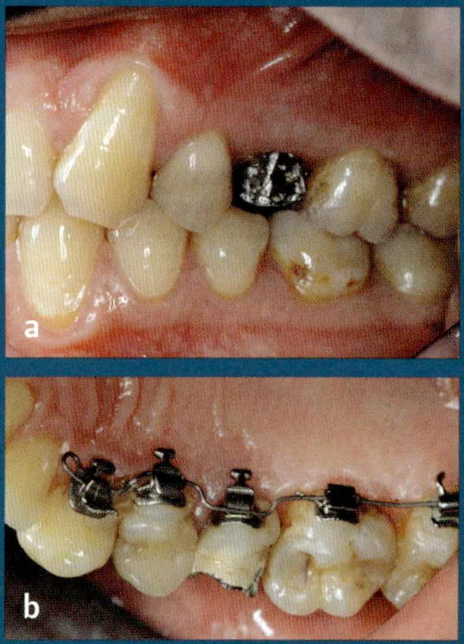

8.226 Lingual mechanics, .016 β-titanium sectional, extrusive steps, 1.5 mm activations.

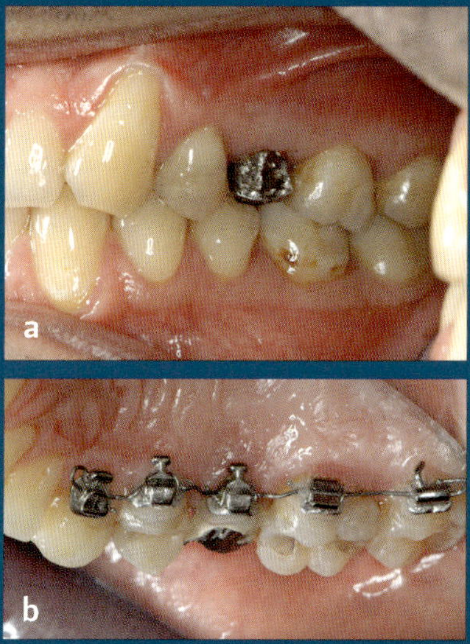

8.227 Lingual mechanics, .016 β-titanium sectional, extrusive steps.

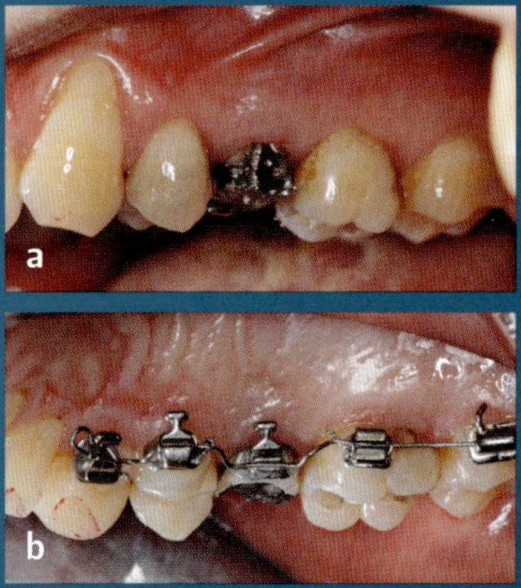

8.228 Lingual mechanics, .016 β-titanium sectional, extrusive steps, 1.5 mm activations.

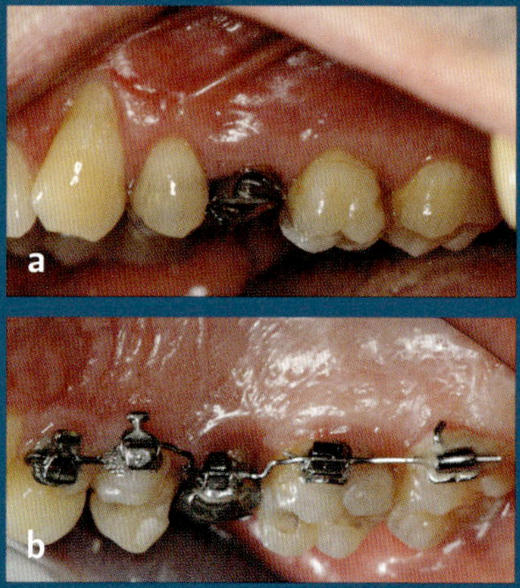

8.229 Lingual mechanics, .017x.017 β-titanium sectional, extrusive steps, 1.5 mm activations.

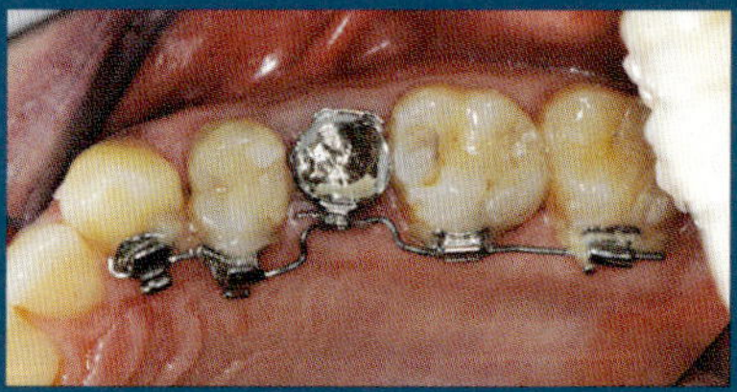

8.230 Lingual mechanics, .017x.017 β-titanium sectional, occlusal view, vestibulo-lingual inset bend to compensate the reduced vestibulo-lingual radicular anatomy with respect to the coronal one and to center the root fragment in the alveolar ridge.

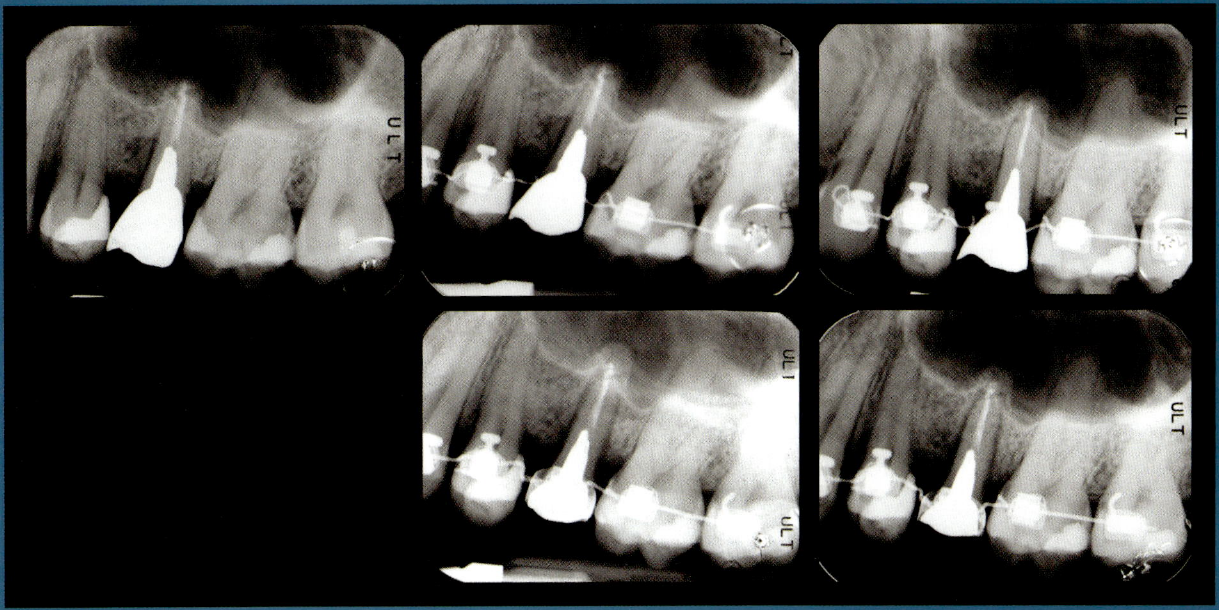

8.231 X-ray monthly follow-up.

At the end of the extrusion, the root fragment is extracted, minimizing the risk of fracture of the buccal cortical plate (8.232). With flapless technique[130] (8.233 and 8.234) the implant (4.5/15 mm Xive®, Dentsply) is placed with maxillary sinus elevation using osteotomes with the LMSF[131,132] technique (see 8.241a). After evaluating the primary stability, the immediate loading temporary crown is applied (8.235 and 8.236).

At the end of the tissue healing (8.237), the final cemented metal ceramic restoration is placed together with the restorations of the adjacent teeth (8.238). Clinical and X-ray follow-up at 1 year and 5 years can be seen in 8.239-8.241. In 8.242 the emergence profile of the peri-implant tissues at the 6-year follow-up can be seen.

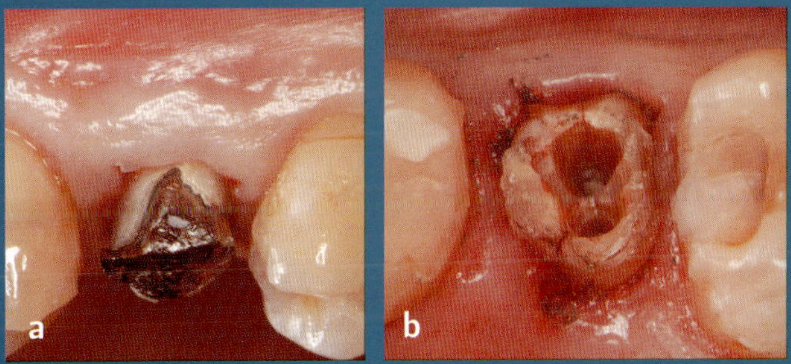

8.232 Detail of the root after extrusion (**a**); the removed post with the fracture line (**b**).

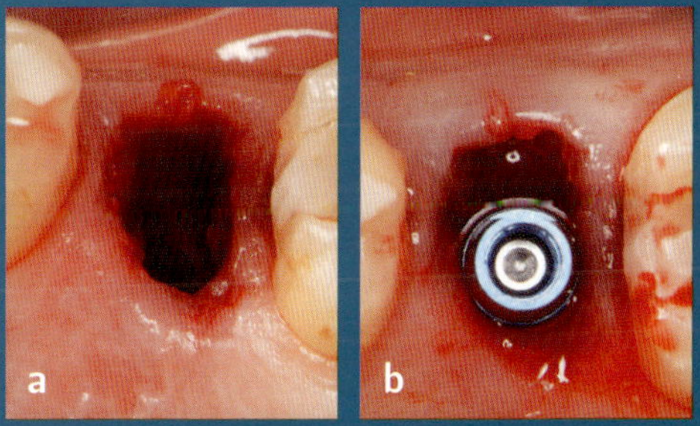

8.233 Post-extraction socket (**a**) and the implant just placed in the socket (**b**).

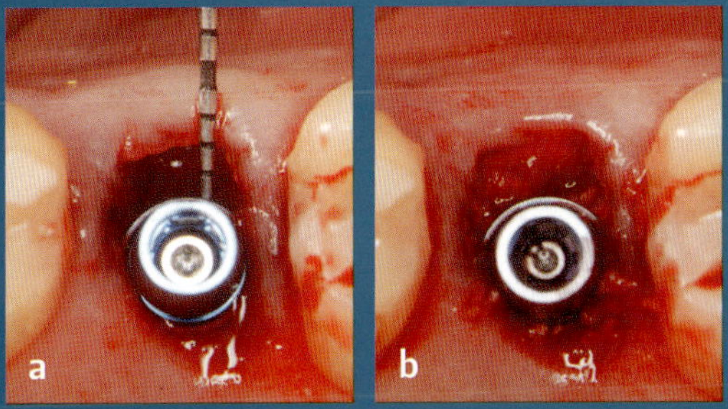

8.234 Measurement of the per-implant space (**a**) filled with the graft material (**b**).

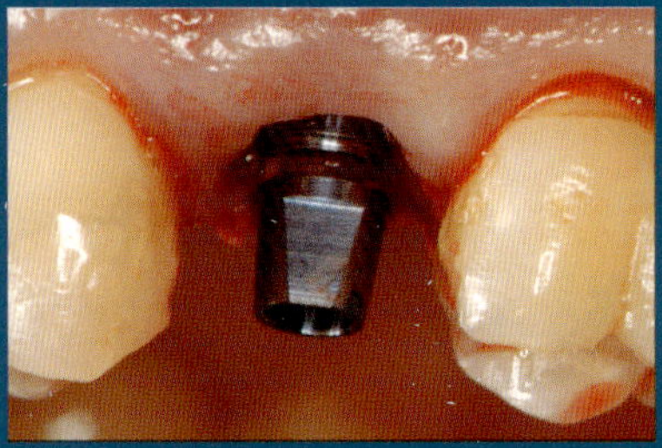

8.235 Temporary abutment for immediate loading in relationship with soft tissue.

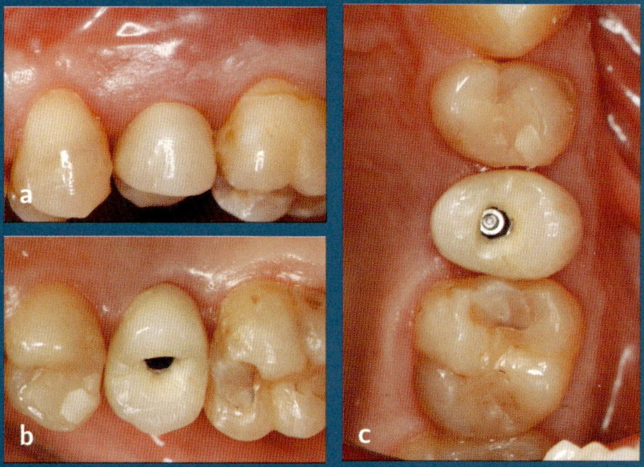

8.236 Temporary crown for immediate loading, just placed.

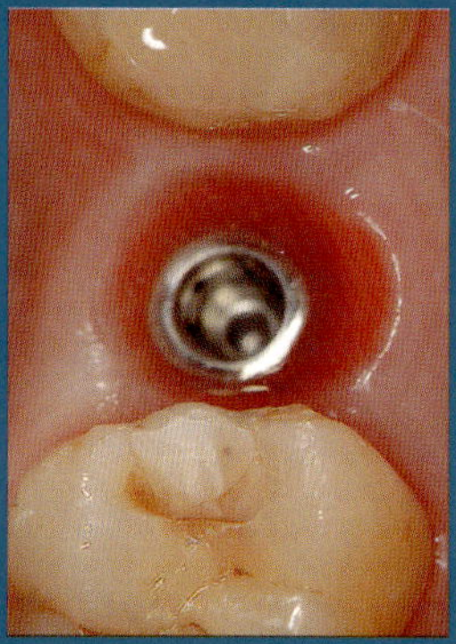

8.237 Soft tissue view before the definitive cementation after the maturation of the tissue.

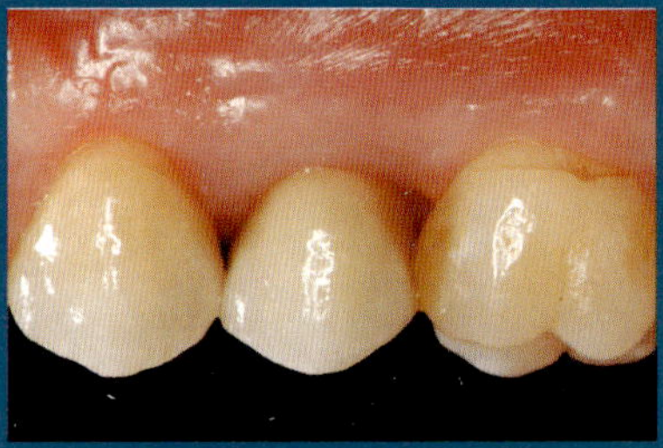

8.238 Vestibular view of the just cemented definitive crown.

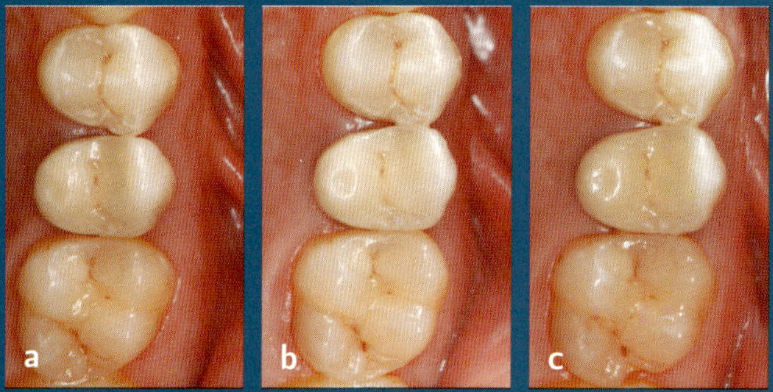

8.239 Occlusal view of the restoration (just cemented [**a**]; 1 year [**b**]; 5 years [**c**]).

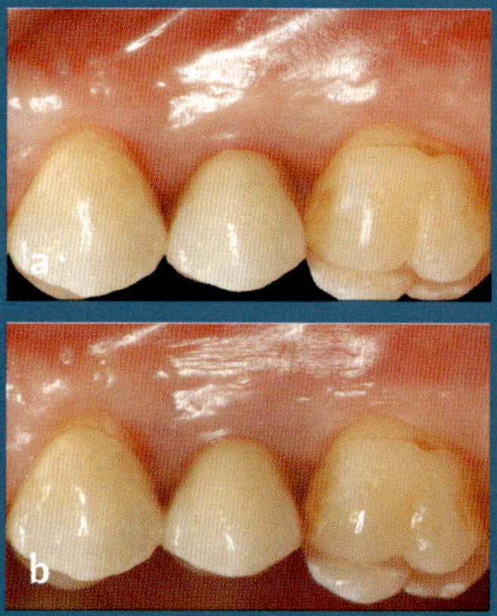

8.240 Vestibular follow-up (1 year [**a**]; 5 years [**b**]).

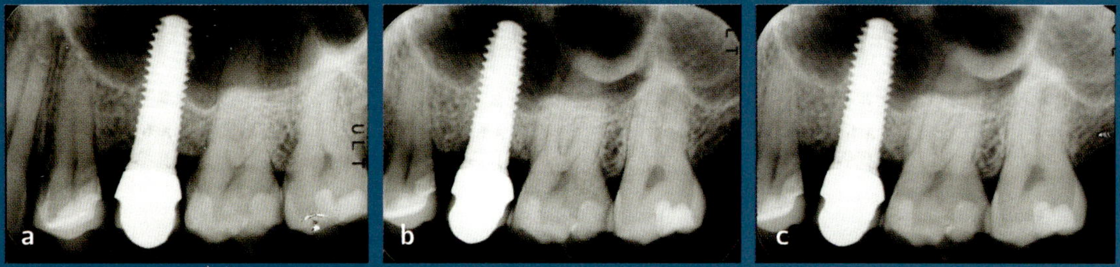

8.241 X-ray follow-up (just cemented [**a**]; 1 year [**b**]; 5 years [**c**]).

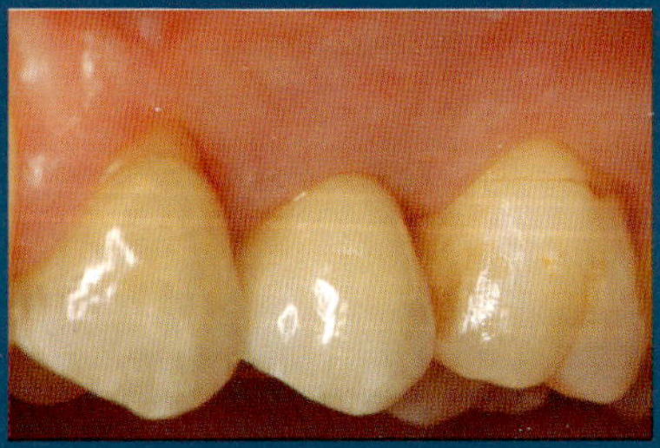

8.242 Soft tissue profile after 6 years.

REFERENCES

1. **Alsahhaf A, Att W.** Orthodontic extrusion for pre-implant site enhancement: Principles and clinical guidelines. *J Prosthodont Res.* 2016;60(3):145-155.
2. **Borzabadi-Farahani A, Zadeh HH.** *Orthodontic therapy in implant dentistry: orthodontic implant site development.* In: Tolstunov L. *Vertical alveolar ridge augmentation in implant dentistry. A surgical manual.* Hoboken, NewJersey. Wiley Blackwell; 2016:30-37.
3. **de Barros LA, de Almeida Cardoso M, de Avila ED et al.** Six-year follow-up of maxillary anterior rehabilitation with forced orthodontic extrusion: achieving esthetic excellence with a multidisciplinary approach. *Am J Orthod Dentofacial Orthop.* 2013;144(4):607-615.
4. **Heithersay GS.** Combined endodontic-orthodontic treatment of transverse root fractures in the region of the alveolar crest. *Oral Surg Oral Med Oral Pathol.* 1973;36(3):404-415.
5. **Brown IS.** The effect of orthodontic therapy on certain types of periodontal defects. I. Clinical findings. *J Periodontol.* 1973;44(12):742-756.
6. **Ingber JS.** Forced eruption. I. A method of treating isolated one and two wall infrabony osseous defects-rationale and case report. *J Periodontol.* 1974;45(4):199 206.
7. **Ingber JS.** Forced eruption: part II. A method of treating nonrestorable teeth - Periodontal and restorative considerations. *J Periodontol.* 1976;47(4):203-216.
8. **Magkavali-Trikka P, Kirmanidou Y, Michalakis K et al.** Efficacy of two site-development procedures for implants in the maxillary esthetic region: a systematic review. *Int J Oral Maxillofac Implants.* 2015;30(1):73-94.
9. **Reitan K.** Clinical and histologic observations on tooth movement during and after orthodontic treatment. *Am J Orthod.* 1967;53(10):721-745.
10. **van Venrooy JR, Yukna RA.** Orthodontic extrusion of single-rooted teeth affected with advanced periodontal disease. *Am J Orthod.* 1985;87(1):67-74.
11. **Hasson JN, Hasson B.** Implant site development by orthodontic forced eruption for esthetic restoration of adjacent implants. *Clin Adv Periodontics.* 2016;6(3):146-152.
12. **Ziskind D, Sharon E, Hirschfeld Z, Becker A.** Analysis of lateral tooth movement during forced orthodontic eruption. *J Prosthet Dent.* 2000; 84(4):462-466.
13. **Salama H, Garber DA, Salama MA et al.** Fifty years of interdisciplinary site development: lessons and guidelines from periodontal prosthesis. *J Esthet Dent.* 1998;10(3):149-156.
14. **Mirmarashi B, Torbati A, Aalam A, Chee W.** Orthodontically assisted vertical augmentation in the esthetic zone. *J Prosthodont.* 2010;19(3):235-239.
15. **Holst S, Hegenbarth EA, Schlegel KA, Holst AI.** Restoration of a nonrestorable central incisor using forced orthodontic eruption, immediate implant placement, and an all-ceramic restoration: a clinical report. *J Prosthet Dent.* 2007;98(4):251-255.
16. **Brindis MA, Block MS.** Orthodontic tooth extrusion to enhance soft tissue implant esthetics. *J Oral Maxillofac Surg.* 2009;67(Suppl 11):49-59.
17. **Pikdoken L, Erkan M, Usumez S.** Gingival response to mandibular incisor extrusion. *Am J Orthod Dentofacial Orthop.* 2009;135(4):432.e1-433.
18. **Kajiyama K, Murakami T, Yokota S.** Gingival reactions after experimentally induced extrusion of the upper incisors in monkeys. *Am J Orthod Dentofacial Orthop.* 1993;104(1):36-47.
19. **Paolone MG, Kaitsas R.** Orthodontic-periodontal interactions: orthodontic extrusion in interdisciplinary regenerative treatments. *Int Orthod.* 2018;16(2):217-245.
20. **Paolone MG, Kaitsas R, Paolone G, Kaitsas V.** Lingual orthodontics and forced eruption: a means for osseous and tissue regeneration. *Prog Orthod.* 2008;9(2):46-57.
21. **Kaitsas R, Paolone MG, Paolone G.** Guided orthodontic regeneration: A tool to enhance conventional regenerative techniques in implant surgery. *Int Orthod.* 2015;13(4):539-554.
22. **Jepsen S, Caton JG, Albandar JM et al.** Periodontal manifestations of systemic diseases and developmental and acquired conditions: Consensus report of workgroup 3 of the 2017 World Workshop on the Classification of Periodontal and Peri-Implant Diseases and Conditions. *J Clin Periodontol.* 2018;(Suppl 45)20:S219-S229.
23. **Fakhry A.** Enhancing restorative, periodontal, and esthetic outcomes through orthodontic extrusion. *Eur J Esthet Dent.* 2007;2(3):312-320.
24. **Durham TM, Goddard T, Morrison S.** Rapid forced eruption: a case report and review of forced eruption techniques. *Gen Dent.* 2004;52(2):167-176.
25. **Mihram WL, Murphy NC.** The orthodontist's role in 21st century periodontic-prosthodontic therapy. *Semin Orthod.* 2008;14(4):272-289.
26. **Heij DG, Opdebeeck H, van Steenberghe D et al.** Facial development, continuous tooth eruption, and mesial drift as compromising factors for implant placement. *Int J Oral Maxillofac Implants.* 2006;21(6):867-878.
27. **Op Heij DG, Opdebeeck H, van Steenberghe D, Quirynen M.** Age as compromising factor for implant insertion. *Periodontol 2000.* 2003;33(1):172-184.
28. **Oesterle LJ, Cronin RJ Jr.** Adult growth, aging, and the single-tooth implant. *Int J Oral Maxillofac Implants.* 2000;15(2):252-260.
29. **Borzabadi-Farahani A, Zadeh HH.** Adjunctive orthodontic applications in dental implantology. *J Oral Implantol.* 2015;41(4):501-508.
30. **Schwartz-Arad D, Levin L, Ashkenazi M.** Treatment options of untreatable traumatized anterior maxillary teeth for future use of dental implantation. *Implant Dent.* 2004;13(2):120-128.
31. **Potashnick SR, Rosenberg ES.** Forced eruption: principles in periodontics and restorative dentistry. *J Prosthet Dent.* 1982;48(2):141-148.
32. **Hamasni FM, Majzoub ZAK.** Effect of patient- and surgery-related factors on supracrestal tissue reestablishment after crown lengthening procedure. *Quintessence Int.* 2019;50(10):792-801.
33. **Zenóbio EG, Moreira RC, Soares RV et al.** A mixed-model study assessing orthodontic tooth extrusion for the reestablishment of biologic width. A systematic review and exploratory randomized trial. *Int J Periodontics Restorative Dent.* 2015;35(1):19-27.

34. Biggerstaff RH, Sinks JH, Carazola JL. Orthodontic extrusion and biologic width realignment procedures: methods for reclaiming nonrestorable teeth. *J Am Dent Assoc.* 1986;112(3):345-348.

35. Pontoriero R, Celenza F Jr, Ricci G, Carnevale G. Rapid extrusion with fiber resection: a combined orthodontic-periodontic treatment modality. *Int J Periodontics Restorative Dent.* 1987;7(5):30-43.

36. da Silva VC, de Molon RS, Martins RP et al. Effects of orthodontic tooth extrusion produced by different techniques, on the periodontal tissues: a histological study in dogs. *Arch Oral Biol.* 2020;116:104768.

37. Schwimer CW, Rosenberg ES, Schwimer DH. Rapid extrusion with fiberotomy. *J Esthet Dent.* 1990;2(3):82-88.

38. Kozlovsky A, Tal H, Lieberman M. Forced eruption combined with gingival fiberotomy. A technique for clinical crown lengthening. *J Clin Periodontol.* 1988;15(9):534-538.

39. Levine HL, Stahl SS. Repair following periodontal flap surgery with the retention of gingival fibers. *J Periodontol.* 1972;43(2):99-103.

40. Carvalho CV, Bauer FP, Romito GA et al. Orthodontic extrusion with or without circumferential supracrestal fiberotomy and root planing. *Int J Periodontics Restorative Dent.* 2006;26(1):87-93.

41. Bach N, Baylard JF, Voyer R. Orthodontic extrusion: periodontal considerations and applications. *J Can Dent Assoc.* 2004;70(11):775-780.

42. Ngan P, Knobloch L. Multidisciplinary and esthetic approach to clinical crown lengthening: report of a case. *Quintessence Int.* 1993;24(12):835-839.

43. Malmgren O, Malmgren B, Frykholm A. Rapid orthodontic extrusion of crown root and cervical root fractured teeth. *Endod Dent Traumatol.* 1991;7(2):49-54.

44. Addy LD, Durning P, Thomas MB, McLaughlin WS. Orthodontic extrusion: an interdisciplinary approach to patient management. *Dent Update.* 2009;36(4):212-218.

45. Kim SH, Tramontina VA, Papalexiou V, Luczyszyn SM. Orthodontic extrusion and implant site development using an interocclusal appliance for a severe mucogingival deformity: a clinical report. *J Prosthet Dent.* 2011;105(2):72-77.

46. Koyuturk AE, Malkoc S. Orthodontic extrusion of subgingivally fractured incisor before restoration. A case report: 3-years follow-up. *Dent Traumatol.* 2005;21(3):174-178.

47. Roth A, Yildirim M, Diedrich P. Forced eruption with microscrew anchorage for preprosthetic leveling of the gingival margin. Case report. *J Orofac Orthop.* 2004;65(6):513-519.

48. Brown GJ, Welbury RR. Root extrusion, a practical solution in complicated crown-root incisor fractures. *Br Dent J.* 2000;189(9):477-478.

49. Ivey DW, Calhoun RL, Kemp WB et al. Orthodontic extrusion: its use in restorative dentistry. *J Prosthet Dent.* 1980;43(4):401-407.

50. Kwon EY, Lee JY, Choi J. Effect of slow forced eruption on the vertical levels of the interproximal bone and papilla and the width of the alveolar ridge. *Korean J Orthod.* 2016;46(6):379-385.

51. Wehr C, Roth A, Gustav M, Diedrich P. Forced eruption for preservation of a deeply fractured molar. *J Orofac Orthop.* 2004;65(4):343-354.

52. Reichert C, Hagner M, Jepsen S, Jäger A. Interfaces between orthodontic and periodontal treatment: their current status. *J Orofac Orthop.* 2011;72(3):165-186.

53. Gölz L, Reichert C, Dirk C, Jäger A. Retrospective investigation of gingival invaginations: Part II: microbiological findings and genetic risk profile. *J Orofac Orthop.* 2012;73(5):387-396.

54. Robertson P, Schultz L, Levy B. Occurrence and distribution of interdental gingival clefts following orthodontic movement into bicuspid extraction sites. *J Periodontol.* 1977;48(4):232-235.

55. Diedrich P, Fritz U, Kinzinger G. Interrelationship between periodontics and adult orthodontics. *J Periodontol.* 2004;1(3):143-149.

56. Janson M, Janson G, Murillo-Goizueta OE. A modified orthodontic protocol for advanced periodontal disease in Class II division 1 malocclusion. *Am J Orthod Dentofacial Orthop.* 2011;139(4 Suppl):S133-S144.

57. Soolari A, Erickson D, Soolari A. Orthodontic forced eruption: a team approach in aesthetic treatment. *Dent Today.* 2014;33(7):112-117.

58. Capri D, Albehbehani Y, Smukler H. Augmentation of an anterior edentulous ridge for fixed prosthodontics with combined use of orthodontics and surgery: a clinical report. *J Prosthet Dent.* 2003;90(2):111-115.

59. Bertl K, Neuner H, Meran A et al. Does the time-point of orthodontic space closure initiation after tooth extraction affect the incidence of gingival cleft development? A randomized controlled clinical trial. *J Periodontol.* 2020;91(5):572-581.

60. Zere E, Einy S, Asbi T et al. Orthodontic extraction space closure with and without socket preservation: a comparative case analysis. *Quintessence Int.* 2019;50(4):306-314.

61. Stappert D, Geiman R, Zadi ZH, Reynolds MA. Gingival clefts revisited: Evaluation of the characteristics that make one more susceptible to gingival clefts. *Am J Orthod Dentofacial Orthop.* 2018;154(5):677-682.

62. Reichert C, Götz W, Smeets R et al. The impact of nonautogenous bone graft on orthodontic treatment. *Quintessence Int.* 2010;41(8):665-672.

63. Pinheiro ML, Moreira TC, Feres-Filho EJ. Guided bone regeneration of a pronounced gingivo-alveolar cleft due to orthodontic space closure. *J Periodontol.* 2006;77(6):1091-1095.

64. Carvalho RS, Nelson D, Kelderman H, Wise R. Guided bone regeneration to repair an osseous defect. *Am J Orthod Dentofacial Orthop.* 2003;123(4):455-467.

65. Tiefengraber J, Diedrich P, Fritz U, Lantos P. Orthodontic space closure in combination with membrane supported healing of extraction sockets (MHE) a pilot study. *J Orofac Orthop.* 2002;63(5):422-428.

66. Mayer T, Basdra EK, Komposch G, Staehle HJ. Localized alveolar ridge augmentation before orthodontic treatment. A case report. *Int J Oral Maxillofac Surg.* 1994;23(4):226-228.

67. Rivera Circuns AL, Tulloch JF. Gingival invagination in extraction sites of orthodontic patients: their incidence, effects on periodontal health,

and orthodontic treatment. *Am J Orthod.* 1983;83(6):469-476.

68. **Reichert C, Gölz L, Dirk C, Jäger A.** Retrospective investigation of gingival invaginations: Part I: Clinical findings and presentation of a coding system. *J Orofac Orthop.* 2012;73(4):307-316.

69. **Diedrich P, Wehrbein H.** Orthodontic retraction into recent and healed extraction sites. A histologic study. *J Orofac Orthop.* 1997;58(2):90-99.

70. **Rönnerman A, Thilander B, Heyden G.** Gingival tissue reactions to orthodontic closure of extraction sites. Histologic and histochemical studies. *Am J Orthod.* 1980;77(6):620-625.

71. **Helm S, Petersen PE.** Causal relation between malocclusion and periodontal health. *Acta Odontol Scand.* 1989;47(4):223-228.

72. **Gölz L, Reichert C, Jäger A.** Gingival invagination - A systematic review. *J Orofac Orthop.* 2011;72(6):409-420.

73. **Van der Weijden F, Dell'Acqua F, Slot DE.** Alveolar bone dimensional changes of post-extraction sockets in humans: a systematic review. *J Clin Periodontol.* 2009;36(12):1048-1058.

74. **Araújo MG, Lindhe J.** Dimensional ridge alterations following tooth extraction. An experimental study in the dog. *J Clin Periodontol.* 2005;32(2):212-218.

75. **Wehrbein H, Bauer W, Diedrich PR.** Gingival invagination area after space closure: a histologic study. *Am J Orthod Dentofacial Orthop.* 1995;108(6):593-598.

76. **Tolstunov L, Hamrick JFE, Broumand V et al.** Bone augmentation techniques for horizontal and vertical alveolar ridge deficiency in oral implantology. *Oral Maxillofac Surg Clin North Am.* 2019;31(2):163-191.

77. **Esposito M, Grusovin MG, Felice P et al.** The efficacy of horizontal and vertical bone augmentation procedures for dental implants - A Cochrane systematic review. *Eur J Oral Implantol.* 2009;2(3):167-184.

78. **Butler B, Kinzer GA.** Managing esthetic implant complications. *Compend Contin Educ Dent.* 2012;33(7):514-522.

79. **Tondelli PM, Kay FA, Kuabara MR.** Orthodontic extrusion as an aid in oral rehabilitation. *Oral Health Dent Manag.* 2014;13(2):223-228.

80. **Somar M, Mohadeb JV, Huang C.** Predictability of orthodontic forced eruption in developing an implant site: a systematic review. *J Clin Orthod.* 2016;50(8):485-492.

81. **Salama H, Salama M.** The role of orthodontic extrusive remodeling in the enhancement of soft and hard tissue profiles prior to implant placement: a systematic approach to the management of extraction site defects. *Int J Periodontics Restorative Dent.* 1993;13(4):312-333.

82. **Mantzikos T, Shamus I.** Forced eruption and implant site development: an osteophysiologic response. *Am J Orthod Dentofacial Orthop.* 1999;115(5):583-591.

83. **Zachrisson BU.** JCO/interviews Dr. Bjorn U. Zachrisson on excellence in finishing. Part 2. *J Clin Orthod.* 1986;20(8):536-556.

84. **Mantzikos T, Shamus I.** Case report: forced eruption and implant site development. *Angle Orthod.* 1998;68(2):179-186.

85. **Mantzikos T, Shamus I.** Forced eruption and implant site development: soft tissue response. *Am J Orthod Dentofacial Orthop.* 1997;112(6):596-606.

86. **Celenza F.** The development of forced eruption as a modality for implant site enhancement. *Alpha Omegan.* 1997;90(2):40-43.

87. **Papadopoulou AK, Papageorgiou SN, Hatzopoulos SA et al.** Alveolar ridge alterations in the maxillary anterior region after tooth extraction through orthodontic forced eruption for implant site development: a clinical CBCT study. *Eur J Orthod.* 2020;42(3):295-304.

88. **Amato F, Mirabella AD, Macca U, Tarnow DP.** Implant site development by orthodontic forced extraction: a preliminary study. *Int J Oral Maxillofac Implants.* 2012;27(2):411-420.

89. **Conserva E, Fadda M, Ferrari V, Consolo U.** Predictability of a new orthodontic extrusion technique for implant site development: a retrospective consecutive case-series study. *Scientific World Journal.* 2020;2020:4576748.

90. **Hochman MN, Chu SJ, Tarnow DP.** Orthodontic extrusion for implant site development revisited: A new classification determined by anatomy and clinical outcomes. *Semin Orthod.* 2014;20(3):208-227.

91. **Kan JY, Kim YJ, Rungcharassaeng K, Kois JC.** Accuracy of bone sounding in assessing facial osseous-gingival tissue relationship in maxillary anterior teeth. *Int J Periodontics Restorative Dent.* 2017;37(3):371-375.

92. **Kois JC.** The restorative-periodontal interface: biological parameters. *Periodontol 2000.* 1996;11(1):29-38.

93. **Korayem M, Flores-Mir C, Nassar U, Olfert K.** Implant site development by orthodontic extrusion. A systematic review. *Angle Orthod.* 2008;78(4):752-760.

94. **Bauer C, Boileau MJ, Bazert C.** Implementation of orthodontic extraction for pre-implant soft tissue management: a systematic review. *Int Orthod.* 2019;17(1):20-37.

95. **Zuccati G, Bocchieri A.** Implant site development by orthodontic extrusion of teeth with poor prognosis. *J Clin Orthod.* 2003;37(6):307-313.

96. **Joo JY, Son S, Lee JY.** Implant site development for enhancing esthetics of soft and hard tissue and simplification of implant surgery using a forced eruption. *Int J Periodontics Restorative Dent.* 2016;36(4):583-589.

97. **González López S, Olmedo Gaya MV, Vallecillo Capilla M.** Esthetic restoration with orthodontic traction and single-tooth implant: case report. *Int J Periodontics Restorative Dent.* 2005;25(3):239-245.

98. **Chou YH, Du JK, Chou ST et al.** An interdisciplinary treatment approach combining orthodontic forced eruption with immediate implant placement to achieve a satisfactory treatment outcome: a case report. *Clin Implant Dent Relat Res.* 2013;15(1):113-120.

99. **Hayashi J, Shin K.** Implant site development by orthodontic extrusion and buccal root torque at a site showing severe gingival recession with periodontitis: a case report. *Int J Periodontics Restorative Dent.* 2019;39(4):589-594.

100. **Nozawa T, Sugiyama T, Yamaguchi S et al.** Buccal and coronal bone augmentation using forced eruption and buccal root torque: a case report. *Int J Periodontics Restorative Dent.* 2003;23(6):585-591.

101. **Uribe F, Taylor T, Shafer D, Nanda R.** A novel approach for implant site development through root tipping. *Am J Orthod Dentofacial Orthop.* 2010;138(5):649-655.

102. **Hinds KF.** Alveolar ridge development with forced eruption and distraction of retained natural dentition. *Oral Maxillofac Surg Clin North Am.* 2004;16(1):75-89.

103. **Watanabe T, Marchack BW, Takei HH.** Creating labial bone for immediate implant placement: a minimally invasive approach by using orthodontic therapy in the esthetic zone. *J Prosthet Dent.* 2013;110(6):435-441.

104. **Holst AI, Nkenke E, Blatz MB et al.** Prosthetic considerations for orthodontic implant site development in the adult patient. *J Oral Maxillofac Surg.* 2009;67(11 Suppl):82-88.

105. **Rokn AR, Saffarpour A, Sadrimanesh R et al.** Implant site development by orthodontic forced eruption of nontreatable teeth: a case report. *Open Dent J.* 2012;6:99-104.

106. **Lee EA.** Tridimensional reconstruction of a complex iatrogenic defect using orthodontic forced eruption and minimally invasive bone grafting. *Compend Contin Educ Dent.* 2017;38(7):447-456.

107. **Erkut S, Arman A, Gulsahi A et al.** Forced eruption and implant treatment in posterior maxilla: a clinical report. *J Prosthet Dent.* 2007;97(2):70-74.

108. **Paolone MG, Kaitsas R, Kaitsas F.** Lingual orthodontics in an adult patient with upper premolar extraction: Case report. *Int Orthod.* 2020;18(1):165-177.

109. **Park JH, Shin SW, Lee JY.** Two-step immediate loading of mandibular overdentures retained by mini-implants: a prospective clinical study. *Int J Prosthodont.* 2018;31(5):446-450.

110. **Chambrone L, Chambrone LA.** Forced orthodontic eruption of fractured teeth before implant placement: case report. *J Can Dent Assoc.* 2005;71(4):257-261.

111. **Keceli HG, Guncu MB, Atalay Z, Evginer MS.** Forced eruption and implant site development in the aesthetic zone: a case report. *Eur J Dent.* 2014;8(2):269-275.

112. **Proffit WR.** *Contemporary Orthodontics.* 6th ed., Philadelphia: Elsevier; 2019.

113. **Minsk L.** Orthodontic tooth extrusion as an adjunct to periodontal therapy. *Compend Contin Educ Dent.* 2000; 21(9):768-770.

114. **Garlock DT, Buschang PH, Araujo EA et al.** Evaluation of marginal alveolar bone in the anterior mandible with pretreatment and posttreatment computed tomography in nonextraction patients. *Am J Orthod Dentofacial Orthop.* 2016;149(2):192-201.

115. **Buskin R, Castellon P, Hochstedler JL.** Orthodontic extrusion and orthodontic extraction in preprosthetic treatment using implant therapy. *Pract Periodontics Aesthet Dent.* 2000;12(2):213-220.

116. **de Molon RS, de Avila ED, de Souza JA et al.** Forced orthodontic eruption for augmentation of soft and hard tissue prior to implant placement. *Contemp Clin Dent.* 2013;4(2):243-247.

117. **Ribeiro G, Maciel J, Pereira J, Tanaka O.** Forced eruption for all four maxillary incisors prior to implant rehabilitation. *Eur J Gen Dent.* 2012;1(2):99-103.

118. **Braga G, Bocchieri A.** A new flapless technique for crown lengthening after orthodontic extrusion. *Int J Periodontics Restorative Dent.* 2012;32(1):81-90.

119. **Rasner SL.** Orthodontic extrusion: an adjunct to implant treatment. *Dent Today.* 2011;30(3):104-109.

120. **Fadda M, Cortesi R.** Estrusione ortodontica preprotesica: un metodo semplice per sviluppare il sito implantare. *Ortodonzia Clinica.* 2009;2(1):21-29.

121. **Owman-Moll P.** Orthodontic tooth movement and root resorption with special reference to force magnitude and duration. A clinical and histological investigation in adolescents. *Swed Dent J Suppl.* 1995;105:1-45.

122. **Turley PK, Joiner MW, Hellstrom S.** The effect of orthodontic extrusion on traumatically intruded teeth. *Am J Orthod.* 1984;85(1):47-56.

123. **Von Böhl M, Maltha J, Von den Hoff H, Kuijpers-Jagtman AM.** Changes in the periodontal ligament after experimental tooth movement using high and low continuous forces in beagle dogs. *Angle Orthod.* 2004;74(1):16-25.

124. **Sterr N, Becker A.** Forced eruption: biological and clinical considerations. *J Oral Rehabil.* 1980;7(5):395-402.

125. **Paolone MG, Kaitsas V.** I materiali dell'ortodonzia. *Il Dentista Moderno.* 1992;(Suppl 8):33-42.

126. **Hiro T, Iglesia FD, Andreu P.** Indirect bonding technique in lingual orthodontics: the HIRO system. *Prog Orthod.* 2008;9(2):34-45.

127. **Tinti C, Benfenati SP.** The ramp mattress suture: a new suturing technique combined with a surgical procedure to obtain papillae between implants in the buccal area. *Int J Periodontics Restorative Dent.* 2002;22(1):63-69.

128. **Kaitsas R, Alfonsi F.** *Lembi e suture.* In: Barone A, Bianchi E. *Manuale di chirurgia orale.* Milano: Elsevier Masson; 2011:213-269.

129. **Bassetti RG, Stähli A, Bassetti MA, Sculean A.** Soft tissue augmentation procedures at second-stage surgery: a systematic review. *Clin Oral Investig.* 2016;20(7):1369-1387.

130. **Divakar TK, Gidean Arularasan S, Baskaran M et al.** Clinical evaluation of placement of implant by flapless technique over conventional flap technique. *J Maxillofac Oral Surg.* 2020;19(1):74-84.

131. **Bruschi GB, Crespi R, Capparè P et al.** Localized management of sinus floor technique for implant placement in fresh molar sockets. *Clin Implant Dent Relat Res.* 2013;15(2):243-250.

132. **Bruschi GB, Scipioni A, Calesini G, Bruschi E.** Localized management of sinus floor with simultaneous implant placement: a clinical report. *Int J Oral Maxillofac Implants.* 1998;13(2):219-226.

Ortho–perio timing

Introduction

Patients that need combined ortho-periodontal treatments need a synergic action among specialties. The main questions are: 1) at what stage of periodontal treatment can orthodontic treatment take place? 2) When is it the best time for orthodontics to be started after surgery? 3) Should different orthodontic timing and approaches be foreseen according to the various types of surgery? 4) How can orthodontics and periodontology be coordinated? 5) Can surgery be reduced or avoided with orthodontic therapy and, therefore, can orthodontics forego surgical treatment?

The timing of the orthodontic treatment of the patient undergoing active periodontal therapy is a topic where the available literature is still small. While many clinicians agree that orthodontic movement should begin after the end of active periodontal therapy, there is no real protocol that can be applied to the ortho-perio patient[1] and various studies suggest that orthodontic movement may have an impact on the morphology of the bone defect, reduce pocket depth, improve connective tissue healing[1] and modify the surgical approach. Historically, several Authors have analysed the feasibility of orthodontic movement after periodontal surgery. There are many histological studies on animals. Nemcovsky et al.[2,3] and Murakami et al.[4] described the benefits of orthodontic movement in rats started 1 week after surgery in experimentally created periodontal defects, demonstrating positive effects on the stop of epithelial apical growth, reduction of pocket depth and improvement of defects bone healing. Positive effects were observed on the formation of new attachment without damaging effects on the periodontium after early movement[5], even after regenerative therapy[7]. Therefore, the orthodontic tooth movement has no negative effects on the periodontium, if started immediately after periodontal surgery or before the complete healing of the periodontal wound. Clinically, in humans, the literature has analysed orthodontic movement started 7-10 days after periodontal surgery[6-9], showing successful results whereby patients with chronic periodontitis and angular defects on migrated incisors[6] had stable effects on periodontal health and on the level of the interdental papilla, with clinical periodontal attachment gain[7]. The feasibility of orthodontic treatment after periodontal surgery requires an analysis of the timing of the orthodontic movement in relation to the various types of periodontal surgery.

Surgical timing

After performing periodontal surgery, it is necessary to understand whether it is appropriate to undertake orthodontic treatment immediately or whether it is better to wait for the surgical wound to heal. In the absence of tooth movement, complete histological healing of the periodontal wound can be observed 3-6 months after conservative surgical therapy[10] and 12 months after regenerative surgical therapy[11]. Literature is not univocal about the protocol of when it is better to start orthodontic movement after periodontal surgery, ranging from 7 days up to 1 year[12]. It is not even well defined and clear how the surgical mechanisms of osteoinduction have synergic effects with orthodontic movement[13]. What it is sure is that orthodontic movement tends to increase the mitotic activity of the cells of the periodontal ligament[14]. Some Authors[15], however, have discouraged early movement, because healing of the reparative wound establishes an unfavourable condition for orthodontic movements of intrusion and translation [15]. After an appropriate periodontal surgical therapy has been performed, other Authors[16] state that teeth can be moved in the intrabony defects achieving in one single time the closure of the space and the radiological filling of the defect, the reduction of the probing depth and the gain of the clinical attachment level[16]. In the following pages we will analyse the data reported by the literature for what concerns timing in relation to the various types of periodontal surgery.

Conservative surgery and bone surgery

Concerning open flaps, many Authors advise not to wait for healing before starting orthodontic treatment[17]. Various case reports have described the start of the orthodontic movement 10 days after open flap debridment[18] up to 4 months[19].

The matter changes when we take into consideration bone surgery, either corrective during the open flap surgery, or resective, because these techniques could have a partial contraindication, due to the fact that the extension of bone removal with surgery can be reduced and therefore improved by the bone remodeling process induced by the orthodontic movement, which can have a positive influence on the bone topography[15]. In fact, often periodontal defects that initially require surgery may become non-surgical after orthodontic treatment[20]. This consideration is valid in the esthetic area too. The individual segmental extrusion of the teeth, through the bone level guided movement (as we have seen in Chapter 6), can modify the morphology of the defect, create physiological bone and gingival topography, preserve the greatest amount of periodontal attachment available and therefore prepare the patient for long-term maintenance[21] without reducing, or even performing, osteoplasty and/or ostectomy surgery. Thus, orthodontic treatment can reduce the extent of removal of healthy bone for resective surgery by levelling and aligning the teeth to re-establish a new alveolar ridge topography[15] and improve bone development[13].

Regenerative surgery

The application of light orthodontic force stimulates bone apposition and promotes repair of the periodontal lesion[22]. Therefore, the orthodontic movement would aim to facilitate healing. However, when the treatment plan foresees a periodontal regenerative surgery, it is necessary to program the clinical sequence: is it convenient to perform the surgery before the orthodontic movement or vice versa? Can orthodontics change the defect environment to improve the predictability of surgery so that must tooth movement be performed before? Or, if GTR is performed earlier, when should the orthodontic movement start (*early movement* or *after healing*)? Can the bone graft placed into the defect create problems to the movement itself?

FIRST GTR OR FIRST ORTHODONTICS?

The sequence of procedures, in the lack of scientific evidence, is mainly based on personal clinical experience[23]. Some clinicians agree with orthodontic movement started immediately after initial periodontal therapy even in the presence of severe periodontal disease. These Authors justify this clinical approach by stating that, bringing the roots closer together, the defect can be modified making it narrower, facilitating the regenerative treatment and its prognosis. Improving the dental position in the early stages of treatment also increases the patient's compliance to hygiene care; this reality is also encouraged by the esthetic change[17], and the tooth movement creates a better predictability of the surgical technique itself[24,25]. Some Authors suggest that intrusion can deepen the bone defect improving vascularization and creating better conditions for the predictability of GTR[26] (as already described in Chapter 5, paragraph *Intrusive movements*). Rabie et al.[25] used intrusive movement before regenerative surgery to modify the anatomy of the defect changing a suprabony defect into an intrabony defect that could be regenerated with surgical therapy (see 5.5). These Authors justify this approach stating that, in their opinion, early alignment incorporates a greater portion of the root within the bone, increases the crown/root ratio, modifies a horizontal defect in a vertical one and increases vascularization in the defect, increasing the regenerative response during bone regeneration. Cao et al.[27], starting from a suprabony defect, using an intrusion movement associated with supracrestal circumferential fibrotomy, created an intrabony defect which then they regenerated by GTR showing, in their opinion, that the orthodontic movement before surgery can improve some types of periodontal defects.

The opposite approach involves periodontal surgery before that orthodontic movement begins. This leads to a reduction of periodontal problems before orthodontic treatment and better results of the regenerative treatment. The positive effect of GTR on the bone makes the adaptation of soft tissues easier, reducing the size of the "black triangles" and the papilla reconstruction with the root approaching. This movement, when performed before the regenerative surgery, can reduce the blood support to the papilla and make tissue manipulation difficult[17]. In vertical bone defects, the orthodontic movement performed after the regenerative treatment allows the tooth to move into a satisfactory bone environment[28]. Positive results of orthodontic movement after GTR have been confirmed by clinical reports with surgical re-entry[29]. For what concerns cases that require intrusion, there are no clear indications for the timing of the GTR. Some case reports state that GTR surgical procedures prior to intrusion lead to new bone formation and attachment gain[29-31]. The main concept behind the surgery before orthodontic movement is to obtain regeneration (with the formation of new cement, new fibers, new alveolar bone) and not a repair (with the formation of long junctional epithelium, connective repair, partial bone formation)[1,32]. GTR procedures, according to Vanarsdall[21], when they are necessary to recreate a new periodontal attachment on the root, must always precede the tooth orthodontic movement and should be part of the initial therapy before starting the active orthodontic treatment.

EARLY MOVEMENT – AFTER HEALING

In literature there are various controversies regarding the relationship between the timing of orthodontics in relation to the regenerative surgery[24,31,33,34]. In the case of surgical regenerative techniques, the beginning of orthodontic movement could influence the regenerative result[21]. As a consequence, two approaches are taken into consideration: *early movement*, which begins according to several Authors from 10 days to 4 months after surgery to create favorable conditions for orthodontics[29,31,33,35-37] and the approach to start movement when healing has occurred (*after healing*)[23,28,36,38,39]. Regarding the immediate approach, some clinical studies[34,37] have shown excellent results with orthodontic treatment started 10-14 days after regenerative surgery, without showing side effects on regeneration, with new bone formation on the scaled root surface[40]. The choice of 14 days is also due to the fact that the realignment of the tooth at an early stage of the surgical wound healing determines a more favourable anatomical environment for the healing of hard and soft tissues, resulting in a complete filling of the interdental papilla, reduction of the probing, radiographic bone filling, tooth realignment and esthetic improvement[37,41]. The positive effects may justify the clinical choice that tooth movement in the regenerated areas can be performed without detrimental effects on the new level of periodontal support apparatus[16]. Within 4 weeks[32] the mitotic activity of periodontal cells is increased and the orthodontic movement occurs in immature bone, justifying the early starting of the orthodontic movement[42,43], up to 6 weeks, when the interaction between healing and remodeling with the orthodontic movement could lead to an additional attachment gain[15]. Attia et al.[44,45], evaluating the efficacy of various timing plans for the beginning of active orthodontic treatment after GTR, suggest that significant improvements in periodontal regeneration can be observed after 1 year in defects treated with immediate application of orthodontic forces after surgery. Diedrich et al.[32], starting the movement 1 month after GTR, showed histologically regeneration in animals with extensive cementoneogenesis and osteoneogenesis. After 6 months, the experimental bone pockets were no longer detectable after orthodontics and substantial cement and bone formation were observed. Hence, regenerative periodontal procedures provide favorable pre-conditions for tooth movement. In addition, this neo-apposition of connective fibers also improves dental intrusion/extrusion movements, because the new supracrestal and periodontal fibers transmit orthodontic forces by stimulating the alveolar bone[15]. In the presence of a membrane, according to some authors[17], the tooth movement should not start before the beginning of the resorption of the membrane and the maturation of the soft tissue above the site to be regenerated. Starting the orthodontic movement too early could accelerate the resorption of the resorbable membrane and jeopardize the regenerative result.

Some Authors prefer the *after healing* approach. Jepsen et al.[38] started orthodontic treatment 1 year after GTR; Maeda et al.[39], after 16 months. Ghezzi et al.[36] state that orthodontic treatment, carried out 1 year after GTR, after hard and soft tissues are mature, does not affect the results of periodontal regeneration, with an average reduction in PD of 5.57 ± 1.55 mm in 14 patients. Reichert et al.[28] report that the patient treated with GTR must be re-evaluated again no earlier than 6 months after the last intervention and that orthodontic treatment can be considered no earlier than this re-evaluation.

BONE GRAFT

In cases where the defect regeneration requires a bone graft, it is necessary to evaluate whether this material can negatively affect the subsequent tooth movement. In the past, the periodontist cautiously delayed the orthodontic movement until the regenerated tissue maturation occured[13]. Recent studies[46], however, have shown that movement in the graft during healing is not only possible but actually improves orthodontic clinical outcomes and the bone graft does not prevent tooth movement. Araujo et al.[47] confirmed on Beagle dogs that not only was the movement possible in all the cases, but also that the rate of the graft degradation and bone turnover was accelerated by orthodontic stimulation and that, by orthodontic movement, it is possible to move the tooth in a previously grafted area. Hossain et al.[48], on dogs with autologous bone graft or β-tricalcium phosphate, demonstrated changes in grafted sites similar to those with native bone when undergoing orthodontic movement. Ahn et al.[49] observed on Beagle dogs that, starting orthodontic movement immediately after the application of the graft, favourable regeneration results were found, with a better bone density and a reduced risk of inhibition of movement in case of delayed forces after surgery. Da Silva et al.[50] confirmed the same result in degree II furcations too in which the graft did not create problems to tooth movement. Kawamoto et al.[51] demonstrated that the histological response of orthodontic movement in regenerated areas with morphogenetic proteins and spongiosa is the same to the movement performed in native bone. Even in areas grafted with synthetic materials[52,53] tooth movement was carried out without problems. Some Authors, however, have expressed doubts, obtaining discouraging results. Da Silva et al.[50] found that teeth with class II furcations after GTR (60 days after surgery) could be moved with bodily movement without jeopardising the regenerative process, but in teeth with class III furcations with intrusive movement after GTR (1 month after surgery)[43] movement did not improve bone formation; it has been hypothesized that there was an unfavourable interaction between the degradation of the biomaterial and the orthodontic movement; this situation did not occur, however, if a simple *open flap debridement*, always accompanied by orthodontic movement was performed. Probably these results are due to regenerative difficulties correlated with GTR of class III furcations instead of to the difficulties of the orthodontic movement with the graft material.

Clinical case reports with orthodontic movements in regenerated sites with graft material have also been described in which it has been confirmed by surgical re-entries that the orthodontic movement does not affect the regeneration outcomes[37,54]. Surgical re-entries confirmed complete filling of the bone defect with a bone-like hard tissue and interdental papillae, reduction of probing, radiographic bone filling, dental alignment and improvement in esthetics[37,41]. Dental alignment (leveling), and in general orthodontic tooth movement, at an early stage of surgical wound healing determines a more favorable anatomic environment for hard and soft tissues[37].

Mucogingival surgery

The timing and indication for surgery of mucogingival defects are still widely debated. The optimal timing to enhance such preventive surgery, as well as the time of starting the force application (during the healing phase or 6 months after surgery), are not yet clear[26].

Wennström[55] states that the need for periodontal intervention should be assessed after the completion of orthodontic treatment. Literature suggests however, as a preventive measure[12] where the periodontal tissues are thin, to increase the thickness of the soft tissue before starting the tooth movement if the development of bone dehiscence is suspected[55-57] or when the necessary orthodontic movement may occur in a compromised dental housing[58]. A simple preventive gingival tissue augmentation, in fact, can be recommended especially in patients with thin periodontal phenotype[13]. Reichert et al.[28], when mucogingival surgery has been performed, suggest that orthodontic treatment can begin not before 6 months after the execution of a further periodontal re-evaluation. In conclusion, although clinical experience shows that soft tissue augmentation of the bucco-lingual gingival dimension before orthodontic treatment can be considered a feasible clinical option, there is no solid scientific evidence on the best timing for an increase in soft tissues when planning a change in the inclination of the incisors[59]; this implies that this treatment cannot be considered generalizable in every patient, because the assessment of the quality and quantity of the soft tissue is personal and subjective and, therefore, not standardizable.

Phases of treatment

We will now examine the various combined phases of the periodontal/orthodontic treatment. From a periodontal point of view, the treatment plan[60] is developed in three phases (9.1):

1. Initial phase, in which the patient undergoes initial periodontal therapy and periodontal re-evaluation.
2. Corrective phase, in which periodontal surgery is performed before orthodontic treatment. Start of orthodontic treatment, implant placement where necessary, and orthodontic detailing. Further surgery of residual defects after orthodontic movement.
3. Maintenance phase: SPT (Supportive Periodontal Therapy).

In *Clinical case 2* in Chapter 11 we will see a "step-by-step" application of this integrated orthodontic-periodontal timing in the various phases of treatment.

Integrating periodontal data with orthodontic ones from an ortho-perio point of view, we can outline the following phases.

1. Pre-orthodontic phase (9.1)

In this first phase, periodontal treatment is performed and completed before orthodontic treatment[61-63]. After re-evaluation, if necessary, conservative and/or bone surgery is performed if defects are not expected to improve with orthodontic therapy[5,64]. It must be waited from 2[22] up to 6 months before starting orthodontic movement[65,66] to evaluate the tissues response to treatment and their remodeling, healing and stabilization[26]. Patient compliance and motivation continue to be assessed[26,28,67,68], and kept to a high level. In some cases of aggressive periodontitis[64], it must be necessary to wait even longer, up to about 2 years[69]. Initial periodontal treatment should be performed before orthodontic treatment to restore and maintain the health of the supporting tissues[22]. In fact, orthodontics performed after obtaining periodontal stability does not complicate the disease, as long as there is the active cooperation of the patient[68].

2. Orthodontic phase (9.2)

The opportunity to share the interdisciplinary treatment plan gives the orthodontist the possibility to re-evaluate the periodontal status and the interdisciplinary plan before the beginning of the active orthodontic mechanics. The task for the periodontist during the active phase of orthodontic treatment is to support the orthodontist in the interception and early diagnosis of the development of new active sites of periodontal disease exacerbation[70] and to share these assessments with the orthodontist. During orthodontic treatment, professional hygiene sessions and periodontal tissue checks must be performed routinely[26,28,62,66]. Specific intervals must vary for each patient according to the orthodontic-periodontal risk factors and the planned tooth movements[26], so that any form of tissue inflam-

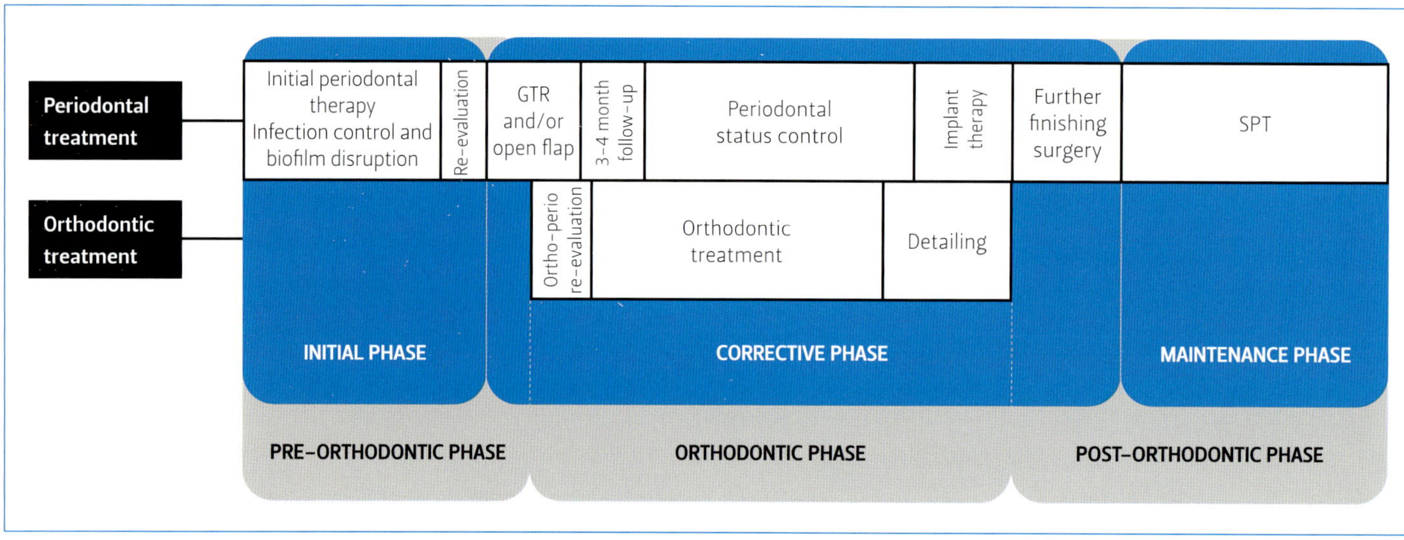

9.1 Schematic diagram of the timing in the orthodontic-periodontal treatment with phases. GTR: Guided Tissue Regeneration; SPT: Supportive Periodontal Therapy.

Tab. 9.1 Pre-orthodontic phase

Preliminary periodontal evaluation
Initial periodontal therapy (reduction of the inflammation; Infection control and elimination of the bacterial biofilm with patient compliance and hygiene care evaluation; smoking cessation)
Re-evaluation
Pre-orthodontic surgery: open flap, improvement of the soft tissues and GTR (where and if necessary)
Endodontic and restorative treatment

mation can be early diagnosed[71]. This approach allows for orthodontic therapy to be performed safely[72]. In case of an aggressive form of periodontal disease is detected or any worsening or breakdown of periodontal disease[71] is suspected, orthodontic treatment must be stopped[64].

3. Post-orthodontic phase (9.3)

The periodontal treatment plan must be re-evaluated during the final phase of the orthodontic treatment, when the position of the hard and soft tissues can be determined in a definitive way. However, this re-evaluation must depend on the clinical characteristics of the case and on the general treatment plan[26,70,73]. Periodontal maintenance must be present from the beginning of the periodontal therapy and throughout the whole orthodontic treatment[63], and must be maintained during the entire patient's dental life[1,67]; periodontal disease must be kept under control before, during and after orthodontic treatment[68]. Close monitoring is a key factor for successful treatment, because it allows to identify and treat any sign of aggravation in order to restore proper periodontal health[17]. The patient should be aware that failure in the control after treatment contributes to the reactivation of the previously treated disease[68].

One thing is certain: periodontal treatment before any orthodontic treatment must achieve complete periodontal stability and periodontal health conditions must be maintained in the long term with a proper supportive therapy program[74].

Operative timing

"*First Perio – Then Ortho*" or "*First Ortho – Then Perio*"? At a clinical level we must distinguish whether

Tab. 9.2 Orthodontic phase

Re-evaluation of the orthodontic treatment plan in relationship with interdisciplinary plan and periodontal status
Biomechanical control of the movement and anchorages in the periodontal patient
Continuous monitoring of the periodontal health, rehevaluation every month, every 2 months, every 3 months

Tab. 9.3 Post-orthodontic phase

Re-evaluation of the periodontal treatment plan (if necessary)
Re-evaluation of the mucogingival defects
Final restorative-prosthetic treatment plan
SPT (Supportive Periodontal Therapy) and regular periodontal and orthodontic follow-up

orthodontic treatment is part of a primarily periodontal request or if the patient's initial request was orthodontics and the orthodontist asked for an evaluation and therefore for periodontal therapy. The choice is performed at the re-evaluation time, in which it is necessary to evaluate the morphology of the defects and must be shared between the periodontist and the orthodontist.

First Perio – Then Ortho

If, after periodontal re-evaluation, it has been established that the periodontal surgical solution to be performed before the orthodontic therapy produces a better prognosis *per se*, we will proceed first to the periodontal surgery and then to the orthodontic movement. This eventuality occurs in:

- *bone craters*: the bone craters do not improve with orthodontic treatment, except for shallow defects. The main choice is resective surgery for the treatment of areas that are intended for orthodontic therapy (see Chapter 11, *Clinical case 2*);
- *bone defects in which GTR alone is able to improve the environment* allowing a more predictable orthodontic treatment (9.2-9.10, see Chapter 11, *Clinical case 2*; 9.11-9.17);
- *furcation involvement:* furcations require special attention and need to be treated because they can worsen during some orthodontic movements being their periodontal maintenance very difficult. They often require resective surgical treatment with root separation or root resection (see 5.13 and 5.14) or regenerative therapy (see 5.15);
- *mucogingival surgery* to cover recessions or to perform soft tissue augmentation (see 7.24-7.29) in the case that the defects have been assessed as uncontrollable during orthodontic therapy.

First Ortho – Then Perio

If it is estimated that the resolution of the defects may not be a pure surgical periodontal treatment or if orthodontics can modify the defect creating a more maintainable environment over time or favor a more predictable three-dimensional morphology for tissue regeneration or resective bone surgery to the point to eliminate this completely, we proceed first to the orthodontic movement and then to the periodontal surgery, if this last one is still necessary. This happens in:

- *Emiseptal defects*: this defect can be modified or eliminated by an appropriate orthodontic treatment. In the case of a tilted tooth, an uprighting and extrusive tooth movement levels the bone defect (9.18-9.23).
- *Bone levelling*: bone remodeling during flap surgery with a resective approach may be a second choice to orthodontically induced remodeling, which can have a positive influence on bone topography. The surgical corrective phase of periodontal therapy could be delayed until the end of orthodontic therapy because the tooth movement could modify the gingival and bone morphology[75]. Many of these problems can be corrected using the bone level as a guide for placing brackets with bone level repositioning (see Chapter 6, *Clinical case 1*).
- *GTR and implant site development*: surgery should be postponed if orthodontics can modify the anatomy of the defect improving predictability and/or in the case of implant placement if orthodontic extrusion can regenerate soft or hard tissue (see Chapter 8, *Clinical cases 4-6*).
- *Orthodontics as a recessions treatment*: surgery is postponed after re-evaluation of the soft tissues following the bucco-lingual movement of the tooth within the alveolar envelope (see 7.8-7.10) or after the analysis of the phenotypic post-orthodontics appearance (9.24; see Chapter 7, *Clinical case 1*).
- *Root proximity*: if necessary, surgical treatment is performed after the orthodontic movement has created space between the roots improving the interproximal septa (see Chapter 6, *Clinical case 4;* 3.15).
- *Dental extrusion*: to recover tooth substance which was lost because of decays or fractures without performing a more destructive resective surgery[76] which must be realized only if necessary after orthodontic repositioning (see Chapter 8, *Clinical cases 1 and 2*).

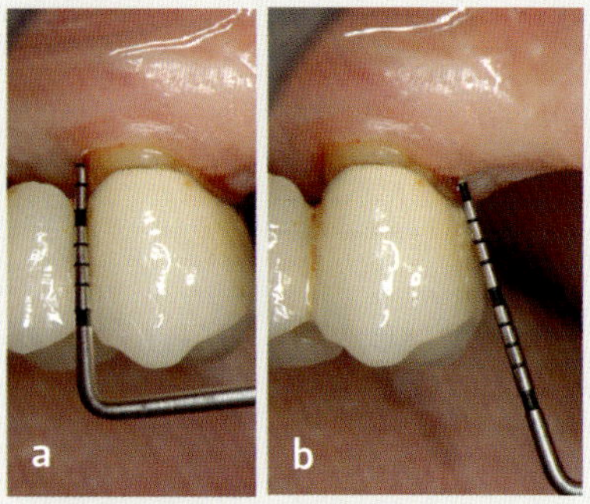

9.2 Periodontal probing of the distal defect of 1.5.

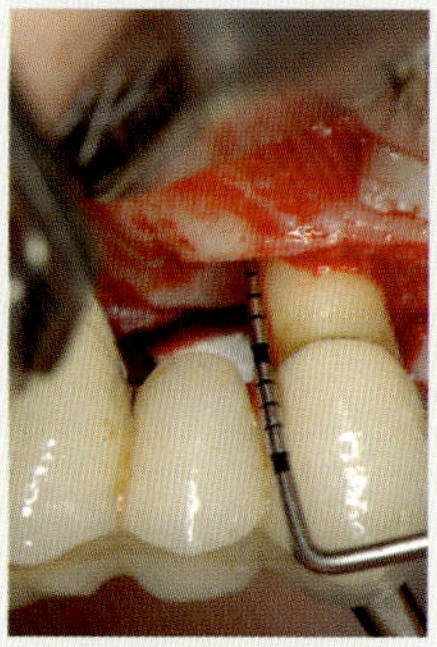

9.3 Surgical view of the intrabony defect of 1.5.

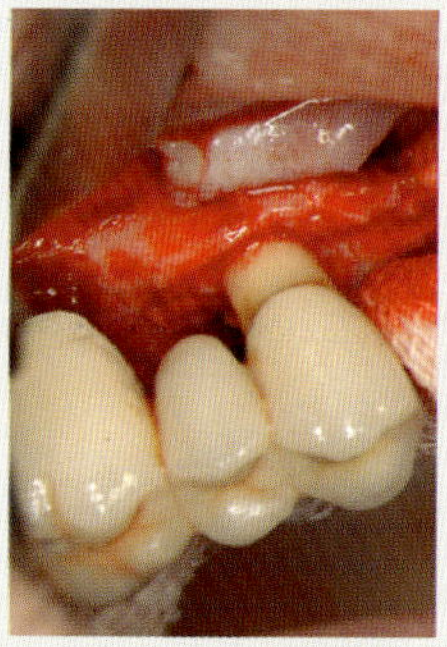

9.4 Autologous bone graft in the defect.

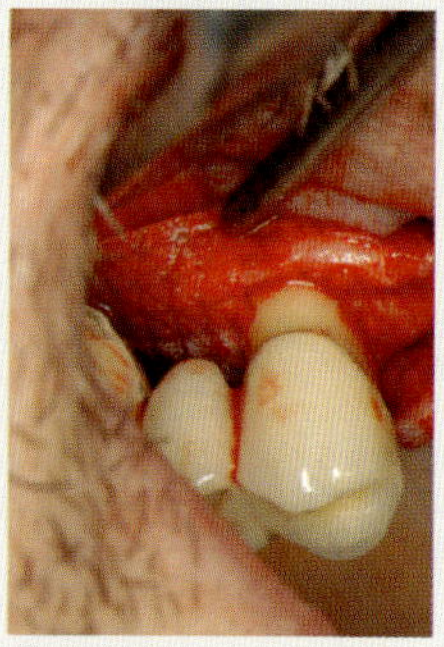

9.5 Setting of the resorbable membrane

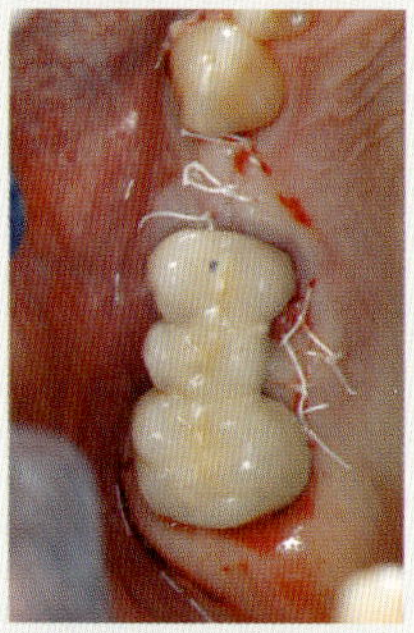

9.6 ePTFE suture: occlusal view.

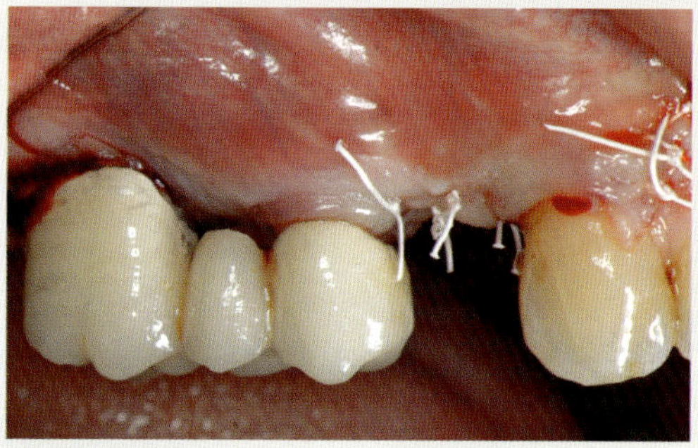

9.7 ePTFE suture: vestibular view.

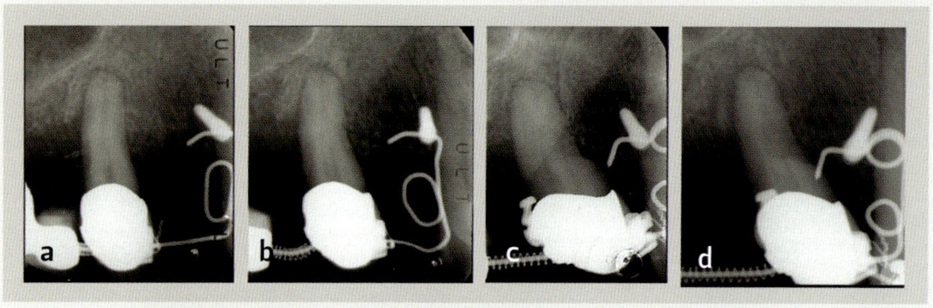

9.8 X-ray check of the bodily movement of 1.5.

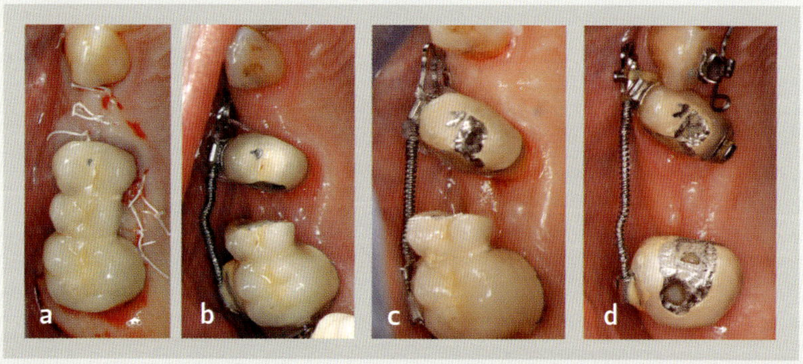

9.9 Phases of the orthodontic movement of 1.5 where it can be seen the bone crest regularization next to the tooth (occlusal view).

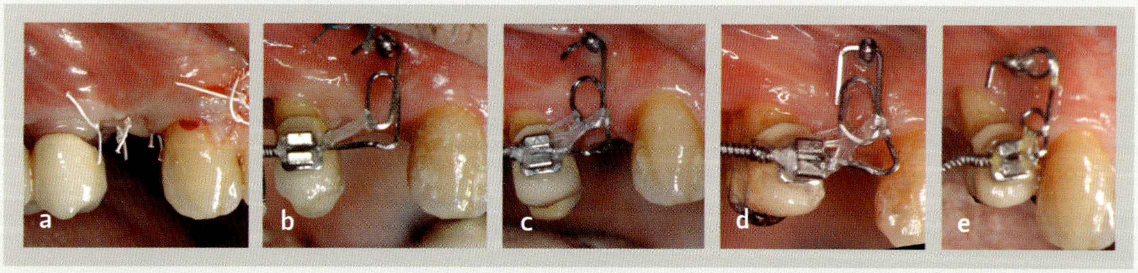

9.10 Phases of the orthodontic movement of 1.5 (vestibular view).

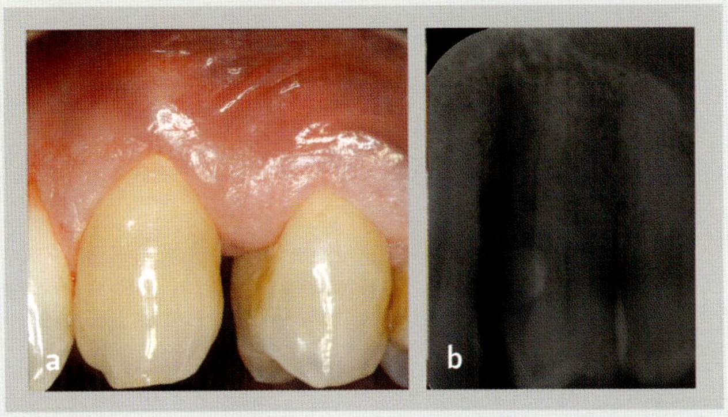

9.11 Tissue aspect of the 2.4 (**a**) and X-ray check of the intrabony defect mesial to 2.4 (**b**).

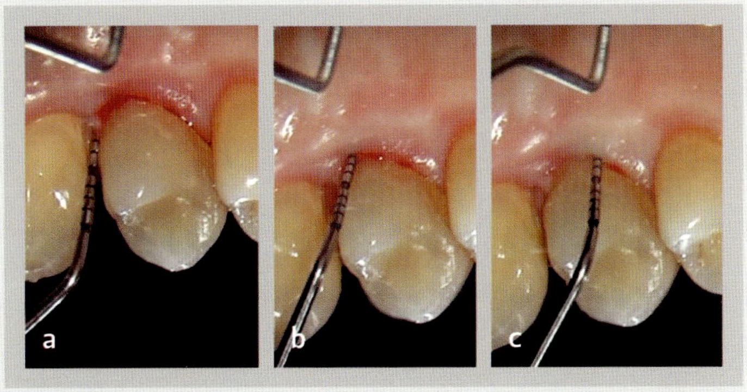

9.12 Bone defect probing.

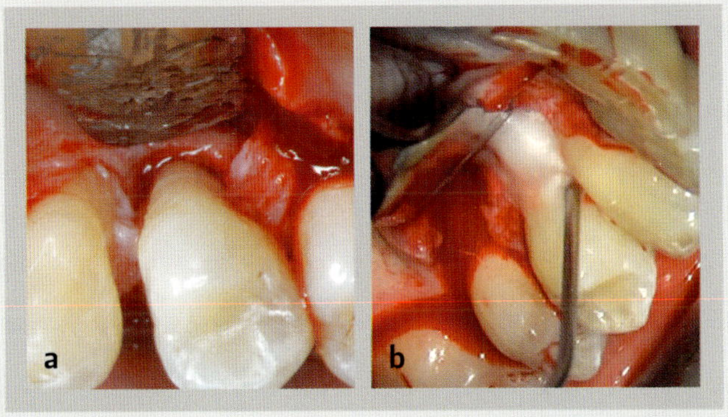

9.13 Surgical view of the defect after root scaling (**a**) and application of regeneration material (**b**).

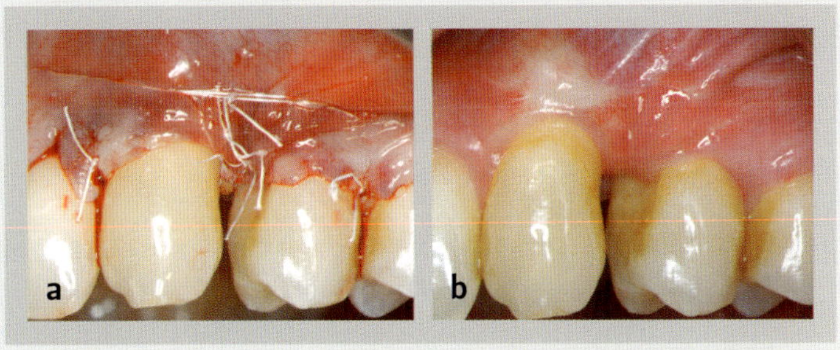

9.14 Suture (**a**) and tissue aspect before starting the orthodontic movement (**b**).

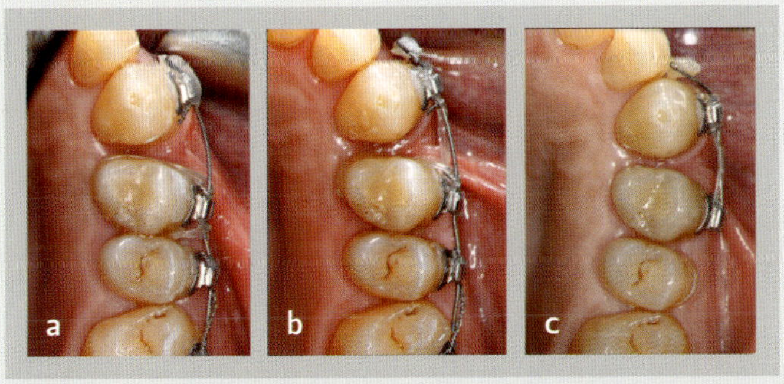

9.15 Phases of the movement of the 2.4 towards the defect (movement starts 1 month after GTR).

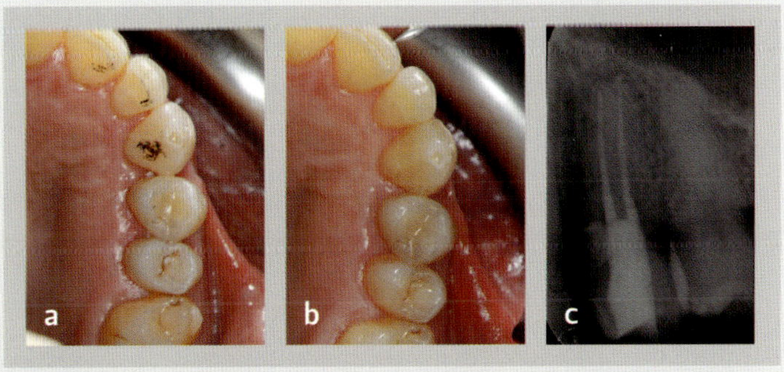

9.16 Occlusal view of the sector after restoration of the contact point (**a**). Clinical (**b**) and X-ray (**c**) 1-year follow-up showing the complete defect filling.

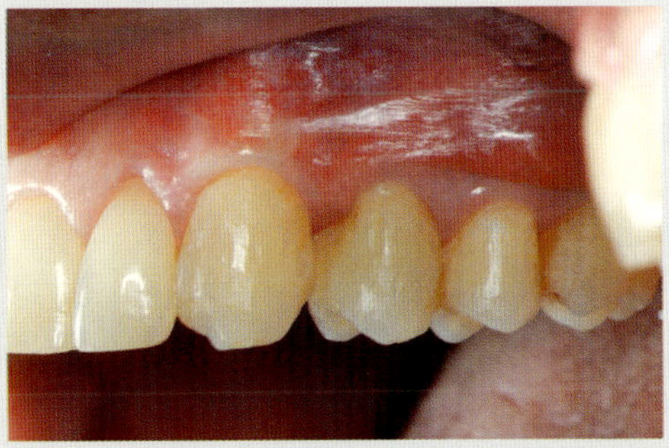

9.17 1-year vestibular follow-up.

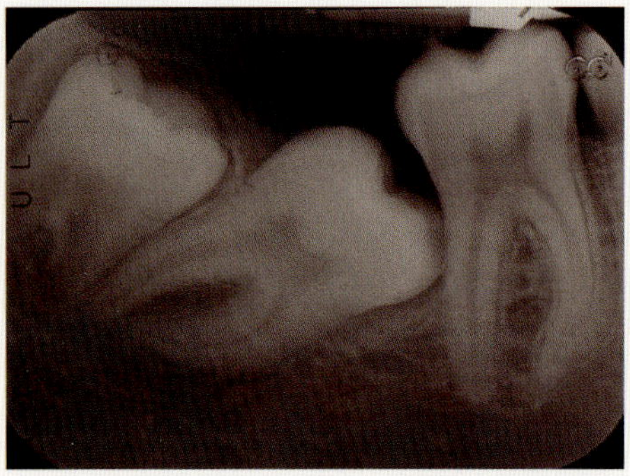

9.18 X-ray that shows the 4.7 in horizontal retention with the 4.6 distal defect.

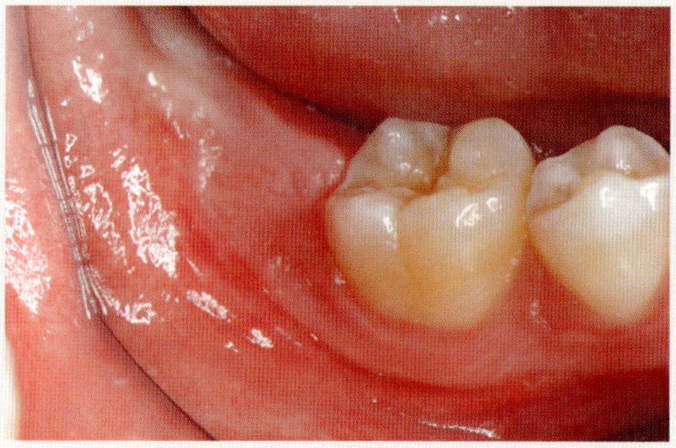

9.19 Clinical view of the tissues before the surgery of the second molar.

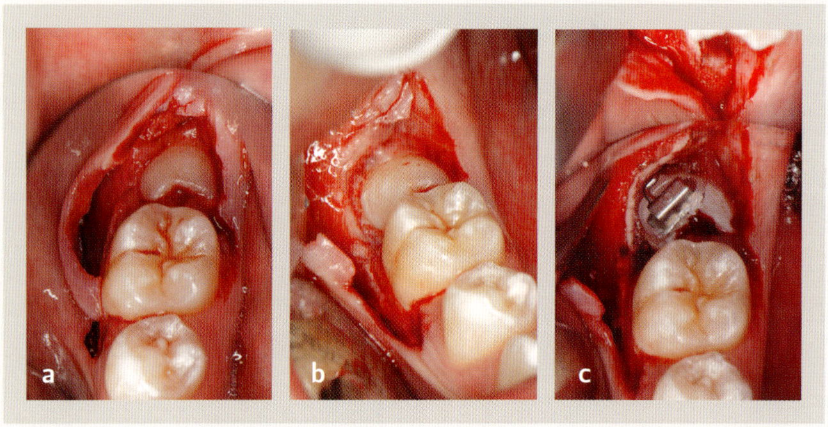

9.20 Flap elevation (**a**) and coronal osteotomy (**b**) with intrasurgical view of the brackets placed on the tooth (**c**).

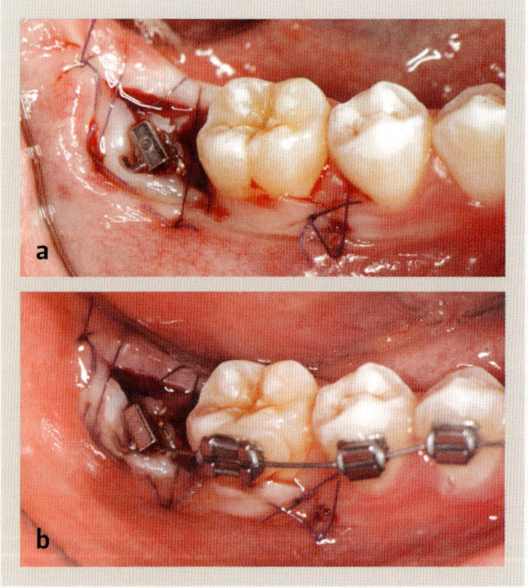

9.21 Apically repositioned flap suture for the maintenance of the keratinized tissue (**a**) and orthodontic mechanics application (**b**).

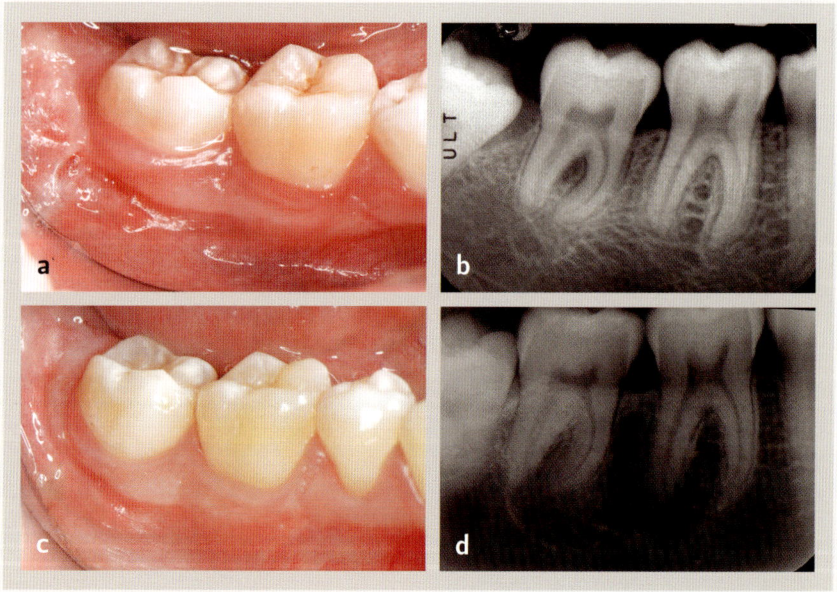

9.22 Clinical view (**a**) and X-ray check (**b**) at the end of the treatment and 10-year follow-up (**c,d**) where it is possible to see the maintenance of the soft tissue and the interproximal bone crest perfectly mineralized.

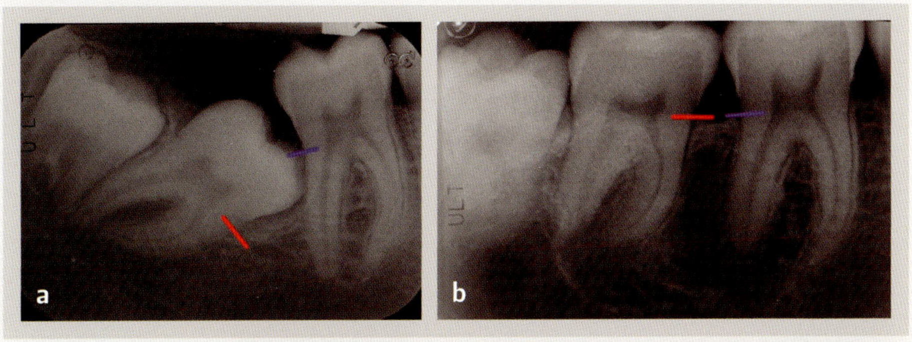

9.23 Relationship of the cemento-enamel junction before the orthodontic movement (**a**) and after 10 years (**b**).

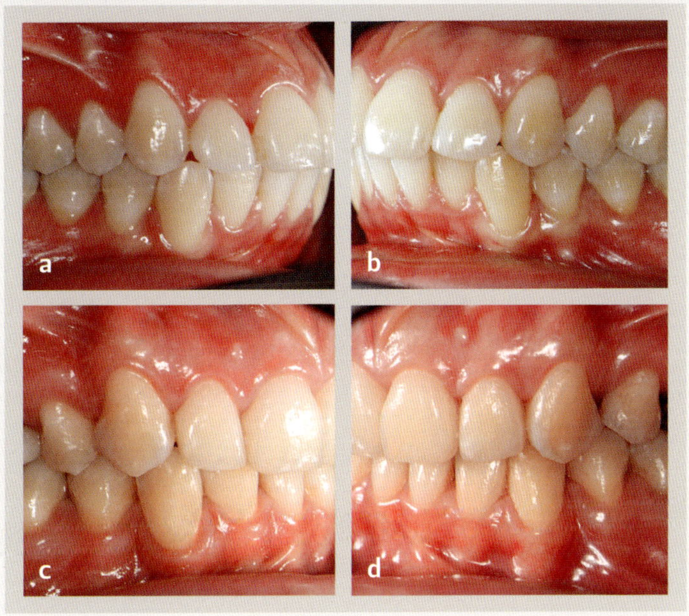

9.24 Comparison between the initial (**a,b**) and final (**c,d**) gingival tissues after orthodontic treatment (see Chapter 7, *Clinical case 1*) where an apparent "thickening" of the gingival tissues is clinically observed.

REFERENCES

1. Gorbunkova A, Pagni G, Brizhak A et al. Impact of orthodontic treatment on periodontal tissues: a narrative review of multidisciplinary literature. *Int J Dent*. 2016;2016:4723589.
2. Nemcovsky CE, Sasson M, Beny L et al. Periodontal healing following orthodontic movement of rat molars with intact versus damaged periodontia towards a bony defect. *Eur J Orthod*. 2007;29(4):338-344.
3. Nemcovsky CE, Beny L, Shanberger S et al. Bone apposition in surgical bony defects following orthodontic movement: a comparative histomorphometric study between root- and periodontal ligament-damaged and periodontally intact rat molars. *J Periodontol*. 2004;75(7):1013-1019.
4. Murakami T, Yokota S, Takahama Y. Periodontal changes after experimentally induced intrusion of the upper incisors in Macaca fuscata monkeys. *Am J Orthod Dentofacial Orthop*. 1989;95(2):115-126.
5. Cardaropoli D, Gaveglio L, Abou-Arraj RV. Orthodontic movement and periodontal bone defects: rationale, timing, and clinical implications. *Semin Orthod* 2014;20(3):177-187.
6. Re S, Cardaropoli D, Abundo R, Corrente G. Reduction of gingival recession following orthodontic intrusion in periodontally compromised patients. *Orthod Craniofac Res*. 2004;7(1):35-39.
7. Cardaropoli D, Re S, Corrente G, Abundo R. Reconstruction of the maxillary midline papilla following a combined orthodontic-periodontic treatment in adult periodontal patients. *J Clin Periodontol*. 2004;31(2):79-84.
8. Corrente G, Abundo R, Re S et al. Orthodontic movement into infrabony defects in patients with advanced periodontal disease: a clinical and radiological study. *J Periodontol*. 2003;74(8):1104-1109.
9. Cardaropoli D, Re S, Corrente G, Abundo R. Intrusion of migrated incisors with infrabony defects in adult periodontal patients. *Am J Orthod Dentofacial Orthop*. 2001;120(6):671-677.
10. Wikesjö UM, Nilvéus RE, Selvig KA. Significance of early healing events on periodontal repair: a review. *J Periodontol*. 1992;63(3):158-165.

11. **Cortellini P, Tonetti MS.** Focus on intrabony defects: guided tissue regeneration. *Periodontol 2000.* 2000;22(1):104-132.

12. **Harshita N, Kamath DG, Kadakampally D.** Perio-ortho interactions. A review. *J Pharm Sci & Res.* 2018; 10(5):1053-1056.

13. **Palomo L, Palomo JM, Bissada NF.** Salient periodontal issues for the modern biologic orthodontist. *Semin Orthod.* 2008;14(4):229-245.

14. **Roberts WE, Chase DC.** Kinetics of cell proliferation and migration associated with orthodontically-induced osteogenesis. *J Dent Res.* 1981;60(2):174-181.

15. **Diedrich P, Fritz U, Kizinger G.** Interrelationship between periodontics and adult orthodontics. *Perio.* 2004;1(3):143-149.

16. **Cardaropoli D.** Orthodontics for the adult periodontal patient: first or second choice treatment? *Prog Orthod.* 2009;10(2):88-96.

17. **Chackartchi T, Chaushu S, Stabholz A.** *Orthodontic treatment in patients with severe periodontal disease.* In: Eliades T, Katsaros C. *The ortho-perio patient: clinical evidence & therapeutic guidelines.* Batavia, IL. Quintessence Publishing Co; 2019:189-210.

18. **Feu D, Menezes FC, Augusto Mendes Miguel J, Cardoso Abdo Quintão C.** Orthodontic treatment in the severely compromised periodontal patient. *J Orthod.* 2012;39(4):303-313.

19. **Machuca G, Martínez F, Machuca C, Bullón P.** A combination of orthodontic, periodontal, and prosthodontic treatment in a case of advanced malocclusion. *Int J Periodontics Restorative Dent.* 2003;23(5):499-505.

20. **Mathews DP, Kokich VG.** Managing treatment for the orthodontic patient with periodontal problems. *Semin Orthod.* 1997;3(1):21-38.

21. **Vanarsdall RL.** Orthodontics and periodontal therapy. *Periodontol 2000.* 1995;9(1):132-149.

22. **Kruk H, Bensaid X, Chevalier G et al.** Severe periodontitis and orthodontics: How far should we go? *Int Orthod.* 2018;16(3):450-462.

23. **Roccuzzo M, Marchese S, Dalmasso P, Roccuzzo A.** Periodontal regeneration and orthodontic treatment of severely periodontally compromised teeth: 10-year results of a prospective study. *Int J Periodontics Restorative Dent.* 2018;38(6):801-809.

24. **Passanezi E, Janson M, Janson G et al.** Interdisciplinary treatment of localized juvenile periodontitis: a new perspective to an old problem. *Am J Orthod Dentofacial Orthop.* 2007;131(2):268-276.

25. **Rabie ABM, Gildenhuys R, Boisson M.** Management of patients with severe bone loss: bone induction and orthodontics. *World J Orthod.* 2001;2(2):142-153.

26. **Gkantidis N, Christou P, Topouzelis N.** The orthodontic-periodontic interrelationship in integrated treatment challenges: a systematic review. *J Oral Rehabil.* 2010;37(5):377-390.

27. **Cao T, Xu L, Shi J, Zhou Y.** Combined orthodontic-periodontal treatment in periodontal patients with anteriorly displaced incisors. *Am J Orthod Dentofacial Orthop.* 2015 Nov;148(5):805-13.

28. **Reichert C, Hagner M, Jepsen S, Jäger A.** Interfaces between orthodontic and periodontal treatment: their current status. *J Orofac Orthop.* 2011;72(3):165-186.

29. **Re S, Corrente G, Abundo R, Cardaropoli D.** Orthodontic movement into bone defects augmented with bovine bone mineral and fibrin sealer: a reentry case report. *Int J Periodontics Restorative Dent.* 2002;22(2):138-145.

30. **Jang I, Lee JK, Song GS et al.** Application of enamel matrix derivative and intrusive orthodontic movement in the treatment of vertical bony defects: a case report. *Int J Periodontics Restorative Dent.* 2019;39(1):73-81.

31. **Diedrich PR.** Guided tissue regeneration associated with orthodontic therapy. *Semin Orthod.* 1996;2(1):39-45.

32. **Diedrich P, Fritz U, Kinzinger G, Angelakis J.** Movement of periodontally affected teeth after guided tissue regeneration (GTR)-an experimental pilot study in animals. *J Orofac Orthop.* 2003;64(3):214-227.

33. **Ogihara S, Marks MH.** Enhancing the regenerative potential of guided tissue regeneration to treat an intrabony defect and adjacent ridge deformity by orthodontic extrusive force. *J Periodontol.* 2006;77(12):2093-2100.

34. **Re S, Corrente G, Abundo R, Cardaropoli D.** Orthodontic treatment in periodontally compromised patients: 12-year report. *Int J Periodontics Restorative Dent.* 2000;20(1):31-39.

35. **Derton N, Derton R, Perini A et al.** Orthodontic treatment in periodontal patients: a case report with 7 years follow-up. *Int Orthod.* 2011;9(1):92-109.

36. **Ghezzi C, Masiero S, Silvestri M et al.** Orthodontic treatment of periodontally involved teeth after tissue regeneration. *Int J Periodontics Restorative Dent.* 2008;28(6):559-567.

37. **Cardaropoli D, Re S, Manuzzi W et al.** Bio-Oss collagen and orthodontic movement for the treatment of infrabony defects in the esthetic zone. *Int J Periodontics Restorative Dent.* 2006;26(6):553-559.

38. **Jepsen K, Jaeger A, Jepsen S.** Esthetic and functional rehabilitation of a severely compromised central incisor: an interdisciplinary approach. *Int J Periodontics Restorative Dent.* 2015;35(3):e35-e43.

39. **Maeda S, Ono Y, Nakamura K, Kuwahara T.** Molar uprighting with extrusion for implant site bone regeneration and improvement of the periodontal environment [published correction appears in *Int J Periodontics Restorative Dent.* 2008 Oct;28(5):451]. *Int J Periodontics Restorative Dent.* 2008;28(4):375-381.

40. **Tsai HC, Yao CJ, Wong MY.** Early orthodontic tooth movement into regenerative bony defects: a case report. *Int J Periodontics Restorative Dent.* 2017;37(4):581-589.

41. **Cardaropoli D, Re S.** Interdental papilla augmentation procedure following orthodontic treatment in a periodontal patient. *J Periodontol.* 2005;76(4):655-661.

42. **Ogihara S, Wang HL.** Periodontal regeneration with or without limited orthodontics for the treatment of 2- or 3-wall infrabony defects. *J Periodontol.* 2010;81(12):1734-1742.

43. **da Silva VC, Cirelli CC, Ribeiro FS et al.** Intrusion of teeth with class III furcation: a clinical, histologic and histometric study in dogs. *J Clin Periodontol.* 2008;35(9):807-816.

44. **Attia MS, Shoreibah EA, Ibrahim**

SA, NASSAR HA. Histological evaluation of osseous defects combined with orthodontic tooth movement. *J Int Acad Periodontol.* 2012;14(1):7-16.

45. ATTIA MS, SHOREIBAH EA, IBRAHIM SA, NASSAR HA. Regenerative therapy of osseous defects combined with orthodontic tooth movement. *J Int Acad Periodontol.* 2012;14(1):17-25.

46. WILCKO WM, WILCKO T, BOUQUOT JE, FERGUSON DJ. Rapid orthodontics with alveolar reshaping: two case reports of decrowding. *Int J Periodontics Restorative Dent.* 2001;21(1):9-19.

47. ARAÚJO MG, CARMAGNOLA D, BERGLUNDH T ET AL. Orthodontic movement in bone defects augmented with Bio-Oss. An experimental study in dogs. *J Clin Periodontol.* 2001;28(1):73-80.

48. HOSSAIN MZ, KYOMEN S, TANNE K. Biologic responses of autogenous bone and beta-tricalcium phosphate ceramics transplanted into bone defects to orthodontic forces. *Cleft Palate Craniofac J.* 1996;33(4):277-283.

49. AHN HW, OHE JY, LEE SH ET AL. Timing of force application affects the rate of tooth movement into surgical alveolar defects with grafts in beagles. *Am J Orthod Dentofacial Orthop.* 2014;145(4):486-495.

50. DA SILVA VC, CIRELLI CC, RIBEIRO FS ET AL. Orthodontic movement after periodontal regeneration of class II furcation: a pilot study in dogs. *J Clin Periodontol.* 2006;33(6):440-448.

51. KAWAMOTO T, MOTOHASHI N, KITAMURA A ET AL. A histological study on experimental tooth movement into bone induced by recombinant human bone morphogenetic protein-2 in beagle dogs. *Cleft Palate Craniofac J.* 2002;39(4):439-448.

52. MACHIBYA FM, ZHUANG Y, GUO W ET AL. Effects of bone regeneration materials and tooth movement timing on canine experimental orthodontic treatment. *Angle Orthod.* 2018;88(2):171-178.

53. RU N, LIU SS, BAI Y ET AL. BoneCeramic graft regenerates alveolar defects but slows orthodontic tooth movement with less root resorption. *Am J Orthod Dentofacial Orthop.* 2016;149(4):523-532.

54. NAGY P, MOLNAR B, NEMES B ET AL. Histologic evaluation of human intrabony periodontal defects treated with deproteinized bovine bone mineral in combination with orthodontic tooth movement: a case series [published online ahead of print, 2019 Nov 11]. *Int J Periodontics Restorative Dent.* 2019;40(3):321-330.

55. WENNSTRÖM JL. Mucogingival considerations in orthodontic treatment. *Semin Orthod.* 1996;2(1):46-54.

56. MELSEN B, ALLAIS D. Factors of importance for the development of dehiscences during labial movement of mandibular incisors: a retrospective study of adult orthodontic patients. *Am J Orthod Dentofacial Orthop.* 2005;127(5):552-625.

57. THILANDER B, NYMAN S, KARRING T, MAGNUSSON I. Bone regeneration in alveolar bone dehiscences related to orthodontic tooth movements. *Eur J Orthod.* 1983;5(2):105-114.

58. KAO RT, CURTIS DA, KIM DM ET AL. American Academy of Periodontology best evidence consensus statement on modifying periodontal phenotype in preparation for orthodontic and restorative treatment. *J Periodontol.* 2020;91(3):289-298.

59. KLOUKOS D, ELIADES T, SCULEAN A, KATSAROS C. Indication and timing of soft tissue augmentation at maxillary and mandibular incisors in orthodontic patients. A systematic review. *Eur J Orthod.* 2014;36(4):442-449.

60. SANZ M, HERRERA D, KEBSCHULL M ET AL. Treatment of stage I-III periodontitis-The EFP S3 level clinical practice guideline. *J Clin Periodontol.* 2020;47 Suppl 22:4-60.

61. AHN JC, LEE JH, YOON JH ET AL. Interdisciplinary treatment of a patient with multiple missing teeth and periodontitis. *Am J Orthod Dentofacial Orthop.* 2018;153(2):278-289.

62. LEVIN L, EINY S, ZIGDON H ET AL. Guidelines for periodontal care and follow-up during orthodontic treatment in adolescents and young adults. *J Appl Oral Sci.* 2012;20(4):399-403.

63. WENNSTRÖM JL, STOKLAND BL, NYMAN S, THILANDER B. Periodontal tissue response to orthodontic movement of teeth with infrabony pockets. *Am J Orthod Dentofacial Orthop.* 1993;103(4):313-319.

64. HAZAN-MOLINA H, LEVIN L, EINY S, AIZENBUD D. Aggressive periodontitis diagnosed during or before orthodontic treatment. *Acta Odontol Scand.* 2013;71(5):1023-1031.

65. ZACHRISSON BU. Clinical implications of recent orthodontic-periodontic research findings. *Semin Orthod.* 1996;2(1):4-12.

66. JOHAL AS, LEE RT. The periodontal-orthodontic interface: a simple solution to a difficult problem. *Br J Orthod.* 1998;25(2):95-99.

67. CZOCHROWSKA EM, ROSA M. The orthodontic/periodontal interface. *Semin Orthod.* 2015;21(1):3-14.

68. SABATOSKI CV, BUENO RC, REYES PACHECO AA ET AL. Combined periodontal, orthodontic, and prosthetic treatment in an adult patient. *Case Rep Dent.* 2015;2015:716462.

69. ZAFIROPOULOS GG, DI PRISCO MO, DELI G ET AL. Maintenance after a complex orthoperio treatment in a case of generalized aggressive periodontitis: 7-year result. *J Int Acad Periodontol.* 2010;12(4):112-122.

70. JOHAL A, IDE M. Orthodontics in the adult patient, with special reference to the periodontally compromised patient. *Dent Update.* 1999;26(3):101-108.

71. BOYER S, FONTANEL F, DANAN M ET AL. Severe periodontitis and orthodontics: evaluation of long-term results. *Int Orthod.* 2011;9(3):259-273.

72. CERRONI S, PASQUANTONIO G, CONDÒ R, CERRONI L. Orthodontic fixed appliance and periodontal status: an updated systematic review. *Open Dent J.* 2018;12(1):614-622.

73. HAN JY. A comparative study of combined periodontal and orthodontic treatment with fixed appliances and clear aligners in patients with periodontitis. *J Periodontal Implant Sci.* 2015;45(6):193-204.

74. AIMETTI M, GARBO D, ERCOLI E ET AL. Long-term prognosis of severely compromised teeth following combined periodontal and orthodontic treatment: a retrospective study. *Int J Periodontics Restorative Dent.* 2020;40(1):95-102.

75. ONG MA, WANG HL, SMITH FN. Interrelationship between periodontics and adult orthodontics. *J Clin Periodontol.* 1998;25(4):271-277.

76. KAITSAS R. *La posizione sub-gengivale del margine.* In: Scolavino S, Paolone G. *Restauri diretti nei settori posteriori.* Milano. Quintessence Publishing Ed.; 2019:148-149.

Orthodontics and restorative dentistry. Considerations in the periodontal patient

Gaetano Paolone and Maria Giacinta Paolone

The restorative and esthetic treatments in the periodontal patient that need a restorative contribution often require an interdisciplinary and individualized approach[1-3]. In the patient with periodontal disease the interproximal cervical area is increased (the so-called "black triangles") for the interdental alveolar ridge impairment because of the radicular and crown divergence due to pathological dental migration. The contact point is totally lost[4] or becomes minimal, and reduced to a more incisally placed point. The esthetic resolution therefore involves a combination of restorative therapies, such as modification of the interproximal anatomy with reductive ameloplasty[5,6], recontouring of the interproximal surfaces and flattening of the contact area to lengthen the interproximal contact towards the papilla[7], additive reconstructive solutions and orthodontic movements that can have different objectives: correcting root divergence, bringing teeth closer in order to contribute to the papillary modification[8], leveling the residual periodontal support or obtaining a marginal and esthetic, correction of the gingival scalloping[9] (10.1).

From an esthetic point of view, the anterior diastema closure and the interdental papilla reconstruction represent one of the most complex problems during periodontal treatment[10,11]. Approaching teeth with orthodontic movement changes the topography of the alveolar ridge and, consequently, the position of the interdental papilla integrating with a reshaping aimed at the apical displacement of the contact point[3,12-14]. The increased space of the papilla in the "black hole" effect is usually due to one of these three causes: tooth shape, divergence with root angulation, or periodontal bone loss. Orthodontics can work on these last two factors and, for this reason, assumes a role in the rehabilitation of interdental support loss with an esthetic defect in the anterior teeth and helps to restore a correct dental shape and relationship[13,15-17]. If the patient has black triangles, the

Tab. 10.1 Orthodontic contributions to restorative treatment in the periodontal patient

Correction of 3D position of the teeth
Correction of root divergence
Approach of the teeth to contribute to the papillae modification
Modification of the gingival emergence
Correction of the morphology of the residual periodontal support

first aspect that must be evaluated is to observe whether the problem concerns the papilla or the tooth contact point. If the problem is at the concerns the papilla, a lack of supporting bone due to a periodontal problem may be one of the causes. In some situations orthodontics can offer a contribution to the resolution and improvement of a papilla deficit. Closing the contact point, the interproximal gingiva can be squeezed and consequently moved incisally. Another possibility is a sectorial extrusion of adjacent teeth when the interproximal bone level is positioned apically[18] or it is asymmetrical.

The diagnostic and therapeutic sequence, already extensively described by Kokich[17], takes into account at first, always after initial periodontal therapy, the assessment of the exposure of the gingival margin of the anterior group while smiling and at rest[19], the periodontal assessment of the amount of extension, quality and residual morphology of the periodontal support, the residual crown/root ratio to define the eventual possibility of an extrusive correction and the evaluation of the presence of wear that can reveal an extrusion after an abrasion that occurred over time[8,11,20-22]. The control of the tooth position must not only take into account the correction of the derotations and the apico-coronal leveling of the periodontal support and the gingival scalloping, but also the torque movement, the symmetry of the lateral segments of the dentition and of the anterior group itself, contributing to the exposure of the incisors at rest[23-27].

Clinical case 1

The patient is affected by agenesis of the lower second premolars and reports a previous orthodontic treatment and a previous implant treatment at the 4.7 site. The patient's request is the rehabilitation of the edentoulous 4.5 site without having an implant-prosthetic solution. The patient has a tendency to class III, facial symmetry, normal nasolabial angle, normal neck-chin length and slight lower lip tension (10.1), absence of 3.5 and 4.5, implant in 4.7 site, canine class I and molar class III on the right, molar and canine class III on the left, reduced OVJ and OVB (10.2), biprotrusion, normodivergence, tendency to skeletal class III, incisive vestibuloversion (10.3; 10.2).

The patient has a small intrabony defect on 2.1 (10.4) which, after the initial periodontal therapy (10.5), will be treated with orthodontics without surgical therapy through sectorial extrusions. The space of the 3.5 is closed with a sliding mechanics and loops with lingual orthodontic technique. At the beginning lingual orthodontics (Kurz 7th Generation®, Ormco) is applied with set-up and indirect bonding on the lower arch, at first the alignment was performed with a .016 CuNiTi archwire, then a .016 β-titanium archwire was applied and then a .017×.017 β-titanium archwire. Only in this phase the upper lingual appliance is bonded, always with an indirect set-up that pre-incorporates the extrusion of 2.1 with a .016 CuNiTi (10.6) archwire. Subsequently a .017×.017 β-titanium archwire (10.7) is used with the aim of achieving an orthodontic correction of the intraosseous defect of 2.1 by means of sectorial extrusion, always bending on the .017×.017 β-titanium archwire progressive extrusive steps with tipping and torque aimed at leveling the mesial defect of 2.1 at the level of the mesial bone peak of 1.1 (10.8). The patient needs a 2.1 restorative procedure, being conscious from the very beginning of the limit of the emergence profile due to the reduced root conicity of the extruded root, as described in Chapter 8. The patient, after the removal of the orthodontic mechanics, shows a reduction of labial tension (10.9), canine class I and molar class III, normalization of OBJ and OVB (10.10), correction of incisive inclination and skeletal sagittal and vertical control, slight apical root resorption, which is already present before the start of treatment (10.11; see 10.2).

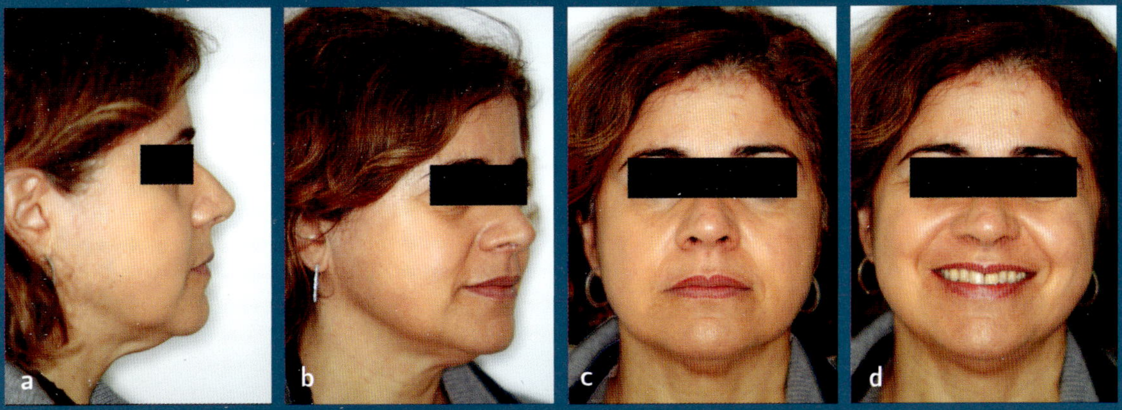

10.1 Extraoral pre-treatment photos.

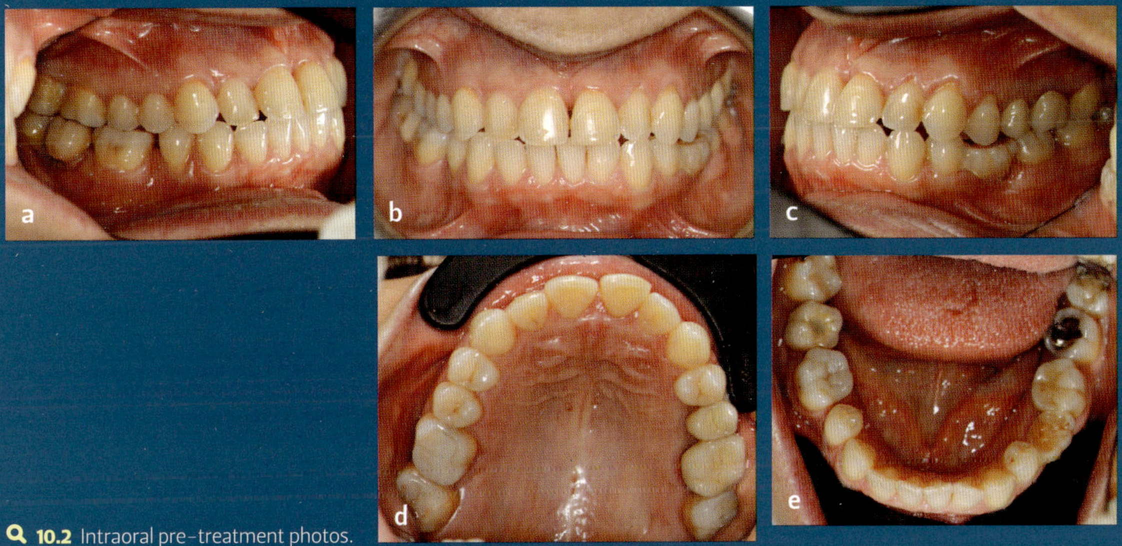

10.2 Intraoral pre-treatment photos.

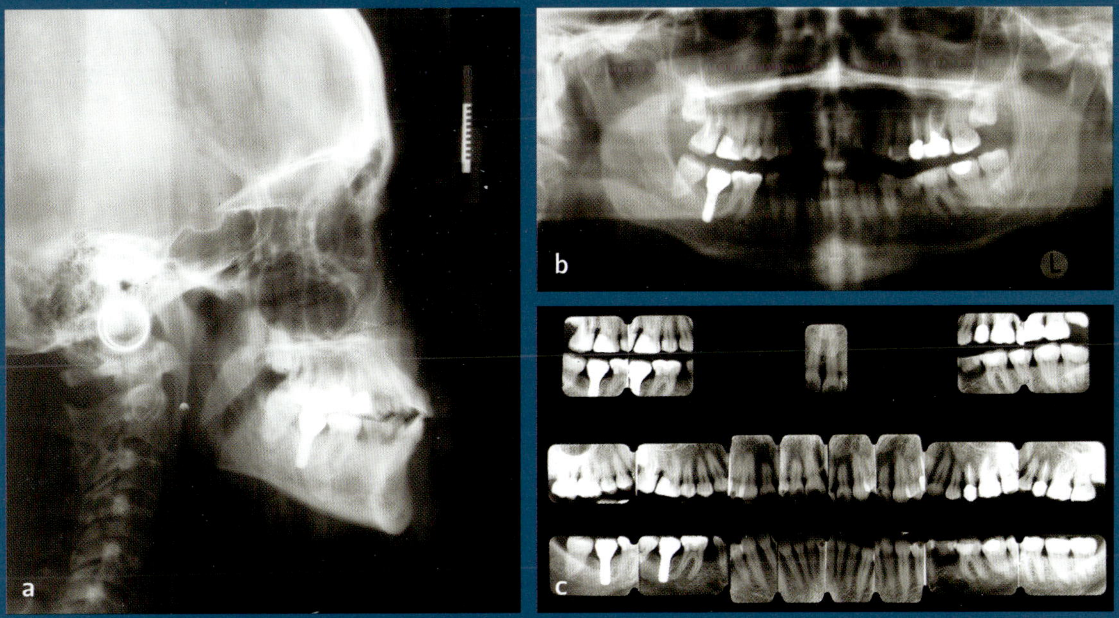

10.3 Pre-treatment cephalometric Rx (**a**), panoramic Rx (**b**), full radiographic periodontal status (**c**).

Tab. 10.2 Cephalometric values

Sagittal skeletal relationships	Pre-treatment	Post-treatment	Retention	Mean	DS
Maxillary sagittal relationship SNA	86°	87°	86°	82°	3.5°
Mandibular sagittal relationship SNPg	86°	86°	85°	80°	3.5°
Intermaxillary sagittal relationship ANPg	0°	1°	1°	2°	2.5°
Vertical skeletal relationships					
Maxillary vertical relationship SN / ANS-PNS	8°	6°	6°	8°	3.0°
Mandibular vertical relationship SN / Go-Gn	30°	28°	27°	33°	2.5°
Intermaxillary vertical relationship ANS-PNS / Go-Gn	22°	22°	21°	25°	6.0°
Dento-basal relationships					
Upper incisor inclination $\underline{1}$ - ANS-PNS	128°	123°	122°	110°	6.0°
Lower incisor inclination $\overline{1}$ - Go-Gn	95°	90°	90°	94°	7.0°
Lower incisor compensation $\overline{1}$ - A-Pg (mm)	+5	+2	+2	2	2.0
Dental relationships					
Overjet (OVJ, mm)	1	3	3	3,5	2.5
Overbite (OVB, mm)	1	2	2	2	2.5
Interincisal angle $\underline{1}/\overline{1}$	122°	123°	122°	132°	6.0°

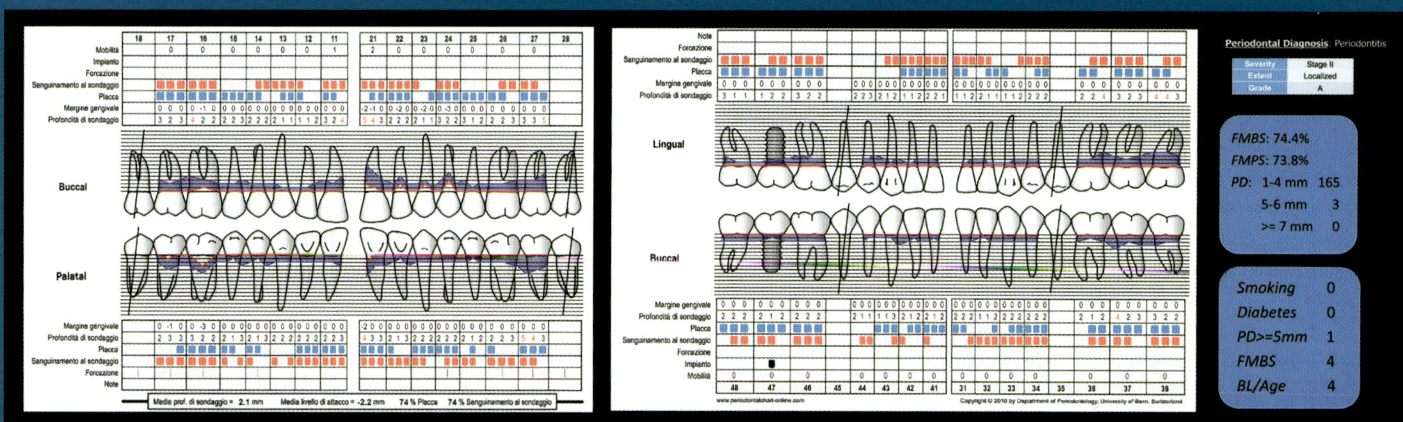

10.4 Initial periodontal probing, periodontal diagnosis, periodontal indexes, risk assessment (Online periodontal charting tool, www.perio-tools.com).

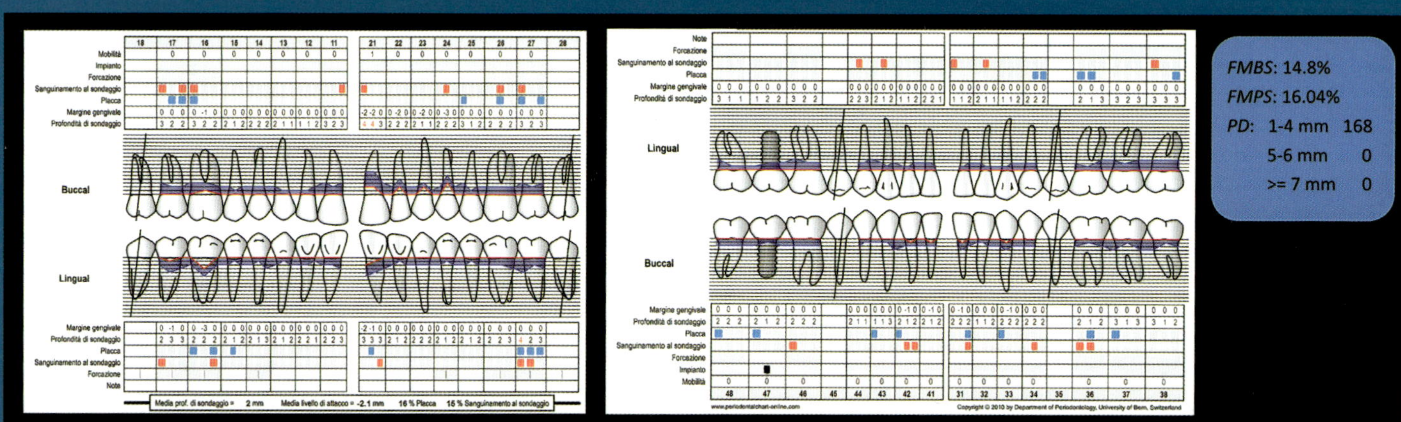

10.5 Re-evaluation periodontal probing and periodontal indexes (Online periodontal charting tool, www.perio-tools.com).

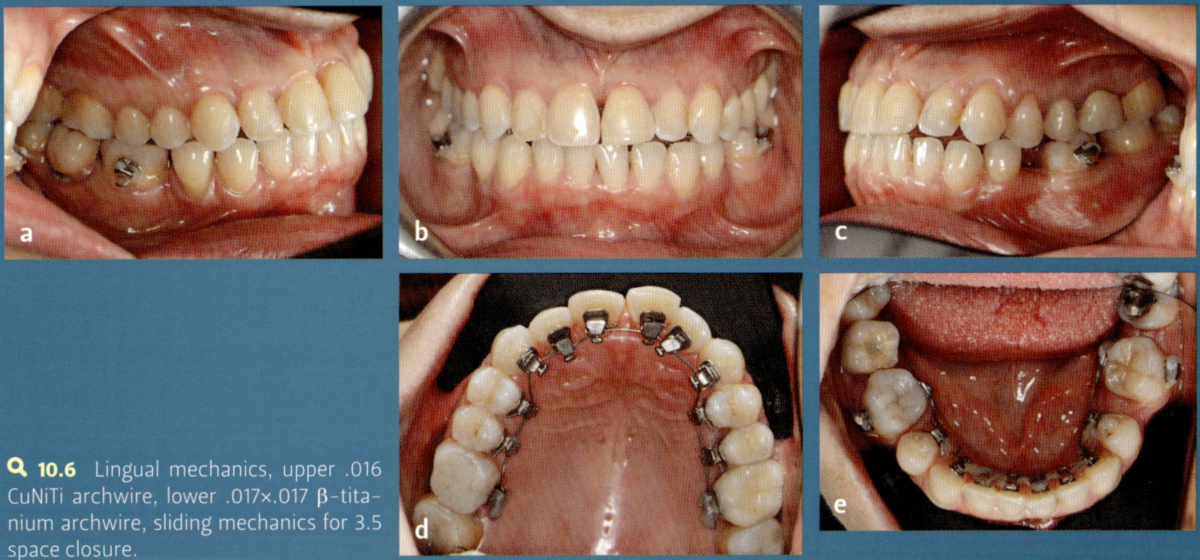

10.6 Lingual mechanics, upper .016 CuNiTi archwire, lower .017×.017 β-titanium archwire, sliding mechanics for 3.5 space closure.

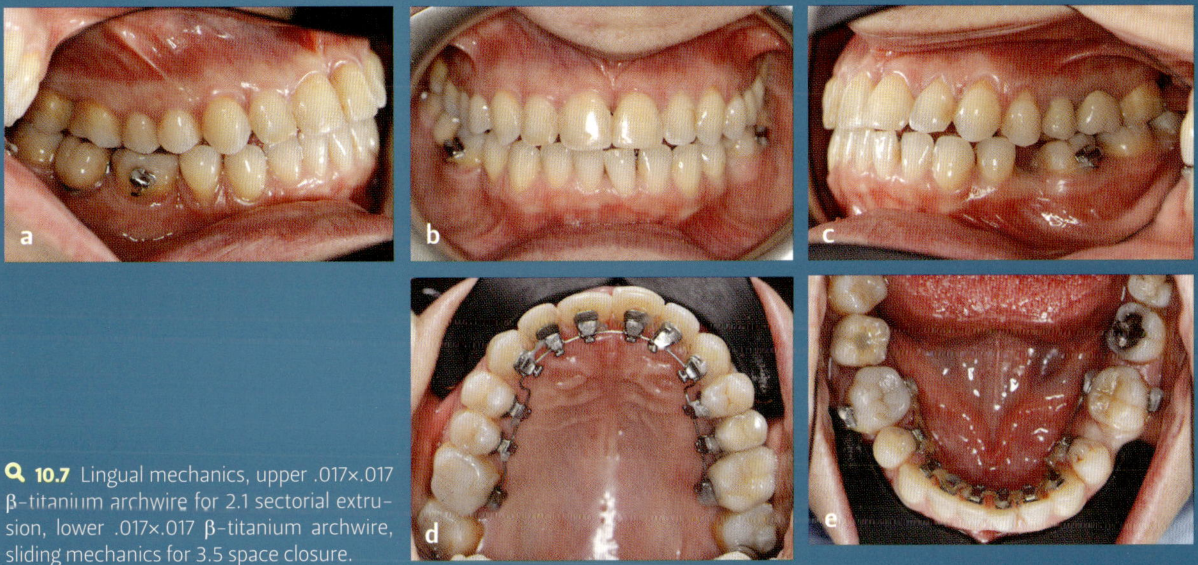

10.7 Lingual mechanics, upper .017×.017 β-titanium archwire for 2.1 sectorial extrusion, lower .017×.017 β-titanium archwire, sliding mechanics for 3.5 space closure.

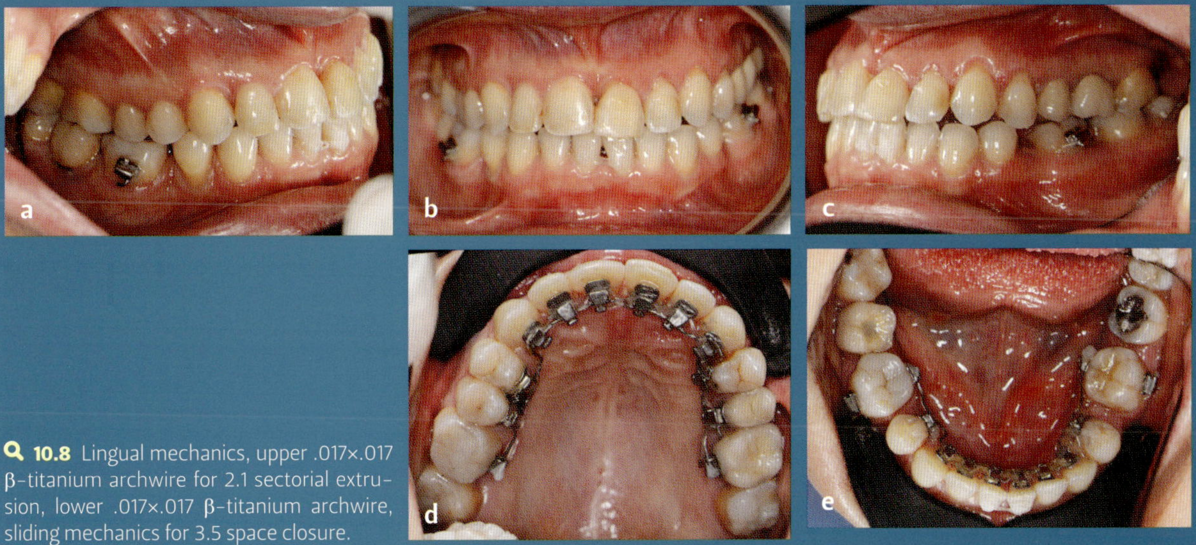

10.8 Lingual mechanics, upper .017×.017 β-titanium archwire for 2.1 sectorial extrusion, lower .017×.017 β-titanium archwire, sliding mechanics for 3.5 space closure.

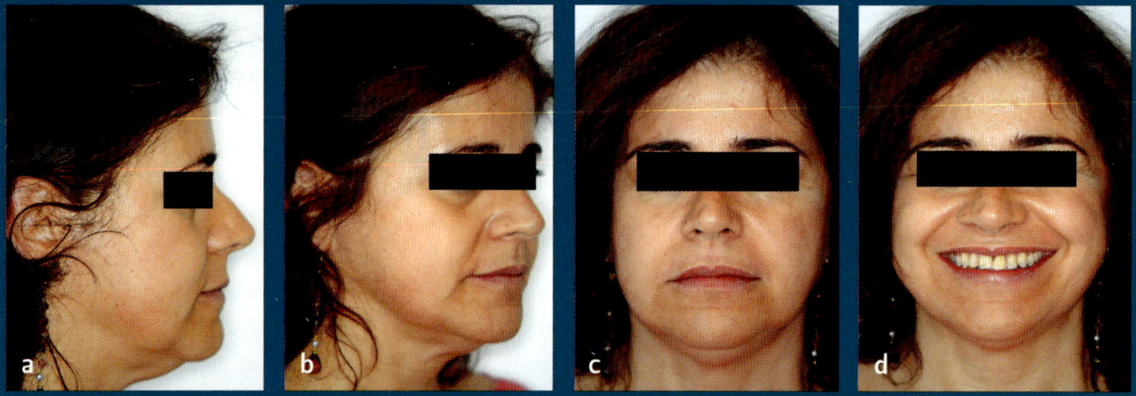

10.9 Extraoral post-orthodontic treatment photos, pre-restorative situation.

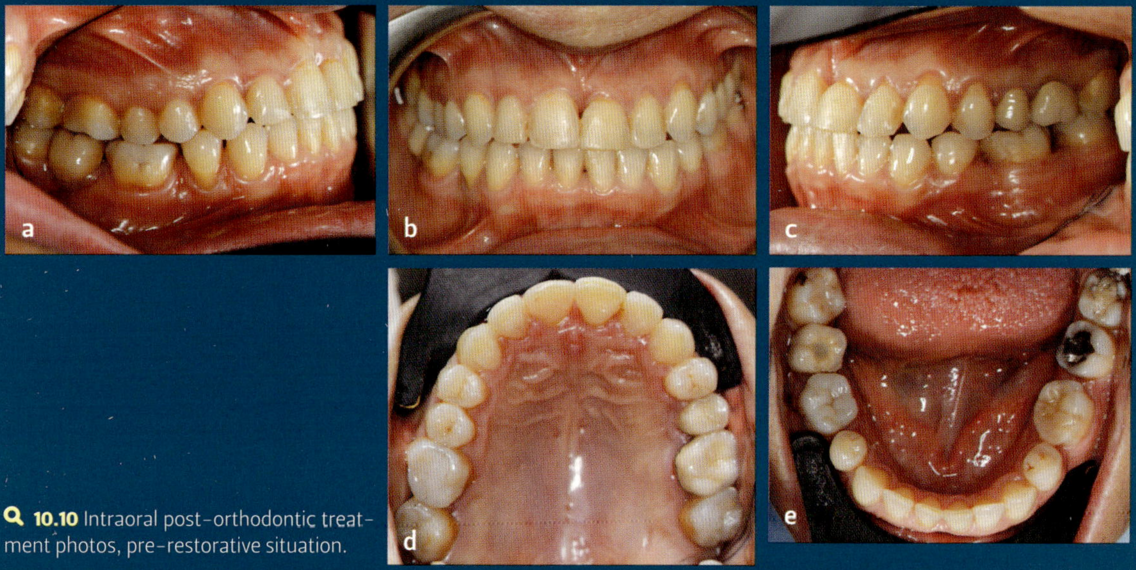

10.10 Intraoral post-orthodontic treatment photos, pre-restorative situation.

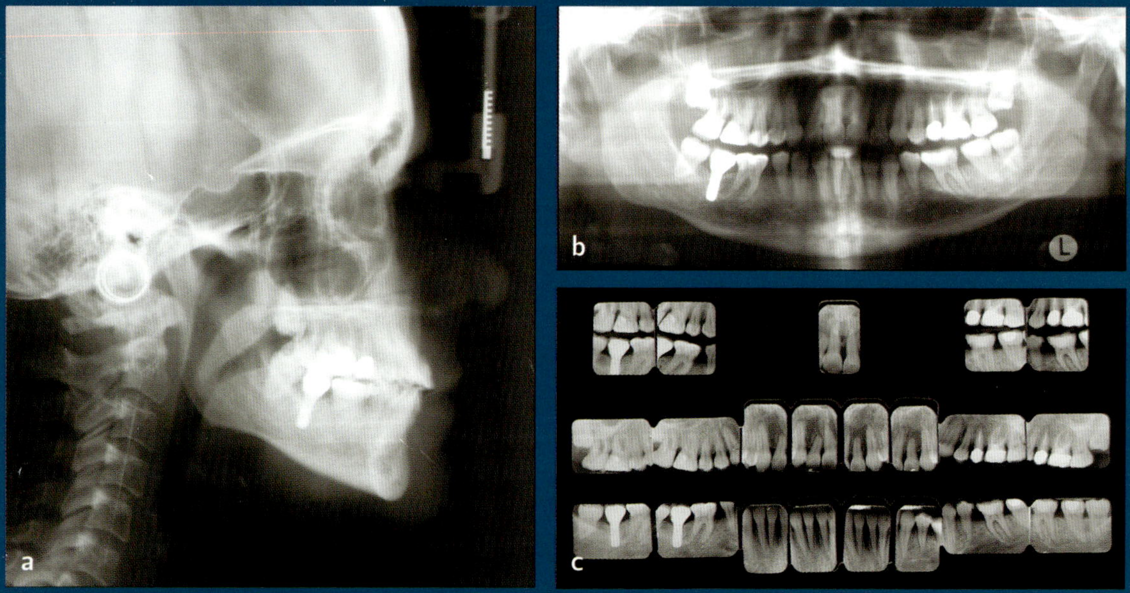

10.11 Post-orthodontic treatment cephalometric Rx (**a**), panoramic Rx (**b**), full radiographic periodontal status (**c**), pre-restorative situation.

The patient is now ready for the restorative procedures. Once the orthodontic treatment is finished, a long-term additive restorative rehabilitation in resin based composite is planned. This will allow to evaluate the behavior of the temporary rehabilitation and plan a definitive one in ceramic. This composite restoration, although has to be considered temporary, has however a multiple purpose: esthetic previsualization of the shapes, occlusal and interdental stability and monitoring of periodontal tissues in the cervical area. In clinical situations where there has been an orthodontic extrusion, the challenge very often is the management of the different cervical diameter of the extruded elements, as can be seen from the initial clinical situation (10.12). In these clinical situations, the correct approach lays between an ideal cervical shape and the available emergence from a reduced cervical diameter. The composite, allowing additive and subtractive modifications, is suitable as a material of excellence for developing and monitoring cervical emergencies that can be more or less steep. Following silicone impressions, a diagnostic wax-up was performed to preview the final shapes. After isolation with rubber dam (10.13), the silicone index (10.14) is checked for passivity and adaptation. The elements are sandblasted with aluminum oxide 50 µm, 2 atm, 2 cm. Etching is carried out with phosphoric acid and the adhesive system is applied. The palatal surface and the incisal margin are placed on the silicone index and printed in the mouth after repositioning. The interproximal surfaces are restored with sectional matrices and, finally, the buccal surface is modelled with high diffusion materials[28]. The cervical portion is first idealized to provide, as much as possible, a mirror-like symmetry between the two dental elements (10.15) and then it is modified to reduce the overhangs (10.16). After the completion of the lateral incisors, the final clinical situation is appreciable in 10.17.

At the 2-year follow-up, the patient shows facial balance (10.18), dental (10.19) and skeletal stability (10.20 and 10.21; see 10.2), harmonization of the interincisal bone peak (10.22) and harmonious smile (10.23).

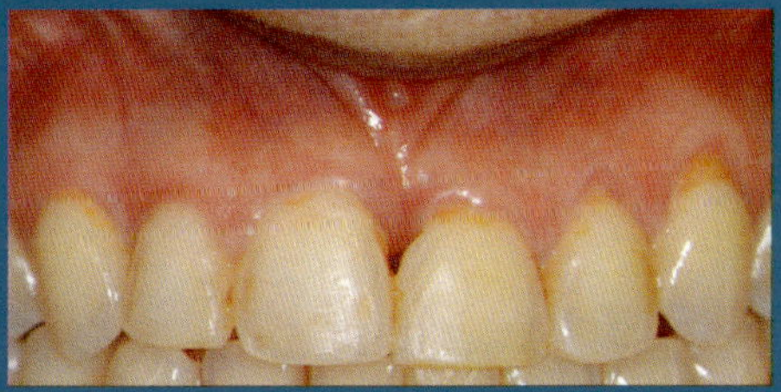

10.12 Clinical aspect before the restorative procedure.

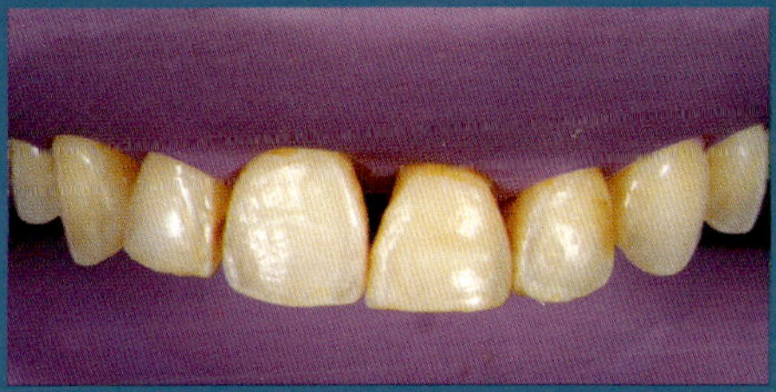

10.13 Isolation with rubber dam.

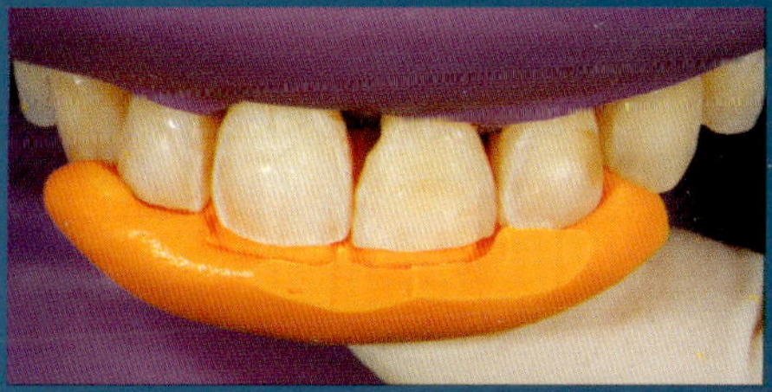

10.14 Silicone index try-in.

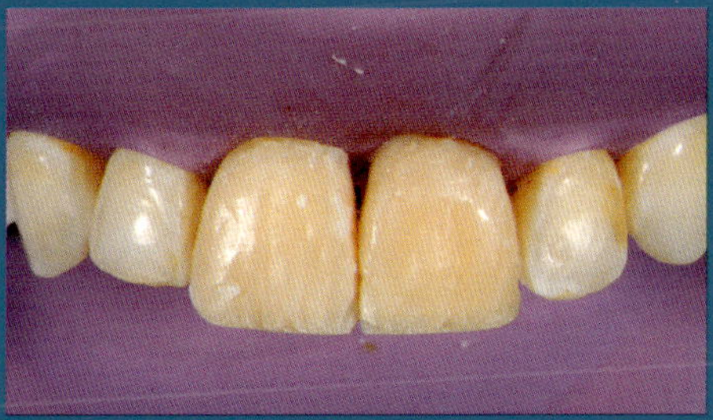

10.15 Composite layering on both incisors.

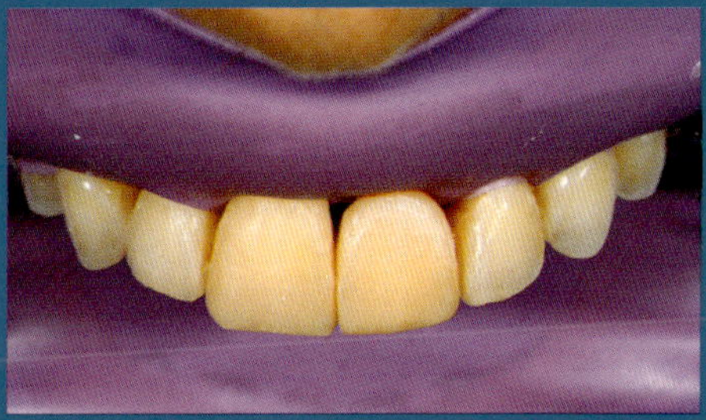

10.16 Horizontal over-hangs reduction.

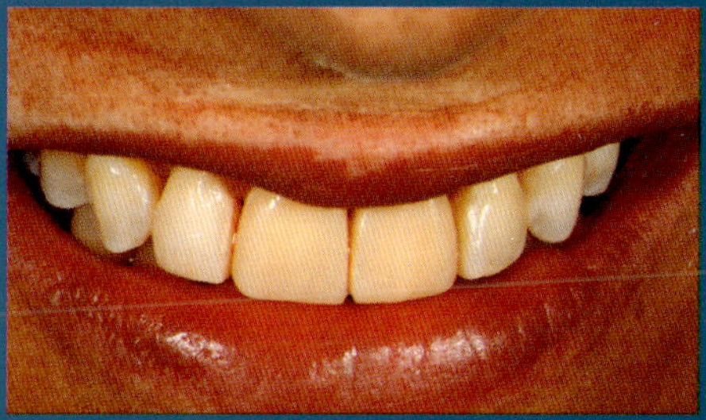

10.17 The smile of the patient at the end of the long-term temporary restorative procedure.

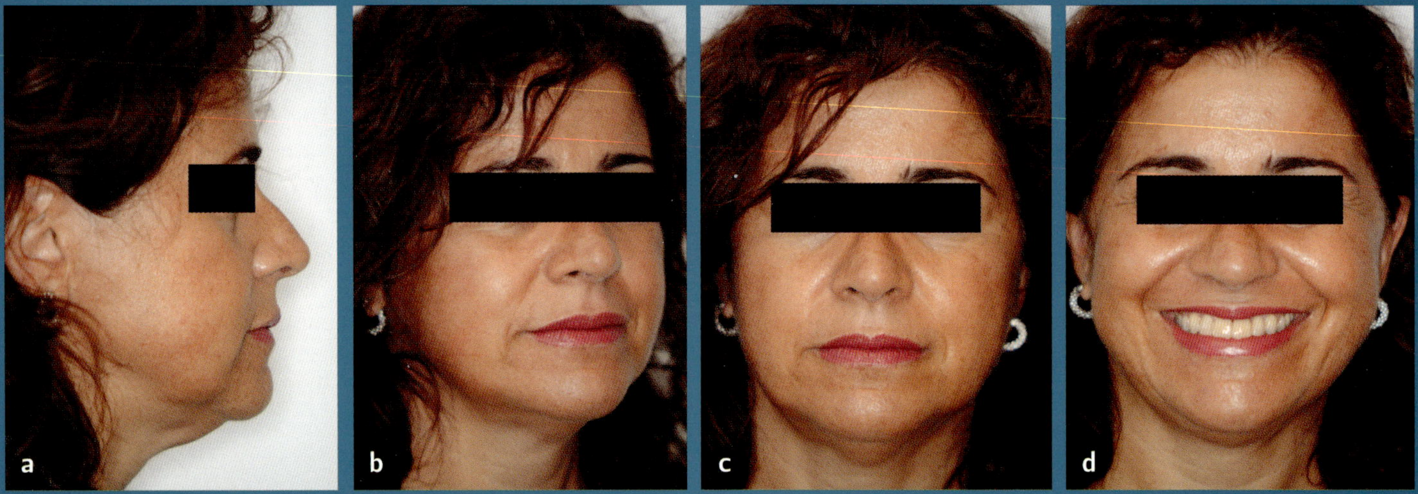

10.18 Extraoral post-treatment photos.

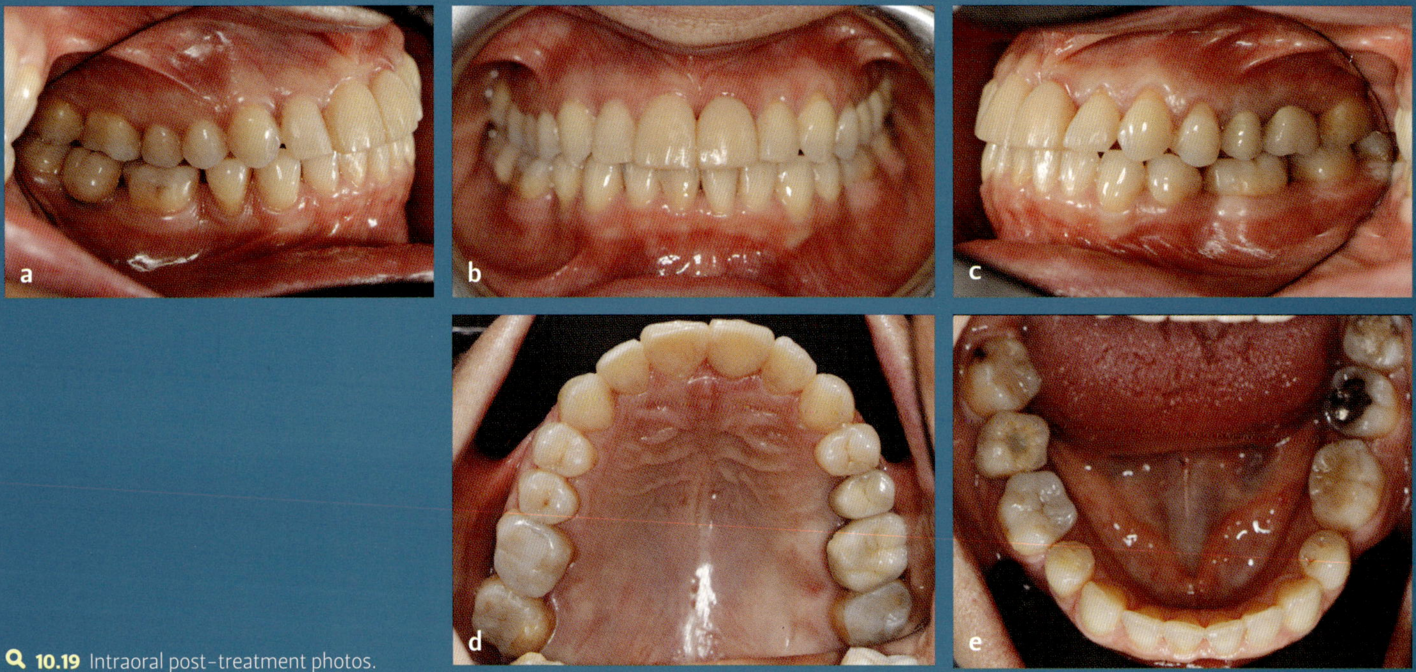

10.19 Intraoral post-treatment photos.

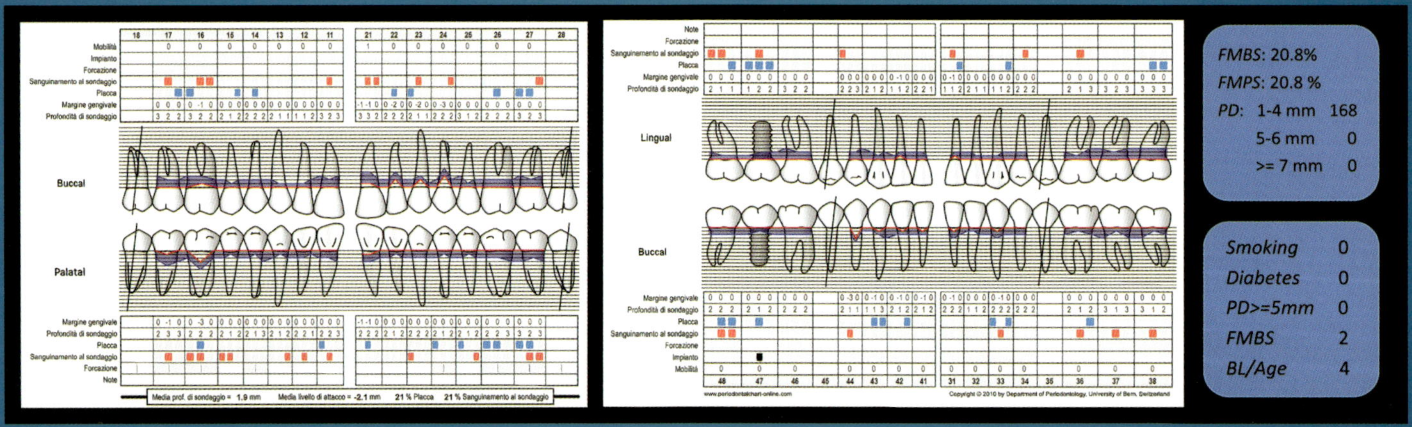

10.20 Periodontal probing, periodontal indexes, risk assessment at 2-year follow-up (Online periodontal charting tool from www.perio-tools.com).

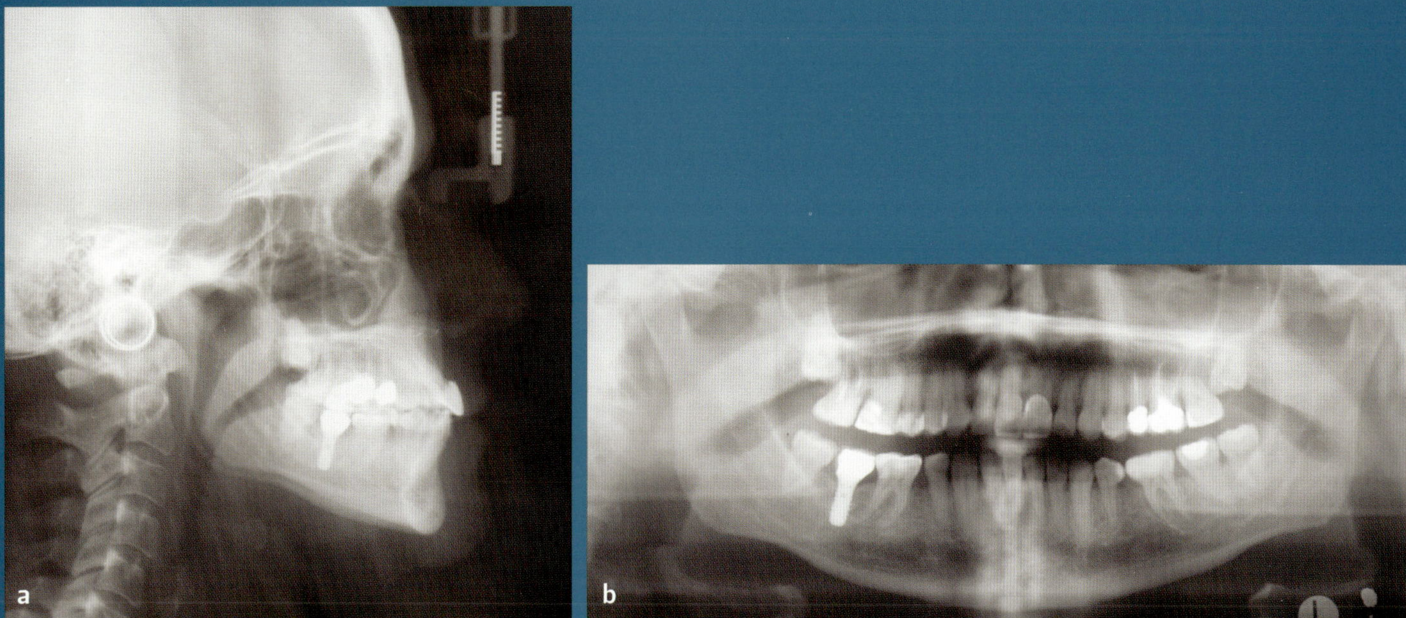

10.21 Post-treatment cephalometric Rx (**a**), panoramic Rx (**b**).

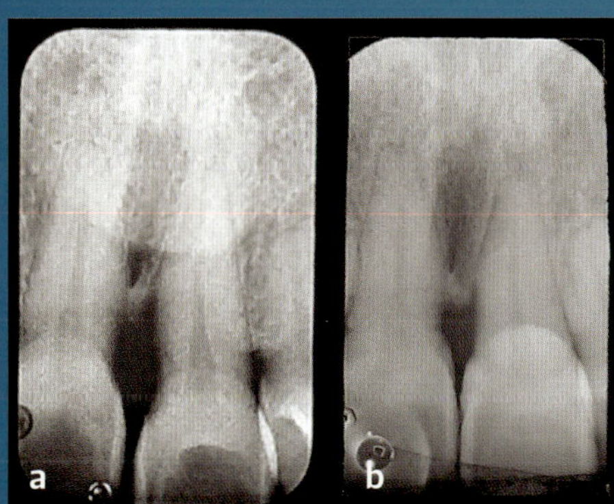

10.22 X-ray comparison pre- and post-orthodontic-restorative treatment where the elimination of the intrabony defect of the 2.1 by orthodontic movement can be seen.

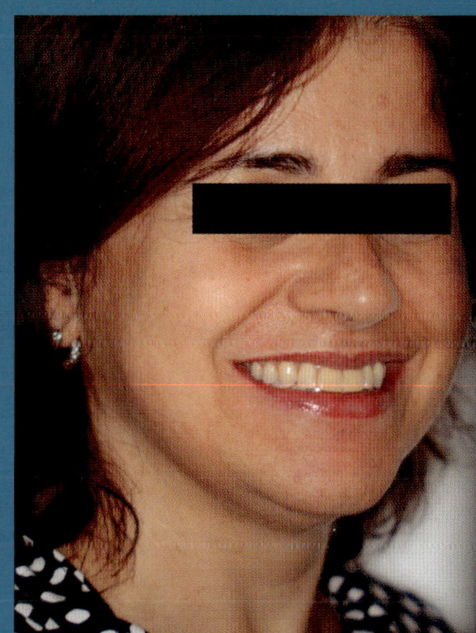

10.23 The smile of the patient at the end of treatment.

REFERENCES

1. Lyons KM, Darby I. Interdisciplinary periodontics: the multidisciplinary approach to the planning and treatment of complex cases. *Periodontol 2000*. 2017;74(1):7-10.
2. de Barros LA, de Almeida Cardoso M, de Avila ED et al. Six-year follow-up of maxillary anterior rehabilitation with forced orthodontic extrusion: achieving esthetic excellence with a multidisciplinary approach. *Am J Orthod Dentofacial Orthop*. 2013;144(4):607-615.
3. Diedrich P, Fritz U, Kizinger G. Interrelationship between periodontics and adult orthodontics. *Perio*. 2004;1(3):143-149.
4. Wise RJ, Nevins M. Anterior tooth site analysis (Bolton Index): how to determine anterior diastema closure. *Int J Periodontics Restorative Dent*. 1988;8(6):8-23.
5. Zachrisson BU, Minster L, Ogaard B, Birkhed D. Dental health assessed after interproximal enamel reduction: caries risk in posterior teeth. *Am J Orthod Dentofacial Orthop*. 2011;139(1):90-98.
6. Zachrisson BU, Nyøygaard L, Mobarak K. Dental health assessed more than 10 years after interproximal enamel reduction of mandibular anterior teeth. *Am J Orthod Dentofacial Orthop*. 2007;131(2):162-169.

7. Janson M, Janson G, Murillo-Goizueta OE. A modified orthodontic protocol for advanced periodontal disease in Class II division 1 malocclusion. *Am J Orthod Dentofacial Orthop.* 2011;139(4 Suppl):S133-S144.

8. Gkantidis N, Christou P, Topouzelis N. The orthodontic-periodontic interrelationship in integrated treatment challenges: a systematic review. *J Oral Rehabil.* 2010;37(5):377-390.

9. Roth A, Yildirim M, Diedrich P. Forced eruption with microscrew anchorage for preprosthetic leveling of the gingival margin. Case report. *J Orofac Orthop.* 2004;65(6):513-519.

10. Machuca G, Martínez F, Machuca C, Bullón P. A combination of orthodontic, periodontal, and prosthodontic treatment in a case of advanced malocclusion. *Int J Periodontics Restorative Dent.* 2003;23(5):499-505.

11. Keim RG. Aesthetics in clinical orthodontic-periodontic interactions. *Periodontol 2000.* 2001;27(1):59-71.

12. Gorbunkova A, Pagni G, Brizhak A et al. Impact of orthodontic treatment on periodontal tissues: a narrative review of multidisciplinary literature. *Int J Dent.* 2016;2016:4723589.

13. Reichert C, Hagner M, Jepsen S, Jäger A. Interfaces between orthodontic and periodontal treatment: their current status. *J Orofac Orthop.* 2011;72(3):165-186.

14. Ghezzi C, Masiero S, Silvestri M et al. Orthodontic treatment of periodontally involved teeth after tissue regeneration. *Int J Periodontics Restorative Dent.* 2008;28(6):559-567.

15. Kokich VG. Excellence in finishing: modifications for the perio-restorative patient. *Semin Orthod.* 2003;9(3):184-203.

16. Kokich VO Jr, Kiyak HA, Shapiro PA. Comparing the perception of dentists and lay people to altered dental esthetics. *J Esthet Dent.* 1999;11(6):311-324.

17. Kokich VG. Esthetics: the orthodontic-periodontic restorative connection. *Semin Orthod.* 1996;2(1):21-30.

18. Kapoor A, Singhai L, Kapoor S, Kapoor A. Ortho-perio interrelationships: an overview. *Int J Prev Clinic Dent Res.* 2016;3(3):206-212.

19. Harshita N, Kamath DG, Kadakampally D. Perio-ortho interactions. A review. *J Pharm Sci & Res.* 2018; 10(5):1053-1056.

20. Rosa M, Lucchi P, Ferrari S et al. Agénésie congénitale des incisives latérales maxillaires: évaluation parodontale et fonctionnelle à long terme après fermeture orthodontique de l'espace avec ingression de la première prémolaire et égression de la canine [Congenitally missing maxillary lateral incisors: long-term periodontal and functional evaluation after orthodontic space closure with first premolar intrusion and canine extrusion]. *Orthod Fr.* 2017;88(4):319-332.

21. Rosa M, Lucchi P, Ferrari S et al. Congenitally missing maxillary lateral incisors: long-term periodontal and functional evaluation after orthodontic space closure with first premolar intrusion and canine extrusion. *Am J Orthod Dentofacial Orthop.* 2016;149(3):339-348.

22. Zachrisson BU. Interdental papilla reconstruction in adult orthodontics. *World J Orthod.* 2004;5(1):67-73.

23. Zachrisson BU, Amat P. La recherche de l'excellence en orthodontie de l'adulte: entretien avec Bjørn U. Zachrisson [The search for excellence in adult orthodontics; an interview with Bjørn U. Zachrisson]. *Orthod Fr.* 2014;85(4):301-326.

24. Artun J, Kokich VG, Osterberg SK. Long-term effect of root proximity on periodontal health after orthodontic treatment. *Am J Orthod Dentofacial Orthop.* 1987;91(2):125-130.

25. Artun J, Osterberg SK, Kokich VG. Long-term effect of thin interdental alveolar bone on periodontal health after orthodontic treatment. *J Periodontol.* 1986;57(6):341-346.

26. Tuverson DL. Anterior interocclusal relations. Part II. *Am J Orthod.* 1980;78(4):371-393.

27. Tuverson DL. Anterior interocclusal relations. Part I. *Am J Orthod.* 1980;78(4):361-370.

28. Paolone G., Scolavino S. *Restauri diretti nei settori anteriori.* Milano. Quintessence Publishing Ed.; 2020.

Orthodontics in interdisciplinary treatment

Orthodontics, treating an increasing number of patients that have not only periodontal challenges, but also restorative and prosthetic impairement, needs to be in relationship with all the other specialties, such as restorative, prosthetic dentistry and implant surgery modifying, simplifying or solving the adult interdisciplinary rehabilitation problems. Adding orthodontic treatment to a complete rehabilitation plan that includes periodontology, implant rehabilitation, oral surgery and restorative treatments changes the clinician's point of view through the observation of problems that, without orthodontics, could lead to more invasive resolutions. In 11.1 we observe a case that, to a non-orthodontically trained group, could appear to be resolvable, albeit correctly, with a "classic" therapy through periodontal surgery and conventional prosthetic rehabilitation. Introducing orthodontics, however, the perspective changes, offering new solutions and integrated therapies (11.2).

Rehabilitative treatment of patients with periodontal support loss and teeth loss is a challenge and requires integration with other specialties to achieve optimal results. In the same way orthodontists who join these treatments must share the modern available surgical and rehabilitation techniques. This allows various specialists to plan and perform the best possible treatment for the patient. The goal of adult interdisciplinary treatment should be individualized and shared and the whole team should stick to the plan. In these cases, the aim of orthodontic therapy is to create the necessary conditions for the rehabilitation and replacement of missing teeth[1].

The use of orthodontics in the interdisciplinary, restorative and prosthetic patient and the application of an orthodontic appliance allow an enhancement of the prosthetic treatment *in toto* using additional dental movements such as the optimal distribution of the teeth, the parallelism of the abutments, the spaces for the pontics and the soft tissue remodeling in the edentulous site for their adaptation through orthodontic extrusion[2,3], the correction of mucogingival and bone defects. It allows then an improvement of the crown/root relationships, the closing of the spaces and the movement of the teeth which need serious uprighting[4]. Modern orthodontics with the use of TADs allows to provide mechanics that were previously difficult to manage even in patients with severe edentulousness or with reduced anchorage sites[5].

Below are reported two complete clinical cases in which we will examine how orthodontics takes part to complex rehabilitative cases: *Clinical case 1* starts from an orthodontic request, *Clinical case 2* from a rehabilitative request. In this second case, we will outline a complete workflow of an ortho-perio treatment from the very beginning to the end of the therapy and to the long-term re-evaluation, applying the correct timing procedure as described in 9.1.

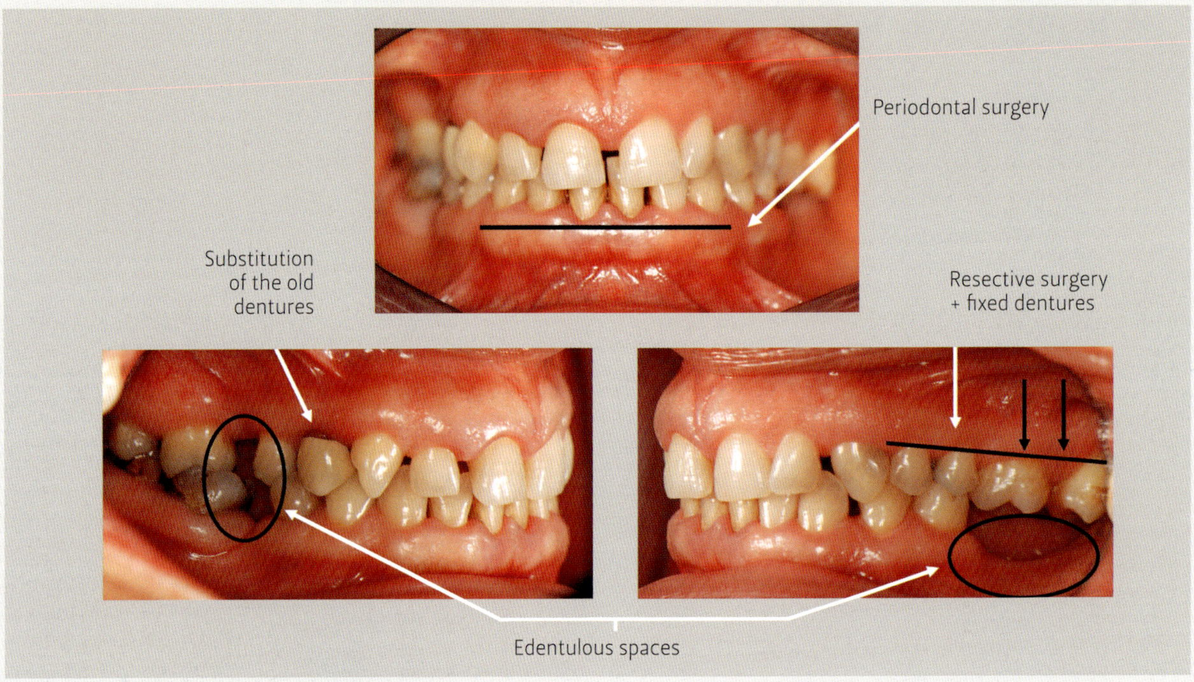

11.1 Treatment of an interdisciplinary case with "classic" therapy.

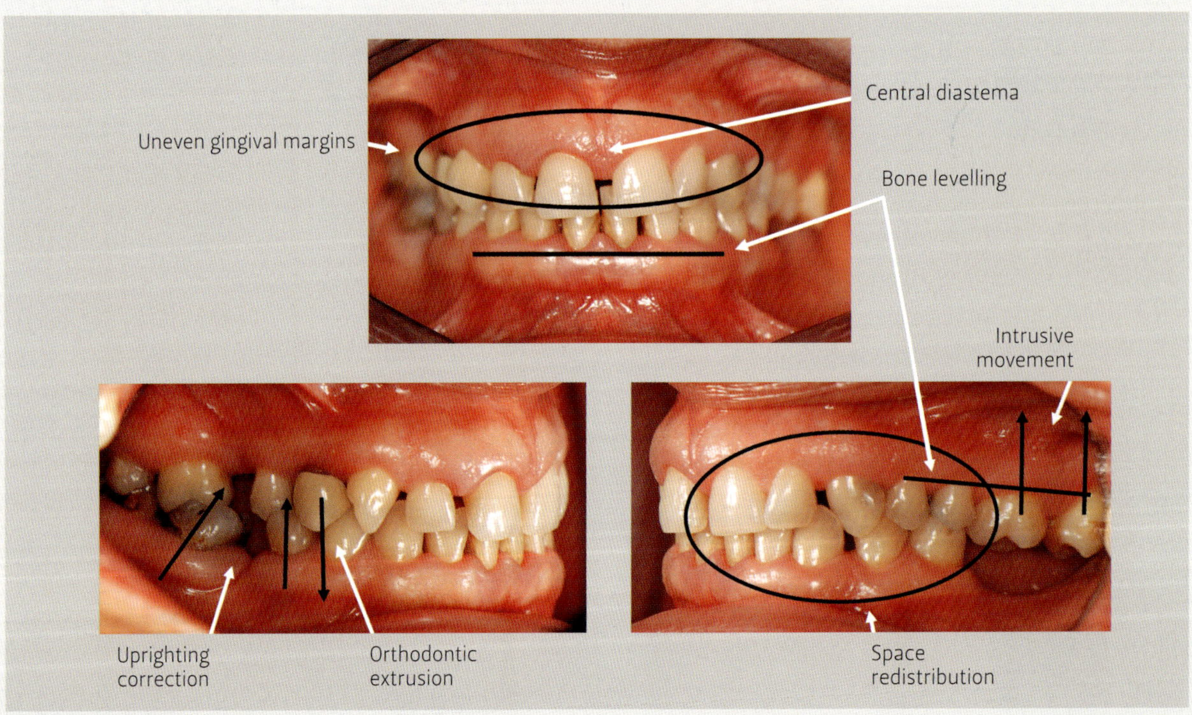

11.2 Integrated orthodontic-periodontal-surgical-restorative treatment.

Clinical case 1

The patient's request includes the resolution of the recurrent abscesses on 4.2-4.3 and of the lower anterior crowding with the preparation of the dentition for a complete implant-prosthetic rehabilitation. The treatment of the 4.2-4.3 lesion is described in detail as orthodontic extraction treatment in Chapter 8, *Clinical Case 3.*

The patient has facial symmetry, slightly open nasolabial angle, normal chin-neck length, and competent lips (11.3), absence of 1.4, 1.6, 1.8, 2.5, 2.8, 3.8, 4.8, molar and canine class I, normal OVJ, increased OVB (11.4), biretrusion, normodivergence (11.5; 11.1). The periodontal diagnosis after periodontal evaluation (11.6) is periodontitis stage III generalized grade C[6,7] with high FMPS and FMBS values with medium-high risk (Perio Risk: 13)[8-10]. After initial periodontal therapy, the re-evaluation (11.7) shows a reduction of FMBS and FMPS <20% and of the probing values. Residual pockets are treated in 4.2-4.3 site with an orthodontic extraction, as described in Chapter 8, and in 1.5-1.7 site with an orthodontic movement after a GTR procedure on 1.5 (as described in Chapter 9) and a subsequent extraction together with the 1.7 extraction after movement in the edentulous area in order to regularize the ridge to allow implant placement (such as described in Chapter 6).

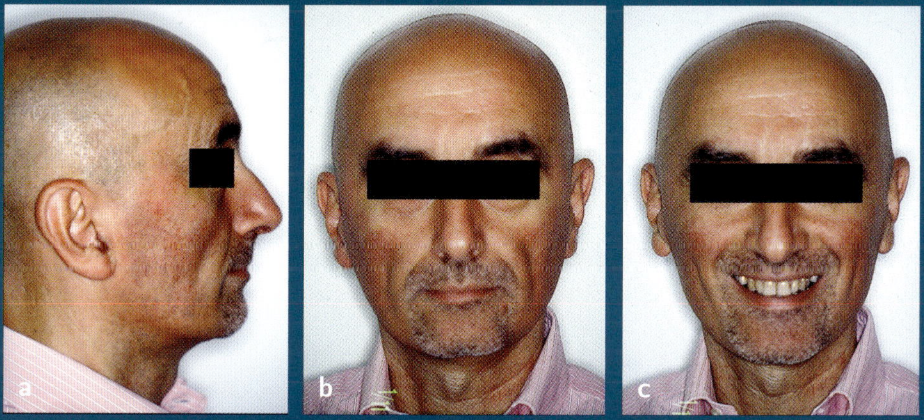

11.3 Extraoral pre-treatment photos.

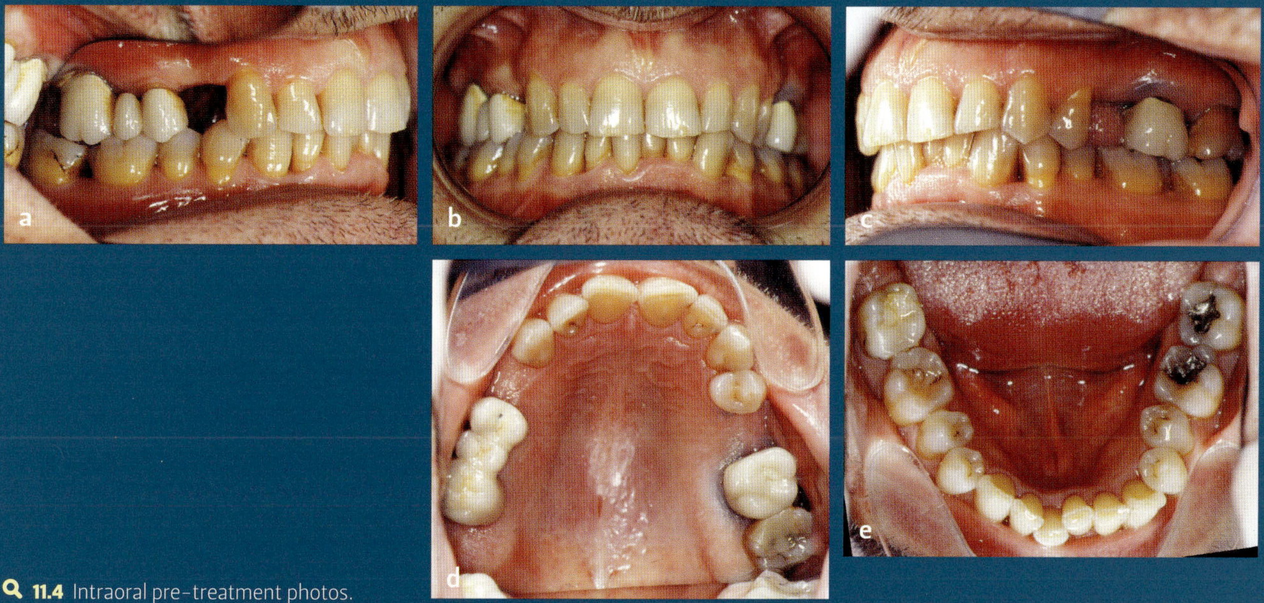

11.4 Intraoral pre-treatment photos.

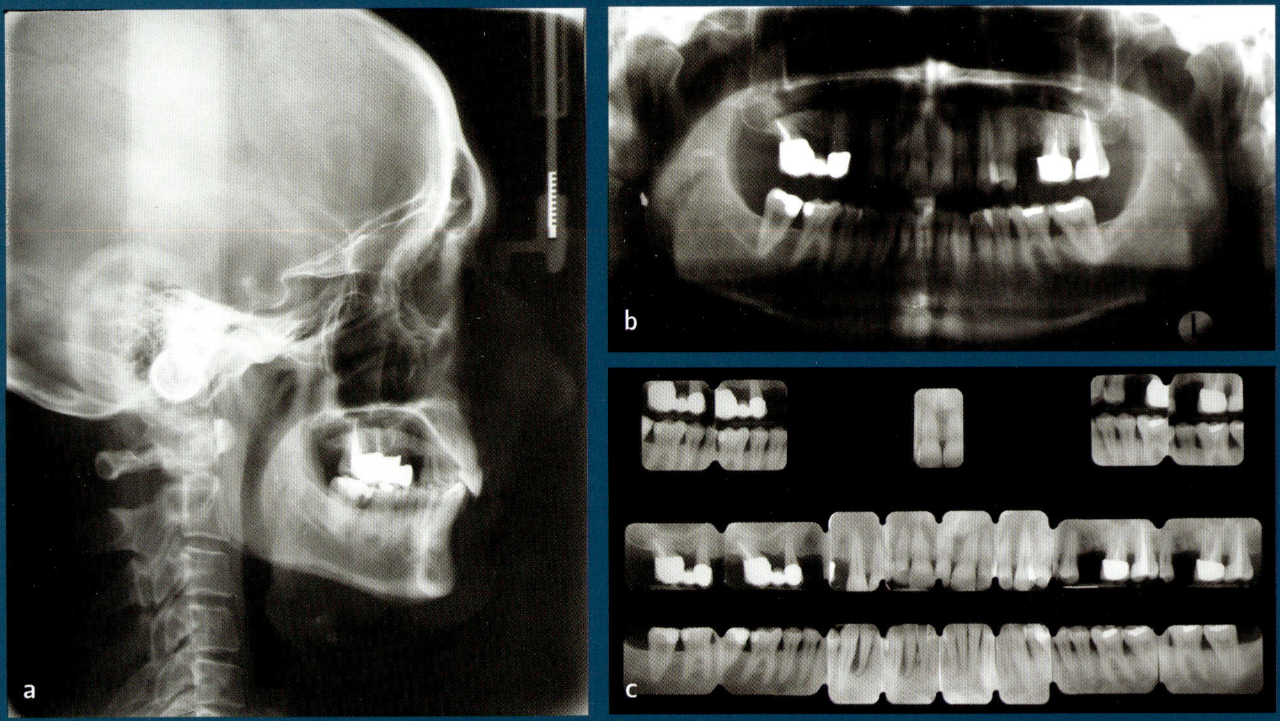

11.5 Pre-treatment cephalometric Rx (**a**), panoramic Rx (**b**), full radiographic periodontal status (**c**).

Tab. 11.1 Cephalometric values

Sagittal skeletal relationships	**Pre-treatment**	**Post-treatment**	**Mean**	**DS**
Maxillary sagittal relationship SNA	73°	73°	82°	3.5°
Mandibular sagittal relationship SNPg	71°	72°	80°	3.5°
Intermaxillary sagittal relationship ANPg	2°	1°	2°	2.5°
Vertical skeletal relationships				
Maxillary vertical relationship SN / ANS-PNS	9°	10°	8°	3.0°
Mandibular vertical relationship SN / Go-Gn	29°	28°	33°	2.5°
Intermaxillary vertical relationship ANS-PNS / Go-Gn	20°	18°	25°	6.0°
Dento-basal relationships				
Upper incisor inclination $\underline{1}$ - ANS-PNS	101°	97°	110°	6.0°
Lower incisor inclination $\overline{1}$ - Go-Gn	102°	98°	94°	7.0°
Lower incisor compensation $\overline{1}$ - A-Pg (mm)	0	-1	2	2.0
Dental relationships				
Overjet (OVJ, mm)	4	3	3,5	2.5
Overbite (OVB, mm)	6	3	2	2.5
Interincisal angle $\underline{1}/\overline{1}$	137°	140°	132°	6.0°

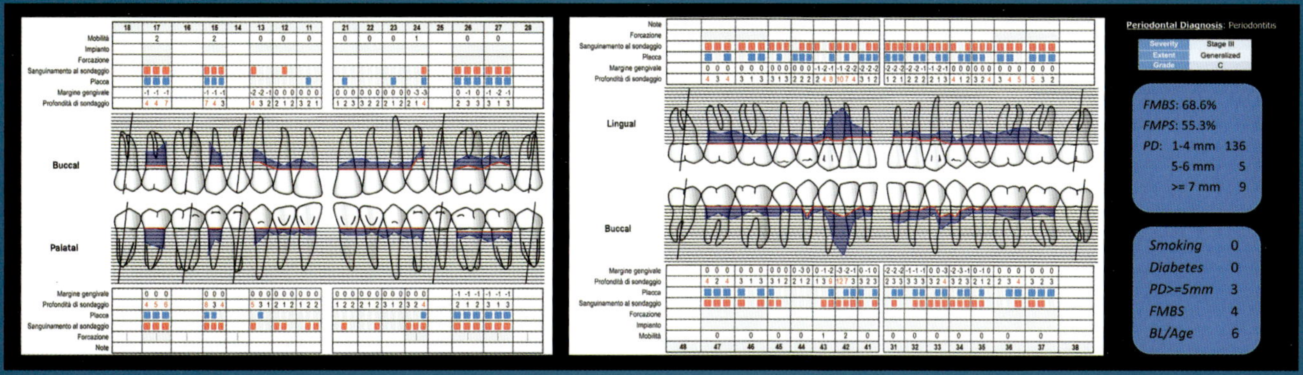

11.6 Initial periodontal probing, periodontal diagnosis, periodontal indexes, periodontal diagnosis, risk assessment (Online periodontal charting tool from www.perio-tools.com).

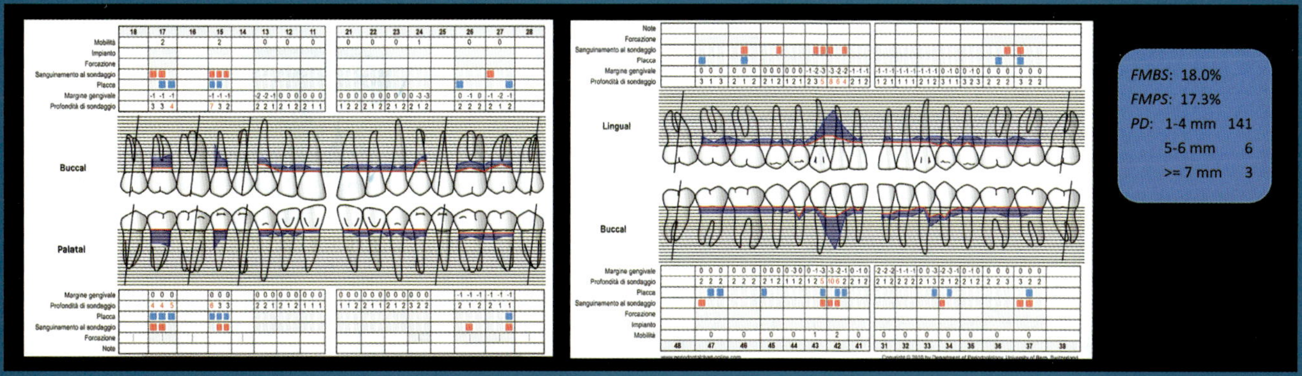

11.7 Re-evaluation periodontal probing and periodontal indexes (Online periodontal charting tool from www.perio-tools.com).

Orthodontic phase

At first the lingual mechanics (Kurz 7th Generation, ®Ormco) is applied with set-up and indirect bonding on the lower arch; for details and images of the extrusive extraction phase of 4.2, see Chapter 8. Towards the end of the extrusion of 4.2, in the vestibular area between 1.3 and 1.5 a miniscrew is positioned as an anchoring system for a sectional designed to stimulate the site for the implant's insertion in the upper right sector by extrusion and mesialization of 1.5 and distalization of 1.7 with loops and NiTi compressed spring (11.8; see 9.2-9.10; 6.35-6.37). In the upper arch, alignment is realized with a .016 CuNiTi archwire

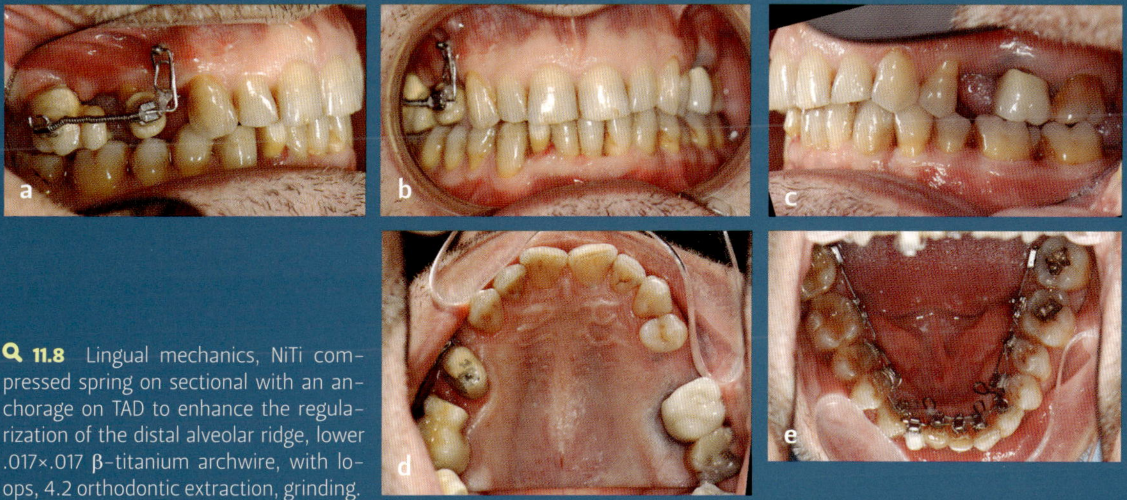

11.8 Lingual mechanics, NiTi compressed spring on sectional with an anchorage on TAD to enhance the regularization of the distal alveolar ridge, lower .017×.017 β-titanium archwire, with loops, 4.2 orthodontic extraction, grinding.

during the first month (11.9), then with a .016 β-titanium archwire and then with a .017×.017 β-titanium archwire with loops (see 11.15), after the application of the temporary crowns on the osseointegrated implants, and finally with an arch .017×.025 β-titanium archwire. In the lower arch the alignment is carried out with a 017×.017 β-titanium archwire with loops, detailed with a .017×.025 β-titanium archwire.

Surgical phase

During the last part of the orthodontic phase, the implants are placed in the upper right and left sectors. In the right area (11.10 and 11.11), after regularization of the crest with the movement of 1.5 in the edentulous area, teeth are extracted and implants (Frialit-2®, Dentsply) placed by LMSF[11,12] technique at the 1.5 and 1.7 sites and by ERE[13] technique at the 1.4 site. An implant (Frialit-2®, Dentsply) is placed in 2.5 site (11.12)

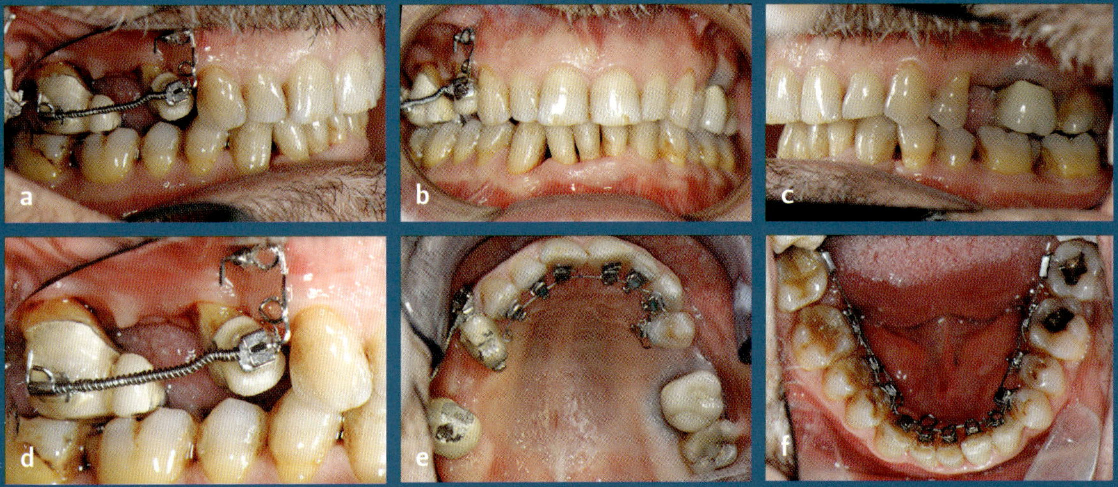

11.9 Lingual mechanics, NiTi compressed spring on sectional with an anchorage on TAD, tipping and extrusion to regularize the alveolar distal ridge, lower .017×.017 β-titanium archwire, with closing loops post- 4.2 orthodontic extraction.

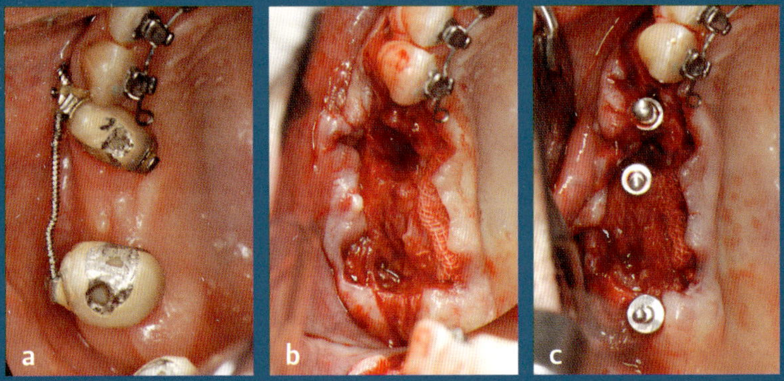

11.10 Clinical view of the bone ridge on the distal site of the 1.5 after bodily mesializationmovement towards 1.3 (**a**); bone ridge after teeth extraction (**b**); implant probe to evaluate the implant placement (**c**).

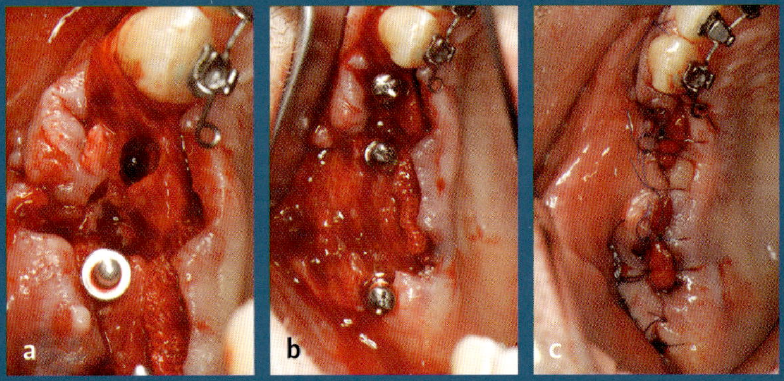

11.11 Detail of the E.R.E. used for implant placement in 1.4 site (**a**); implant on site (**b**); suture (**c**).

where a small vestibular fenestration, present at the level of the implant site, is regenerated by autologous bone. At the end of osseointegration in the right upper sector (11.13), in the second surgical phase an apical repositioning flap is performed to keep the amount of keratinized tissue intact. The second surgical phase on 2.5 implant site is associated with a surgical crown lengthening on 2.6 and 2.7 (11.14). In 11.16, it can be observed tissues before final cementation. At the end of the treatment the patient has facial balance, molar and canine class I, normalization of OVJ and OVB and cephalometric values (11.17 -11.19; see 11.1). At the periodontal level the values at the end of treatment (11.20) indicate a good stability of periodontal indexes, with FMBS and FMPS <20%, elimination of all periodontal probing >4 mm and the risk evaluation reached a medium-low grade (Perio Risk: 5)[8-10], thanks to the treatment on the 4.2 defect and the elimination of all periodontal probing >5 mm.

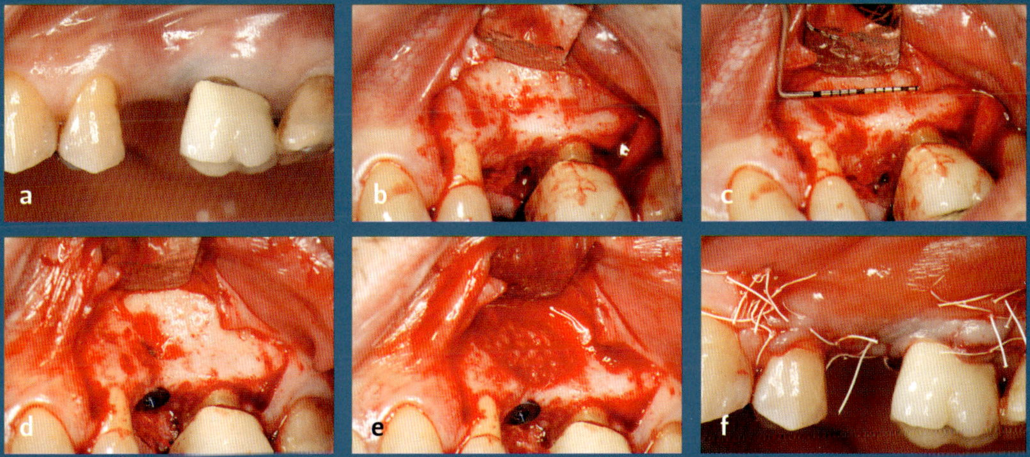

11.12 Implant placement on 2.4 site, with the bone fenestration regenerated by autologous bone (**e**) and the flap suture.

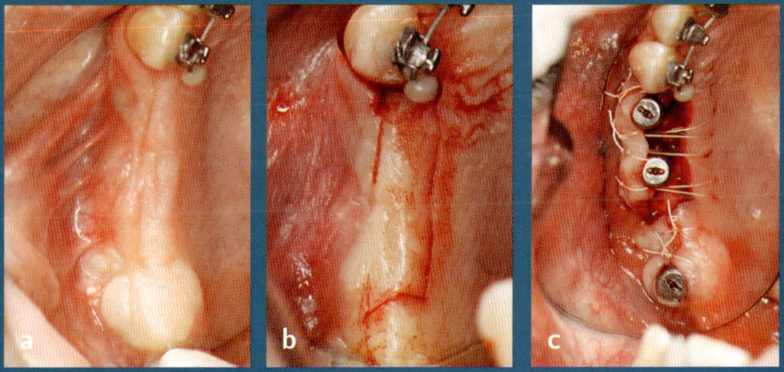

11.13 Second stage surgery on upper right sector; palatal keratinized tissue and its vestibular repositioning with ePTFE suture.

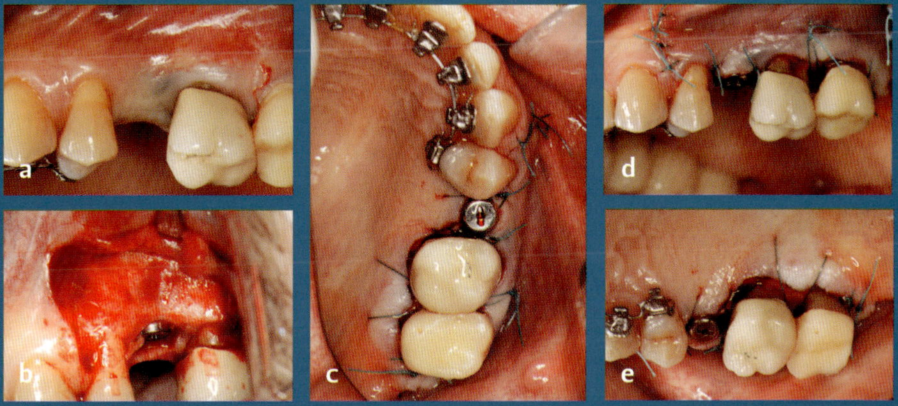

11.14 Second stage surgery on upper left sector; detail of the fenestration of the 11.12 regenerated by autologous bone (**b**); vertical and horizontal mattress suture after surgical crown lengthening of 2.6 and 2.7 (**d**,**e**).

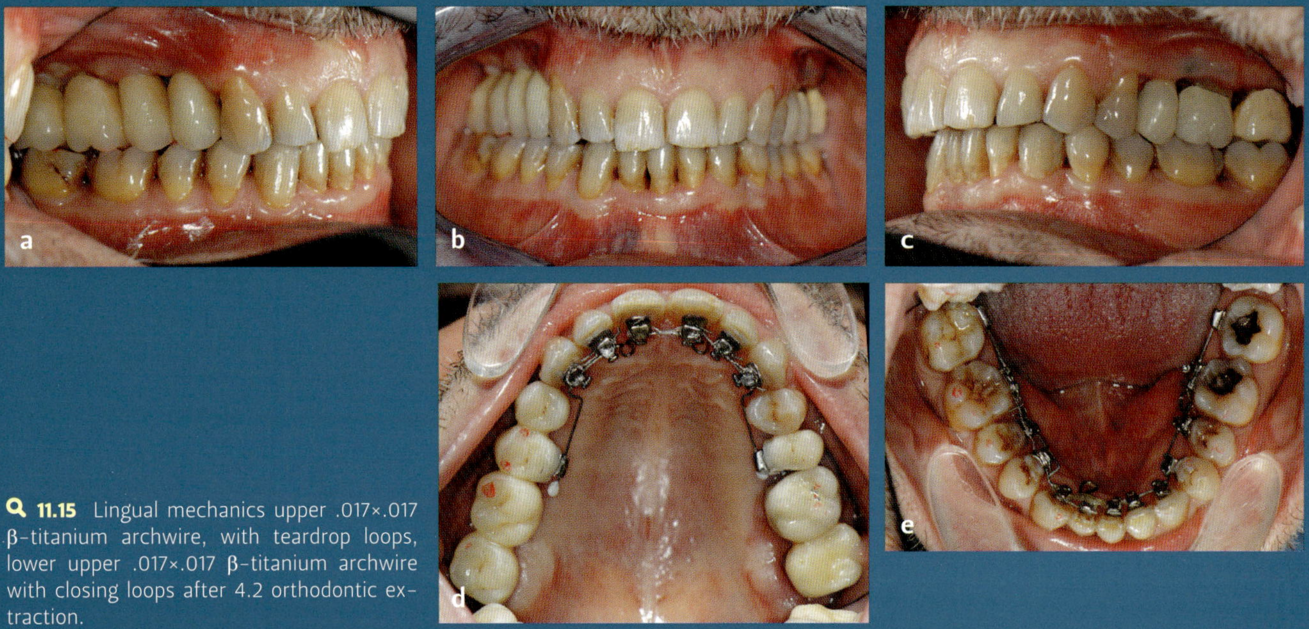

11.15 Lingual mechanics upper .017×.017 β-titanium archwire, with teardrop loops, lower upper .017×.017 β-titanium archwire with closing loops after 4.2 orthodontic extraction.

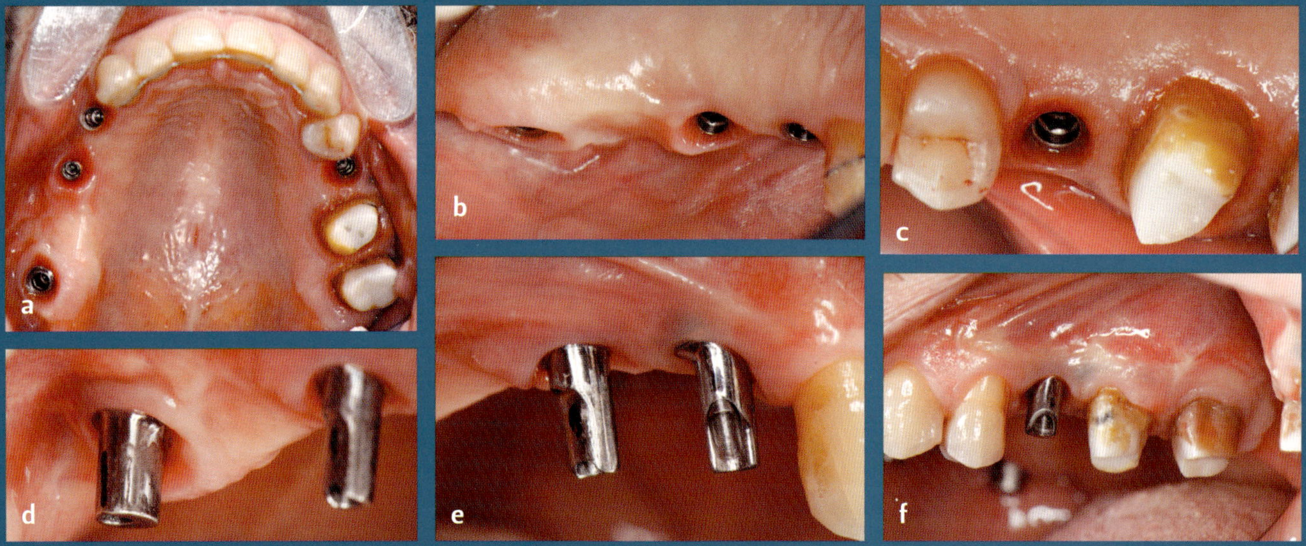

11.16 Final view of the soft tissues before the cementation of the fixed crowns (on teeth and on implants), with their abutments.

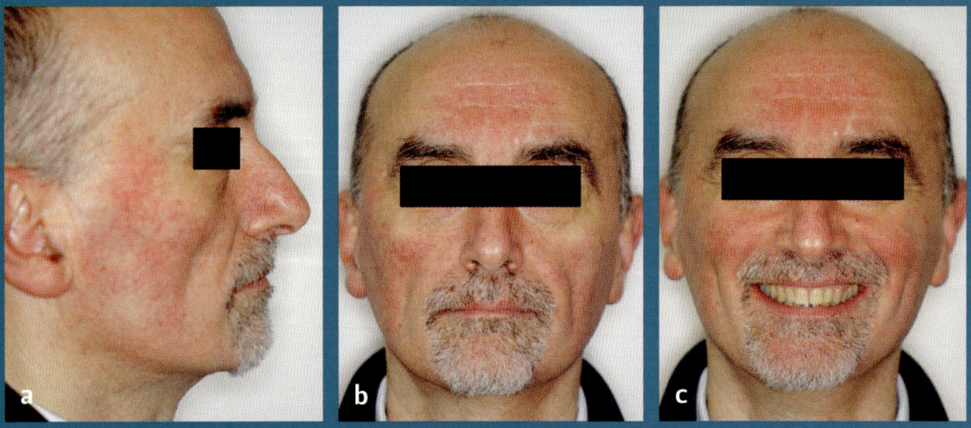

11.17 Extraoral post-treatment photos.

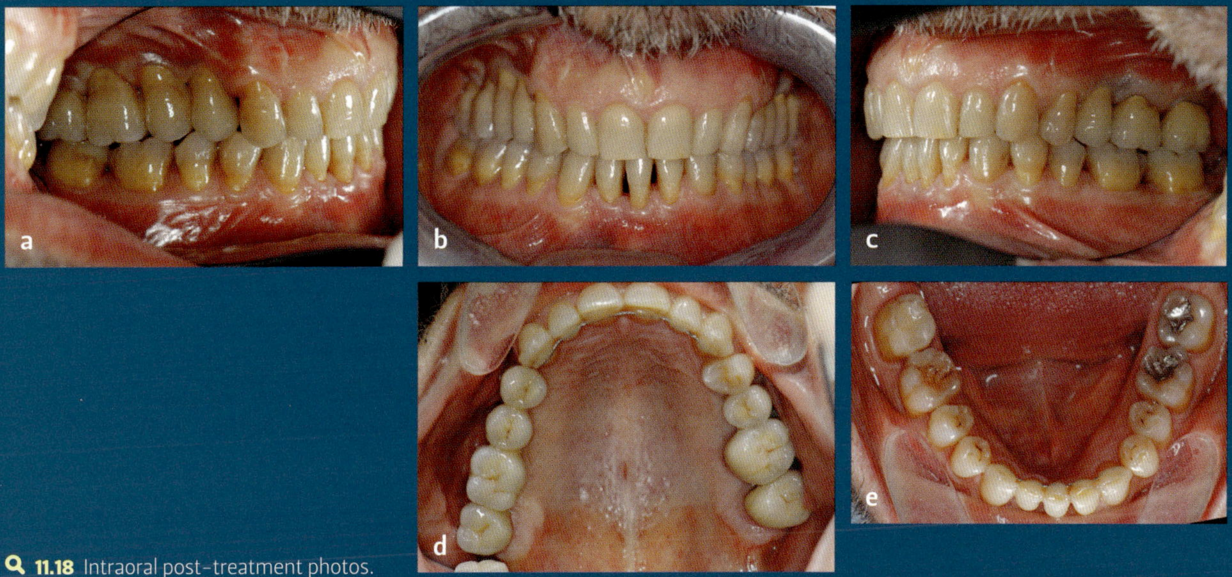

11.18 Intraoral post-treatment photos.

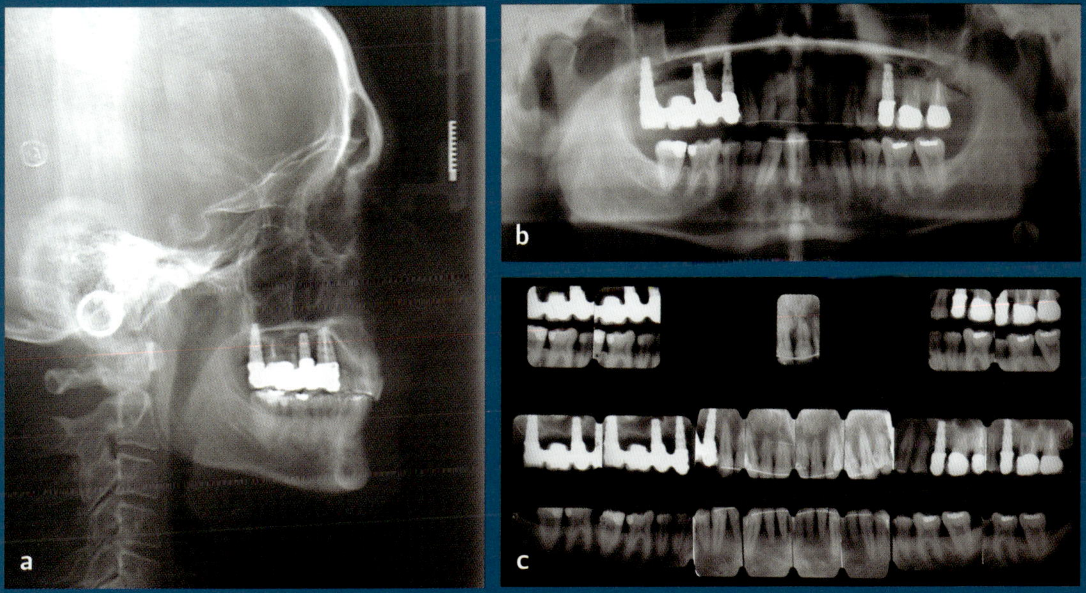

11.19 Post-treatment cephalometric Rx (**a**), panoramic Rx (**b**), full radiographic periodontal status (**c**).

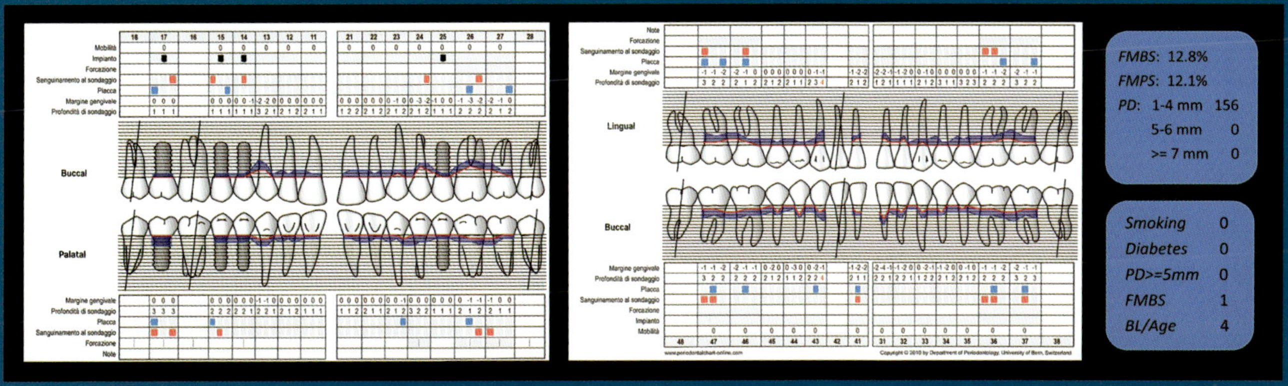

11.20 Post-treatment periodontal probing, periodontal indexes, risk assessment (Online periodontal charting tool from www.perio-tools.com).

Clinical case 2

Pre-orthodontic phase (phase 1 ortho-perio timing, see 9.1)

The patient's request is to completely rehabilitate her mouth, solve edentulous areas and periodontal problems and improve the esthetics of her smile. She complains about esthetic dissatisfaction for the superior anterior group, for the diastema and for the lack of teeth. She does not report pain or bleeding during oral hygiene manoeuvres. She reports stress from work and she's a former smoker (about 8-10 cigarettes/day), a habit stopped 10 years before. She reports her last dental visit about 5 years before, during which the lower left molars were extracted and various endo-restorative and prosthetic treatments were performed. She reports that the missing elements were extracted over the years due to decays. Although not aware of optimal oral hygiene, she is determined to carry out a complete rehabilitation, therefore she would not refuse orthodontic treatment, if necessary. For this reason we evaluate the patient at the very beginning also from the orthodontic point of view. The patient has facial symmetry and sagittal harmony, mild labial incompetence, slight gingival smile (11.21), canine and premolar class I (the absence of 1.6, 3.6 and 4.6 makes molar class non evaluable), normal OVJ and increased OVB, lingual inclination of incisors, absence of several dental elements (1.6, 2.8, 3.6, 3.7, 3.8, 4.6), extrusion of 2.6, 2.7, superior interincisal diastema (11.22), skeletal normodivergent class I (11.23; 11.2). The patient is examined from a periodontal point of view with the execution of a complete

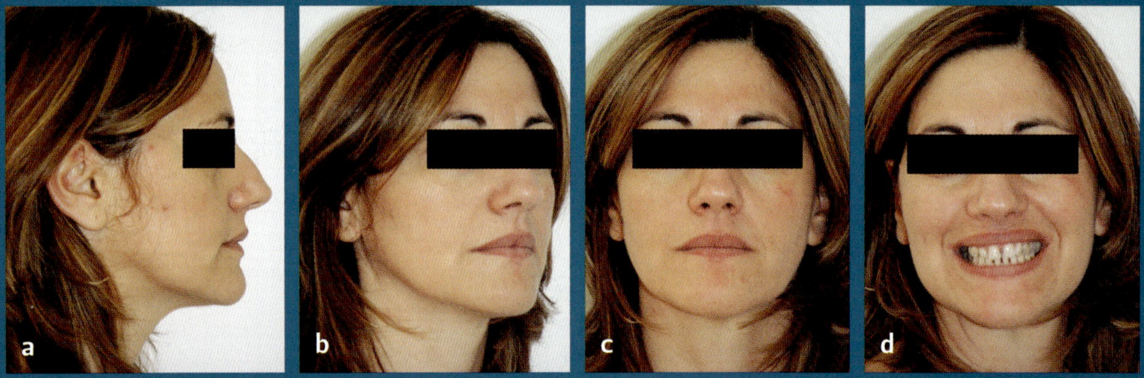

11.21 Extraoral pre-treatment photos.

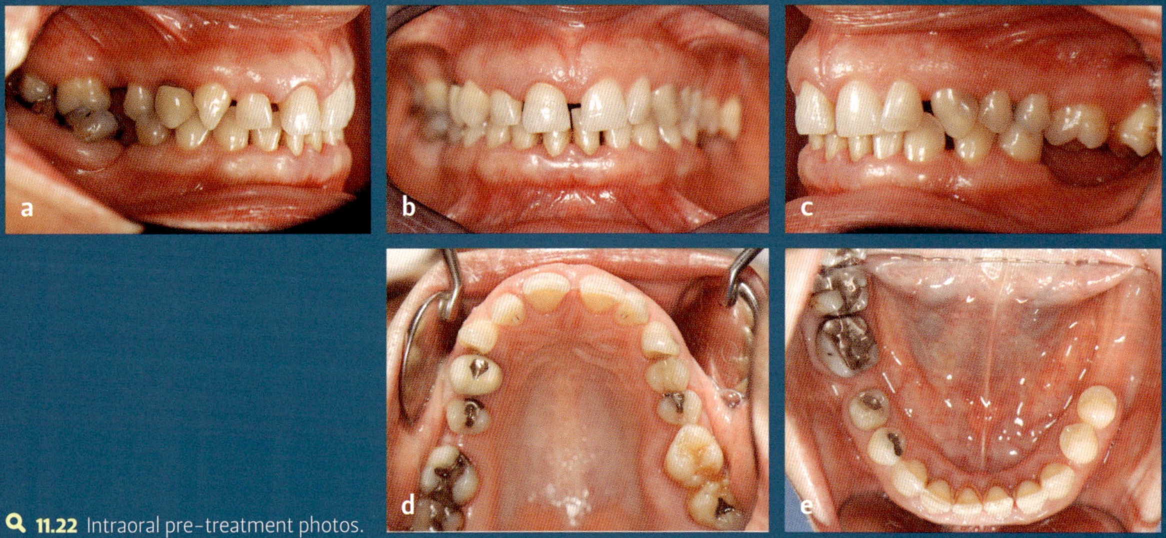

11.22 Intraoral pre-treatment photos.

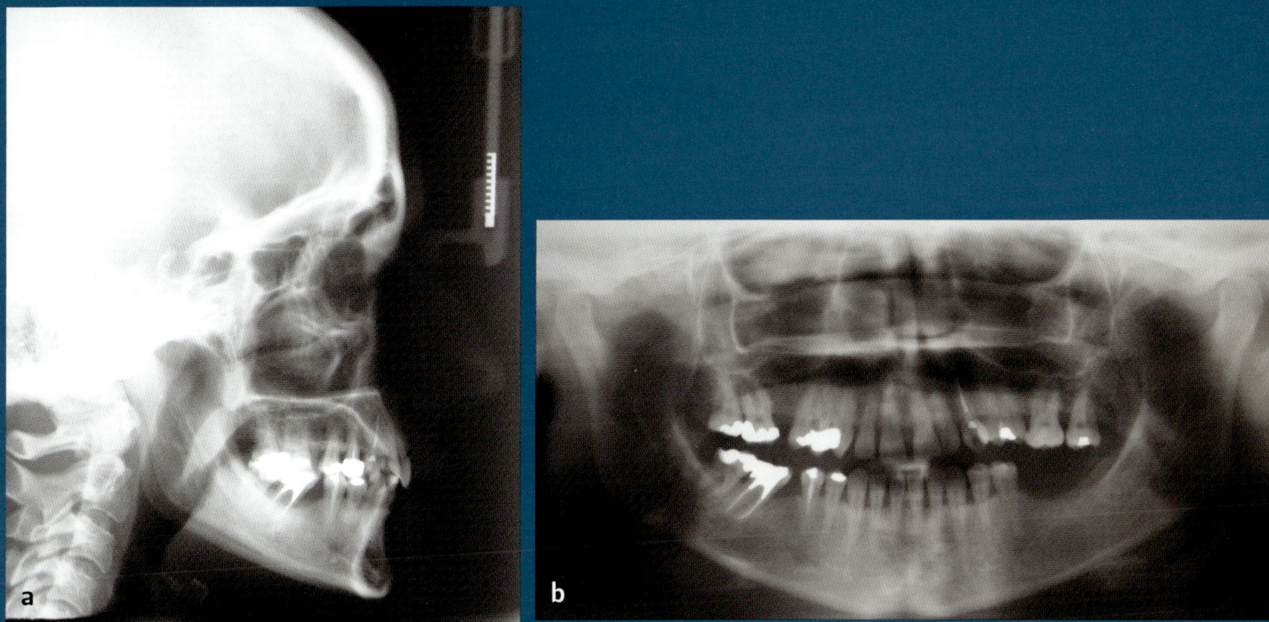

11.23 Pre-treatment cephalometric Rx (**a**) panoramic Rx (**b**).

Tab. 11.2 Cephalometric values

Sagittal skeletal relationships	Pre-treatment	Post-treatment	Media	Mean
Maxillary sagittal relationship SNA	83°	81°	82°	3.5°
Mandibular sagittal relationship SNPg	81°	80°	80°	3.5°
Intermaxillary sagittal relationship ANPg	2°	1°	2°	2.5°
Vertical skeletal relationships				
Maxillary vertical relationship SN / ANS-PNS	9°	7°	8°	3.0°
Mandibular vertical relationship SN / Go-Gn	34°	33°	33°	2.5°
Intermaxillary vertical relationship ANS-PNS / Go-Gn	25°	26°	25°	6.0°
Dento-basal relationships				
Upper incisor inclination 1 - ANS-PNS	104°	107°	110°	6.0°
Lower incisor inclination 1 - Go-Gn	86°	85°	94°	7.0°
Lower incisor compensation 1 - A-Pg (mm)	-1	-1	2	2.0
Dental relationships				
Overjet (OVJ, mm)	3	3	3.5	2.5
Overbite (OVB, mm)	5	3	2	2.5
Interincisal angle 1 / 1	144°	146°	132°	6.0°

radiographic status (11.24) and periodontal probing (11.25) showing gingival and generalized tissue inflammation. Deposits of plaque and calculus are present, particularly on the lower incisors and on the lingual side of the lower molars, as it can be seen in the photographs of the various sectors (11.26). The patient's periodontal diagnosis is a periodontitis stage III generalized grade B[6,7] with a medium-high risk (Perio Risk: 13)[8-10]. After having performed the initial periodontal therapy and the endodontic treatment with the restoration of 2.3, the patient is re-evaluated after 8 weeks[14]. The effect of the initial periodontal therapy is expressed with a reduction of the clinical signs of inflammation: FMBS (11.5%) and FMPS (8.9%) (11.27). The compliance has improved and the patient radically has changed her hygiene habits. For what concerns 1.4, due to the response failure to initial therapy, to the persistence of grade 2 mobility, high BOP and PI rate, unfavourable crown/root ratio, the need for endodontic retreatment and new prosthetic restoration, and taking into account the cost/benefit ratio, we decided for the extraction of 1.4 and its substitution with an osseointegrated implant. At some sites, however, there are still defects with a probing >4 mm, positive BOP and inverse architecture. In 11.28 the situation of the sectors can be observed at the time of the re-evaluation.

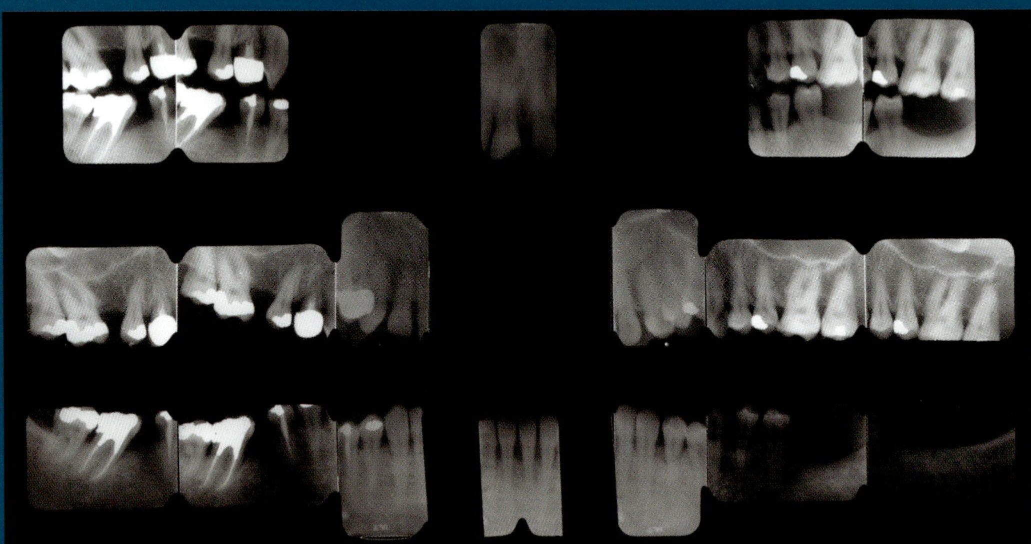

11.24 Pre-treatment full radiographic periodontal status.

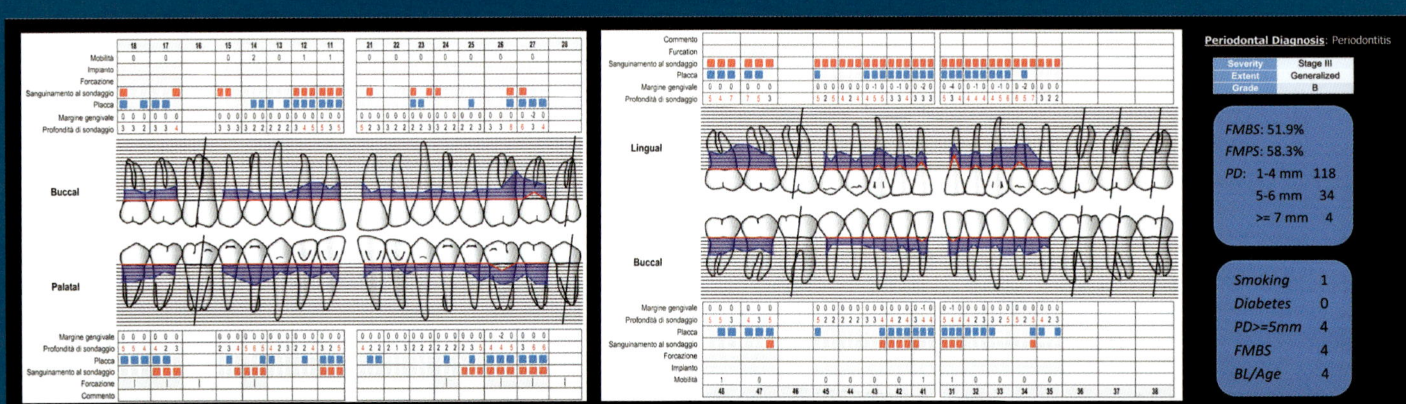

11.25 Initial periodontal probing, periodontal diagnosis, periodontal indexes, risk assessment (Online periodontal charting tool from www.perio-tools.com).

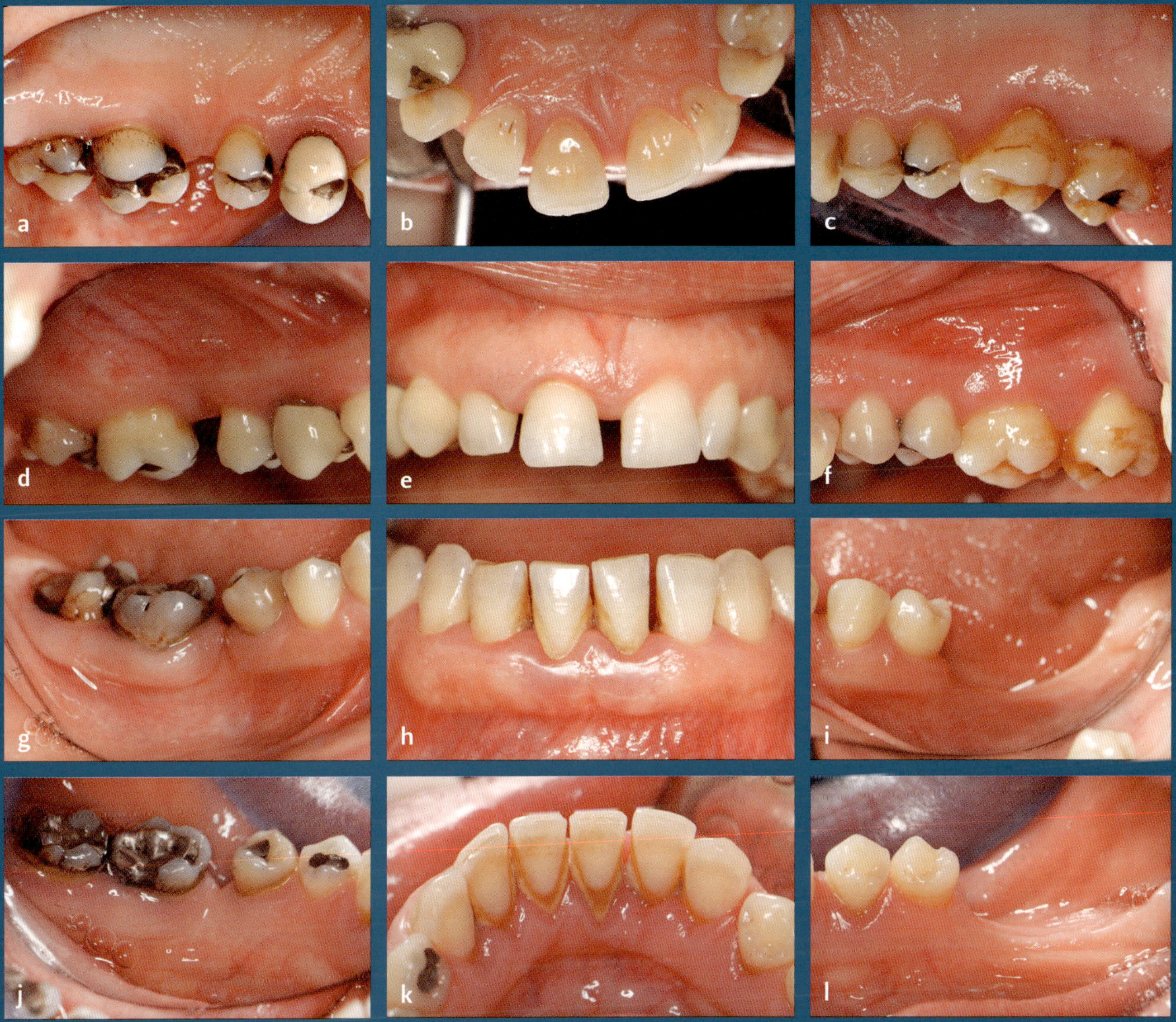

11.26 Pre-treatment vestibular and palatal/lingual general view of the six sectors.

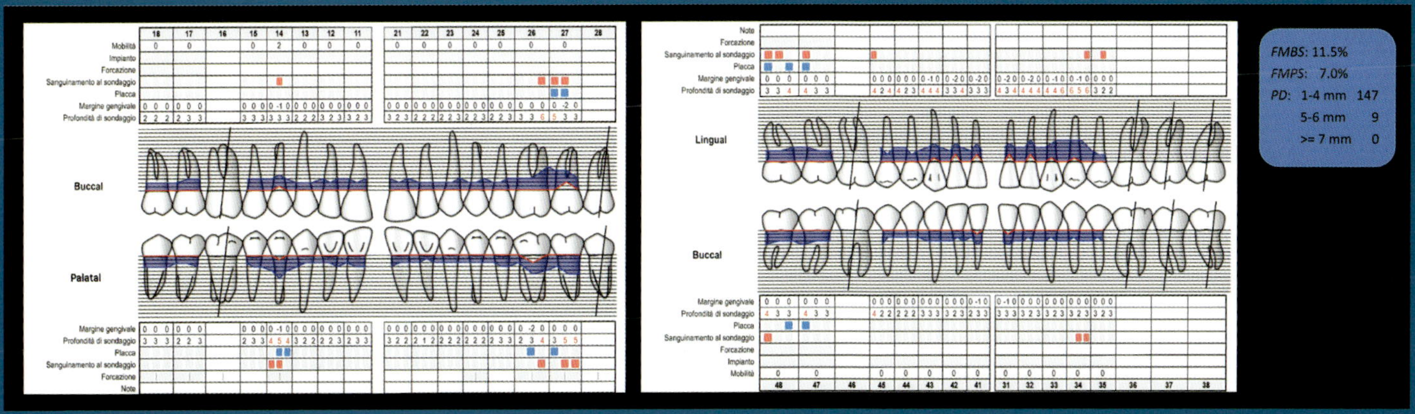

11.27 Re-evaluation periodontal probing and periodontal indexes (Online periodontal charting tool from www.perio-tools.com).

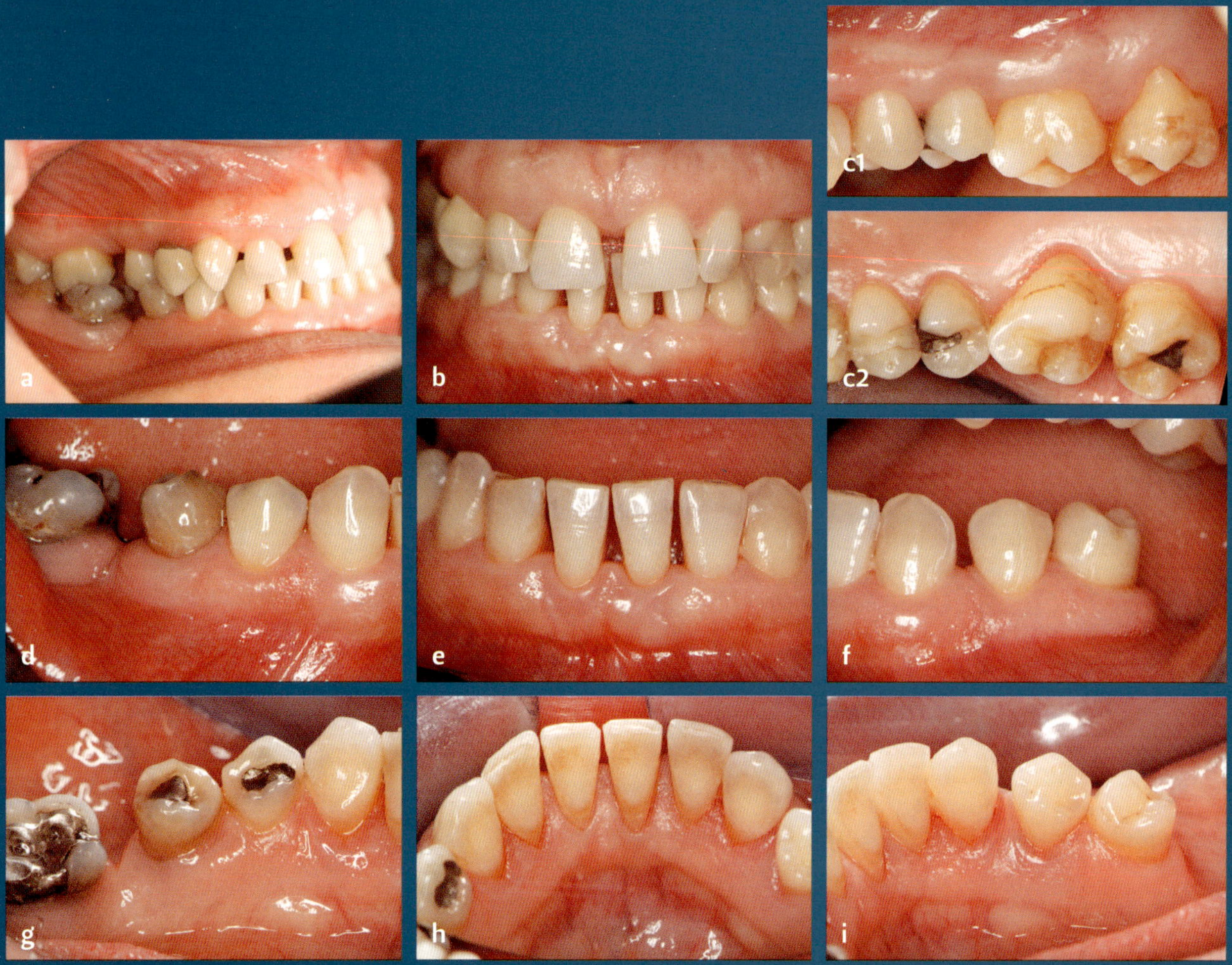

11.28 Re-evaluation vestibular and palatal/lingual general view of the six sectors.

PERIODONTAL SURGICAL THERAPY

Two osseous resective surgeries are performed in the III and V sectors to restore a physiological anatomy of the alveolar bone, resulting in a tissue morphology that facilitates the home and professional oral care and preparing the patient for the subsequent orthodontic treatment. A Fibre Retention Osseous Resective Surgery (FibReORS) in the left upper sector[15-18] (11.29-11.31) and an osseous resective surgery with lingual ramping in the lower central sector[19] (11.32-11.35) are performed. The treatment of the III sector is justified taking into account that the anatomy of the bone crater cannot be modified by orthodontic movement (see Chapter 9, paragraph *Operative timing*), while in the V sector, although there are present periodontal probings that are maintainable with SPT (Supportive Periodontal Therapy), we have preferred to minimize the gingival sulcus by surgical treatment, in prevision of a lingual orthodontic appliance application (OPRA, see Chapter 2, page 14).

SECOND RE-EVALUATION

After the corrective periodontal surgical phase, the patient undergoes a second re-evaluation with a new complete radiographic status (11.36) and a periodontal probing in which clinical signs of inflammation are further reduced (FMBS and FMPS 6%) (11.37). Patient compliance always remains high. The surgical therapy has completely eliminated pathological periodontal probings >3 mm. Having stabilized the periodontal situation on our schedule, the orthodontic treatment can be started.

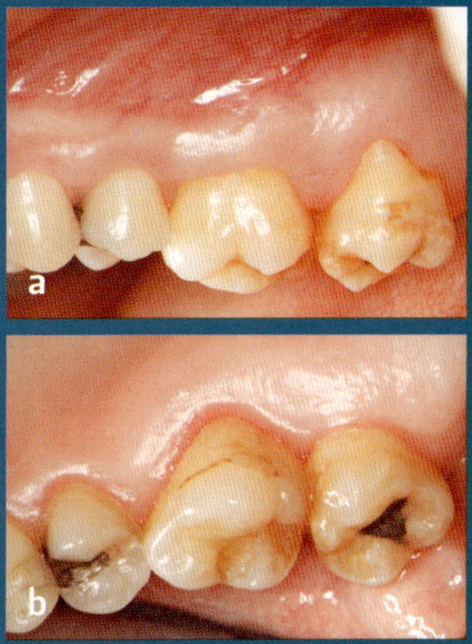

11.29 Clinical view of the III sectors before the osseous resective surgery.

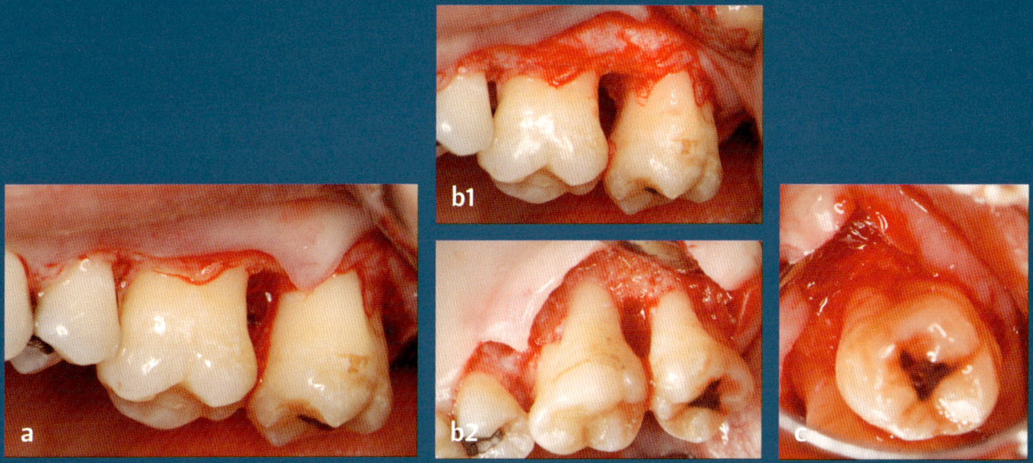

11.30 Flap design for the Fibre Retention Osseous Resective Surgery (FibReORS) and distal wedge (**a**,**c**); view of the physiologic contour of alveolar bone after bone surgery (**b1**,**b2**).

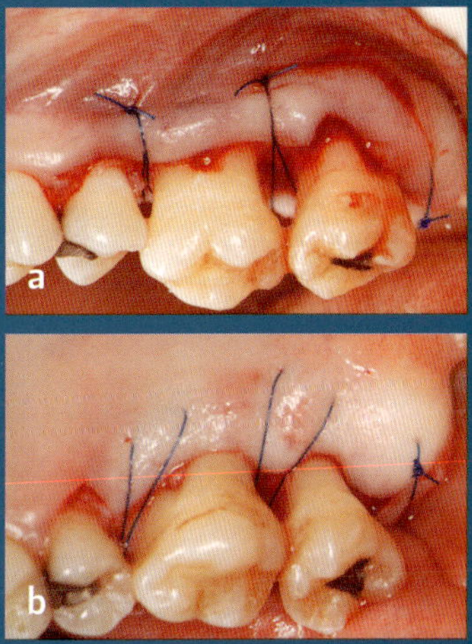

11.31 Flap suture with vertical mattress on vestibular and horizontal mattress on palatal aspect and the distal suture.

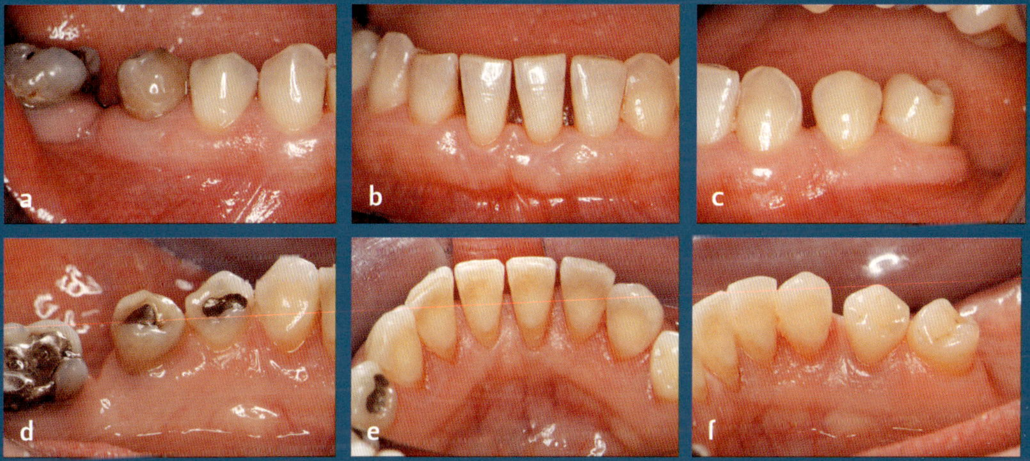

11.32 Clinical view of the lower arch before the osseous resective surgery.

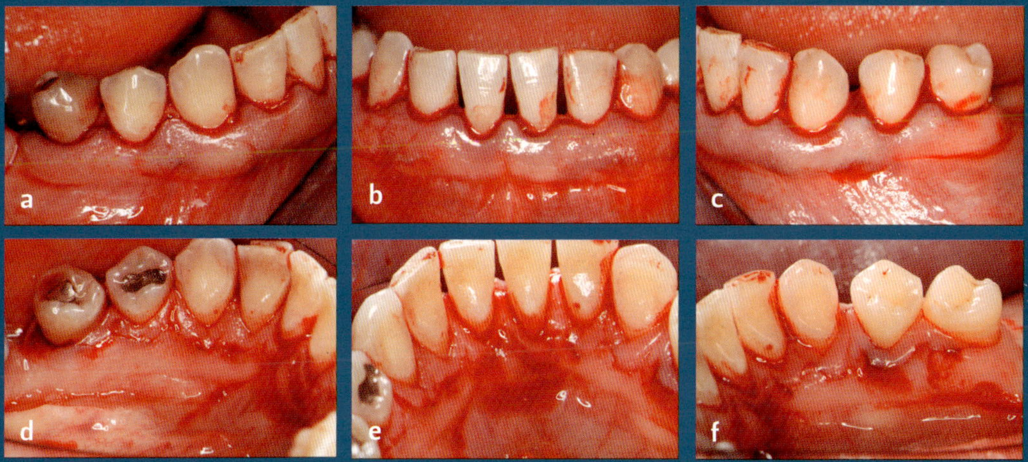

11.33 Intrasulcular vestibular incision and paramarginal incision on the lingual aspect.

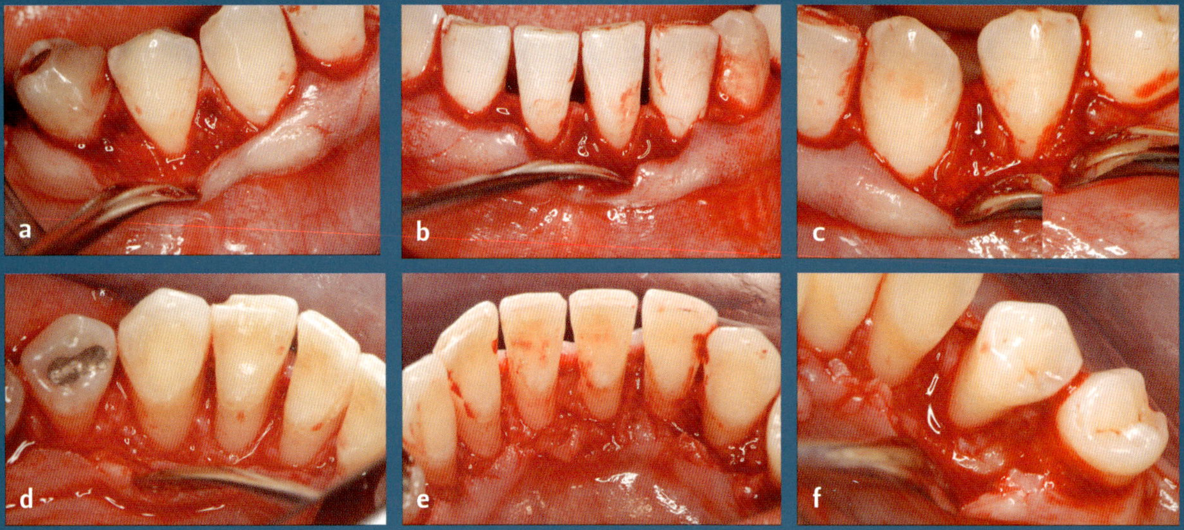

11.34 Clinical view of the bone level after the lingual ramping bone surgery.

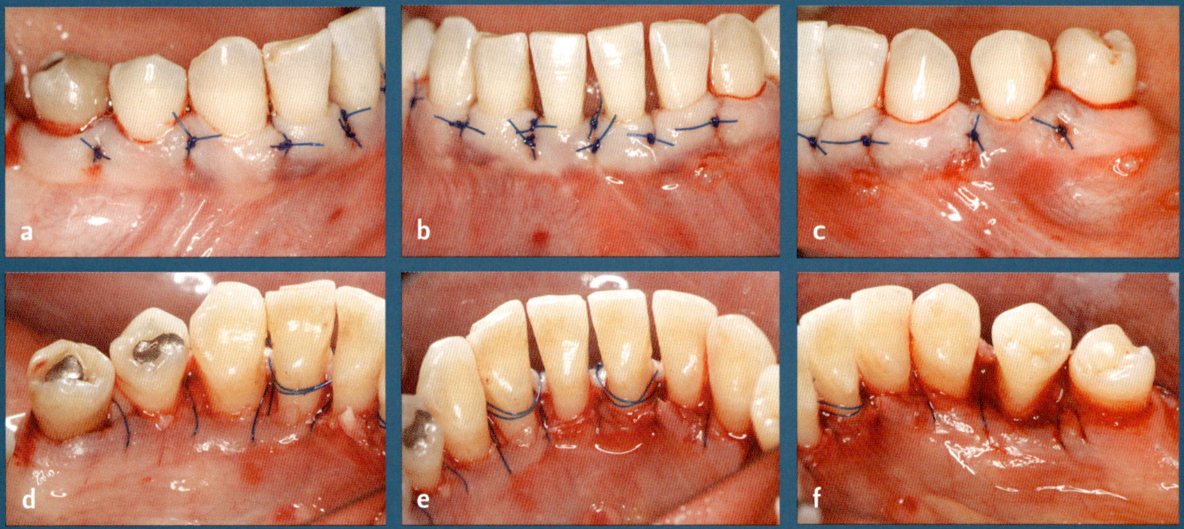

11.35 Flap suture after surgery.

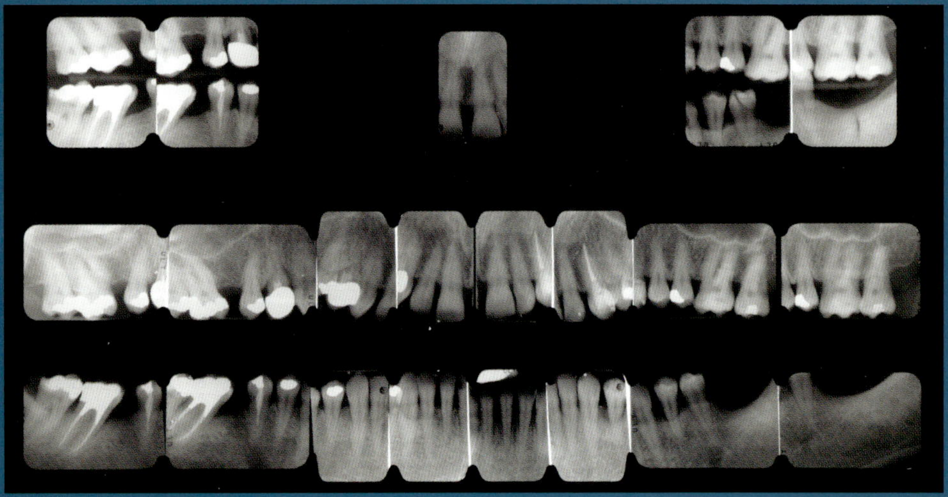

11.36 Radiographic periodontal status after the second re-evaluation, after the tissues healing before the orthodontic treatment.

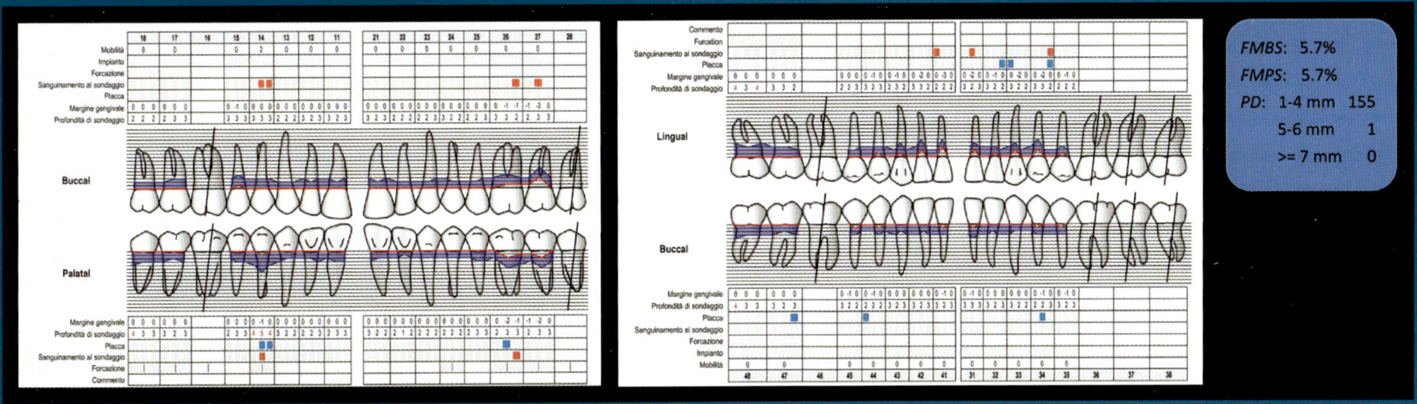

11.37 Second re-evaluation periodontal probing and periodontal indexes after periodontal surgery and before orthodontic treatment (Online periodontal charting tool from www.perio-tools.com).

Orthodontic phase (phase 2 ortho-perio timing, see 9.1)

The orthodontic mechanics is realized in lingual technique (Kurz 7th Generation, ®Ormco) with indirect bonding. The first arch is a .016 CuNiTi archwire during the first month; then a .016 β-titanium archwire, at first simple, then with loops to make sectorial movements of distalization and extrusion, aimed to level the residual bone defects (11.38); then a rectangular .017×.017 β-titanium archwire with extrusive steps (11.39); finally, a .017×.025 β-titanium archwire. The mechanics, in addition to the correction and detailing of the occlusion, the alignment and the correction of rotations, contributes to the levelling of the bone architecture, in particular of the upper anterior group before closing the diastema with sectorial microextrusions, and with an extrusion finalized to the development of the 1.4 implant site, as described in Chapter 8. Subsequently, together with the derotation, an intrusion of 2.6 is performed, which becomes legitimated thanks to the elimination of the residual crater obtained by periodontal surgery.

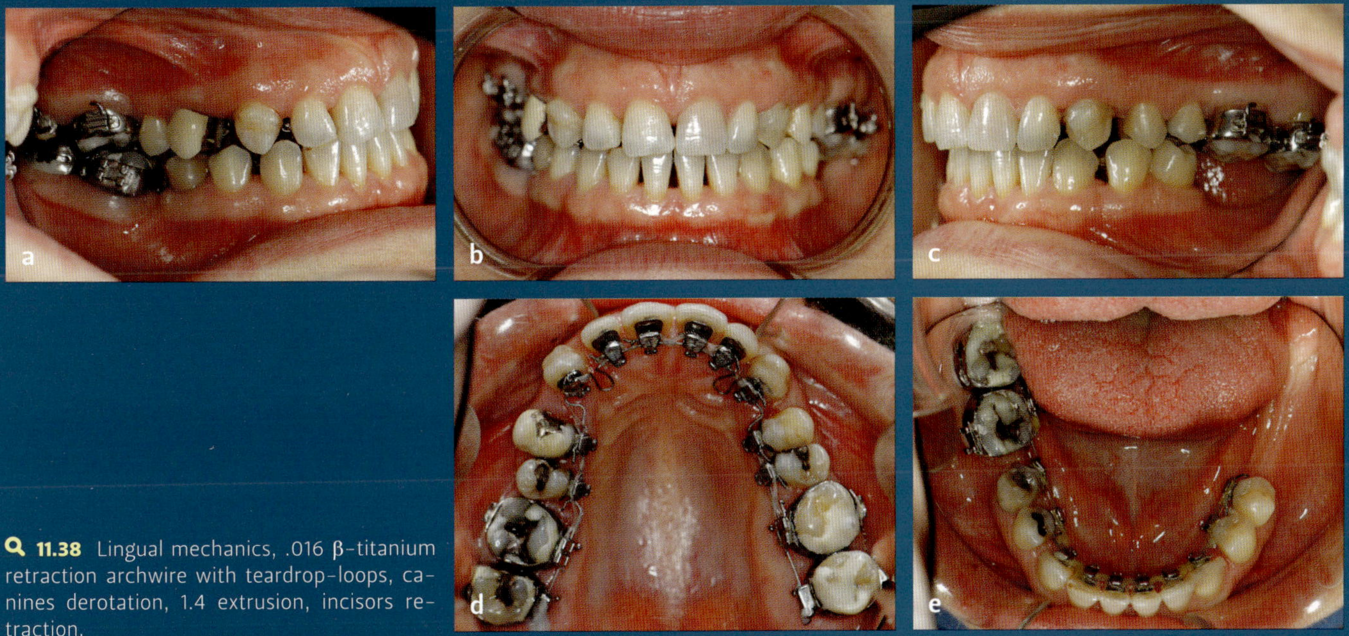

11.38 Lingual mechanics, .016 β-titanium retraction archwire with teardrop-loops, canines derotation, 1.4 extrusion, incisors retraction.

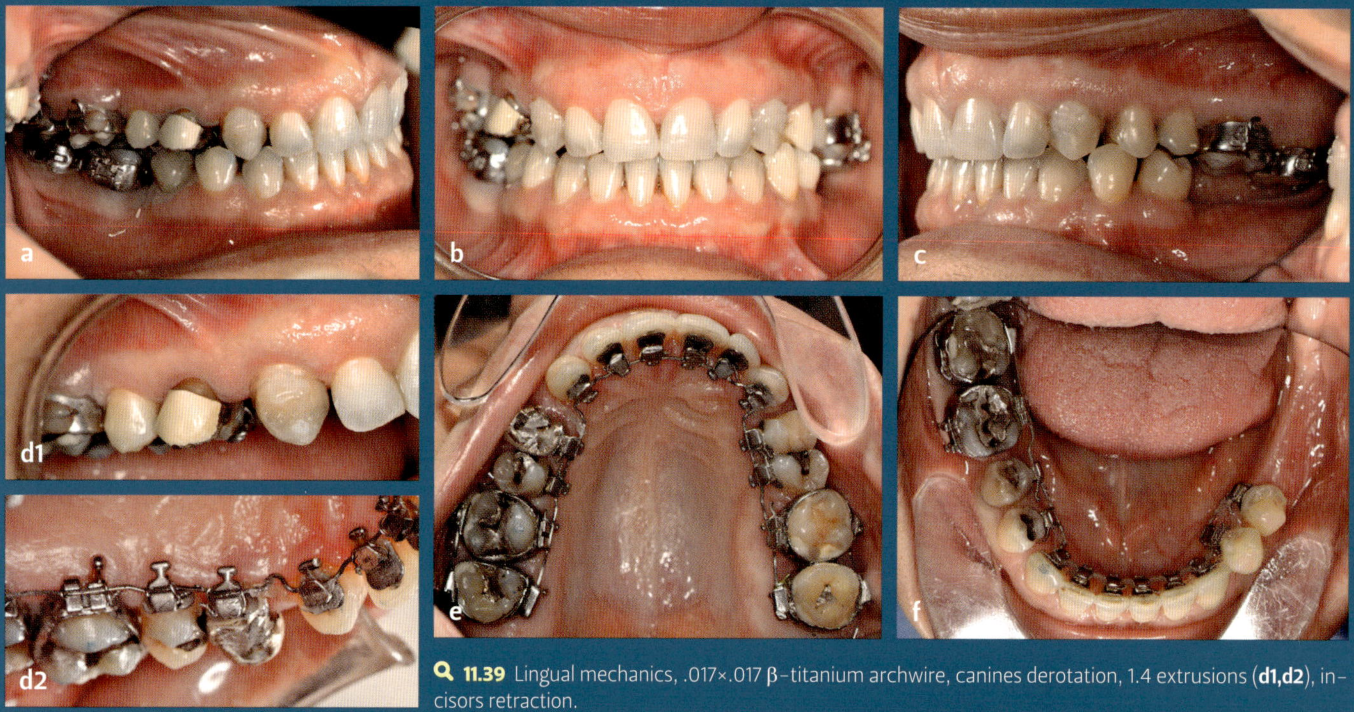

11.39 Lingual mechanics, .017×.017 β-titanium archwire, canines derotation, 1.4 extrusions (**d1,d2**), incisors retraction.

IMPLANTS – LOWER LEFT AREA

During the orthodontic detailing phase, two implants are placed in the lower left sector. After careful planning of clinical and radiographic parameters, implant placement in 3.6 and 3.7 sites is planned (Xive®, Dentsply) while a GBR is performed with a non-resorbable membrane in ePTFE[20,21]. Since the peri-implant bone defect has both a horizontal and vertical component, and since the distal attachment level at 3.5 is preserved, a technique that involves only one surgical time guarantees a less invasive and more predictable approach (11.40-11.46).

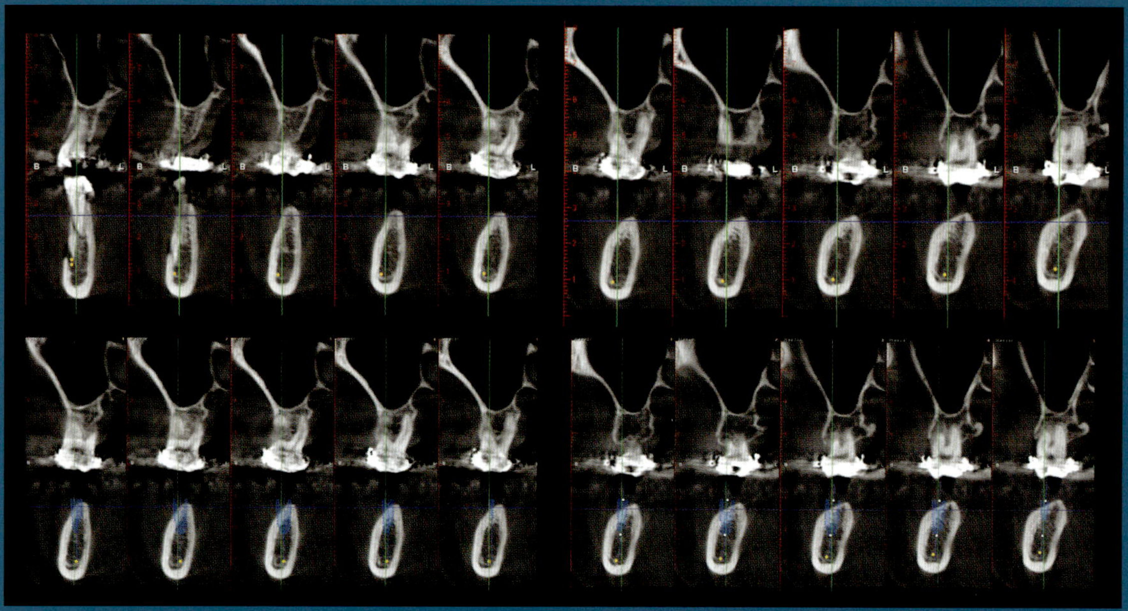

11.40 CBCT study for implant surgery in the lower left edentulous sector.

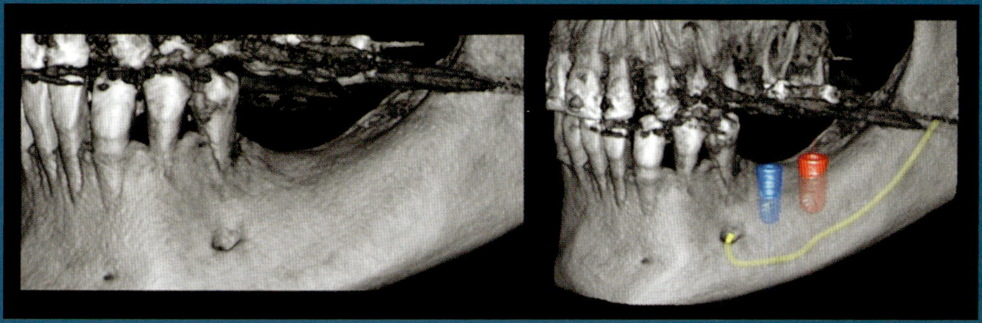

11.41 Planning of the implant positioning in the edentulous crest by CBCT with 3D recon- struction of the lower jaw.

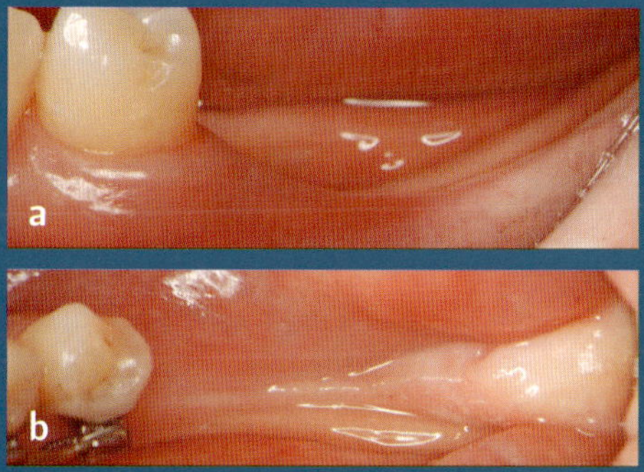

11.42 View of the edentulous crest at the sur- gery time.

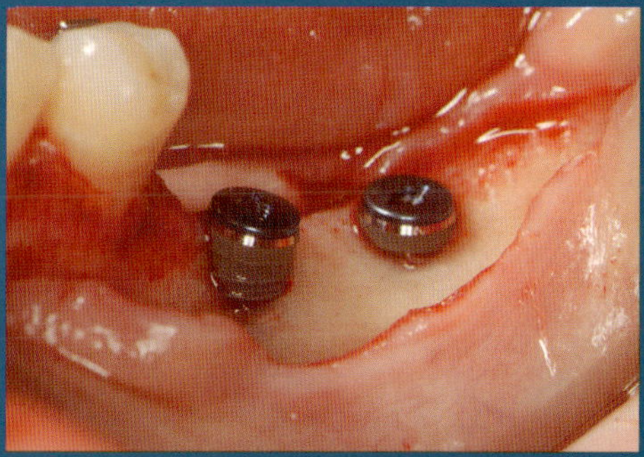

11.43 Implant placement in the lower left site where it can be seen the amount of vertical bone re- generation.

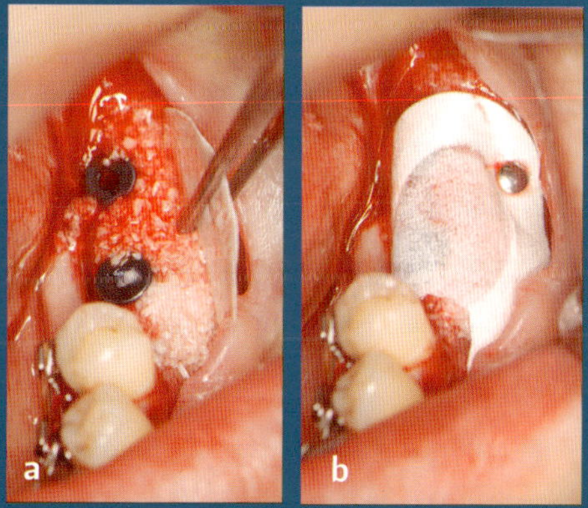

11.44 Bone graft: autologous 50% + xeno- graft 50% covered by a non-resorbable not reinforced ePTFE membrane and fixed with pin.

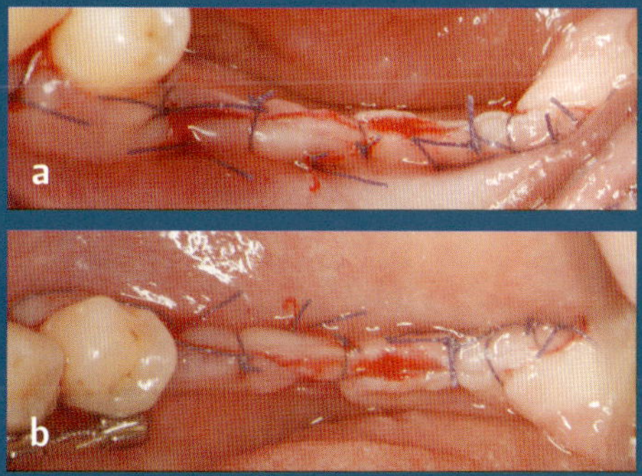

11.45 Flap suture with 2 types of sutures (ho- rizontal mattress + interrupted sutures) with re- sorbable material.

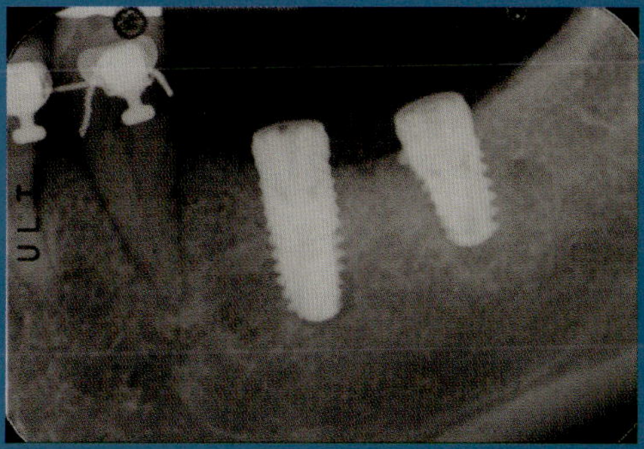

11.46 Post-surgical X-ray check.

IMPLANT – SITE 1.4

An orthodontic extrusion is used as a bone and tissue regenerative means, as it is widely described in Chapter 8, followed by an immediate post-extraction implant placement (Xive®, Dentsply)[22] (11.47-11.50).

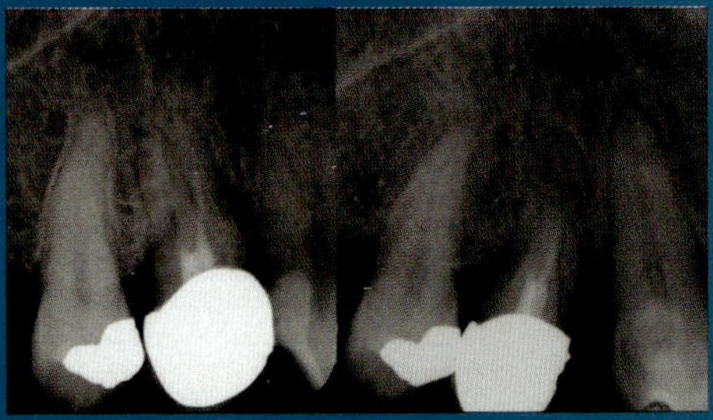

11.47 Pre-treatment 1.4 X-ray and after extrusion for implant site development, where it can be seen the elimination of the mesial bone defect.

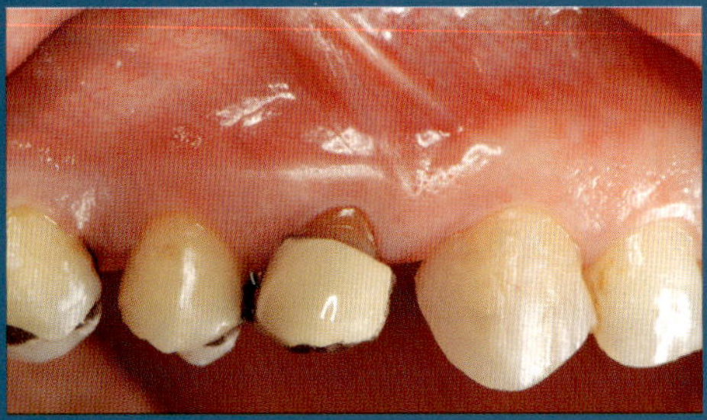

11.48 Soft tissue aspect at the end of extrusion.

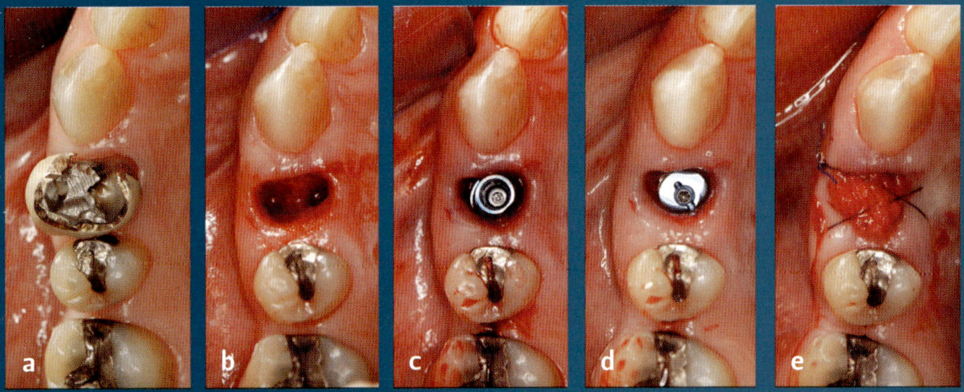

11.49. 49 Steps of the implant placement (fragment extraction [b],immediate post-extraction implant [c,d]; covering of the socket with fibrin sponge and resorbable X suture [e]).

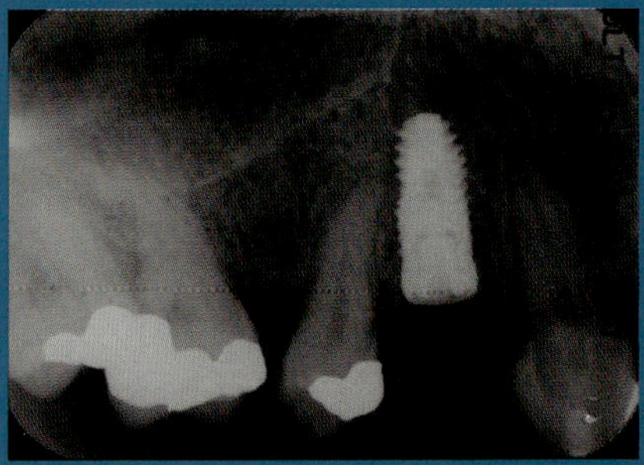

11.50 Post-surgical X-ray check.

Post-orthodontic phase (phase 3 ortho-perio timing, see 9.1)

SECOND IMPLANT SURGICAL PHASE

In the 3.6 3.7 site, after 9 months from the lower GBR, the membrane is removed with a partial thickness flap, two healing abutments are applied and a periosteal suture is performed to stabilize the flap (11.51 and 11.52). In the 1.4 site, 4 months after the implant placement, the implant is uncovered by removing crestal soft tissue in excess due to the large amount of keratinized tissue, and a healing abutment is applied.

PROSTHETIC FINALIZATION

Subsequently the lower implants are finalized with cemented dentures (11.53-11.55) and the upper implant is finalized together with a composite inlay on 1.5, with cemented denture (11.56-11.60).

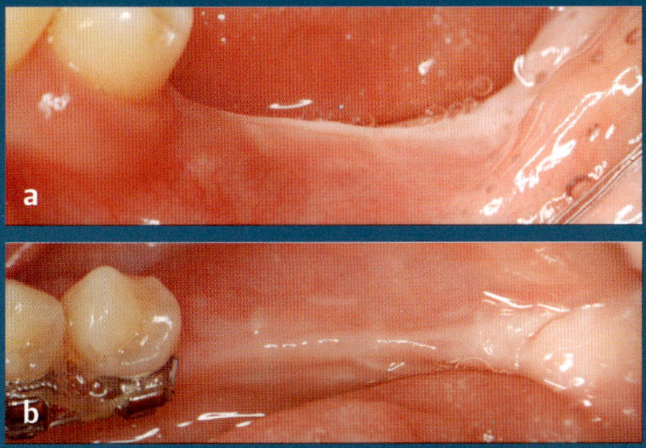

11.51 Soft tissue appearance of the edentulous lower left ridge at the second stage surgery, where it can be seen the perfect healing without inflammation.

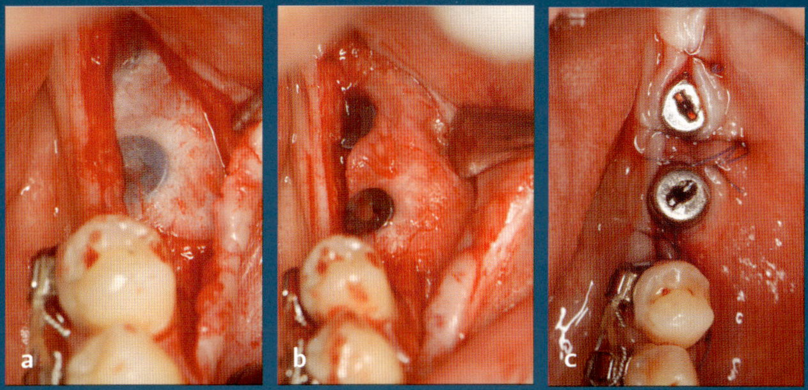

11.52 Flap elevation for membrane undercovering without inflammation (**a**); newly formed bone around implants (**b**); repositioned flap suture with the same amount of keratinized gingiva maintained on the vestibular and lingual aspect around the healing abutment (**c**).

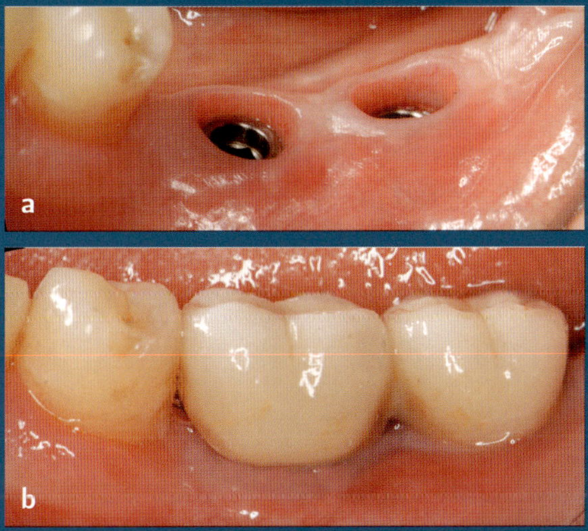

◀ **11.53** Peri-implant soft tissues at the cementation time and with the fixed partial denture *in situ*.

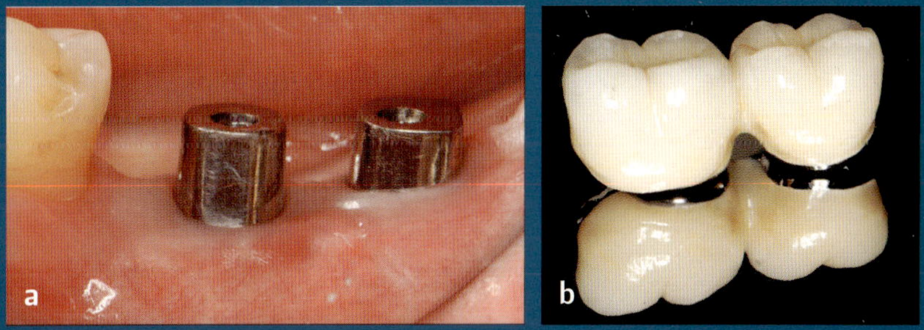

11.54 Customized abutment AMA style and prosthetic appliance.

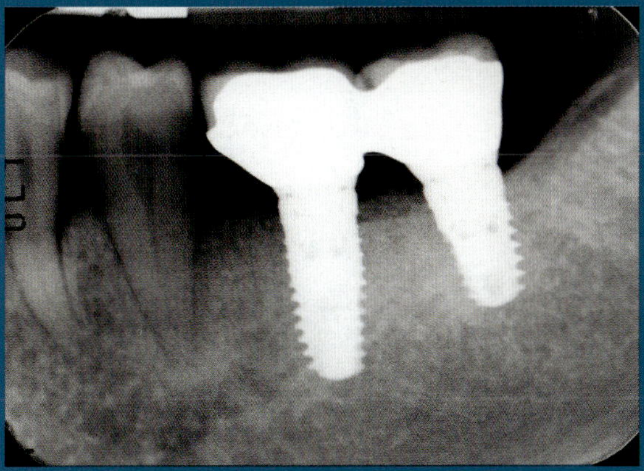

11.55 Radiographic check at cementation time.

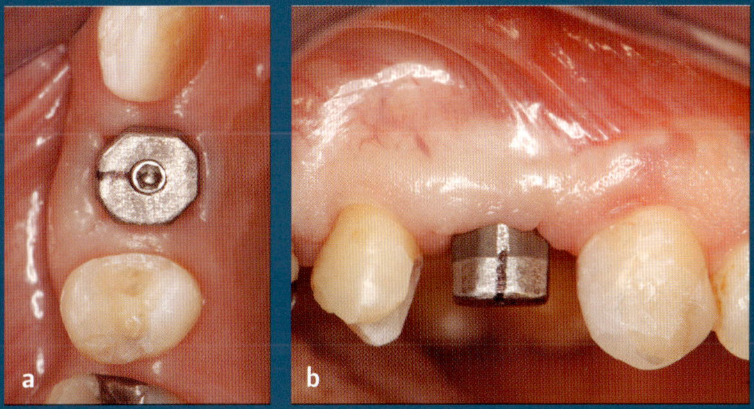

11.56 Soft tissue aspect on 1.4 site at the definitive impression with customized abutment, where it can be seen the amount of the vestibular keratinized tissue.

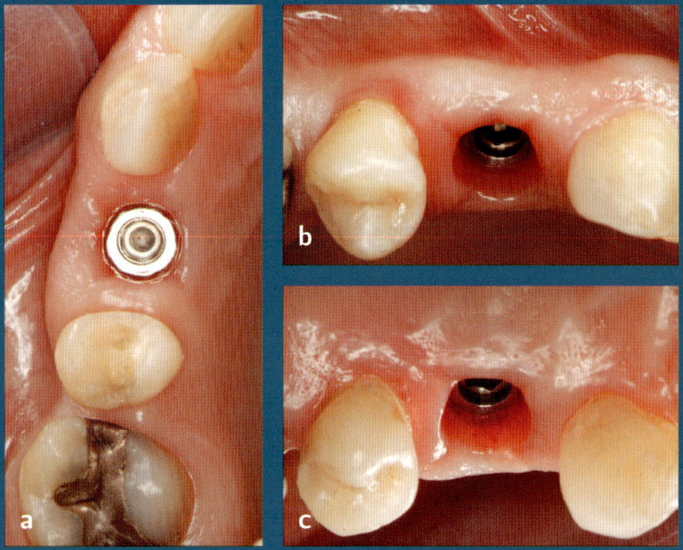

11.57 Peri-implant soft tissue aspect before the definitive cementation.

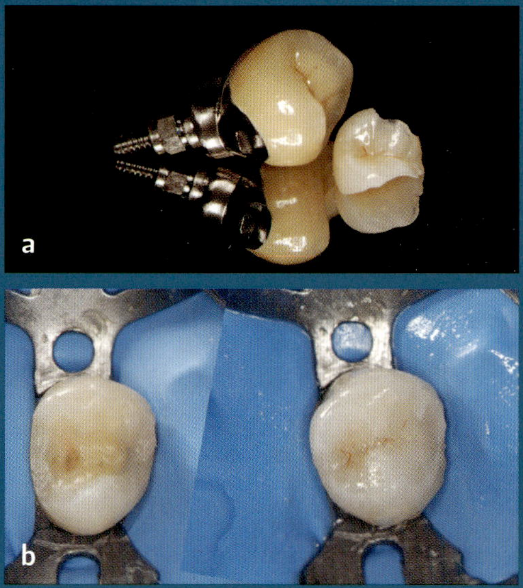

11.58 Fixed denture and steps of the simultaneous adhesive cementation of composite inlay on 1.5.

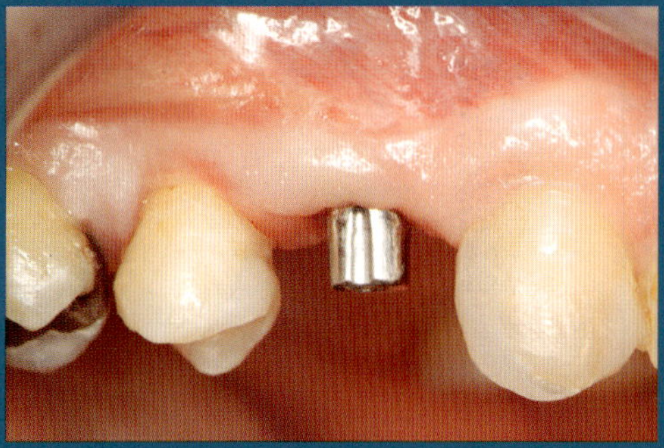

11.59 Customized abutment of the 1.4 according the AMA technique.

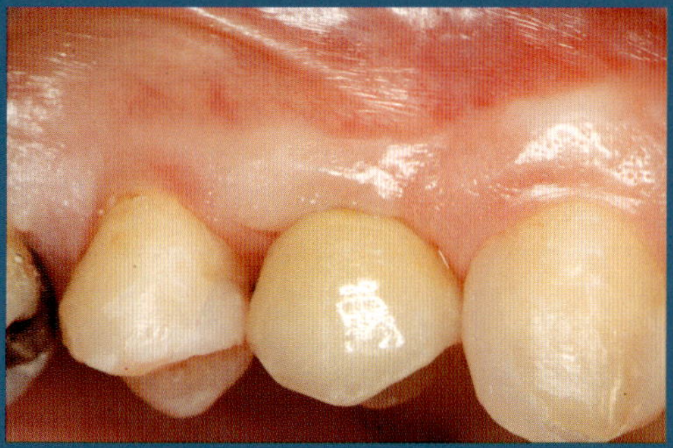

11.60 Definitive cementation of the 1.4 fixed denture.

FINAL RE-EVALUATION

At the end of the combined periodontal-orthodontic-implant treatment, the patient presents facial harmony (11.61), dental class I with normalization of OVJ and OVB (11.62) and skeletal class I (11.63 and 11.64; see 11.2); these values are stable after 10 years (11.65 and 11.66). From a periodontal point of view, the treatment achieves the planned objectives, with substantial improvement in the level of oral hygiene and FMBS (5.3%) and FMPS (4.7%), that remain stable up to the 10 year follow-up (11.67). The patient continues to demonstrate excellent compliance, which has been increasing in time. She now has a medium-low risk level (Perio Risk: 5)[8-10] and she takes part to a maintenance program with periodic SPT sessions every 4 months. The reduction of the PPD and the almost total absence of the BOP are positive prognostic parameters for the long-term as observed from the quality of the tissues (11.68), at a radiographic level (11.69) and in the perfect osseointegration of the implants (11.70).

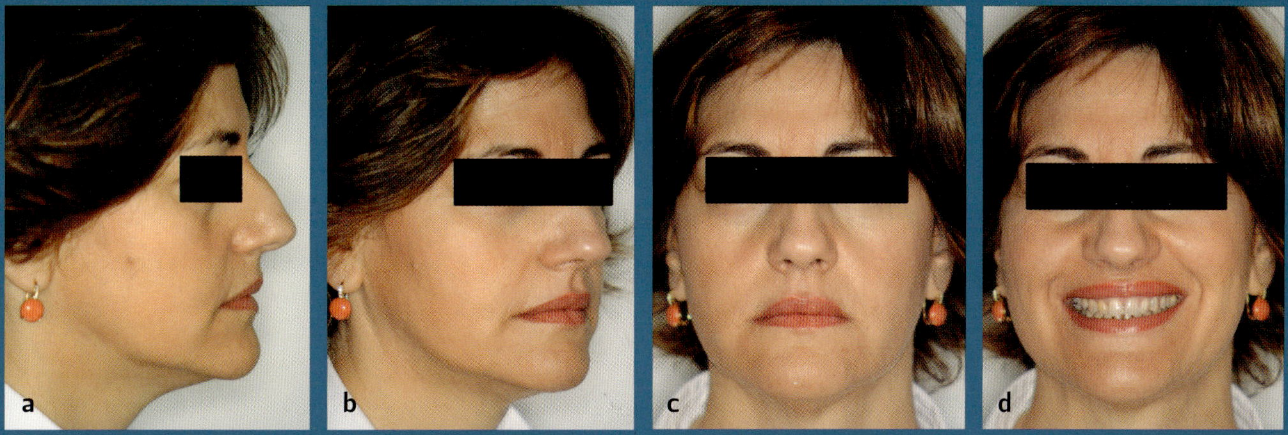

11.61 Extraoral post-treatment photos.

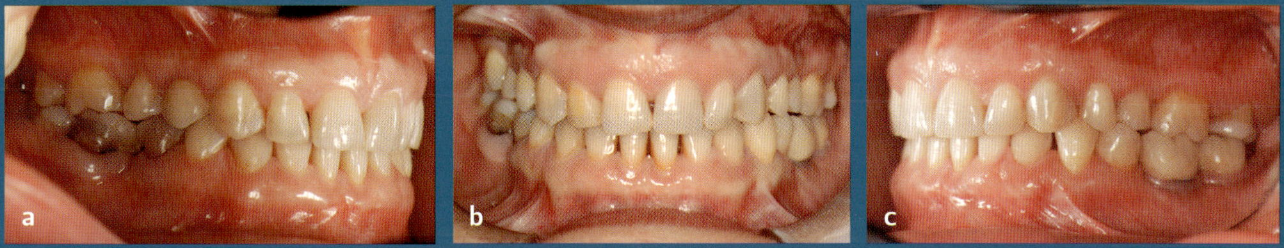

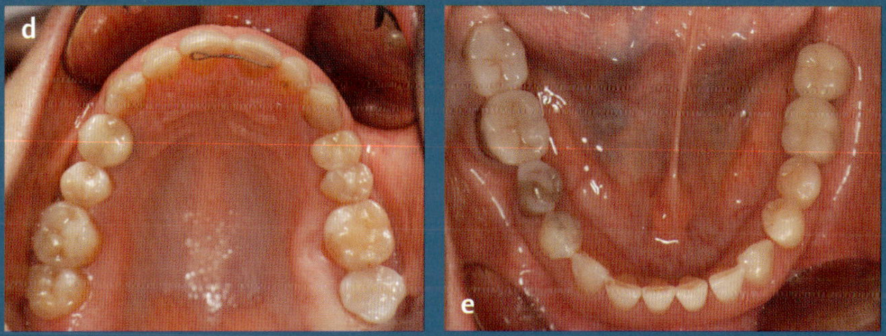

11.62 Intraoral post-treatment photos.

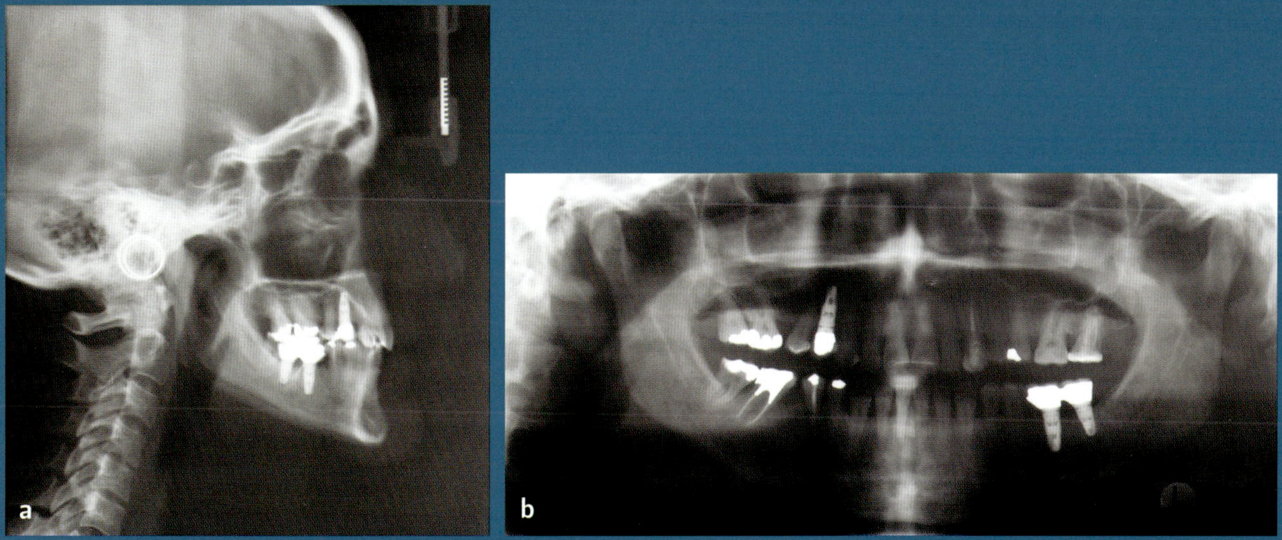

11.63 Post-treatment cephalometric Rx (**a**) panoramic Rx (**b**).

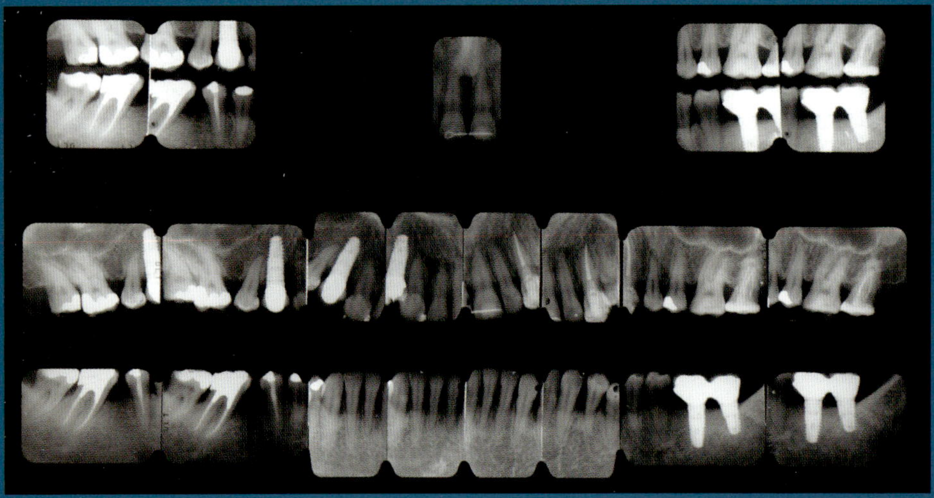

11.64 Post-treatment full radiographic periodontal status.

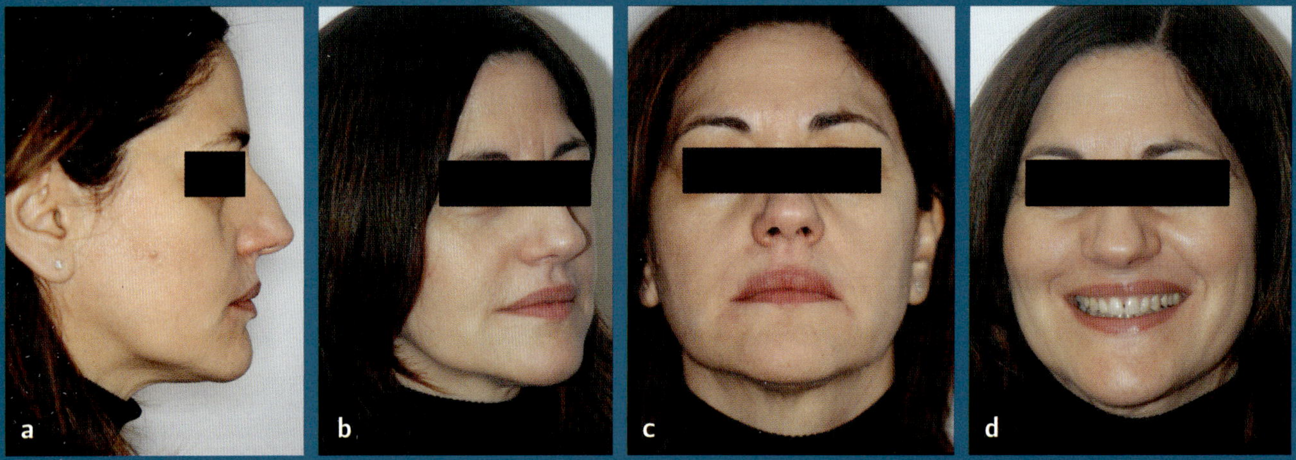

11.65 Extraoral 10-year follow-up photos.

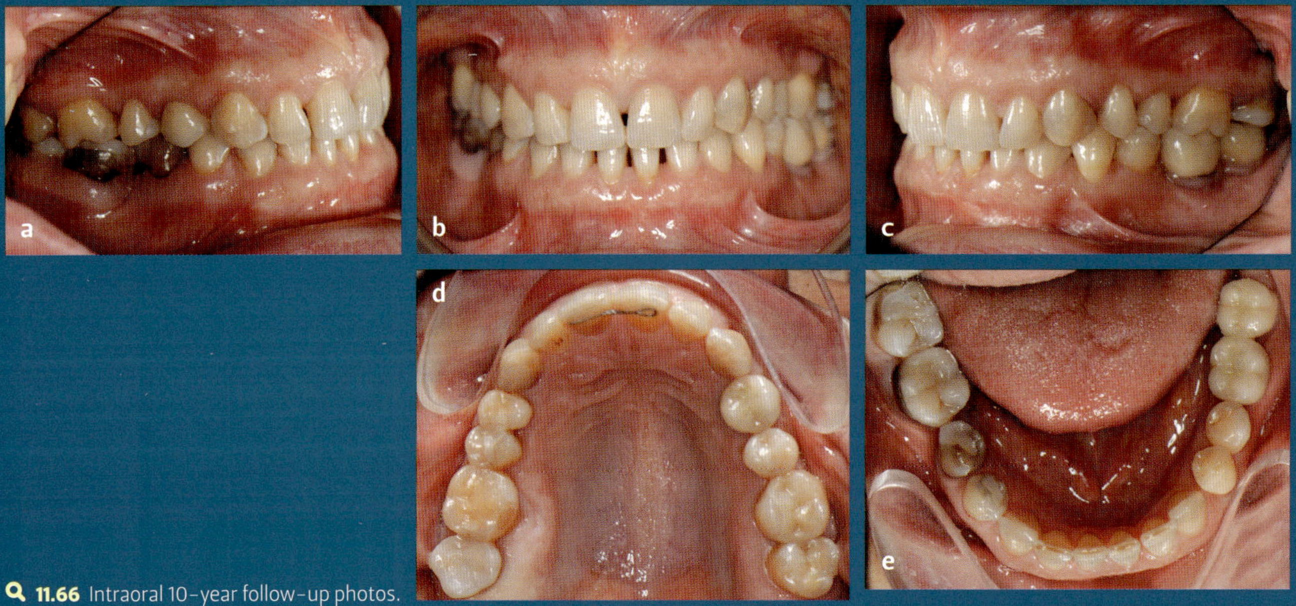

11.66 Intraoral 10-year follow-up photos.

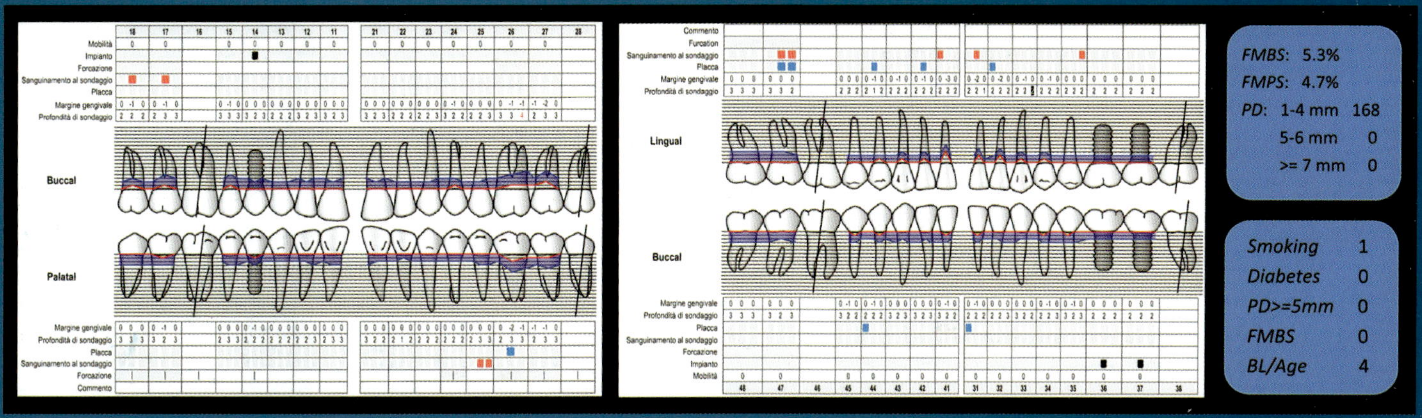

11.67 10-year follow-up periodontal probing, periodontal indexes, risk assessment (Online periodontal charting tool from www.perio-tools.com).

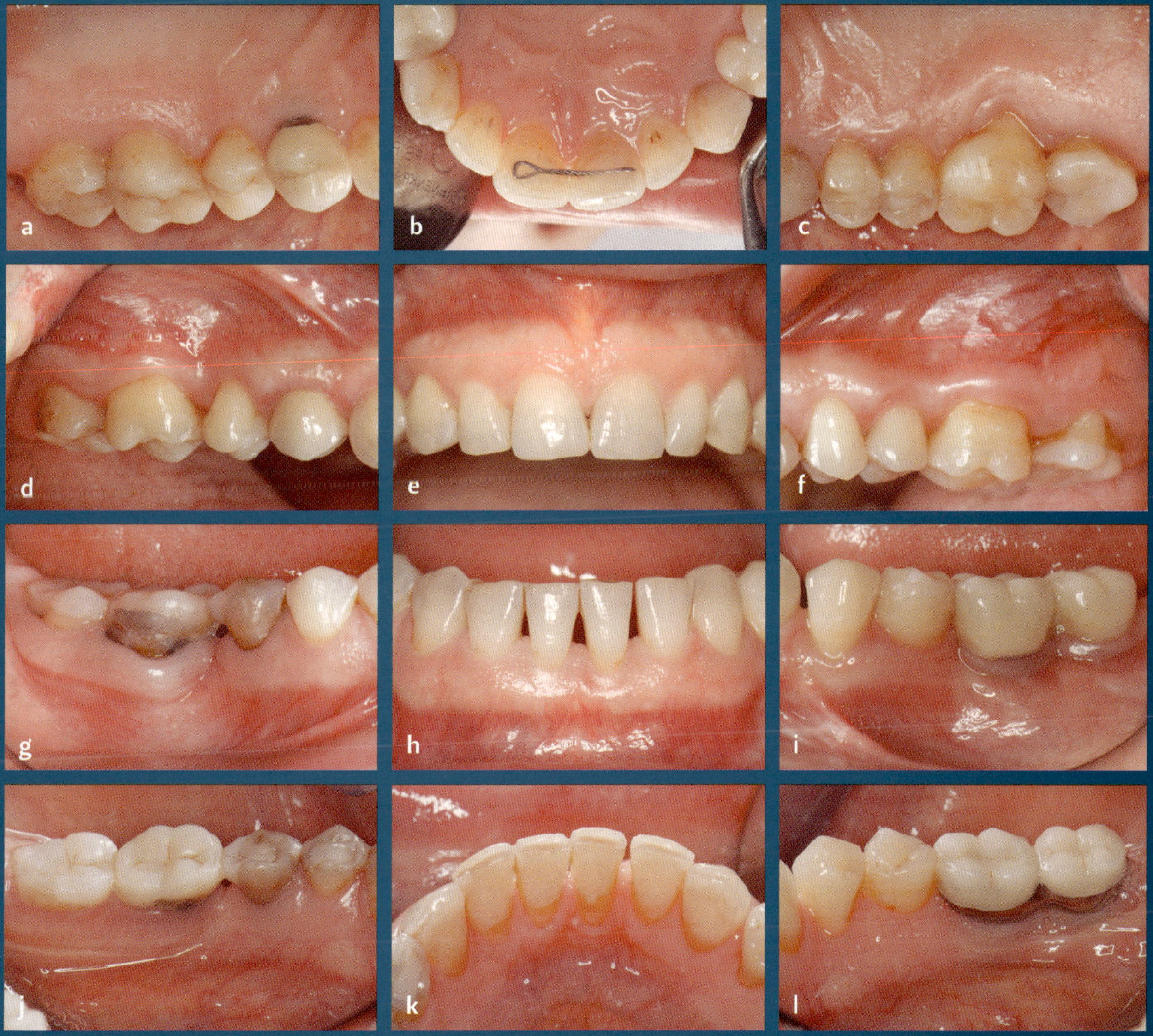

11.68 10-year follow-up vestibular and palatal/lingual general view of the six sectors.

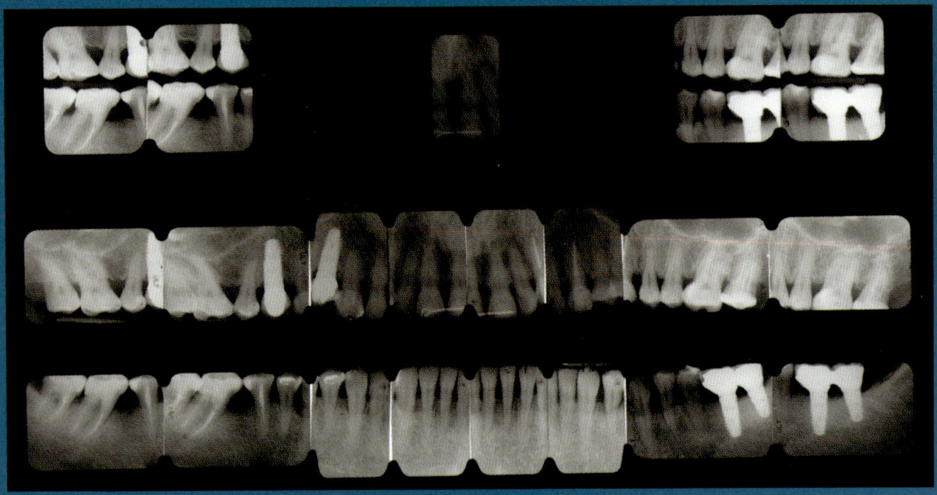

11.69 10-year follow-up full radiographic periodontal status.

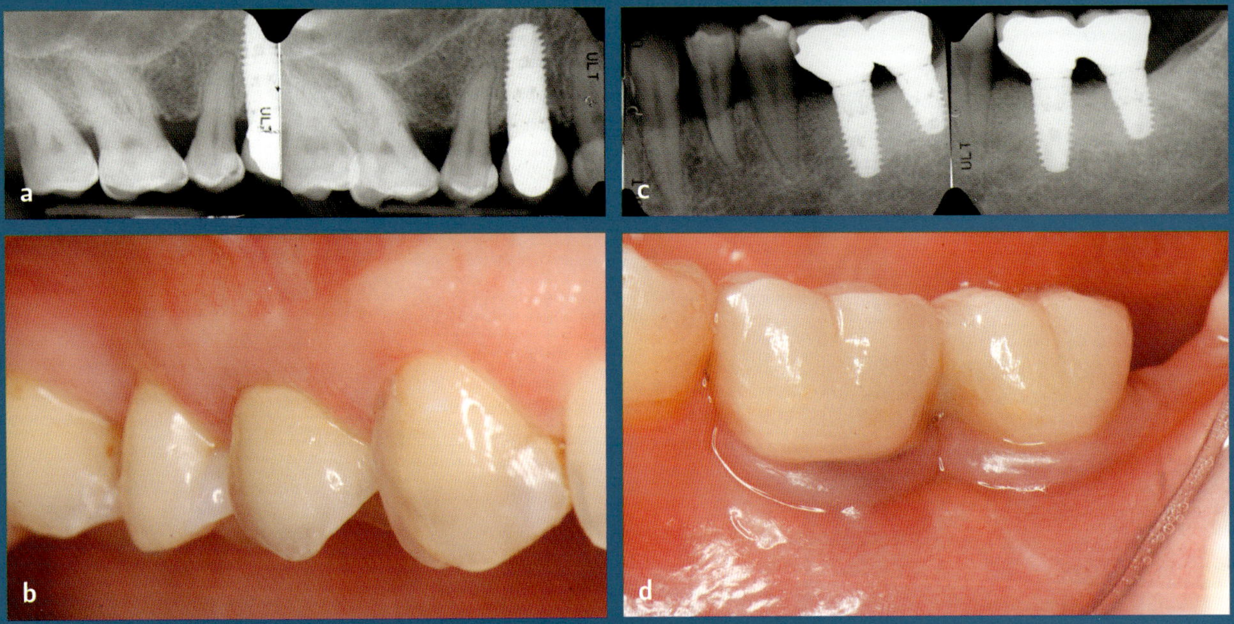

11.70 10-year follow-up clinical view and radiographic images of the implant areas.

REFERENCES

1. de Barros LA, de Almeida Cardoso M, de Avila ED et al. Six-year follow-up of maxillary anterior rehabilitation with forced orthodontic extrusion: achieving esthetic excellence with a multidisciplinary approach. *Am J Orthod Dentofacial Orthop.* 2013;144(4):607-615.
2. Capri D, Albehbehani Y, Smukler H. Augmentation of an anterior edentulous ridge for fixed prosthodontics with combined use of orthodontics and surgery: a clinical report. *J Prosthet Dent.* 2003;90(2):111-115.
3. Soolari A, Erickson D, Soolari A. Orthodontic forced eruption: a team approach in aesthetic treatment. *Dent Today.* 2014;33(7):112-117.
4. Chambrone L, Chambrone LA. Forced orthodontic eruption of fractured teeth before implant placement: case report. *J Can Dent Assoc.* 2005;71(4):257-261.
5. Ahn JC, Lee JH, Yoon JH et al. Interdisciplinary treatment of a patient with multiple missing teeth and periodontitis. *Am J Orthod Dentofacial Orthop.* 2018;153(2):278-289.
6. Kornman KS, Tonetti MS. Proceedings of the World Workshop on the Classification of Periodontal and Peri-Implant Diseases and Conditions. *J Periodontol.* 2018;89 Suppl 1:S1-S291.
7. Kornman KS, Tonetti MS. Proceedings of the World Workshop on the Classification of Periodontal and Peri-Implant Diseases and Conditions. *J Clin Periodontol.* 2018;45 Suppl 20:S1-S291.
8. Trombelli L, Minenna L, Toselli L et al. Prognostic value of a simplified method for periodontal risk assessment during supportive periodontal therapy. *J Clin Periodontol.* 2017;44(1):51-57.
9. Trombelli L, Farina R, Ferrari S et al. Comparison between two methods for periodontal risk assessment. *Minerva Stomatol.* 2009;58(6):277-287.
10. Farina R, Ferrari S, Pasetti P et al. Comparison between two methods for periodontal risk assessment. Abstracts of the 6th International Congress of the European Federation of Periodontology (Europerio 6), Stockholm June 4-6 2009. *J. Clin Periodontol.* 2009;36(S9):82(abstr. #157).
11. Bruschi GB, Crespi R, Capparè P et al. Localized management of sinus floor technique for implant placement in fresh molar sockets. *Clin Implant Dent Relat Res.* 2013;15(2):243-250.
12. Bruschi GB, Scipioni A, Calesini G, Bruschi E. Localized management of sinus floor with simultaneous implant placement: a clinical report. *Int J Oral Maxillofac Implants.* 1998,13(2):219-226.
13. Scipioni A, Bruschi GB, Calesini G. The edentulous ridge expansion technique: a five-year study. *Int J Periodontics Restorative Dent.* 1994;14(5):451-459.
14. Segelnick SL, Weinberg MA. Reevaluation of initial therapy: when is the appropriate time? *J Periodontol.* 2006;77(9):1598-1601.
15. Cairo F, Carnevale G, Nieri M et al. Benefits of fibre retention osseous resective surgery in the treatment of shallow infrabony defects: a double-blind, randomized, clinical trial describing clinical, radiographic and patient-reported outcomes. *J Clin Periodontol.* 2013;40(2):163-171.
16. Carnevale G, Cairo F, Nieri M, Tonetti MS. Fibre retention osseous resective surgery: how deep is the infrabony component of the osseous-resected defects?. *J Clin Periodontol.* 2008;35(2):133-138.
17. Carnevale G. Fibre retention osseous resective surgery: a novel conservative approach for pocket elimination. *J Clin Periodontol.* 2007; 34(2):182-187.
18. Carnevale G, Kaldahl WB. Osseous resective surgery. *Periodontol 2000.* 2000;22(1):59-87.
19. Ochsenbein C, Bohannan HM. The palatal approach to osseous surgery. I. Rationale. *J Periodontol.* 1963; 34(1):60-68.
20. Tinti C, Parma-Benfenati S. Vertical ridge augmentation: surgical protocol and retrospective evaluation of 48 consecutively inserted implants. *Int J Periodontics Restorative Dent.* 1998;18(5):434-443.
21. Simion M, Jovanovic SA, Tinti C, Benfenati SP. Long-term evaluation of osseointegrated implants inserted at the time or after vertical ridge augmentation. A retrospective study on 123 implants with 1-5 year follow-up. *Clin Oral Implants Res.* 2001;12(1):35-45.
22. Hämmerle CH, Chen ST, Wilson TG Jr. Consensus statements and recommended clinical procedures regarding the placement of implants in extraction sockets. *Int J Oral Maxillofac Implants.* 2004;(Suppl 19):26-28.